THIRD EDITION

PDR®

Drug Guide for Mental Health Professionals

THOMSON™

Publisher's Note

Contents

PDR® Drug Guide
for Mental Health Professionals

THIRD EDITION

Senior Director, Editorial & Publishing: Bette LaGow
Manager, Professional Services: Michael Deluca, PharmD, MBA
Drug Information Specialists: Anila Patel, PharmD; Nermin Shenouda, PharmD; Greg Tallis, RPh
Contributing Editors: Kris Minne, RPh; Harris B. Stratyner, PhD, CASAC
Project Editors: Kathleen Engel, Lori Murray
Associate Editors: Sabina Borza, Elise Philippi
Senior Director, Client Services: Stephanie Struble
Project Manager: Christina Klinger
Manager, Production Purchasing: Thomas Westburgh
Manager, Art Department: Livio Udina
Electronic Publishing Designers: Deana DiVizio, Carrie Faeth, Jamie Pinedo
Production Associate: Joan K. Akerlind
Traffic Assistant: Kim Condon
Cover design: Thomson Healthcare Creative Services, Greenwood Village, CO

Senior Director, Copy Sales: Bill Gaffney
Senior Product Manager: Richard Buchwald

THOMSON PDR

Executive Vice President, PDR: Kevin D. Sanborn
Vice President, Products & Solutions: Christopher Young
Vice President, Clinical Relations: Mukesh Mehta, RPh
Vice President, Operations: Brian Holland
Vice President, Strategic Marketing: Valerie E. Berger
Vice President, Pharmaceutical Sales: Anthony Sorce

Officers of Thomson Healthcare Inc.: *President and Chief Executive Officer:* Robert Cullen; *Chief Medical Officer:* Alan Ying, MD; *Senior Vice President and Chief Technology Officer:* Frank Licata; *Chief Strategy Officer:* Courtney Morris; *Executive Vice President, Payer Decision Support:* Jon Newpol; *Executive Vice President, Provider Markets:* Terry Cameron; *Executive Vice President, Marketing and Innovation:* Doug Schneider; *Senior Vice President, Finance:* Phil Buckingham; *Vice President, Human Resources:* Pamela M. Bilash; *General Counsel:* Darren Pocsik

ISBN: 1-56363-679-0   Printed in Canada

Foreword

PDR® Drug Guide for Mental Health Professionals can easily be the key publication for the psychotherapist who wants to understand the patient and his environment. Today's therapy involves not only the patient's original worries, but may also include the immense number of drugs that come into the patient's system through the health food store; misguided neighbors and other acquaintances; the local pusher of "recreational drugs;" the seller of herbs and primitive concoctions; the international commerce of "miracle drugs;" and many other sources. Americans today spend billions of dollars on "natural" and other alternative medications. A book such as this one—which examines chemical compounds that any patient may use on his own or on the advice of people who know little more than he does—becomes a must for the therapist.

Knowledge of approved therapies is also necessary. Gone are the days when some physicians and many patients believed that every tablet purchased at a drug store had a single target, that each effect of a prescription was beneficial, and that each medication helped restore health.

Today people take pills to try to eliminate symptoms, control side effects of other pills, get intoxicated, satisfy their curiosity about the arcane, imitate their friends and neighbors, or try to achieve qualities or powers they never had. The search for eternal youth, limitless vitality, or unusual powers continues to entice far too many, whereas not enough take medications that will restore their health.

The effects of medications vary a great deal depending on the patient, the medication, and many other factors. Any patient differs from many others according to age, sex, medical history, and variables that affect metabolism and reactivity to external agents.

A major challenge in current medicine is that patients with similar symptoms may have completely different disorders. The hyperactive child may suffer a gamut of disorders, from a syndrome resulting from brain injury, to bipolar disorder, to intoxication from a self-administered substance, to the beginning of a schizophreniform disorder.

In this day and age when there is a large multiplicity of generic agents that are sold as if they were the same as the original medication, the clinician not only needs to examine the patient but also the medications dispensed for him.

The variables to consider when trying to prescribe the most effective medication for a given patient now extend to ethnic and cultural considerations. The same metabolic pathways that distinguish people of different ethnic origins also affect the responsiveness to chemicals used to treat psychiatric disorders, meaning that the same medication may have unexpected effects in these different patients. Additionally, cultural traditions impacting the use and the effects of most medications may also come into play.

Children have finally come to the attention of those who investigate diseases and their treatment. Their presentation is often controlled by genetic and family factors, problems associated with growth and development, the presence of other illnesses, and the confusion generated by illnesses that share the same symptoms. All of this requires a health practitioner to keep at his or her fingertips as much information as possible about what we know and would like to know about medications for children. Recent debates about the use of antidepressants in children show that we are far from consensus on the danger of suicide, and we may facilitate rather than prevent suicide if we do not use antidepressants when necessary.

Psychotropic medications are not used as often as they are necessary to help the adult population with psychiatric disorders. Prejudices, fear, ignorance, and plain neglect may combine with lack of health financing to produce limited treatment or no treatment for patients who otherwise could regain their health. This book states the reasons that may convert the skeptical into advocates for the use of medications for mental disorders that can be properly diagnosed, can be treated effectively, and have often been lethal. Every mental health professional needs to remember that mental illness is well on its way to becoming the most important cause of disability in the world.

The general population is getting older and affected by groups of illnesses that are progressively more common, and often attack the same individuals at the same time. Today it is not unusual to see a patient who suffers from obesity, diabetes, high cholesterol, high blood pressure, anxiety, and depression. When we obtain the list and dosage of his medications, we get to understand why many older patients may have to decide whether they eat or use that same money to try to buy some of their medications. The astute clinician has to be prepared to offer knowledge that promotes effective, sensible, and hopefully affordable medication strategies.

Most physicians are in favor of establishing partnerships with our patients, so that the next prescription is given to an informed patient who knows and understands his diagnosis, who has information about the reasons for his treatment and the potential results, who has access to more and better information about medications, and who can be the first one to detect any therapeutic problem. In my opinion, *PDR® Drug Guide for Mental Health Professionals* helps create this atmosphere of sharing and offering mutual support.

Rodrigo A. Muñoz, M.D., F.A.P.A.
Clinical Professor of Psychiatry
University of California, San Diego
Medical Director, Outpatient Psychiatric Services
Scripps Mercy Hospital, San Diego
Past President, American Psychiatric Association

Section 1

Psychotropic Drug Profiles

In this section you'll find detailed overviews of more than 100 medications commonly used in the treatment of mental and emotional disorders. The drug profiles are organized alphabetically by brand name and cross-referenced by generic name. When no brand name is available, the profile is titled by the generic name. The information is drawn from the drug's government-approved product labeling. Included are the drug's potential side effects, reasons the drug should *not* be prescribed, necessary precautions, typical dosage regimens, and signs of overdose. A detailed review of each drug's possible interactions with other medications can be found in Section 2.

ABILIFY

Aripiprazole
Other brand name: Abilify Discmelt

Why is this drug prescribed?

Abilify is used in the treatment of schizophrenia and bipolar disorder. The drug is thought to work by modifying sensitivity to two of the brain's chief chemical messengers, serotonin and dopamine.

Most important fact about this drug

Abilify may cause tardive dyskinesia, a condition marked by involuntary muscle spasms and twitches in the face and body. This condition can become permanent and is most common among older people, especially women. Patients should see their doctor immediately if they begin to have any involuntary movements. They may need to discontinue Abilify therapy.

In addition, elderly patients with dementia who are treated with antipsychotic drugs such as Abilify have an increased risk of stroke and death. Abilify is not approved to treat dementia-related psychosis.

How should this medication be taken?

Abilify should be taken once a day; it may be taken with or without food. Abilify is available as a tablet, oral solution, and an orally disintegrating tablet (Discmelt). After removal from the package, the Discmelt should be placed on the tongue immediately and allowed to dissolve. It is best not to take the Discmelt with liquid; however, if necessary, patients can drink liquid once the tablet has dissolved. The Discmelt should not be split.

• *Missed dose...*
  Generally, forgotten doses should be taken as soon as remembered. However, if it is almost time for the next dose, patients should skip the one they missed and return to their regular schedule. Doses should never be doubled.

• *Storage instructions...*
  Store at room temperature.

What side effects may occur?

Side effects cannot be anticipated. If any develop or change in intensity, patients should inform their doctor as soon as possible.

• *Side effects may include:*
  Anxiety, blurred vision, constipation, cough, headache, insomnia, light-headedness, nausea, rash, restlessness, runny nose, sleepiness, tremors, vomiting, weakness

A variety of other reactions have been reported on extremely rare occasions. Any new or unusual symptom should be checked with the doctor.

Why should this drug not be prescribed?
If Abilify causes an allergic reaction, the patient will be unable to use it.

Special warnings about this medication
In rare cases, Abilify has been known to cause a potentially fatal condition called neuroleptic malignant syndrome. Symptoms include high fever, rigid muscles, irregular pulse or blood pressure, rapid heartbeat, excessive perspiration, altered mental status, and changes in heart rhythm. Patients who develop these symptoms need to alert their doctor immediately. Abilify should be discontinued.

Certain antipsychotic drugs are associated with an increased risk of developing high blood sugar, which on rare occasions has led to coma or death. To date, there have been only a few reports of blood sugar problems during treatment with Abilify. Even so, all patients taking this drug should be monitored closely by their doctor for signs of high blood sugar, especially those with risk factors for diabetes.

Because Abilify tends to make some people sleepy, patients should be cautious about operating hazardous machinery such as cars until they are certain the drug will not impair their ability.

In a few people, Abilify can cause an abrupt drop in blood pressure when they stand up, leading to light-headedness or even fainting. Abilify should be used with caution by anyone with a heart or circulatory problem, people who take blood pressure medication, and those who tend to become dehydrated.

Abilify has triggered seizures in a very small number of patients, and can also interfere with the swallowing mechanism. The risk of either problem is greater among older adults. If a patient has ever had a seizure, the doctor should be made aware of it. Abilify should be used with caution.

Drugs such as Abilify can cause the body to overheat. Patients should be cautious in hot weather and when exercising strenuously, and should be sure to get plenty of liquids.

Patients who must watch their sugar intake should be aware that Abilify oral solution contains sugar. In addition, patients who have phenylketonuria and cannot metabolize the amino acid phenylalanine should be aware that Abilify Discmelt contains this substance.

Abilify has not been tested in children or teenagers. Older adults should use the drug with caution.

Caution is advised when taking Abilify with blood pressure medications classified as alpha-adrenergic blockers (such as Hytrin and Cardura) and when combining it with drugs that act on the brain, including tranquilizers, antidepressants, sleeping pills, narcotic painkillers, and other schizophrenia medications.

Although Abilify does not interact with alcohol, the manufacturer recommends avoiding the combination.

Possible food and drug interactions when taking this medication

See the entry for the generic name aripiprazole on page 285.

Special information about pregnancy and breastfeeding

The effects of Abilify during pregnancy have not been adequately studied. The drug is recommended only if its benefits are thought to outweigh the potential risk to the baby. If a patient is pregnant or planning to become pregnant, she should inform her doctor immediately.

Breastfeeding is not recommended during Abilify therapy.

Recommended dosage

SCHIZOPHRENIA

Adults: The usual dose is 10 or 15 milligrams taken once a day. The doctor will wait at least 2 weeks before prescribing an increased dosage.

BIPOLAR DISORDER

Adults: The usual dose is 30 milligrams taken once a day. Depending on the patient's response, the doctor may decrease the dose to 15 milligrams a day.

Overdosage

Any medication taken in excess can have serious consequences. If an overdose is suspected, seek medical attention immediately.

- *Symptoms of Abilify overdose may include:*
  Sleepiness, vomiting

Acamprosate *See Campral, page 33*

ADDERALL

Amphetamines
Other brand name: Adderall XR

Why is this drug prescribed?

Adderall is prescribed in the treatment of attention deficit hyperactivity disorder (ADHD). It is used as part of a broader treatment plan that includes psychological, educational, and social measures. An extended-release form of the drug, called Adderall XR, is available for once-daily treatment of ADHD.

The regular form of Adderall is also prescribed for narcolepsy.

Most important fact about this drug

Adderall, like all amphetamines, has a high potential for abuse. If used in large doses over long periods of time, it can cause dependence and addiction. It's important for patients to use Adderall only as prescribed.

How should this medication be taken?

Adderall can be taken with or without food. Patients should use no more than the prescribed amount of Adderall. It should not be taken for a longer time or for any other purpose than prescribed.

The first dose should be taken upon awakening. If additional doses are prescribed, they should be taken at intervals of 4 to 6 hours. Patients should avoid late-evening doses, which can interfere with sleep.

Adderall XR extended-release capsules can be taken whole, or the contents can be sprinkled on applesauce. The applesauce should be eaten immediately, without chewing or crushing the medicine. Patients should be sure to use the entire contents of the capsule.

- *Missed dose...*
  If the patient is taking 1 dose a day, and at least 6 hours remain before bedtime, the dose should be taken as soon as remembered. If it's not remembered until the next day, the patient should skip the dose and go back to the regular schedule.

  If the patient is taking more than 1 dose a day, and remembers within an hour or so of the scheduled time, the missed dose should be taken immediately. Otherwise, the patient should skip the dose and go back to the regular schedule.

  Patients should never take 2 doses at once.

- *Storage instructions...*
  Adderall should be stored at room temperature in a tight, light-resistant container.

What side effects may occur?

Side effects cannot be predicted. If any develop or change in intensity, patients should inform their doctor as soon as possible.

- *Side effects of Adderall may include:*
  Dry mouth, high blood pressure, hives, impotence, overstimulation, rapid or pounding heartbeat, stomach and intestinal disturbances, weight loss

- *Side effects of Adderall XR may include:*
  Abdominal pain, diarrhea, dizziness, fever, infection (including viral), insomnia, loss of appetite, mood swings, nausea, nervousness, vomiting, weakness, weight loss

Why should this drug not be prescribed?

Adderall should never be prescribed for patients with any of the following conditions:

Heart disease or hardening of the arteries
High blood pressure
High pressure in the eye (glaucoma)
Overactive thyroid gland

Patients should avoid using Adderall within 14 days of taking a drug classified as an MAO inhibitor, such as the antidepressants Nardil and Parnate. A potentially life-threatening spike in blood pressure could result.

Adderall should not be prescribed for patients who have ever had a reaction to similar stimulant drugs. Adderall is also contraindicated for patients who appear agitated or are prone to substance abuse.

Special warnings about this medication

Before starting Adderall therapy, patients should tell the doctor about all their medical problems, especially if they have a history of heart problems, heart defects, or high blood pressure; mental problems including psychosis, mania, bipolar disorder, or depression; tics or Tourette's syndrome; kidney, liver, or thyroid problems; and seizures or an abnormal brain wave test (EEG).

Adderall should be used with caution if the patient has even a mild case of high blood pressure. Patients should be careful, too, about driving or operating machinery until they know how this drug affects them. It may impair judgment and coordination.

Amphetamines like Adderall may cause heart-related side effects such as increased blood pressure and heart rate. Amphetamines are also associated with life-threatening reactions, including stroke and heart attack in adults and sudden death in patients who have underlying heart problems or defects. Patients should contact their doctor immediately if they develop signs of heart problems such as chest pain, shortness of breath, or fainting while using Adderall.

In addition, amphetamines may cause or worsen certain psychiatric problems such as behavioral and thought disorders, bipolar disorder, and aggressive behavior or hostility. These drugs can also cause new psychotic symptoms (such as delusions, paranoia, and hearing voices) and new manic symptoms in children and teenagers. Patients and their caregivers should be advised to contact their doctor right away if they develop new or worsening mental symptoms.

If the problem is attention deficit disorder, the doctor should do a complete history and evaluation before prescribing Adderall, taking particular account of the severity of the symptoms and the age of the child. If the problem is a temporary reaction to a stressful situation, Adderall is probably not called for.

There are no data on long-term Adderall therapy in children. However, other amphetamine-based medications have been known to stunt growth, so the child should be watched carefully.

Patients should always check with their doctor before combining Adderall with the following types of drugs: antidepressants (including MAO inhibitors and lithium), antipsychotic medication, narcotic pain medicine, anticonvulsants, blood thinners, blood pressure medication, stomach acid medicine, and cold or allergy medicines that contain decongestants.

Possible food and drug interactions when taking this medication

See the entry for the generic name amphetamines on page 284.

Special information about pregnancy and breastfeeding

Heavy use of amphetamines during pregnancy can lead to premature birth or low birth weight. Pregnant women should avoid taking Adderall unless absolutely necessary.

Amphetamines do find their way into breast milk, so patients should not take Adderall while breastfeeding.

Recommended dosage

Whether the problem is attention-deficit disorder or narcolepsy, the dosage should be kept as low as possible.

ATTENTION DEFICIT HYPERACTIVITY DISORDER

Adderall
Children 3 to 5 Years of Age: The usual starting dose is 2.5 milligrams daily. Each week, the daily dosage may be increased by 2.5 milligrams until the condition is under control.

Children 6 Years of Age and Older: The usual starting dose is 5 milligrams once or twice a day. Each week, the daily dosage may be increased by 5 milligrams. Only in rare cases will a child need more than 40 milligrams per day.

Therapy may be interrupted occasionally to see if the drug is still needed.

Adderall XR
Children 6 Years of Age and Older: The usual starting dose for children taking Adderall for the first time is 10 milligrams once daily in the morning. At weekly intervals, the doctor may increase the daily dosage by 5 or 10 milligrams, up to a maximum of 30 milligrams a day.

Children already taking regular Adderall are prescribed a single dose of Adderall XR equal to their previous daily total.

Adderall XR has not been tested on children under 6 years old.

NARCOLEPSY

Adderall
Adults: The usual total daily dose ranges from 5 to 60 milligrams, taken as 2 or more smaller doses.

Children under 12 Years of Age: The usual starting dose is 5 milligrams daily. Each week, the daily dose may be raised by 5 milligrams until the condition is under control.

Children 12 Years of Age and Older: The usual starting dose is 10 milligrams daily, with weekly increases of 10 milligrams daily until the drug takes effect.

Overdosage
A large overdose of Adderall can be fatal. Warning signs of a massive overdose include convulsions and coma.

• *Symptoms of Adderall overdose may include:*
  Abdominal cramps, changes in blood pressure, combative behavior, confusion, diarrhea, hallucinations, heightened reflexes, high fever, irregular heartbeat, nausea, panic, rapid breathing, restlessness, tremor, vomiting

If an overdose is suspected, seek emergency treatment immediately.

Alprazolam *See Xanax, page 260*

Alprazolam orally disintegrating tablet *See Niravam, page 144*

Ambien *See Ambien CR, page 7*

AMBIEN CR
Zolpidem tartrate
Other brand name: Ambien

Why is this drug prescribed?
Ambien CR is used for the short-term treatment of insomnia, including trouble falling sleep and waking up often during the night. Studies show that Ambien CR is effective for up to 7 hours.

Most important fact about this drug
Sleep problems are usually temporary and require medication for a week or two at most. Insomnia that lasts longer could be a sign of another medical problem. Patients should check with their doctor if they find that they need this medicine for more than 7 to 10 days.

How should this medication be taken?

Ambien CR works very quickly, usually within 30 minutes. Patients should take it just before going to bed, and only when they can devote a full 7 to 8 hours to sleep. They should take no more than the prescribed dose.

Because Ambien CR is an extended-release tablet, it should be swallowed whole and never divided, chewed, or crushed. It's best not to take the drug with food, since this may slow its effects.

- *Missed dose...*
  Ambien CR should be taken only as needed. Patients should never double the dose.

- *Storage instructions...*
  Store at room temperature. Protect from extreme heat.

What side effects may occur?

Side effects cannot be predicted. If any develop or change in intensity, patients should inform their doctor as soon as possible.

- *Side effects may include:*
  Back pain, dizziness, drowsiness, fatigue, headache, hallucinations, muscle aches, nausea

Why should this drug not be prescribed?

Patients who have an allergic reaction to Ambien CR will not be able to use the drug.

Special warnings about this medication

When sleep medications are used every night for more than a few weeks, some may lose their effectiveness. People can also become dependent on sleep medications if they are used for a long time or at high doses. Anyone who has had previous problems with addiction to alcohol or drugs should make sure the doctor knows about it.

Before taking this drug, patients should inform the doctor if they have a history of depression.

Some people using Ambien CR have experienced unusual changes in their thinking and/or behavior. Patients should alert the doctor if they notice a change. Ambien CR and other sleep medicines can cause a special type of memory loss. It should not be taken on an overnight airplane flight of less than 7 to 8 hours, since "traveler's amnesia" may occur.

Until patients know whether the medication will have any "carry over" effect the next day, they should use extreme care while doing anything that requires complete alertness, such as driving a car or operating machinery. Older adults, in particular, should be aware that they may be more apt to fall.

Patients with liver problems should use Ambien CR with caution. It will take longer for its effects to wear off.

Sleepwalking—including eating or driving while not fully awake with no memory of the event—has been reported by people taking sleep medicines such as Ambien CR. These behaviors are more likely to occur if the sleep medicine is taken with alcohol or other drugs used to treat depression and anxiety. In addition, rare cases of severe allergic reactions have also been reported. If patients experience any of these events, they should contact their doctor immediately.

Patients should consult with their doctor before stopping Ambien CR if they've taken it for more than 1 or 2 weeks. Sudden discontinuation of a sleep medicine can bring on withdrawal symptoms ranging from unpleasant feelings to vomiting and cramps.

When taking Ambien CR, patients should not drink alcohol. It can increase the drug's side effects.

Patients who have a history of heavy snoring, sleep apnea, or breathing problems such as asthma, bronchitis, or emphysema may find that the condition worsens while they use Ambien CR.

Ambien CR has not been studied in patients less than 18 years old.

Patients should always check with their doctor before combining Ambien CR with drugs that affect the central nervous system, including antidepressants and anti-anxiety medication. Remind patients not to drink alcohol while using Ambien CR.

Possible food and drug interactions when taking this medication

See the entry for the generic name zolpidem on page 425.

Special information about pregnancy and breastfeeding

Patients should inform their doctor immediately if they are pregnant or plan to become pregnant. Babies whose mothers take certain sedative/hypnotic drugs may have withdrawal symptoms after birth and may seem limp and flaccid. Ambien CR is not recommended for use by nursing mothers.

Recommended dosage

ADULTS

Ambien CR extended-release tablets: The recommended dosage for adults is 12.5 milligrams right before bedtime. The doctor will prescribe a smaller dose of 6.25 milligrams if the patient is likely to be sensitive to the drug or has a liver problem.

Ambien tablets: The recommended dosage for adults is 10 milligrams right before bedtime. The doctor will prescribe a smaller dose of 5 milligrams if the patient is likely to be sensitive to the drug or has a liver problem.

Overdosage

People who take too much Ambien CR may become excessively sleepy or even go into a light coma. The symptoms of overdose are more severe if the person is also taking other drugs that depress the central nervous system. Some cases of overdose have been fatal. If an overdose is suspected, seek medical attention immediately.

AMITRIPTYLINE HYDROCHLORIDE

Why is this drug prescribed?

Amitriptyline is prescribed for the relief of symptoms of mental depression. It is a member of the group of drugs called tricyclic antidepressants. Some doctors also prescribe amitriptyline to treat bulimia (an eating disorder), to control chronic pain, to prevent migraine headaches, and to treat a pathological weeping and laughing syndrome associated with multiple sclerosis.

Most important fact about this drug

Amitriptyline must be taken regularly for several weeks before it becomes fully effective. It's important that patients not skip any doses, even if they seem to make no difference or don't seem necessary.

How should this medication be taken?

Amitriptyline must be taken exactly as prescribed. Patients may experience side effects, such as mild drowsiness, early in therapy. However, these problems usually disappear after a few days. Beneficial effects may take as long as 30 days to appear.

Amitriptyline may cause dry mouth. Sucking a hard candy, chewing gum, or melting bits of ice in the mouth can provide relief.

- *Missed dose...*
  Generally, the forgotten dose should be taken as soon as remembered. However, if it is almost time for the patient's next dose, they should skip the dose they missed and go back to their regular schedule. Doses should never be doubled.

  Patients who take a single daily dose at bedtime should not make up for it in the morning. It may cause side effects during the day.

- *Storage instructions...*
  Amitriptyline should be stored at room temperature in a tightly closed container, and protected from light and excessive heat.

What side effects may occur?

Side effects cannot be predicted. If any develop or change in intensity, patients should inform their doctor as soon as possible.

Older adults are especially liable to experience certain side effects of amitriptyline, including rapid heartbeat, constipation, dry mouth, blurred vision, sedation, and confusion, and are in greater danger of sustaining a fall.

* *Side effects may include:*
  Blurred vision, bone marrow depression, bowel problems, breast enlargement (in males and females), constipation, dry mouth, hair loss, heart attack, high body temperature, problems urinating, rash, seizure, stroke, swelling of the testicles, water retention

* *Side effects due to rapid decrease in dose or abrupt withdrawal from amitriptyline may include:*
  Headache, nausea, vague feeling of bodily discomfort

* *Side effects due to gradual dosage reduction may include:*
  Dream and sleep disturbances, irritability, restlessness

These side effects do not signify an addiction to the drug.

Why should this drug not be prescribed?

Anyone who is sensitive to or has ever had an allergic reaction to amitriptyline or similar drugs such as Norpramin and Tofranil should not take this medication. Patients should be careful to make the doctor aware of any drug reactions they have experienced.

Amitriptyline cannot be used by anyone taking an MAO inhibitor such as the antidepressants Nardil and Parnate. Unless the doctor says otherwise, it should also be avoided by patients recovering from a heart attack.

Special warnings about this medication

In clinical studies, antidepressants increased the risk of suicidal thinking and behavior in children and adolescents with depression and other psychiatric disorders. Anyone considering the use of amitriptyline, or any other antidepressant in a child or adolescent, must balance the risk with the clinical need. Amitriptyline is not approved for treating children less than 12 years old.

Additionally, the progression of major depression is associated with a worsening of symptoms and/or the emergence of suicidal thinking or behavior in both adults and children, whether or not they are taking antidepressants. Patients and caregivers should watch for any change in symptoms or any new symptoms that appear suddenly—especially agitation, anxiety, hostility, panic, restlessness, extreme hyperactivity, and suicidal thinking or behavior—and report them to the doctor immediately. Be especially observant at the beginning of treatment or whenever there is a change in dose.

Amitriptyline should not be stopped abruptly, especially if the patient has been taking large doses for a long time. The doctor will schedule a gradual reduction in dosage that will help prevent a possible relapse and will reduce the possibility of withdrawal symptoms.

Amitriptyline may make the skin more sensitive to sunlight. Patients should stay out of the sun, wear protective clothing, and apply a sunblock.

Amitriptyline can make patients drowsy or less alert. They should avoid driving, operating dangerous machinery, or participating in any hazardous activity that requires full mental alertness until they know how this drug affects them.

While taking this medication, patients may feel dizzy or light-headed or actually faint when getting up from a lying or sitting position. If getting up slowly doesn't help or if this problem continues, the doctor should be notified.

Amitriptyline should be used with caution in patients with a history of seizures, urinary retention, glaucoma or other chronic eye conditions, a heart or circulatory system disorder, or liver problems. Caution is also warranted in patients who are receiving thyroid medication. The doctor should be apprised of all the patient's medical problems before the start of amitriptyline therapy.

Patients should tell doctors they are taking amitriptyline before having surgery, dental treatment, or any diagnostic procedure. Certain drugs used during surgery, such as anesthetics and muscle relaxants, and drugs used in certain diagnostic procedures may react badly with amitriptyline.

Amitriptyline may intensify the effects of alcohol. Patients should avoid drinking alcohol while taking this medication.

Possible food and drug interactions when taking this medication

See the entry for amitriptyline on page 278.

Special information about pregnancy and breastfeeding

The effects of amitriptyline during pregnancy have not been adequately studied. Patients should inform their doctor immediately if they are pregnant or are planning to become pregnant.

This medication appears in breast milk. If amitriptyline is essential to a patient's health, the doctor may advise her to discontinue breastfeeding until treatment is finished.

Recommended dosage

ADULTS

The usual starting dosage is 75 milligrams per day divided into 2 or more smaller doses. The doctor may gradually increase this dose to 150 milligrams per day. The total daily dose is generally never higher than 200 milligrams.

Alternatively, the doctor may start patients with 50 milligrams to 100 milligrams at bedtime. This bedtime dose may be gradually increased by 25 or 50 milligrams up to a total of 150 milligrams a day.

For long-term use, the usual dose ranges from 40 to 100 milligrams taken once daily, usually at bedtime.

CHILDREN

Use of amitriptyline is not recommended for children under 12 years of age.

The usual dose for adolescents 12 years of age and over is 10 milligrams, 3 times a day, with 20 milligrams taken at bedtime.

OLDER ADULTS

The usual dose is 10 milligrams taken 3 times a day, with 20 milligrams taken at bedtime.

Overdosage

An overdose of amitriptyline can prove fatal. If an overdose is suspected, seek medical attention immediately.

- *Symptoms of amitriptyline overdose may include:*
  Abnormally low blood pressure, confusion, convulsions, dilated pupils and other eye problems, disturbed concentration, drowsiness, hallucinations, impaired heart function, rapid or irregular heartbeat, reduced body temperature, stupor, unresponsiveness, or coma

- *Symptoms contrary to the usual effect of this medication are:*
  Agitation, extremely high body temperature, overactive reflexes, rigid muscles, vomiting

Amitriptyline with chlordiazepoxide *See Limbitrol, page 114.*

AMITRIPTYLINE WITH PERPHENAZINE

Why is this drug prescribed?

Amitriptyline with perphenazine is used to treat anxiety, agitation, and depression. It is a combination of a tricyclic antidepressant (amitriptyline) and a tranquilizer (perphenazine).

Amitriptyline with perphenazine can also help people with schizophrenia who are depressed and people with insomnia, fatigue, loss of interest, loss of appetite, or a slowing of physical and mental reactions.

Most important fact about this drug

Amitriptyline with perphenazine may cause tardive dyskinesia—a condition marked by involuntary muscle spasms and twitches in the face and body. This condition may be permanent and appears to be most common among the elderly, especially women.

How should this medication be taken?

Amitriptyline with perphenazine may be taken with or without food. It should not be taken with alcohol. Amitriptyline with perphenazine should not be taken within 2 hours of antacids or diarrhea medication.

- *Missed dose...*
  Generally, a forgotten dose should be taken as soon as remembered. However, if it is within 2 hours of the next dose, patients should skip the missed dose and go back to their regular schedule. Doses should never be doubled.

- *Storage instructions...*
  Amitriptyline with perphenazine should be stored at room temperature in a tightly closed container. Amitriptyline with perphenazine 2 to 10 milligrams tablets should be protected from light.

What side effects may occur?

Side effects cannot be predicted. If any develop or change in intensity, patients should inform their doctor as soon as possible.

- *Side effects may include:*
  Disorientation, dry mouth, high or low blood pressure, nervous system disorders, sedation

Why should this drug not be prescribed?

Amitriptyline with perphenazine must never be combined with drugs that slow down the central nervous system, including alcohol, barbiturates, analgesics, antihistamines, or narcotics.

It should not be used by anyone who is recovering from a recent heart attack or has an abnormal bone marrow condition. It should be avoided by patients who have had an allergic reaction to phenothiazines or amitriptyline.

People who are taking antidepressant drugs known as MAO inhibitors (including Nardil and Parnate) should not take amitriptyline with per-phenazine.

Special warnings about this medication

In clinical studies, antidepressants increased the risk of suicidal thinking and behavior in children and adolescents with depression and other psy-chiatric disorders. Anyone considering the use of amitriptyline with per-phenazine, or any other antidepressant in a child or adolescent, must bal-ance the risk with the clinical need. Amitriptyline with perphenazine is not approved for use in children.

Additionally, the progression of major depression is associated with a worsening of symptoms and/or the emergence of suicidal thinking or behavior in both adults and children, whether or not they are taking anti-depressants. Patients and caregivers should watch for any change in symp-toms or any new symptoms that appear suddenly—especially agitation, anxiety, hostility, panic, restlessness, extreme hyperactivity, and suicidal thinking or behavior—and report them to the doctor immediately. Be especially observant at the beginning of treatment or whenever there is a change in dose.

Amitriptyline with perphenazine should be used with caution by anyone who has ever had glaucoma; difficulty urinating; breast cancer; breathing problems; seizures; or heart, liver, kidney, or thyroid disease. Caution is also in order if the patient is exposed to extreme heat or pesticides. Be aware that amitriptyline with perphenazine may mask signs of brain tumor, intestinal blockage, and overdose of other drugs.

Drugs such as amitriptyline with perphenazine have been known to trigger a potentially fatal condition known as neuroleptic malignant syndrome. Symptoms include high fever, muscle rigidity, unstable blood pressure, rapid or irregular heartbeat, and excessive sweating. If any of these symptoms develop, patients should see their doctor immediately. Amitriptyline with perphenazine therapy will need to be discontinued.

If a patient develops a fever without a cause, they should stop taking amitriptyline with perphenazine and call their doctor.

Amitriptyline with perphenazine could make patients more sensitive to sunlight. Encourage them to stay out of the sun, wear protective clothing, and use sunblock.

Amitriptyline with perphenazine could also trigger a manic episode in bipolar patients, although the drug's tranquilizing effects seem to reduce this risk.

While taking this medication, patients may feel dizzy or light-headed or actually faint when getting up from a lying or sitting position. If getting up more slowly doesn't help or if the problem continues, patients should alert the doctor.

Patients should tell the doctor or dentist they're taking amitriptyline with perphenazine before having any surgery, dental work, or diagnostic procedure. Amitriptyline with perphenazine could interact with anesthetics, muscle relaxants, and other drugs used during surgical procedures.

Nausea, headache, and a general ill feeling can result if amitriptyline with perphenazine is stopped abruptly. Patients need to follow the doctor's instructions closely when discontinuing amitriptyline with perphenazine. If the dose is gradually reduced, they may still experience irritability, restlessness, and dream and sleep disturbances, but these effects will not last.

This drug may impair the ability to drive a car or operate potentially dangerous machinery. Patients should not participate in any activities that require full alertness if they are unsure about their ability.

Amitriptyline with perphenazine contains the same active ingredients as amitriptyline and perphenazine and should not be used with these drugs.

Extreme drowsiness and other potentially serious effects can result if amitriptyline with perphenazine is combined with alcohol or other central nervous system depressants such as narcotics, painkillers, and sleep medications.

Possible food and drug interactions when taking this medication

See the entry for the generic names amitriptyline and perphenazine on pages 278 and 372.

Special information about pregnancy and breastfeeding

Amitriptyline with perphenazine may cause false-positive results on pregnancy tests. Amitriptyline with perphenazine should not be used by pregnant women or mothers who are breastfeeding.

Recommended dosage

Each patient's dose must be individualized. The maximum dose is 8 tablets a day. It may be a few days to a few weeks before the patient notices any improvement.

The following dosages are for adults; older patients and adolescents usually take lower doses. Amitriptyline with perphenazine is not recommended for use in children since the proper dosage has not been established.

NONPSYCHOTIC ANXIETY AND DEPRESSION

The usual dose is 1 tablet of amitriptyline with perphenazine 2-25 milligrams or 4-25 milligrams taken 3 or 4 times a day.

ANXIETY IN PEOPLE WITH SCHIZOPHRENIA

The usual dose is 2 tablets of amitriptyline with perphenazine 4-25 milligrams taken 3 times a day. The doctor may prescribe another tablet of amitriptyline with perphenazine 4-25 milligrams at bedtime, if needed.

For patients who continue taking amitriptyline with perphenazine, the doctor will probably reduce the dosage to 1 tablet a day.

Overdosage

Any medication taken in excess can have serious consequences. An overdose of amitriptyline with perphenazine can be fatal. If an overdose is suspected, seek medical help immediately.

- *Symptoms of amitriptyline with perphenazine overdose may include:*
  Abnormalities of posture and movements, agitation, coma, convulsions, dilated pupils, drowsiness, extreme low body temperature, eye movement problems, high fever, heart failure, overactive reflexes, rapid or irregular heartbeat, rigid muscles, stupor, very low blood pressure, vomiting

AMOXAPINE

Why is this drug prescribed?

Amoxapine relieves the symptoms of depression. It belongs to the class of antidepressants known as tricyclics and is believed to work by balancing certain natural chemicals in the brain.

Most important fact about this drug

Serious, sometimes fatal, reactions can occur when drugs such as amoxapine are taken with another type of antidepressant called an MAO inhibitor. Drugs in this category include Nardil and Parnate. Amoxapine should be avoided within 2 weeks of taking one of these drugs.

How should this medication be taken?

It's not unusual for a patient to feel no immediate effect from this medication. However, relief of symptoms usually begins within 2 weeks, and sometimes in as few as 4 to 7 days.

Amoxapine can cause dry mouth. Sucking hard candy or chewing gum can help this problem.

- *Missed dose...*

    Patients who usually take amoxapine once a day at bedtime, but forget to take it until morning, should skip the missed dose. If a patient takes several doses per day, the forgotten dose should be taken as soon as it's remembered. If it is almost time for the next dose, the patient should skip the one they missed and return to their regular schedule. Doses should never be doubled.

- *Storage instructions...*

    Amoxapine can be stored at room temperature. It should be protected from excessive heat.

What side effects may occur?

Side effects cannot be predicted. If any develop or change in intensity, patients should inform their doctor as soon as possible.

- *Side effects may include:*

    Anxiety, blurred vision, confusion, constipation, difficulty sleeping, dizziness, drowsiness, dry mouth, excessive appetite, excitement, fatigue, fluid retention, fluttery heartbeat, headache, increased perspiration, lack of muscle coordination, nausea, nervousness, nightmares, restlessness, skin rashes, tremors, weakness

Why should this drug not be prescribed?

Amoxapine must be avoided by anyone taking an MAO inhibitor. (See "Most important fact about this drug.") Patients should also avoid this medication if recovering from a heart attack or if they are sensitive to or have ever had an allergic reaction to amoxapine or dibenzoxazepine medications.

Special warnings about this medication

Amoxapine may cause facial and body twitching known as tardive dyskinesia. This happens more often in older adults, especially older women. Patients who develop involuntary facial or body movements should see their doctor immediately.

Neuroleptic malignant syndrome (NMS) has also occurred in people using amoxapine. NMS is characterized by extremely high body temperature; rigid muscles; excessive perspiration; altered mental state; and irregular pulse, blood pressure, and heartbeat. If any of these symptoms develop, they should be reported to the doctor immediately.

Amoxapine should be used with care in patients who have difficulty urinating, and in those who suffer from angle-closure glaucoma, or increased pressure within the eye. It should also be used cautiously by anyone who has a seizure disorder or has had one in the past.

The antidepressant drug Prozac (fluoxetine) can increase the effects of amoxapine. If the patient is switching from Prozac to amoxapine, the doctor may wait 5 weeks or more before starting the new drug.

Patients with a heart condition should use amoxapine with caution. There have been reports of heart attack and stroke in patients taking this type of antidepressant.

Antidepressants can cause allergic reactions such as skin rashes or fever in some people. This usually occurs during the first few days of treatment. Patients should stop taking the medication and consult their doctor if these symptoms develop.

Amoxapine may cause drowsiness. Caution is warranted when driving, operating machinery or appliances, or doing any activity that requires full mental alertness until it's known how the patient reacts on amoxapine.

Amoxapine may increase the effects of alcohol. Patients should not drink alcohol while taking this medication.

Possible food and drug interactions when taking this medication

See the entry for amoxapine on page 282.

Special information about pregnancy and breastfeeding

Although the effects of amoxapine during pregnancy have not been adequately studied, stillbirths and decreased birth weight have appeared in animal studies. Amoxapine should be used only if the potential benefits outweigh the potential risks. Patients should inform their doctors immediately if they are pregnant or plan to become pregnant.

Amoxapine appears in breast milk and could affect a nursing infant. If this medication is essential to the patient's health, her doctor may advise her to stop breastfeeding until her treatment is finished.

Recommended dosage

Effective dosages of amoxapine may vary from one person to another.

ADULTS

The usual starting dosage is 50 milligrams 2 or 3 times daily. If the patient tolerates the drug well, the doctor may increase the dosage to 100 milligrams 2 or 3 times daily by the end of the first week. If that dose is not effective after 2 weeks, the doctor may increase the dose even further.

When the effective dosage has been established, the doctor may prescribe a single dose (not to exceed 300 milligrams) at bedtime.

CHILDREN

Safety and effectiveness have not been established in children under the age of 16.

OLDER ADULTS

In general, lower dosages are recommended for older people. The recommended starting dosage of amoxapine is 25 milligrams 2 or 3 times daily. If this is well tolerated, the doctor may increase the dosage by the end of the first week to 50 milligrams 2 or 3 times daily. A daily dosage of 100 to 150 milligrams may be enough for many older people, but some may need up to 300 milligrams.

Overdosage

Any medication taken in excess can have serious consequences. If an overdose is suspected, seek medical treatment immediately.

- *Symptoms of amoxapine overdose may include:*
  Coma; convulsions; kidney failure; severe, protracted epileptic seizures

Amphetamines *See Adderall, page 3*

ANAFRANIL
Clomipramine hydrochloride

Why is this drug prescribed?
Anafranil, a chemical cousin of tricyclic antidepressant medications such as Tofranil and amitriptyline, is used in the treatment of obsessive-compulsive disorder.

Most important fact about this drug
Serious, even fatal, reactions have been known to occur when drugs such as Anafranil are taken along with drugs classified as MAO inhibitors. Drugs in this category include the antidepressants Nardil and Parnate. Anafranil must never be combined with one of these drugs.

How should this medication be taken?

Anafranil should be taken with meals at first, to avoid stomach upset. After a regular dosage has been established, patients can take 1 dose at bedtime to avoid sleepiness during the day.

This medicine may cause dry mouth. Hard candy, chewing gum, or bits of ice may relieve this problem.

* *Missed dose...*
  Patients who take 1 dose at bedtime should consult their doctor if they miss a dose. The missed dose should not be taken in the morning. Patients who take 2 or more doses a day can take the missed dose as soon as they remember. If it is almost time for the patient's next dose, they should skip the one they missed and go back to their regular schedule. Doses should never be doubled.

* *Storage instructions...*
  Anafranil should be stored at room temperature in a tightly closed container, away from moisture.

What side effects may occur?

Side effects cannot be predicted. If any develop or change in intensity, patients should inform their doctor as soon as possible.

The most significant risk is that of seizures. Headache, fatigue, and nausea can also be problems. Men are likely to experience problems with sexual function. Unwanted weight gain is a potential problem for many people who take Anafranil, although a small number actually lose weight.

* *Side effects may include:*
  Constipation, dizziness, dry mouth, impotence, increased appetite, increased sweating, indigestion, libido change, nausea, nervousness, sleepiness, tremor, twitching, visual changes, weight gain, weight loss

Why should this drug not be prescribed?

This medication cannot be used by patients who are sensitive to or have ever had an allergic reaction to a tricyclic antidepressant such as Tofranil, amitriptyline, or Tegretol.

Anafranil must be avoided if the patient is taking, or has taken within the past 14 days, an MAO inhibitor such as the antidepressants Parnate or Nardil. Combining Anafranil with one of these medications could lead to fever, seizures, coma, and even death.

Patients who have recently had a heart attack should not take Anafranil.

Special warnings about this medication

This drug should be used with caution in children with depression. In clinical studies, antidepressants increased the risk of suicidal thinking and behavior in children and adolescents with depression and other psychiatric disorders. Anyone considering the use of Anafranil or any other antidepressant in a child or adolescent must balance this risk with the clinical need. In children, Anafranil is only approved to treat obsessive-compulsive disorder.

Additionally, the progression of major depression is associated with a worsening of symptoms and/or the emergence of suicidal thinking or behavior in both adults and children, whether or not they are taking anti-depressants. Patients and caregivers should watch for any change in symptoms or any new symptoms that appear suddenly—especially agita-tion, anxiety, hostility, panic, restlessness, extreme hyperactivity, and suicidal thinking or behavior—and report them to the doctor immediately. Be especially observant at the beginning of treatment or whenever there is a change in dose.

If the patient has narrow-angle glaucoma (increased pressure in the eye) or is having difficulty urinating, Anafranil could make these condi-tions worse. Anafranil should also be used with caution in patients with abnormal kidney function.

If the patient has a tumor of the adrenal gland, this medication could cause blood pressure to rise suddenly and dangerously.

Because Anafranil poses a possible risk of seizures, and because it may impair mental or physical ability to perform complicated tasks, patients should take special precautions if they need to drive a car, oper-ate complicated machinery, or take part in activities such as swimming or climbing, in which suddenly losing consciousness could be dangerous. Note that the risk of seizures is increased if the patient:

Has ever had a seizure
Has a history of brain damage or alcoholism
Is taking another medication that increases the risk of seizures

As with Tofranil, amitriptyline, and other tricyclic antidepressants, an overdose of Anafranil can be fatal. To minimize the risk of overdose, the doctor may prescribe only a small quantity of Anafranil at a time.

Anafranil may cause the skin to become more sensitive to sunlight. Prolonged exposure to sunlight should be avoided.

Before any kind of surgery involving the use of general anesthesia, the doctor or dentist should be informed that the patient is taking Anafranil. The drug may have to be temporarily discontinued.

When it is time to stop taking Anafranil, patients should not quit abruptly. Their doctor will have them taper off gradually to avoid with-drawal symptoms such as dizziness, fever, general feeling of illness, headache, high fever, irritability or worsening of emotional or mental problems, nausea, sleep problems, and vomiting.

Patients should avoid alcoholic beverages while taking Anafranil.

Possible food and drug interactions when taking this medication

See the entry for the generic name clomipramine on page 306.

Special information about pregnancy and breastfeeding

The doctor should be informed immediately if the patient is pregnant or plans to become pregnant. Some babies born to women who took Anafranil have had withdrawal symptoms such as jitteriness, tremors, and seizures. Anafranil should be used during pregnancy only if absolutely necessary.

Anafranil appears in breast milk. The patient's doctor may advise her to stop breastfeeding while she is taking this medication.

Recommended dosage

ADULTS

The usual recommended initial dose is 25 milligrams daily. The doctor may gradually increase this dosage to 100 milligrams during the first 2 weeks. During this period, the patient should take this drug divided into smaller doses, with meals. The maximum daily dosage is 250 milligrams. After the ideal dose has been determined, the doctor may switch the patient to a single dose at bedtime, to avoid sleepiness during the day.

CHILDREN

The usual recommended initial dose is 25 milligrams daily, divided into smaller doses and taken with meals. Within 2 weeks, the doctor may gradually increase the dose to 100 milligrams or 3 milligrams per 2.2 pounds (1 kilogram) of body weight per day, whichever is smaller. The maximum dose is 200 milligrams or 3 milligrams per 2.2 pounds of body weight, whichever is smaller. Once the dose has been determined, the child can take it in a single dose at bedtime.

Overdosage

An overdose of Anafranil can be fatal. If an overdose is suspected, seek medical attention immediately.

- *Critical signs and symptoms of Anafranil overdose may include:*
  Impaired brain activity (including coma), irregular heartbeat, seizures, severely low blood pressure

- *Other signs and symptoms of overdose may include:*
  Agitation, bluish skin color, breathing difficulty, delirium, dilated pupils, high fever, incoordination, little or no urine output, muscle rigidity, overactive reflexes, rapid heartbeat, restlessness, severe perspiration, shock, stupor, twitching or twisting movements, vomiting

There is a danger of heart malfunction and, in rare cases, heart attack.

ANTABUSE
Disulfiram

Why is this drug prescribed?
Antabuse is prescribed to help treat alcohol dependence. Because the drug is not a cure, the patient must be ready to make a change and be willing to undertake a comprehensive treatment program that includes professional counseling, support groups, and close medical supervision. When Antabuse is used alone, without proper motivation and supportive therapy, it is unlikely to have any effect on drinking patterns.

Antabuse works by producing a sensitivity to alcohol that causes a highly unpleasant reaction when the patient ingests even small amounts of alcohol. To get the most out of Antabuse treatment, the patient must be absolutely committed to abstaining from all types of alcohol.

Most important fact about this drug
Antabuse should never be given to a patient who is already intoxicated with alcohol or without the patient's full knowledge. The prescribing physician should also instruct the patient's relatives accordingly.

How should this medication be taken?
Antabuse should be taken once a day, usually in the morning. If sedation occurs, the patient can take the daily dose at bedtime.

Antabuse should never be given until the patient has abstained from alcohol for at least 12 hours.

- *Missed dose...*
  Generally, forgotten doses should be taken as soon as remembered. However, if it is almost time for the next dose, patients should skip the one they missed and return to their regular schedule. Doses should never be doubled.

- *Storage instructions...*
  Store at room temperature, away from light.

What side effects may occur?
Side effects cannot be anticipated. If any develop or change in intensity, patients should inform their doctor as soon as possible.

- *Side effects may include:*
  Inflammation of the optic nerve (possibly leading to blurred vision or vision loss), liver problems (including hepatitis and, on occasion, liver failure), nerve pain (such as pain and tingling in the hands and feet)

A small number of patients experience temporary symptoms during the first 2 weeks of therapy, including drowsiness, fatigue, impotence, headache, skin reactions such as acne or rashes, and a metallic or garlic-like aftertaste. These usually disappear as therapy continues or with a reduced dosage. Skin reactions can often be controlled by treatment with an antihistamine.

Psychotic reactions have also been reported, attributable in most cases to high dosages, toxic interactions with other drugs, or to the unmasking of underlying psychoses caused by the stress associated with alcohol withdrawal.

Why should this drug not be prescribed?

Antabuse should not be given to patients who have severe cardiovascular disease, psychoses, or a sensitivity to the generic ingredient disulfiram or other thiuram derivatives used in pesticides and rubber manufacturing. Patients with a history of skin reactions caused by rubber should be tested for sensitivity to thiuram derivatives before receiving Antabuse.

In addition, patients should not be given Antabuse if they are receiving or have recently received metronidazole (Flagyl, MetroGel), paraldehyde (an anticonvulsant), or any product containing alcohol, including prepared foods and medications such as cough syrup.

Special warnings about this medication

Patients should be fully informed of the sensitivity reaction that will occur if they drink alcohol—even small amounts—while taking Antabuse. This includes skin flushing, throbbing head and neck pain, breathing problems, vomiting, sweating, chest pain, heart palpitations, fainting, weakness, loss of balance, blurred vision, and confusion. The intensity of the reaction varies by individual but is usually proportional to the amount of Antabuse and alcohol ingested. Severe reactions may lead to life-threatening emergencies including heart attack or heart failure, extremely slowed breathing, loss of consciousness, and convulsions. Death could result if proper medical treatment is not sought quickly.

The duration of the alcohol sensitivity reaction can vary from 30 to 60 minutes up to several hours in the most severe cases, or as long as there is alcohol in the blood. In addition, reactions to alcohol may occur up to 14 days after stopping treatment with Antabuse.

Patients should be warned to avoid all forms of alcohol, including rubbing alcohol and household products that contain even small amounts, such as sauces, vinegars, cough syrups, colognes, and aftershave lotions. Likewise, they should not come in contact with or breathe the fumes of paint, paint thinner, varnish, shellac, ethanol fuel, and similar products containing forms of alcohol.

Antabuse should be used with extreme caution in people with diabetes, underactive thyroid, epilepsy, a history of brain damage, and kidney or liver problems.

It is advisable for patients to carry an identification card that states they are receiving Antabuse and that lists the reactions likely to occur if the drug is combined with alcohol. Identification cards may be requested from the patient's doctor or pharmacist.

In some cases, Antabuse treatment has led to severe liver toxicity, including liver failure that resulted in transplantation or death. This toxicity can occur in people with or without a history of liver problems and may develop even after many months of treatment. Warn patients to notify their doctor immediately if they develop any of the following signs of liver damage: fatigue, muscle weakness, general feeling of discomfort or illness, loss of appetite, nausea, vomiting, dark urine, and jaundice (yellowing of the skin or whites of the eyes).

Animal studies suggest that a toxic interaction may occur between orally administered Antabuse and inhaled ethylene dibromide, a chemical mainly used in gasoline mixtures. This interaction may have increased the risk of tumors and death in rats. Although a similar correlation in humans has not been demonstrated, patients should still be cautioned to avoid exposure to ethylene dibromide and its vapors.

Other animal research has suggested that combining Antabuse with nitrites (a common preservative found in processed meats) increased the risk of tumors, although the relevance of this finding for humans is unknown.

Possible food and drug interactions when taking this medication
See the entry for the generic name disulfiram on page 315.

Special information about pregnancy and breastfeeding
The effects of Antabuse during pregnancy have not been adequately studied. The drug is recommended only if its benefits are thought to outweigh the potential risk to the baby. If a patient is pregnant or planning to become pregnant, she should inform her doctor immediately.

It is not known whether Antabuse appears in breast milk. The manufacturer recommends avoiding this drug while nursing.

Recommended dosage
ADULTS

The initial dose is usually 500 milligrams taken once a day for 1 to 2 weeks. Thereafter, the average maintenance dose is 250 milligrams a day (with a range of 125 to 500 milligrams daily).

Overdosage
No information on overdose is available. However, any medication taken in excess can have serious consequences. If an overdose is suspected, seek medical attention immediately.

ARICEPT

Donepezil hydrochloride
Other brand name: Aricept ODT

Why is this drug prescribed?

Aricept is used to treat the symptoms of early Alzheimer's disease. This progressive, degenerative disorder causes physical changes in the brain that disrupt the flow of information and interfere with memory, thinking, and behavior. Aricept can temporarily improve brain function in some Alzheimer's sufferers, although it does not halt the progress of the underlying disease.

Most important fact about this drug

To maintain any improvement, Aricept must be taken regularly. If the drug is stopped, its benefits will soon be lost. Anyone starting the drug must be patient, because it can take up to 3 weeks for any positive effects to appear.

How should this medication be taken?

Aricept should be taken once a day just before bedtime. Caregivers should make sure it's taken every day. If Aricept is not taken regularly, it won't work. It can be taken with or without food.

• *Missed dose...*
  It should be made up as soon as it's remembered. If it is almost time for the patient's next dose, caregivers should skip the one that was missed and go back to the regular schedule. Doses should never be doubled.

• *Storage instructions...*
  Aricept should be stored at room temperature.

What side effects may occur?

Side effects cannot be predicted. If any develop or change in intensity, the doctor should be informed as soon as possible.

  Side effects are more likely with higher doses. The most common side effects are diarrhea, fatigue, insomnia, loss of appetite, muscle cramps, nausea, and vomiting. When one of these effects occurs, it is usually mild and gets better as treatment continues.

• *Other side effects may include:*
  Abnormal dreams, arthritis, bruising, depression, dizziness, fainting, frequent urination, headache, pain, sleepiness, weight loss

Why should this drug not be prescribed?

There are two reasons to avoid Aricept: an allergic reaction to the drug itself, or an allergy to the group of antihistamines that includes Claritin, Allegra, hydroxyzine hydrochloride (Vistaril), cyproheptadine hydrochloride, and azatadine maleate.

Special warnings about this medication

Aricept can aggravate asthma and other breathing problems, and can increase the risk of seizures. It can also slow the heartbeat, cause heartbeat irregularities, and lead to fainting episodes. The doctor should be contacted if any of these problems occur.

In patients who have had stomach ulcers, and those who take a nonsteroidal anti-inflammatory drug such as Advil, ibuprofen, or Aleve, Aricept can make stomach side effects worse. Aricept should be used with caution in such patients, and all side effects should be reported to the doctor.

Aricept will increase the effects of certain anesthetics. The doctor should be made aware of Aricept therapy prior to any surgery.

Possible food and drug interactions when taking this medication

See the entry for the generic name donepezil on page 316.

Special information about pregnancy and breastfeeding

Since it is not intended for women of childbearing age, Aricept's effects during pregnancy have not been studied, and it is not known whether it appears in breast milk.

Recommended dosage

ADULTS

The usual starting dose is 5 milligrams once a day at bedtime for at least 4 to 6 weeks. The dose should not be increased during this period unless directed. The doctor may then change the dosage to 10 milligrams once a day if response to the drug warrants it.

CHILDREN

The safety and effectiveness of Aricept have not been established in children.

Overdosage

Any medication taken in excess can have serious consequences. If an overdose is suspected, seek medical attention immediately.

- *Symptoms of Aricept overdose may include:*
  Collapse, convulsions, extreme muscle weakness (possibly ending in death if breathing muscles are affected), low blood pressure, nausea, salivation, slowed heart rate, sweating, vomiting

Aripiprazole *See Abilify, page 1*

ATIVAN

Lorazepam
Other brand name: Ativan Injection

Why is this drug prescribed?

Ativan is used in the treatment of anxiety disorders, and for short-term (up to 4 months) relief of the symptoms of anxiety. It belongs to a class of drugs known as benzodiazepines.

Ativan Injection is used in the treatment of status epilepticus (a continuous series of seizures without return to consciousness between them), and as a preanesthetic medication to produce sedation, relieve anxiety, and decrease ability to recall events related to the day of surgery.

Most important fact about this drug

Tolerance and dependence can develop with the use of Ativan. Patients may experience withdrawal symptoms if they stop using it abruptly. A change in dose or discontinuation of the drug should occur only under the supervision of a doctor.

How should this medication be taken?

This medication should be taken exactly as prescribed. Ativan Injection should not be given intra-arterially.

- *Missed dose...*
  If it is within an hour or so of the scheduled time, the forgotten dose should be taken as soon as remembered. Otherwise, it should be skipped and the patient should go back to the regular schedule. Doses should never be doubled.

- *Storage instructions...*
  Ativan should be stored at room temperature in a tightly closed container, away from light.

  Ativan Injection should be stored in a refrigerator and be protected from light.

What side effects may occur?

Side effects cannot be predicted. If any develop or change in intensity, patients should inform their doctor as soon as possible.

If any side effects develop, they will usually surface at the beginning of treatment. They will probably disappear as the patient continues to take the drug, or if the dosage is reduced.

- *Side effects of Ativan may include:*
  Dizziness, memory problems, sedation, transient amnesia, unsteadiness, weakness

- *Side effects due to rapid decrease in dose or abrupt withdrawal from Ativan:*

Abdominal and muscle cramps, convulsions, depressed mood, inability to fall or stay asleep, sweating, tremors, vomiting

* *Side effects of Ativan Injection may include:*
Low blood pressure, respiratory depression or respiratory failure, sleepiness

Why should this drug not be prescribed?

Patients who are sensitive to or have ever had an allergic reaction to Ativan or similar drugs such as Valium should not take this medication.

Ativan should also be avoided if the patient has acute narrow-angle glaucoma (a type of eye disease that causes increased pressure in the eyes).

Anxiety or tension related to everyday stress usually does not require treatment with Ativan. Symptoms should be thoroughly evaluated prior to treatment.

Ativan Injection should not be used in people who have a known sensitivity to benzodiazepines. It should also not be used in patients with sleep apnea syndrome or severe respiratory insufficiency.

Special warnings about this medication

Ativan may cause patients to become drowsy or less alert. Therefore, driving or operating dangerous machinery or participating in any hazardous activity that requires full mental alertness is not recommended.

This drug should be used with caution in patients who are severely depressed or have suffered from severe depression. A risk of suicide exists.

Ativan should also be used cautiously in patients with decreased kidney or liver function.

Older patients and those who have been using Ativan for a prolonged period of time should be closely watched for stomach and upper intestinal problems.

Ativan may intensify the effects of alcohol. Patients should avoid alcohol while taking this medication.

With Ativan Injection, there is a risk of respiratory depression or airway obstruction in heavily sedated patients.

It is possible that the impairment of the ability to operate machinery, drive a motor vehicle, or engage in potentially hazardous activities lasts longer than the suggested 24 to 48 hours. Therefore, patients should not perform these activities until their drowsiness has subsided.

It is important to be especially cautious when giving injections to the elderly, very ill, those with liver or kidney problems, and anyone with limited pulmonary reserve.

Possible food and drug interactions when taking this medication

See the entry for the generic name lorazepam on page 348.

Special information about pregnancy and breastfeeding

Patients who are pregnant or planning to become pregnant should not take Ativan. There is an increased risk of birth defects. Ativan Injection may cause fetal damage during pregnancy.

It is not known whether Ativan appears in breast milk. If this medication is essential to a patient's health, the doctor may advise her to discontinue breastfeeding until her treatment is finished.

Recommended dosage

ATIVAN

Adults

The usual recommended dosage is a total of 2 to 6 milligrams per day divided into smaller doses. The largest dose should be taken at bedtime. The daily dose may vary from 1 to 10 milligrams.

Anxiety: The usual starting dose is a total of 2 to 3 milligrams per day taken in 2 or 3 smaller doses.

Insomnia due to anxiety: A single daily dose of 2 to 4 milligrams may be taken, usually at bedtime.

Children

The safety and effectiveness of Ativan have not been established in children less than 12 years of age.

Older Adults

To avoid oversedation, the usual starting dosage for older adults and those in a weakened condition should not exceed a total of 1 to 2 milligrams per day, divided into smaller doses. This dose can be adjusted by the doctor as needed.

ATIVAN INJECTION

Adults

Status Epilepticus: The usual recommended dose is 4 milligrams given slowly (2 milligrams/minute) as an intravenous injection for patients 18 years and older. If seizures stop, no more Ativan is needed. If seizures continue or recur after a 10- or 15-minute observation period, another 4-milligram intravenous dose may be given slowly.

Preanesthetic: As an intramuscular injection being used as a premedicant, the usual recommended dose is 0.05 milligrams for every 2.2 pounds (1 kilogram) of body weight, up to a maximum of 4 milligrams. As an intravenous injection being used for the purpose of sedation and relief of anxiety, the usual initial dose is 2 milligrams total, or 0.02 milligrams per pound of body weight, whichever is smaller. Larger doses up to a total of 4 milligrams, or 0.05 milligrams per 2.2 pounds of body weight, may be beneficial in some patients.

Children
The safety of Ativan Injection has not been established in pediatric patients with status epilepticus. The use of Ativan Injection as a preanesthetic in patients less than 18 years of age is not recommended.

Overdosage
Any medication taken in excess can have serious consequences. An overdose of Ativan can be fatal, though this is rare. If an overdose is suspected, seek medical attention immediately.

* *Symptoms of Ativan overdose may include:*
  Coma, confusion, drowsiness, hypnotic state, lack of coordination, low blood pressure, sluggishness

Atomoxetine *See Strattera, page 216*

Aventyl *See Pamelor, page 151*

Buprenorphine and Naloxone *See Suboxone, page 219*

Bupropion, for depression *See Wellbutrin, page 255*

Bupropion, for smoking cessation *See Zyban, page 267*

BUSPAR
Buspirone hydrochloride

Why is this drug prescribed?
BuSpar is used in the treatment of anxiety disorders and for short-term relief of the symptoms of anxiety.

Most important fact about this drug
BuSpar should not be used with drugs classified as monoamine oxidase (MAO) inhibitors, such as the antidepressants Nardil and Parnate.

How should this medication be taken?
Patients should not be discouraged if they feel no immediate effect. The full benefit of this drug may not be seen for 1 to 2 weeks.

* *Missed dose...*
  Patients should take a forgotten dose as soon as they remember, unless it is almost time for the next dose. If that's the case, they should skip the dose they missed and go back to their regular schedule. Doses should never be doubled.

• *Storage instructions...*
  BuSpar should be stored at room temperature in a tightly closed container, away from light.

What side effects may occur?
Side effects cannot be predicted. If any develop or change in intensity, patients should inform their doctor as soon as possible.

• *Side effects may include:*
  Dizziness, dry mouth, fatigue, headache, light-headedness, nausea, nervousness, unusual excitement

Why should this drug not be prescribed?
This drug should be avoided by patients who are sensitive to or have ever had an allergic reaction to BuSpar or similar mood-altering drugs. BuSpar is also inappropriate for people with severe kidney or liver damage.

Anxiety or tension related to everyday stress usually does not require treatment with BuSpar. Symptoms should be thoroughly assessed prior to treatment.

Special warnings about this medication
The effects of BuSpar on the central nervous system are unpredictable. Patients should avoid driving, operating dangerous machinery, or participating in any hazardous activity that requires full mental alertness while they are taking BuSpar.

Although BuSpar does not intensify the effects of alcohol, it is best to avoid alcohol while taking this medication.

Possible food and drug interactions when taking this medication
See the entry for the generic name buspirone on page 290.

Special information about pregnancy and breastfeeding
The effects of BuSpar during pregnancy have not been adequately studied. Patients should inform their doctor immediately if they are pregnant or plan to become pregnant.

It is not known whether BuSpar appears in breast milk. If this medication is essential to the patient's health, the doctor may advise her to discontinue breastfeeding until her treatment is finished.

Recommended dosage
ADULTS

The recommended starting dose is a total of 15 milligrams per day divided into smaller doses, usually 5 milligrams 3 times a day. Every 2 to 3 days, the doctor may increase the dosage 5 milligrams per day as needed. The daily dose should not exceed 60 milligrams.

CHILDREN

The safety and effectiveness of BuSpar have not been established in children less than 18 years of age.

Overdosage

Any medication taken in excess can have serious consequences. If an overdose of BuSpar is suspected, seek medical attention immediately.

* *Symptoms of BuSpar overdose may include:*
  Dizziness, drowsiness, nausea or vomiting, severe stomach upset, unusually small pupils

Buspirone *See BuSpar, page 31*

CAMPRAL
Acamprosate calcium

Why is this drug prescribed?

Campral is prescribed to treat alcohol dependence. It helps people who have already stopped drinking alcohol keep from starting again.

Patients must be alcohol-free before taking Campral for it to work. Campral is thought to work by restoring and regulating brain chemicals that have been disrupted by long-term exposure to alcohol. Campral is not used for any type of substance dependence other than alcohol.

Most important fact about this drug

Individuals being treated with Campral, and their caregivers, should be aware that alcohol dependence and mental health problems frequently occur together. Pay special attention to any worsening of depression or any new symptoms that occur while taking Campral—especially agitation, anxiety, hostility, and suicidal thoughts or behavior—and report them to the doctor immediately.

How should this medication be taken?

Campral may be taken with food or on an empty stomach. However, taking it with meals may make it easier for the patient to keep on a regular schedule. Patients should continue taking Campral regularly even if they experience a relapse.

* *Missed dose...*
  The patient should take the forgotten dose as soon as they remember. However, if it is almost time for the next dose, the patient should skip the missed dose and return to the regular schedule. Doses should never be doubled.

- *Storage instructions...*
  Campral should be stored at room temperature.

What side effects may occur?
Side effects cannot be predicted. If any develop or change in intensity, patients should tell their doctor as soon as possible.

- *Side effects may include:*
  Anxiety, body pain or weakness, chest pain, depression, diarrhea, dizziness, headache, heart failure, insomnia, irregular heartbeat, kidney failure, nausea, seizure, sudden death, and suicidal thinking or suicide attempt

Why should this drug not be prescribed?
Patients who have severe kidney disease or have had an allergic reaction to Campral cannot take the drug.

Special warnings about this medication
Patients must completely avoid alcohol while taking Campral. If they begin drinking again, they should keep taking Campral and call their doctor right away to discuss the relapse. Campral does not relieve the symptoms of alcohol withdrawal.

Campral should be used with caution in patients who have kidney problems.

Because mental health problems and alcoholism frequently occur together, the patient should tell their doctor about any change in mood or behavior while using Campral (see "Most important fact about this drug").

Campral may affect judgment, thinking, or motor skills. People taking Campral should not drive, operate dangerous machinery, or participate in hazardous activities until they know how this drug affects them.

Possible food and drug interactions when taking this medication
No significant interactions have been reported at this time. However, patients should always tell the doctor about any medicines they take, including over-the-counter drugs, vitamins, and herbal supplements.

Special information about pregnancy and breastfeeding
Campral has not been studied in pregnant women and should be used only if the benefits outweigh the potential risks. Patients should tell their doctor if they are pregnant or plan to become pregnant.

In lab studies, Campral showed up in the milk of breastfeeding animals. It is not known whether Campral appears in human breast milk. The doctor may advise women not to breastfeed while taking this drug.

Recommended dosage

ADULTS

The usual starting dose is two tablets (each tablet contains 333 milligrams) taken three times a day, for a total of six tablets a day. The doctor may lower the dose as needed.

People with moderate kidney disease take half the regular dose—one tablet three times a day.

CHILDREN

The safety and effectiveness of Campral have not been studied in children.

Overdosage

Any medication taken in excess can have serious consequences. If overdose is suspected, seek emergency treatment immediately. Symptoms of Campral overdose may include diarrhea.

Carbamazepine *See Equetro, page 78*

CELEXA

Citalopram hydrobromide

Why is this drug prescribed?

Celexa is used to treat major depression. Like the antidepressant medications Paxil, Prozac, and Zoloft, Celexa is thought to work by boosting serotonin levels in the brain. Serotonin, one of the nervous system's primary chemical messengers, is known to elevate mood.

Most important fact about this drug

Celexa must not be taken for 2 weeks before or after using an antidepressant known as an MAO inhibitor. Drugs in this category include Nardil and Parnate. Combining Celexa with one of these medications could lead to a serious, even fatal reaction.

How should this medication be taken?

Celexa is available in tablet and liquid forms. The drug is taken once a day, in the morning or evening, with or without food. It's important for the patient to take Celexa regularly, even when feeling better. Depression typically begins to lift in 1 to 4 weeks, but it takes several months for the medication to yield its full benefits.

- *Missed dose...*
  Generally, the forgotten dose should be taken as soon as remembered. However, if it is almost time for the next dose, patients should skip the dose they missed and go back to their regular schedule. Doses should never be doubled.

• *Storage instructions...*
Celexa should be stored at room temperature.

What side effects may occur?
Side effects cannot be predicted. If any develop or change in intensity, patients should inform their doctor as soon as possible.

• *Side effects may include:*
Abdominal pain, agitation, anxiety, diarrhea, drowsiness, dry mouth, ejaculation disorder, fatigue, impotence, indigestion, insomnia, loss of appetite, nausea, painful menstruation, respiratory tract infection, sinus or nasal inflammation, sweating, tremor, vomiting

Why should this drug not be prescribed?
If Celexa gives the patient an allergic reaction, it cannot be used. Also remember that Celexa must never be combined with an MAO inhibitor (see "Most important fact about this drug").

Special warnings about this medication
In clinical studies, antidepressants increased the risk of suicidal thinking and behavior in children and adolescents with depression and other psychiatric disorders. Anyone considering the use of Celexa, or any other antidepressant in a child or adolescent, must balance the risk with the clinical need. Celexa has not been studied in children or adolescents and is not approved for treating anyone less than 18 years old.

Additionally, the progression of major depression is associated with a worsening of symptoms and/or the emergence of suicidal thinking or behavior in both adults and children, whether or not they are taking antidepressants. Patients and caregivers should watch for any change in symptoms or any new symptoms that appear suddenly—especially agitation, anxiety, hostility, panic, restlessness, extreme hyperactivity, and suicidal thinking or behavior—and report them to the doctor immediately. Be especially observant at the beginning of treatment or whenever there is a change in dose.

Serotonin-boosting antidepressants could potentially cause stomach bleeding, especially in older patients or those taking nonsteroidal anti-inflammatory drugs (NSAIDs) such as aspirin, ibuprofen (Advil, Motrin), naproxen (Aleve), and ketoprofen. Advise patients to consult their doctor before combining Celexa with NSAIDs or blood-thinning medications.

In recommended doses, Celexa does not seem to impair judgment or motor skills. However, a theoretical possibility of such problems remains, so caution is advisable when driving or operating dangerous equipment until Celexa's effect is known.

There is a slight chance that Celexa will trigger a manic episode. Celexa should be used with caution in patients who suffer from bipolar disorder. Caution is also warranted in patients who are over 60 years old, have liver or kidney problems, suffer from heart disease or high blood pressure, or have ever had seizures.

Celexa does not increase the effects of alcohol. Nevertheless, it's considered unwise to combine Celexa with alcohol or any other drug that affects the brain. Be particularly careful that the patient avoids MAO inhibitors.

Possible food and drug interactions when taking this medication
See the entry for the generic name citalopram on page 304.

Special information about pregnancy and breastfeeding
The effects of Celexa during pregnancy have not been adequately studied, and the potential for harm has not been ruled out. There have been reports of serious complications in newborns who were exposed to Celexa late in the third trimester. Any patient who becomes pregnant or plans to become pregnant while on Celexa therapy should contact her doctor immediately.

Celexa appears in breast milk and will affect the nursing infant. The patient and doctor should discuss discontinuing either breastfeeding or Celexa.

Recommended dosage
ADULTS

The recommended starting dose of Celexa tablets or oral solution is 20 milligrams once a day. Dosage is usually increased to 40 milligrams once daily after at least a week has passed. Doses should not exceed 40 milligrams a day.

For older adults and those who have liver problems, the recommended dose is 20 milligrams once a day.

Overdosage
Any medication taken in excess can have serious consequences. If an overdose is suspected, seek medical attention immediately.

- *Symptoms of Celexa overdose may include:*
  Amnesia, bluish or purplish discoloration of the skin, coma, confusion, convulsions, dizziness, drowsiness, hyperventilation, nausea, rapid heartbeat, sweating, tremor, vomiting

---

CHANTIX
Varenicline tartrate

Why is this drug prescribed?
Chantix is prescribed to help adults stop smoking. It is thought to work by blocking the pleasant effects of nicotine on the brain. Chantix should be used as part of a comprehensive treatment plan that includes behavior modification and counseling support.

Most important fact about this drug

Remind patients that they must set a date to quit smoking and should begin taking Chantix 1 week before the quit date. It may take several weeks before patients notice the full effects of using Chantix. At the beginning of treatment, some patients may slip up and smoke. If this happens, encourage them to try quitting again, since the medication may need more time to build up in their system.

How should this medication be taken?

Chantix should be taken after eating and with a full glass of water.

- *Missed dose...*
  Generally, forgotten doses should be taken as soon as remembered. However, if it is almost time for the next dose, patients should skip the one they missed and return to their regular schedule. Doses should never be doubled.

- *Storage instructions...*
  Store at room temperature.

What side effects may occur?

Side effects cannot be anticipated. If any develop or change in intensity, patients should inform their doctor as soon as possible.

- *Side effects may include:*
  Constipation, gas, nausea, sleep problems (including insomnia and changes in dreaming), vomiting

Why should this drug not be prescribed?

Chantix should not be used if it causes an allergic reaction. In addition, Chantix has not been studied in children and is not recommended for patients less than 18 years old.

Special warnings about this medication

Advise patients who are bothered by persistent nausea and insomnia while taking Chantix to alert their doctor. They may need to take a lower dose.

Quitting smoking can alter how the body metabolizes certain drugs, including insulin, asthma medications, and blood thinners. Patients who are taking other medications may need to see their doctor for dose adjustments.

Patients should let the doctor know if they are on dialysis or have kidney problems; they may need their dosage reduced.

Caution patients not to drive or operate machinery until they know how quitting smoking and using Chantix affects them.

Possible food and drug interactions when taking this medication

No significant interactions have been reported at this time. However, patients should always tell the doctor about any medicines they take, including over-the-counter drugs, vitamins, and herbal supplements.

Special information about pregnancy and breastfeeding

The effects of Chantix during pregnancy have not been studied. The drug is recommended only if its benefits are thought to outweigh the potential risk to the baby. If a patient is pregnant or planning to become pregnant, she should inform her doctor immediately.

It is not known whether Chantix is excreted in human breast milk. However, studies show that it does appear in the breast milk of animals. Patients should consult their doctor before breastfeeding.

Recommended dosage

ADULTS

Patients must first choose a quit date when they will stop smoking. They should begin taking Chantix 1 week before the quit date. Most patients will be prescribed the following regimen for 12 weeks:

Day 1 to Day 3: One white tablet (0.5 milligram) once a day.
Day 4 to Day 7: One white tablet (0.5 milligram) twice a day, once in the morning and again at night.
Day 8 to end of treatment: One blue tablet (1 milligram) twice a day, once in the morning and again at night.

Patients who successfully quit smoking after 12 weeks of Chantix treatment may be prescribed an additional 12-week course of therapy. Patients who are unsuccessful or relapse after treatment should be encouraged to make another attempt after identifying what may have caused the failure.

Overdosage

No information on overdose is available. However, any medication taken in excess can have serious consequences. If an overdose is suspected, seek medical attention immediately.

Chlordiazepoxide *See Librium, page 111*

CHLORPROMAZINE

Brand name: Thorazine

Why is this drug prescribed?

Chlorpromazine is used to treat schizophrenia. It is also prescribed for the short-term treatment of severe behavioral disorders in children, including explosive hyperactivity and combativeness, and for the manic phase of bipolar disorder.

Chlorpromazine is also used to control nausea and vomiting, and to relieve restlessness and apprehension before surgery. It is used as an aid in the treatment of tetanus, and is prescribed for uncontrollable hiccups and acute intermittent porphyria (attacks of severe abdominal pain sometimes accompanied by psychiatric disturbances, cramps in the arms and legs, and muscle weakness).

Most important fact about this drug

Chlorpromazine may cause tardive dyskinesia—a condition marked by involuntary muscle spasms and twitches in the face and body. This condition may be permanent, and appears to be most common among the elderly, especially women.

How should this medication be taken?

Patients taking chlorpromazine in a liquid concentrate form will need to dilute it with carbonated beverage, coffee, fruit juice, milk, tea, tomato juice, or water. Puddings, soups, and other semisolid foods may also be used. It will taste best if it is diluted immediately prior to use. Chlorpromazine should not be mixed with alcoholic beverages.

Antacids such as Gelusil should not be taken at the same time as chlorpromazine. At least 1 to 2 hours should be allowed between doses of the two drugs.

- *Missed dose...*

  Patients taking 1 dose a day should take the missed dose as soon as they remember. If they do not remember until the next day, they should skip the missed dose and go back to their regular schedule.

  Patients who take more than 1 dose a day should take the missed dose if it is within an hour or so of the scheduled time. If they do not remember until later, they should skip the missed dose and go back to their regular schedule. Doses should never be doubled.

- *Storage instructions...*

  Chlorpromazine should be stored away from heat, light, and moisture. The liquid should not be frozen. Since the liquid concentrate form of chlorpromazine is light-sensitive, it should be stored in a dark place, but it does not need to be refrigerated.

What side effects may occur?

Side effects cannot be predicted. If any develop or change in intensity, patients should inform their doctor as soon as possible.

- *Side effects may include:*

  Anticholinergic effects (such as constipation, dry mouth, rapid heartbeat), drowsiness, involuntary muscle spasms and twitches (tardive dyskinesia), jaundice, low blood pressure, low white-blood-cell count (agranulocytosis), movements similar to Parkinson's disease, physical restlessness, neuroleptic malignant syndrome (see "Special warnings about this medication"), restlessness, vision changes

Why should this drug not be prescribed?

Chlorpromazine should not be combined with substances that slow down mental function, such as alcohol, barbiturates, or narcotics. It should be avoided by anyone who has ever had an allergic reaction to any major tranquilizer containing phenothiazine.

Special warnings about this medication

Chlorpromazine should be used with caution if the patient has asthma; a brain tumor; breast cancer; intestinal blockage; emphysema; glaucoma; heart, kidney, or liver disease; respiratory infections; seizures; or an abnormal bone marrow or blood condition. Caution is also advisable if the patient is exposed to pesticides or extreme heat.

Due to its ability to prevent vomiting, chlorpromazine can mask symptoms of an overdose of other drugs. It could also mask symptoms of brain tumor, intestinal blockage, and the neurological condition known as Reye's syndrome. The drug should be avoided in children and adolescents who have symptoms that could indicate Reye's syndrome, including persistent or recurrent vomiting, listlessness, irritability, combativeness, and disorientation.

Stomach inflammation, dizziness, nausea, vomiting, and tremors may result if chlorpromazine is stopped suddenly. Therapy should be discontinued only under a doctor's supervision.

This drug may impair the ability to drive a car or operate potentially dangerous machinery. Patients should not participate in any activities that require full alertness if they are unsure about their ability.

This drug can increase sensitivity to light. Patients should avoid being out in the sun too long.

Chlorpromazine can suppress the cough reflex, so patients may have trouble vomiting.

Chlorpromazine can cause a potentially fatal group of symptoms called neuroleptic malignant syndrome. Symptoms include extremely high body temperature, high fever, rigid muscles, mental changes, irregular pulse or blood pressure, rapid heartbeat, sweating, and changes in heart rhythm. The doctor should be alerted immediately if these symptoms develop. Chlorpromazine therapy will need to be discontinued.

Patients on chlorpromazine for a prolonged period should see their doctor for regular evaluations, since side effects can get worse over time.

Chlorpromazine may cause false-positive phenylketonuria (PKU) tests.

Extreme drowsiness and other potentially serious effects can result if chlorpromazine is combined with alcohol and other mental depressants such as narcotic painkillers like Demerol.

Possible food and drug interactions when taking this medication

See the entry for chlorpromazine on page 302.

Special information about pregnancy and breastfeeding

The effects of chlorpromazine during pregnancy have not been adequately studied. Patients who are pregnant or plan to become pregnant should notify their doctor. Pregnant women should use chlorpromazine only if clearly needed.

Chlorpromazine appears in breast milk and may affect a nursing infant. If this medication is essential to the mother's health, the doctor may advise her not to breastfeed until treatment is finished.

Recommended dosage

Dosage recommendations shown here are for the oral and rectal forms of the drug. In some cases, chlorpromazine is also given by injection. The following indications and dosages are for adults unless otherwise noted.

SCHIZOPHRENIA AND MANIA

The doctor will gradually increase the dosage until symptoms are controlled. Full improvement may not be seen for weeks or even months.

Initial dosages may range from 30 to 75 milligrams daily. The amount is divided into equal doses and taken 3 or 4 times a day. If needed, the doctor may increase the dosage by 20 to 50 milligrams at semiweekly intervals.

NAUSEA AND VOMITING

The usual tablet dosage is 10 to 25 milligrams, taken every 4 or 6 hours, as needed.

One 100-milligram suppository can be used every 6 to 8 hours.

UNCONTROLLABLE HICCUPS

Dosages may range from 75 to 200 milligrams daily, divided into 3 or 4 equal doses.

ACUTE INTERMITTENT PORPHYRIA

Dosages may range from 75 to 200 milligrams daily, divided into 3 or 4 equal doses.

SEVERE BEHAVIOR PROBLEMS OR NAUSEA AND

VOMITING IN CHILDREN

Dosages are based on the child's weight. Chlorpromazine is generally not prescribed for children younger than 6 months.

Oral: The daily dose is 0.25 milligram for each pound of the child's weight, taken every 4 to 6 hours, as needed.

Rectal: The usual dose is 0.5 milligram per pound of body weight, taken every 6 to 8 hours, as necessary.

OLDER ADULTS

In general, older people take lower dosages of chlorpromazine, and any increase in dosage will be gradual. Because of a greater risk of low blood pressure, the doctor will watch the patient closely. Remember that older people (especially older women) may be more susceptible to tardive dyskinesia.

Overdosage

An overdose of chlorpromazine can be fatal. If an overdose is suspected, seek medical help immediately.

- *Symptoms of chlorpromazine overdose may include:*
  Agitation, coma, convulsions, difficulty breathing, difficulty swallowing, dry mouth, extreme sleepiness, fever, intestinal blockage, irregular heart rate, low blood pressure, restlessness

Citalopram *See Celexa, page 35*

Clomipramine *See Anafranil, page 19*

Clonazepam *See Klonopin, page 102*

Clorazepate *See Tranxene, page 235*

Clozapine *See Clozaril, page 43*

CLOZARIL
Clozapine
Other brand name: FazaClo ODT

Why is this drug prescribed?

Clozaril is prescribed for people with severe schizophrenia who have failed to respond to standard treatments. It is also used to help reduce the risk of suicidal behavior in people with schizophrenia. Like all antipsychotic agents, Clozaril is not a cure, but it can help some people return to more normal lives.

Most important fact about this drug

Even though it does not produce some of the disturbing side effects of other antipsychotic medications, Clozaril may cause agranulocytosis, a potentially lethal disorder of the white blood cells. Because of the risk of agranulocytosis, anyone who takes Clozaril is required to have a blood test once a week for the first 6 months. The drug is carefully controlled so that those taking it must get their weekly blood test before receiving the following week's supply of medication. After 6 months of acceptable blood counts, patients are allowed to switch to an every-other-week testing schedule. Anyone whose blood test results are abnormal will be taken off Clozaril either temporarily or permanently, depending on the results of an additional 4 weeks of testing.

Clozaril is not approved for use in older patients with dementia (including Alzheimer's disease) due to the increased risk of sudden death, heart failure, and pneumonia.

How should this medication be taken?

It is important to take Clozaril exactly as directed. Because of the significant risk of serious side effects associated with this drug, patients should be periodically reassessed for continuation of Clozaril therapy. Clozaril is distributed only through the Clozaril Patient Management System, which ensures regular white blood cell testing, monitoring, and pharmacy services prior to delivery of the next supply.

Clozaril may be taken with or without food.

FazaClo ODT rapidly disintegrates after placement in the mouth. The orally disintegrating tablet should not be pushed through the foil. The tablets should remain in the unopened blister until immediately before use. Just prior to use, the patient should peel the foil from the blister and gently remove the tablet. The tablet should then immediately be placed into the mouth, where it should be allowed to disintegrate and be swallowed with saliva. No water is needed to take FazaClo ODT.

Patients should be advised that if the tablets are split, the half-tablet that is not taken should be destroyed.

- *Missed dose...*
  Generally, the forgotten dose should be taken as soon as remembered. However, if it is almost time for the next dose, patients should skip the dose they missed and go back to their regular schedule. Doses should never be doubled.

  If the patient stops taking Clozaril for more than 2 days, it should not be started again without first consulting the physician.

- *Storage instructions...*
  Clozaril should be stored at room temperature.

What side effects may occur?

Side effects cannot be predicted. If any develop or change in intensity, patients should inform their doctor as soon as possible.

The most feared side effect is agranulocytosis, a dangerous drop in the number of a certain kind of white blood cell. Symptoms include fever, lethargy, sore throat, and weakness. If not caught in time, agranulocytosis can be fatal. That is why all people who take Clozaril must have a blood test every week. About 1 percent develop agranulocytosis and must stop taking the drug.

Seizures are another potential side effect, occurring in some 5 percent of people who take Clozaril. The higher the dosage, the greater the risk of seizures.

- *Other side effects may include:*
  Blood disorders, constipation, drowsiness, dry mouth, fainting, fever, headache, low blood pressure, nausea, rapid heartbeat, salivation, sweating, tremor, vertigo, vision problems

Why should this drug not be prescribed?

Clozaril is considered a somewhat risky medication because of its potential to cause agranulocytosis and seizures. It should be taken only by people whose condition is serious, and who have not been helped by more traditional antipsychotic medications such as haloperidol or thioridazine. Clozaril should not be used if the patient:

Has a bone marrow disease or disorder
Has epilepsy that is not controlled
Has ever developed an abnormal white blood cell count while taking Clozaril
Is currently taking some other drug, such as Tegretol, that could cause a decrease in white blood cell count or a drug that could affect the bone marrow
Has ever had an allergic reaction to any of Clozaril's ingredients

Special warnings about this medication

Clozaril can cause drowsiness, especially at the start of treatment. For this reason, and also because of the potential for seizures, patients should not drive, swim, climb, or operate dangerous machinery while taking this medication, at least in the early stages of treatment.

Even though blood tests are done weekly for the first 6 months of treatment and every other week after that, patients need to stay alert for early symptoms of agranulocytosis: weakness, lethargy, fever, sore throat, a general feeling of illness, a flu-like feeling, or ulcers of the lips, mouth, or other mucous membranes. If any such symptoms develop, they should contact their doctor immediately.

Especially during the first 3 weeks of treatment, a fever may develop. If this happens, the patient should notify the doctor.

Instruct patients to check with their doctor before drinking alcohol or using drugs of any kind, including over-the-counter medicines.

Patients with an enlarged prostate or the eye condition called narrow-angle glaucoma must be closely monitored by the doctor. Clozaril could make these conditions worse.

Certain antipsychotic drugs, including Clozaril, are associated with an increased risk of developing high blood sugar, which on rare occasions has led to coma or death. Patients should see their doctor right away if they develop signs of high blood sugar, including dry mouth, thirst, increased urination, and tiredness. Patients who have diabetes or have a high risk of developing it should see their doctor regularly for blood sugar testing.

On rare occasions, Clozaril can cause intestinal problems—constipation, impaction, or blockage—that can, in extreme cases, be fatal.

In very rare cases, Clozaril has been known to cause a potentially fatal inflammation of the heart. This problem is most likely to surface during the first month of treatment, but has also occurred later. Warning signs include unexplained fatigue, shortness of breath, fever, chest pain, and a rapid or pounding heartbeat. Patients should see their doctor immediately if they develop these symptoms. Even a suspicion of heart inflammation warrants discontinuation of Clozaril.

Especially when starting Clozaril therapy, patients may be troubled by a dramatic drop in blood pressure whenever they first stand up. This can lead to light-headedness, fainting, or even total collapse and cardiac arrest. Clozaril also tends to increase the heart rate. Both problems are more dangerous for someone with a heart problem. If a patient suffers from heart disease, make sure the doctor knows about it.

Patients with kidney, liver, or lung disease, or a history of seizures or prostate problems, should discuss the problem with their doctor before taking Clozaril. Nausea, vomiting, loss of appetite, and a yellow tinge to the skin and eyes are signs of liver trouble. The doctor should be contacted immediately if a patient develops these symptoms.

Drugs such as Clozaril can sometimes cause a set of symptoms called neuroleptic malignant syndrome. Symptoms include high fever, muscle rigidity, irregular pulse or blood pressure, rapid heartbeat, excessive perspiration, and changes in heart rhythm. The patient will be taken off Clozaril while this condition is being treated.

There is also a risk of developing tardive dyskinesia, a condition of involuntary, slow, rhythmical movements. This happens more often in older adults, especially older women.

In very rare instances, Clozaril may also cause a blood clot in the lungs. Patients should call their doctor immediately if they develop severe breathing problems or chest pain.

Patients with phenylketonuria should be aware that FazaClo ODT contains phenylalanine (a component of aspartame).

Possible food and drug interactions when taking this medication

See the entry for the generic name clozapine on page 308.

Special information about pregnancy and breastfeeding

The effects of Clozaril during pregnancy have not been adequately studied. Patients who are pregnant or plan to become pregnant should inform their doctor immediately. Clozaril treatment should be continued during pregnancy only if absolutely necessary.

Breastfeeding is not recommended during Clozaril therapy, since the drug may appear in breast milk.

Recommended dosage

ADULTS

Dosage should be carefully individualized and monitored. The usual recommended initial dose is half of a 25-milligram tablet (12.5 milligrams) 1 or 2 times daily. The doctor may increase the dosage in increments of 25 to 50 milligrams a day to achieve a daily dose of 300 to 450 milligrams by the end of 2 weeks. Dosage increases after that will be made only once or twice a week and will be no more than 100 milligrams each time. Dosage is increased gradually because rapid increases and higher doses are more likely to cause seizures and changes in heart rhythm. The highest recommended dosage is 900 milligrams a day divided into 2 or 3 doses.

Patients taking half of a 25-milligram FazaClo ODT tablet should destroy the other half of the tablet that they do not take.

CHILDREN

Safety and efficacy have not been established for children up to 16 years of age.

Overdosage

Any medication taken in excess can have serious consequences. If an overdose is suspected, seek emergency medical attention immediately.

- *Symptoms of overdose with Clozaril may include:*
  Coma, delirium, drowsiness, excess salivation, faintness, low blood pressure, pneumonia, rapid heartbeat, seizures, shallow breathing or absence of breathing

---

COGNEX

Tacrine hydrochloride

Why is this drug prescribed?

Cognex is used for the treatment of mild to moderate Alzheimer's disease. This progressive, degenerative disorder causes physical changes in the brain that disrupt the flow of information and affect memory, thinking, and behavior. Like other Alzheimer's drugs, Cognex can temporarily improve brain function in some Alzheimer's sufferers, although it does not halt the progress of the underlying disease.

Most important fact about this drug

Cognex treatment should not be stopped, or the dosage reduced, without consulting the doctor. A sudden reduction can cause the patient to become more disturbed and forgetful. Taking more Cognex than the doctor advises can also cause serious problems. Dosage should not be changed without instructions from the doctor.

How should this medication be taken?
This medication will work better if taken at regular intervals, usually 4 times a day. Cognex is best taken between meals. However, if it is irritating to the stomach, the doctor may advise taking it with meals. If Cognex is not taken regularly, as the doctor directs, the condition may get worse.

* *Missed dose...*
  Generally, the forgotten dose should be taken as soon as possible. If it is within 2 hours of the next dose, caregivers should skip the missed dose and go back to the regular schedule. Doses should never be doubled.

* *Storage instructions...*
  Cognex should be stored at room temperature, away from moisture.

What side effects may occur?
Side effects cannot be predicted. If any develop or change in intensity, caregivers should tell the doctor as soon as possible.

* *Side effects may include:*
  Abdominal pain, abnormal thinking, agitation, anxiety, chest pain, clumsiness or unsteadiness, confusion, constipation, depression, diarrhea, dizziness, fatigue, flushing, frequent urination, gas, headache, indigestion, inflamed nasal passages, insomnia, liver function disorders, loss of appetite, muscle pain, nausea, rash, sleepiness, upper respiratory infection, urinary tract infection, vomiting, weight loss

Caregivers should report any symptoms that develop while on Cognex therapy. They should alert the doctor if the patient develops nausea, vomiting, loose stools, or diarrhea at the start of therapy or when the dosage is increased. Later in therapy, they should be on the lookout for rash or fever, yellowing of the eyes and skin, or changes in the color of the stool.

Why should this drug not be prescribed?
People who are sensitive to or have ever had an allergic reaction to Cognex (including symptoms such as rash or fever) should not take this medication. If during previous Cognex therapy the patient developed jaundice (yellow skin and eyes), which signals that something is wrong with the liver, Cognex should not be used again.

Special warnings about this medication
Cognex should be used with caution if the patient has a history of liver disease, certain heart disorders, stomach ulcers, or asthma.

Because of the risk of liver problems when taking Cognex, the doctor will schedule blood tests to monitor liver function every other week from at least the fourth week to the sixteenth week of treatment. After 16 weeks, blood tests will be given monthly for 2 months and every 3 months after that. If the patient develops any liver problems, the doctor may temporarily discontinue Cognex treatment until further testing shows that the liver has returned to normal. If the doctor resumes Cognex treatment, regular blood tests will be conducted again.

Before having any surgery, including dental surgery, caregivers should tell the doctor that the patient is being treated with Cognex.

Cognex can cause seizures, and may cause problems with urination.

Possible food and drug interactions when taking this medication

See the entry for the generic name tacrine on page 398.

Special information about pregnancy and breastfeeding

The effects of Cognex during pregnancy have not been studied, and it is not known whether Cognex appears in breast milk.

Recommended dosage

ADULTS

The usual starting dose is 10 milligrams 4 times a day, for at least 4 weeks. The dose should not be increased during this 4-week period unless the doctor says that it should be.

Depending on the patient's tolerance of the drug, dosage may then be increased at 4-week intervals, first to 20 milligrams, then to 30, and finally to 40, always taken 4 times a day.

CHILDREN

The safety and effectiveness of Cognex have not been established in children.

Overdosage

Any medication taken in excess can have serious consequences. If an overdose is suspected, seek medical attention immediately.

- *Symptoms of Cognex overdose may include:*
  Collapse; convulsions; extreme muscle weakness, possibly ending in death (if breathing muscles are affected); low blood pressure; nausea; salivation; slowed heart rate; sweating; vomiting

Concerta *See Ritalin, page 199*

CYMBALTA
Duloxetine hydrochloride

Why is this drug prescribed?
Cymbalta is used to treat major depression and generalized anxiety disorder. It is also used to treat diabetic peripheral neuropathy, a painful nerve disorder associated with diabetes that affects the hands, legs, and feet.

Cymbalta is thought to work by correcting an imbalance of two brain chemicals known to influence mood—serotonin and norepinephrine. It belongs to a class of antidepressants called selective serotonin and norepinephrine reuptake inhibitors (SNRIs).

Most important fact about this drug
Serious, sometimes fatal reactions can occur if Cymbalta is taken with antidepressants known as MAO inhibitors, including the antidepressants Nardil and Parnate. Cymbalta should never be combined with one of these drugs. Patients should wait at least 14 days after stopping an MAO inhibitor before starting treatment with Cymbalta. Likewise, after stopping therapy with Cymbalta, they must allow at least 5 days before starting treatment with an MAO inhibitor.

How should this medication be taken?
Cymbalta should be taken at about the same time each day. The capsule should be swallowed whole; patients should not chew it or break it open. Cymbalta may be taken with or without food.

It may take several weeks before the drug begins to work. Patients should continue taking Cymbalta even if they begin to feel better. They should not stop taking this drug without the doctor's approval. Abruptly stopping treatment may cause severe side effects.

• *Missed dose...*
The forgotten dose should be taken as soon as it is remembered. However, if it is almost time for the next dose, the patient should skip the missed dose and return to the regular schedule. Doses should never be doubled.

• *Storage instructions...*
Cymbalta should be stored at room temperature.

What side effects may occur?
Side effects cannot be predicted. If any develop or change in intensity, patients should inform their doctor as soon as possible.

• *Side effects may include:*
Appetite changes, constipation, diarrhea, dizziness, dry mouth, fatigue, headache, insomnia, nausea, sexual difficulties, sleepiness, sweating, tremor, urinary difficulties, vomiting, weakness

Why should this drug not be prescribed?

Patients cannot use Cymbalta if it causes them to have an allergic reaction. In addition, people who have uncontrolled narrow-angle glaucoma, a disease that causes increased pressure in the eyes, should not take Cymbalta.

Cymbalta should never be combined with an MAO inhibitor (see "Most important fact about this drug").

Patients should not take the drug thioridazine with Cymbalta, as it could cause fatal heartbeat irregularities.

Special warnings about this medication

In clinical studies, antidepressants increased the risk of suicidal thinking and behavior in children and adolescents with depression and other psychiatric disorders. Anyone considering the use of Cymbalta, or any other antidepressant, in a child or adolescent must balance this risk with the clinical need. Cymbalta has not been studied in children or adolescents and is not approved for treating anyone less than 18 years old.

Additionally, the progression of major depression is associated with a worsening of symptoms and/or the emergence of suicidal thinking or behavior in both adults and children, whether or not they are taking antidepressants. Patients and caregivers should watch for any change in symptoms or any new symptoms that appear suddenly—especially agitation, anxiety, hostility, panic, restlessness, extreme hyperactivity, and suicidal thinking or behavior—and report them to the doctor immediately. Be especially observant at the beginning of treatment or whenever there is a change in dose.

Some medical conditions require careful monitoring during treatment with Cymbalta. Patients should be sure to tell their doctor if they have diabetes, glaucoma, high blood pressure, or a seizure disorder.

Cymbalta can cause episodes of mania (abnormally high feelings of excitement and energy), so be sure the doctor is aware if the patient has this condition.

Using Cymbalta is not recommended if the patient has liver problems or severe kidney disease.

Like other antidepressants, Cymbalta can cause drowsiness and affect judgment or motor skills. Patients taking Cymbalta must use caution when driving, operating dangerous machinery, or participating in hazardous activities until they know how the drug affects them.

Patients should never take Cymbalta with MAO inhibitors (see "Most important fact about this drug) or the drug thioridazine. They should consult the doctor first before taking drugs that act on the central nervous system, such as antipsychotics, narcotic painkillers, sleep inducers, or tranquilizers. Due to the possibility of liver damage, Cymbalta should not be taken by people who use alcohol more than occasionally.

Possible food and drug interactions when taking this medication

See the entry for the generic name duloxetine on page 318.

Special information about pregnancy and breastfeeding

Cymbalta had negative effects during pregnancy when given to animals. There have been no adequate studies in pregnant women. Cymbalta should be used during pregnancy only if the benefits outweigh the potential risks.

Cymbalta appears in the breast milk of animals. It is unknown whether the drug appears in human breast milk. Therefore, it's recommended that women avoid breastfeeding while taking Cymbalta.

Recommended dosage

ADULTS 18 YEARS AND OLDER

Major Depression

The total daily dose ranges from 40 milligrams (taken as one 20-milligram capsule twice a day) to 60 milligrams (taken as a 60-milligram capsule once a day or as a 30-milligram capsule twice a day).

Generalized Anxiety Disorder or Diabetic Peripheral Neuropathy

The usual recommended dose is 60 milligrams taken once daily.

Overdosage

Any medication taken in excess can have serious consequences. If an overdose is suspected, seek emergency treatment immediately.

DALMANE

Flurazepam hydrochloride

Why is this drug prescribed?

Dalmane is used for the relief of insomnia—difficulty falling asleep, waking up frequently at night, or waking up early in the morning. It can be used by people whose insomnia keeps coming back and in those who have poor sleeping habits. It belongs to a class of drugs known as benzodiazepines.

Most important fact about this drug

Tolerance and dependence can occur with the use of Dalmane. Patients may experience withdrawal symptoms if they stop using this drug abruptly. They should discontinue or change their dose only in consultation with their doctor.

How should this medication be taken?

Dalmane is taken in a single dose at bedtime. It is important to take this medication exactly as prescribed.

- *Missed dose...*
  The patient should take the dose that they missed as soon as they remember if it is within an hour or so of the scheduled time. If the patient does not remember until later, they should skip that dose and go back to the regular schedule. Doses should never be doubled.

- *Storage instructions...*
  Dalmane should be stored away from heat, light, and moisture.

What side effects may occur?

Side effects cannot be predicted. If any develop or change in intensity, patients should inform their doctor as soon as possible.

- *Side effects may include:*
  Dizziness, drowsiness, falling, lack of muscular coordination, light-headedness, staggering

- *Side effects due to rapid decrease in dose or abrupt withdrawal from Dalmane:*
  Abdominal and muscle cramps, convulsions, depressed mood, inability to fall asleep or stay asleep, sweating, tremors, vomiting

Why should this drug not be prescribed?

Dalmane cannot be used by anyone who is sensitive to or has had an allergic reaction to it or similar drugs such as Valium.

Special warnings about this medication

Dalmane may cause a patient to become drowsy or less alert. Patients should avoid driving, operating dangerous machinery, or participating in any hazardous activity that requires full mental alertness after taking Dalmane.

This drug should be used with caution in patients who are severely depressed, or have suffered from severe depression.

Caution is also warranted in patients who have decreased kidney or liver function or chronic respiratory or lung disease.

Alcohol intensifies the effects of Dalmane. Patients should avoid drinking alcohol while taking this medication.

Possible food and drug interactions when taking this medication

See the entry for the generic name flurazepam on page 327.

Special information about pregnancy and breastfeeding

Dalmane should not be used by women who are pregnant or plan on becoming pregnant. There is an increased risk of birth defects. This drug may appear in breast milk and could affect a nursing infant. If this medication is essential to the patient's health, the doctor may advise her to discontinue breastfeeding until treatment with Dalmane is finished.

Recommended dosage
ADULTS

The usual recommended dose is 30 milligrams at bedtime; however 15 milligrams may be all that is necessary. The doctor should adjust the dose to the patient's needs.

CHILDREN

Safety and effectiveness of Dalmane have not been established in children less than 15 years of age.

OLDER ADULTS

The doctor will limit the dosage to the smallest effective amount to avoid oversedation, dizziness, confusion, or lack of muscle coordination. The usual starting dose is 15 milligrams.

Overdosage
Any medication taken in excess can have serious consequences. If an overdose is suspected, seek medical attention immediately.

* *Symptoms of Dalmane overdose may include:*
  Coma, confusion, low blood pressure, sleepiness

DAYTRANA
Methylphenidate

Why is this drug prescribed?
Daytrana is a skin patch that contains the stimulant methylphenidate. It is prescribed for attention deficit hyperactivity disorder (ADHD) in children 6 years and older. It should be used as part of a comprehensive treatment plan that includes other measures such as counseling and educational support.

The Daytrana patch provides a continuous release of medication. After the patch is applied, the medication flows through the skin and into the bloodstream. The patch is usually worn during the day for about 9 hours.

Most important fact about this drug
The doctor should be alerted if the child or a family member has any heart conditions, including structural abnormalities. Also, be sure to inform the doctor immediately if the child develops symptoms that suggest heart problems, such as chest pain or fainting.

How should this medication be taken?
Daytrana patches should be applied to a clean, dry area on the hip. The patch should be pressed and held firmly to the skin with the palm of the hand for 30 seconds. The patient should alternate hips each day, making sure there is no redness or areas of irritation where the patch is being applied.

The patch should be applied in the morning, 2 hours before an effect is needed, and it should be removed after the child has worn it for 9 hours. If overstimulation or other side effects occur, the doctor should be informed. The patch may need to be removed earlier in the day.

• *Missed dose...*
  If Daytrana is not applied at the correct time, it can be applied as soon as it is remembered. The patch should be removed at the normally scheduled time, even if it has been less than 9 hours, to avoid side effects later in the day.

• *Storage instructions...*
  Daytrana should be stored at room temperature. Each patch should be kept in its original protective pouch until it is ready to be applied.

What side effects may occur?

Side effects cannot be predicted. If any develop or change in intensity, the doctor should be informed as soon as possible.

• *Side effects of Daytrana may include:*
  Decreased appetite, inflammation of the nasal passages, irritation at the site of application (such as redness or itching), nasal congestion, nausea, sadness/crying, sleeplessness, twitching, vomiting, weight loss

• *Other side effects of methylphenidate may include:*
  Allergic reactions, dizziness, drowsiness, fever, headache, increased blood pressure, nervousness, psychosis (abnormal thinking or hallucinations)

Why should this drug not be prescribed?

Daytrana should not be used if the child has:

• Anxiety, tension, or agitation, since methylphenidate may make these conditions worse.
• Allergies to methylphenidate or any other ingredients in Daytrana.
• Glaucoma, an eye disease marked by elevated pressure in the eye.
• Motion or verbal tics, Tourette's syndrome, or a family history of Tourette's syndrome.

In addition, Daytrana should not be combined with antidepressants known as monoamine oxidase inhibitors (MAOIs), or within 14 days of stopping an MAOI.

Special warnings about this medication

Heating pads or other external sources of heat should not be applied to the patch. Also, patients and caregivers should avoid touching the sticky part of the patch.

Although rare, Daytrana could cause an allergic reaction. If it is suspected that the patch is causing skin irritation or a rash, the doctor should be contacted.

The doctor should be alerted immediately if the child develops blurred vision while taking Daytrana. This could be a sign of a serious problem.

The doctor should be aware of the child's complete medical history, especially if the child has ever had any of the following: depression, bipolar disorder, aggressive behavior or hostility, heart problems, high blood pressure, vision problems, a history of alcohol or drug abuse, motion tics (such as repeated twitching) or verbal tics (such as repeated sounds or words), Tourette's syndrome, seizures, or abnormal brain waves as shown on an EEG. Also, the doctor should be informed if the child has ever had hallucinations (such as hearing voices or seeing abnormal visions) or has been diagnosed with psychosis.

In addition, Daytrana should not be combined with antidepressants known as monoamine oxidase inhibitors (MAOIs), or within 14 days of stopping an MAOI.

Before using Daytrana, the doctor should be informed about all prescription, over-the-counter, and herbal medications the child is taking.

Possible food and drug interactions when taking this medication
See the entry for the generic name methylphenidate on page 357.

Special information about pregnancy and breastfeeding
If the patient is sexually active, pregnant, or breastfeeding, they should talk to the doctor about the effects of Daytrana. It is possible for methylphenidate to pass into breast milk.

Recommended dosage
CHILDREN 6 YEARS AND OLDER

The Daytrana patch should be applied to the skin once a day, generally for a 9-hour period. If side effects occur, the doctor may have the child wear the patch for a shorter period of time.

Overdosage
Any medication taken in excess can have serious consequences. The doctor should be contacted immediately if the child uses more than the prescribed amount of Daytrana, or if it is suspected that the child may have symptoms of an overdose.

- *Symptoms of Daytrana overdose may include:*
  Agitation, confusion, convulsions, dry eyes, dry mouth, fever, flushing, hallucinations, headache, heart problems, muscle twitching, tremors

DEPAKOTE

Divalproex sodium (Valproic acid)
Other brand name: Depakote ER

Why is this drug prescribed?

Depakote is used to treat the manic episodes associated with bipolar disorder. In addition, Depakote and Depakote ER—the extended-release form of the drug—are both used to treat certain types of seizures and convulsions. Both of the drugs are also used for the prevention of migraine headaches in adults. Only Depakote ER is prescribed for the treatment of acute manic or mixed episodes associated with bipolar disorder.

Most important fact about this drug

Depakote can cause serious or even fatal liver damage, especially during the first 6 months of treatment. Children under 2 years of age are the most vulnerable, especially if they are also taking other anticonvulsant medicines and have certain other disorders such as mental retardation. The risk of liver damage decreases with age, but patients should always be alert for the following symptoms: loss of seizure control, weakness, dizziness, drowsiness, a general feeling of ill health, facial swelling, loss of appetite, vomiting, and yellowing of the skin and eyes. The doctor should be alerted immediately if a liver problem is suspected.

Depakote has also been known to cause life-threatening damage to the pancreas. This problem can surface at any time, even after years of treatment. Patients should call the doctor immediately if they develop any of the following warning signs: abdominal pain, loss of appetite, nausea, or vomiting.

How should this medication be taken?

Patients should take the Depakote tablet with water and swallow it whole (don't chew it or crush it). It has a special coating to avoid upsetting the stomach.

The sprinkle capsule can be swallowed whole or opened and sprinkled on a teaspoon of soft food such as applesauce or pudding. The food should be swallowed immediately, without chewing. The sprinkle capsules are large enough to be opened easily.

Depakote can be taken with meals or snacks to avoid stomach upset.

Depakote ER is an extended-release product intended to be taken once a day.

- *Missed dose...*

  If a patient takes Depakote once a day, the missed dose should be taken as soon as remembered. If it isn't remembered until the next day, the patient should skip the missed dose and return to the regular schedule.

  If a patient takes more than one dose a day, the missed dose should be taken right away if it's within 6 hours of the scheduled time, and the rest of the day's doses should be taken at equal intervals during the remainder of the day. Doses should never be doubled.

* *Storage instructions...*
  Depakote should be stored at room temperature.

What side effects may occur?

Side effects cannot be predicted. If any develop or change in intensity, patients should inform their doctor as soon as possible. Because Depakote is often used with other antiseizure drugs, it may not be possible to determine whether a side effect is due to Depakote alone. Only the doctor can determine if it is safe to continue taking Depakote.

* *Side effects of Depakote may include:*
  Abdominal pain, blurred vision, diarrhea, double vision, headache, impaired muscle coordination, indigestion, nausea, rapid eye movement, sleepiness, tremor, vomiting, weakness, weight loss or gain

* *Side effects of Depakote ER may include:*
  Abdominal pain, accidental injury, diarrhea, dizziness, indigestion, infection, nausea, pain, sleepiness, sore throat, vomiting, weakness

Why should this drug not be prescribed?

This medication must be avoided by anyone with liver disease, poor liver function, or the genetic abnormality known as urea cycle disorder (UCD).

It is also contraindicated for those who are sensitive to or have ever had an allergic reaction to Depakote.

Special warnings about this medication

This medication can severely damage the liver (see "Most important fact about this drug"). The doctor should test the patient's liver function before starting therapy with this medication and at regular intervals thereafter.

Also remember that the drug can damage the pancreas (see "Most important fact about this drug"). This problem can worsen very rapidly. Patients should contact their doctor without delay if they develop any symptoms.

In people with a rare set of genetic abnormalities called urea cycle disorder, Depakote may adversely affect the brain. Signs of a developing problem include lack of energy, repeated attacks of vomiting, and mental changes. Patients who suspect a problem should see their doctor immediately. Depakote may have to be discontinued.

Depakote causes some people to become drowsy or less alert. Patients should not drive, operate dangerous machinery, or participate in any hazardous activity that requires full mental alertness until they are certain the drug does not affect them this way.

This medication should not be stopped abruptly. A gradual reduction in dosage is usually required under a physician's supervision.

Depakote prolongs the time it takes blood to clot by decreasing the platelet count, which increases the chances of serious bleeding.

This drug can also increase the effect of painkillers and anesthetics. Before any surgery or dental procedure, the doctor should be informed that the patient is taking Depakote.

Patients taking Depakote to prevent migraine should remember that it will not cure a headache once it has started.

Some coated particles from the capsules may appear in the stool. This is to be expected, and is not a cause for worry.

Depakote depresses activity of the central nervous system, and may increase the effects of alcohol. Patients should not drink alcohol while taking this medication.

Possible food and drug interactions when taking this medication

See the entry for the generic name valproic acid on page 420.

Special information about pregnancy and breastfeeding

Depakote may produce birth defects when taken during pregnancy. Patients who are pregnant or plan to become pregnant should inform their doctor immediately. Depakote should be used during pregnancy only if it is essential for seizure control.

Depakote appears in breast milk and could affect a nursing infant. If Depakote is essential to the patient's health, the doctor may advise her to discontinue breastfeeding until her treatment with this medication is finished.

Recommended dosage

Depakote delayed-release and extended-release tablets work differently and cannot be substituted for each other.

DEPAKOTE

Epilepsy

Dosage for adults and children 10 years of age or older is determined by body weight. The usual recommended starting dose is 10 to 15 milligrams per 2.2 pounds (1 kilogram) per day, depending on the type of seizure. The doctor may increase the dose at 1-week intervals by 5 to 10 milligrams per 2.2 pounds (1 kilogram) per day until the seizures are controlled or the side effects become too severe. The maximum dose is 60 milligrams per 2.2 pounds (1 kilogram) per day. If the total dosage is more than 250 milligrams a day, the doctor will divide it into smaller individual doses.

Older adults usually begin taking this medication at lower dosages, and the dosage is increased more slowly.

Manic Episodes

The usual starting dose for those aged 18 and over is 750 milligrams a day, divided into smaller doses. The doctor will adjust the dose for best results.

Migrane Prevention

The usual starting dose for those aged 16 and over is 250 milligrams twice a day. The doctor will adjust the dose, up to a maximum of 1,000 milligrams a day.

Researchers have not established the safety and effectiveness of Depakote for prevention of migraines in children or in adults over 65.

DEPAKOTE ER

Acute Mania or Mixed Episodes

The recommended initial dose is 25 milligrams per 2.2 pounds (1 kilogram) per day. The dose should be increased as rapidly as possible to achieve desired effects at the lowest possible dose. The maximum recommended dosage of 60 milligrams per 2.2 (1 kilogram) pounds per day.

Migraine Prevention

The usual starting dose is 500 milligrams once a day for 1 week. The dose may then be increased to 1,000 milligrams once a day.

Epilepsy

Dosage for adults and children 10 years of age or older is determined by body weight. The usual recommended starting dose is 10 to 15 milligrams per 2.2 pounds (1 kilogram) per day, depending on the type of seizure. The doctor may increase the dose at 1-week intervals by 5 to 10 milligrams per 2.2 pounds (1 kilogram) per day until the seizures are controlled or the side effects become too severe. The maximum dose is 60 milligrams per 2.2 pounds (1 kilogram) per day.

Overdosage

An overdose of Depakote can be fatal. If an overdose is suspected, seek medical attention immediately.

- *Symptoms of Depakote overdose may include:*
  Coma, extreme sleepiness, heart problems

Desipramine *See Norpramin, page 146*

DESOXYN

Methamphetamine hydrochloride

Why is this drug prescribed?

Desoxyn is used to treat attention deficit hyperactivity disorder (ADHD). This drug is given as part of a total treatment program that includes psychological, educational, and social measures.

Desoxyn also may be used for a short time as part of an overall diet plan for weight reduction. Desoxyn is given only when other weight loss drugs and weight loss programs have been unsuccessful.

Most important fact about this drug?
Excessive doses of this medication can produce addiction. Individuals who stop taking this medication after taking high doses for a long time may suffer withdrawal symptoms, including extreme tiredness, depression, and sleep disorders. Signs of excessive use of Desoxyn include severe skin inflammation, difficulty sleeping, irritability, hyperactivity, personality changes, and psychiatric problems.

Desoxyn can lose its effectiveness in decreasing the appetite after a few weeks. If this happens, the medication should be stopped. Patients should never take more than the recommended dose in an attempt to increase the drug's effect.

How should this medication be taken?
It is important to follow the doctor's directions carefully. The doctor will prescribe the lowest effective dose of Desoxyn; it should never be increased without approval.

Patients should avoid taking this medication late in the evening; it can cause difficulty sleeping.

• *Missed dose...*
Generally, the forgotten dose should be taken as soon as remembered. However, if it is almost time for the next dose, the patient should skip the missed dose and return to the regular schedule. Doses should never be doubled.

• *Storage instructions...*
Desoxyn should be stored at room temperature.

What side effects may occur?
Side effects cannot be predicted. If any develop or change in intensity, patients should inform their doctor as soon as possible.

• *Side effects may include:*
Changes in sex drive, constipation, diarrhea, dizziness, dry mouth, exaggerated feeling of well-being, hives, impaired growth, impotence, increased blood pressure, overstimulation, rapid or irregular heartbeat, restlessness, sleeplessness, stomach or intestinal problems, tremor, unpleasant taste, worsening tics or Tourette's syndrome (severe twitching)

Why should this drug not be prescribed?
Desoxyn must never be combined with a monoamine oxidase (MAO) inhibitor such as Nardil or Parnate. Patients should allow 14 days between stopping an MAO inhibitor and beginning therapy with Desoxyn.

Desoxyn should not be taken by anyone who has high pressure in the eyes (glaucoma), advanced hardening of the arteries, heart disease, moderate to severe high blood pressure, thyroid problems, or sensitivity to this type of drug. This medication should also be avoided by anyone who suffers from tics (repeated, involuntary twitches) or Tourette's syndrome or who has a family history of these conditions.

People who are in an agitated state or who have a history of drug abuse should not take this medication.

Desoxyn should not be used to treat children whose symptoms may be caused by stress or a psychiatric disorder.

Special warnings about this medication

Desoxyn is not appropriate for all children with symptoms of ADHD. The doctor will do a complete history and evaluation before prescribing this medication. The doctor will take into account the duration and severity of the symptoms as well as the child's age.

This type of medication can affect the growth of children, so the doctor will monitor them carefully while they are taking this drug. The long-term effects of this type of medication in children have not been established.

Desoxyn should be used with caution by people with mild high blood pressure.

Desoxyn may affect the patient's ability to perform potentially hazardous activities, such as operating machinery or driving a car. Desoxyn should not be used to combat fatigue or to replace rest.

Possible food and drug interactions when taking this medication

See the entry for the generic name methamphetamine on page 356.

Special information about pregnancy and breastfeeding

Infants born to women taking this type of drug have a risk of prematurity and low birth weight. Drug dependence may occur in newborns when the mother has taken this drug prior to delivery. Patients who are pregnant or plan to become pregnant should tell their doctor immediately.

Desoxyn makes its way into breast milk. Women should not breastfeed while taking this medication.

Recommended dosage

ATTENTION DEFICIT HYPERACTIVITY DISORDER

For children 6 years and older, the usual starting dose is 5 milligrams of Desoxyn taken once or twice a day. The doctor may increase the dose by 5 milligrams a week until the child responds to the medication. The typical effective dose is 20 to 25 milligrams a day, usually divided into two doses.

The doctor may periodically discontinue this drug in order to reassess the child's condition and see whether therapy is still needed.

Desoxyn should not be given to children under 6 years of age to treat attention deficit disorder; the safety and effectiveness in this age group have not been established.

WEIGHT LOSS

For adults and children 12 years and older, the usual starting dose is 5 milligrams taken a half hour before each meal. Treatment should not continue for longer than a few weeks. The safety and effectiveness of Desoxyn for weight loss have not been established in children under age 12.

Overdosage

Any drug taken in excess can have dangerous consequences. If an overdose is suspected, seek medical attention immediately.

- *Symptoms of Desoxyn overdose may include:*
  Abdominal cramps, agitation, blood pressure changes, confusion, convulsions (may be followed by coma), depression, diarrhea, exaggerated reflexes, fatigue, hallucinations, high fever, irregular heartbeat, kidney failure, muscle aches and weakness, nausea, panic attacks, rapid breathing, restlessness, shock, tremor, vomiting

DESYREL
Trazodone hydrochloride

Why is this drug prescribed?

Desyrel is prescribed for the treatment of depression. The drug is thought to work by altering levels of serotonin in the brain; however, it's not chemically related to other serotonin-boosting antidepressants such as Paxil and Prozac.

Most important fact about this drug

Desyrel does not provide immediate relief. It may take up to 4 weeks before its benefits are felt, although most patients notice improvement within 2 weeks.

How should this medication be taken?

Desyrel should be taken shortly after a meal or light snack. Patients are more apt to feel dizzy or light-headed if they take the drug before eating. Desyrel may cause dry mouth. Sucking on a hard candy, chewing gum, or melting bits of ice in the mouth can relieve the problem.

- *Missed dose...*
  Generally, patients should take a forgotten dose as soon as they remember. However, if it is within 4 hours of their next dose, they should skip the dose they missed and go back to their regular schedule. Doses should never be doubled.

- *Storage instructions...*
  Desyrel should be stored at room temperature in a tightly closed container away from light and excessive heat.

What side effects may occur?
Side effects cannot be predicted. If any develop or change in intensity, patients should inform their doctor as soon as possible.

- *Side effects may include:*
  Abdominal or stomach disorder, aches or pains in muscles and bones, anger or hostility, blurred vision, brief loss of consciousness, confusion, constipation, decreased appetite, diarrhea, dizziness or lightheadedness, drowsiness, dry mouth, excitement, fainting, fast or fluttery heartbeat, fatigue, fluid retention and swelling, headache, inability to fall or stay asleep, low blood pressure, nasal or sinus congestion, nausea, nervousness, nightmares or vivid dreams, tremors, uncoordinated movements, vomiting, weight gain or loss

Why should this drug not be prescribed?
Anyone who is sensitive to or has ever had an allergic reaction to Desyrel or similar drugs cannot take this medication.

Special warnings about this medication
In clinical studies, antidepressants increased the risk of suicidal thinking and behavior in children and adolescents with depression and other psychiatric disorders. Anyone considering the use of Desyrel, or any other antidepressant in a child or adolescent, must balance the risk with the clinical need. Desyrel has not been studied in children or adolescents and is not approved for treating anyone less than 18 years old.

Additionally, the progression of major depression is associated with a worsening of symptoms and/or the emergence of suicidal thinking or behavior in both adults and children, whether or not they are taking antidepressants. Patients and caregivers should watch for any change in symptoms or any new symptoms that appear suddenly—especially agitation, anxiety, hostility, panic, restlessness, extreme hyperactivity, and suicidal thinking or behavior—and report them to the doctor immediately. Be especially observant at the beginning of treatment or whenever there is a change in dose.

Desyrel may cause patients to become drowsy or less alert and may affect judgment. They should avoid driving, operating dangerous machinery, or participating in any hazardous activity that requires full mental alertness until they know how this drug affects them.

Desyrel has been associated with priapism, a persistent, painful erection of the penis. Men who experience prolonged or inappropriate erections should stop taking this drug and consult their doctor.

In a medical emergency, and before surgery or dental treatment, patients should notify the doctor or dentist that they are taking this drug.

The doctor will ask them to stop using the drug if they are going to have elective surgery.

Caution is warranted in patients with heart disease. Desyrel can cause irregular heartbeats.

Desyrel may intensify the effects of alcohol. Patients should avoid drinking alcohol while taking this medication.

Possible food and drug interactions when taking this medication

See the entry for the generic name trazodone on page 412.

Special information about pregnancy and breastfeeding

The effects of Desyrel during pregnancy have not been adequately studied. Patients should inform their doctor immediately if they are pregnant or planning to become pregnant. This medication may appear in breast milk. If treatment with this drug is essential to the patient's health, the doctor may advise her to discontinue breastfeeding until her treatment is finished.

Recommended dosage

ADULTS

The usual starting dosage is a total of 150 milligrams per day, divided into 2 or more smaller doses. The doctor may increase the dose by 50 milligrams per day every 3 or 4 days. Total dosage should not exceed 400 milligrams per day, divided into smaller doses. Once a patient has responded well to the drug, the doctor may gradually reduce the dose. Because this medication causes drowsiness, the doctor may schedule the largest dose at bedtime.

CHILDREN

The safety and effectiveness of Desyrel have not been established in children below 18 years of age.

Overdosage

Any medication taken in excess can have serious consequences. An overdose of Desyrel in combination with other drugs can be fatal. If an overdose is suspected, seek medical attention immediately.

- *Symptoms of a Desyrel overdose may include:*
  Breathing failure; drowsiness; irregular heartbeat; prolonged, painful erection; seizures; vomiting

DEXEDRINE
Dextroamphetamine sulfate
Other brand name: DextroStat

Why is this drug prescribed?
Dexedrine, a stimulant drug available in tablet or sustained-release capsule form, is prescribed to help treat the following conditions: narcolepsy (recurrent "sleep attacks") and attention deficit hyperactivity disorder (ADHD). The total treatment program should include social, psychological, and educational guidance.

DextroStat is prescribed to treat the same conditions.

Most important fact about this drug
Because it is a stimulant, this drug has high abuse potential. The stimulant effect may give way to a letdown period of depression and fatigue. Although the letdown can be relieved by taking another dose, this soon becomes a vicious circle.

Patients should be aware that if they habitually take Dexedrine or DextroStat in doses higher than recommended, or if they take these medications over a long period of time, they may eventually become dependent on the drugs and suffer withdrawal symptoms when they are unavailable.

How should this medication be taken?
It is important to take Dexedrine exactly as prescribed. If it is prescribed in tablet form, patients may need up to 3 doses a day. The first dose should be taken upon awakening; the next 1 or 2 doses should be taken at intervals of 4 to 6 hours. The sustained-release capsules are taken only once a day.

It is best to avoid taking Dexedrine late in the day, since this could cause insomnia. If patients experience insomnia or loss of appetite while taking this drug, they should notify their doctor; they may need a lower dosage.

The doctor is likely to periodically take the patient off Dexedrine to determine whether the drug is still needed.

Patients should avoid chewing or crushing the sustained-release form, Dexedrine Spansules. They should never increase the dosage, except on their doctor's advice. Dexedrine should not be used to improve mental alertness or to stay awake. It should not be shared with others.

- *Missed dose...*
  Patients who take 1 dose a day should take it as soon as they remember, but not within 6 hours of going to bed. If they do not remember until the next day, they should skip the missed dose and go back to their regular schedule.

Patients who take 2 or 3 doses a day should take the missed dose immediately if it is within an hour or so of the scheduled time. Otherwise, they should skip the dose and go back to their regular schedule. Warn against taking 2 doses at once.

• *Storage instructions...*
Dexedrine should be stored at room temperature in a tightly closed container, away from light.

What side effects may occur?
Side effects cannot be predicted. If any develop or change in intensity, patients should inform their doctor as soon as possible.

• *Side effects of Dexedrine may include:*
Excessive restlessness, overstimulation

• *Effects of chronic heavy abuse of Dexedrine may include:*
Hyperactivity, irritability, personality changes, schizophrenia-like thoughts and behavior, severe insomnia, severe skin disease

• *Side effects of DextroStat may include:*
Anorexia, changes in sex drive, constipation, diarrhea, dizziness, dry mouth, dysphoria, elevation of blood pressure, euphoria, exacerbation of motor and phonic tics and Tourette's syndrome, gastrointestinal disturbances, headache, impotence, insomnia, overstimulation, rapid heartbeat, rash, restlessness, skipped heartbeat, spasms, tremors, unpleasant taste, weight loss

Why should this drug not be prescribed?
This drug must not be taken by anyone who is sensitive to or has ever had an allergic reaction to it.

It should be avoided for at least 14 days after taking a monoamine oxidase inhibitor (MAO inhibitor) such as the antidepressants Nardil and Parnate. Dexedrine and MAO inhibitors may interact to cause a sharp, potentially life-threatening rise in blood pressure.

Dexedrine must also be avoided by anyone suffering from one of the following conditions:

Agitation
Cardiovascular disease
Glaucoma, an eye disease marked by increased intraocular pressure
Hardening of the arteries
High blood pressure
Overactive thyroid gland
Substance abuse

Special warnings about this medication
Patients should be aware that one of the inactive ingredients in Dexedrine is a yellow food coloring called tartrazine (Yellow No. 5). In a few people,

particularly those who are allergic to aspirin, tartrazine can cause a severe allergic reaction.

Dexedrine may impair judgment or coordination. Patients should avoid driving or operating dangerous machinery until they know how they react to the medication.

There is some concern that Dexedrine may stunt a child's growth. For the sake of safety, any child who takes Dexedrine should have his or her growth monitored.

Amphetamines like Dexedrine and DextroStat have been reported to exacerbate motor and phonic tics and Tourette's syndrome. Also, clinical studies suggest that in psychotic pediatric patients administration of amphetamines may exacerbate symptoms of behavior disturbance and thought disorder.

Possible food and drug interactions when taking this medication

See the entry for the generic name dextroamphetamine on page 313.

Special information about pregnancy and breastfeeding

If a patient is pregnant or plans to become pregnant, she should inform her doctor immediately. Babies born to women taking Dexedrine may be premature or have low birth weight. They may also be depressed, agitated, or apathetic due to withdrawal symptoms. DextroStat should be taken during pregnancy only if the potential benefit justifies the potential risk to the fetus.

Since Dexedrine appears in breast milk, it should not be taken by a nursing mother.

Recommended dosage

Patients should take no more Dexedrine than prescribed. Intake should be kept to the lowest level that proves effective.

NARCOLEPSY

Adults: The usual dose is 5 to 60 milligrams per day, divided into smaller, equal doses.

Children: Narcolepsy seldom occurs in children under 12 years of age; however, when it does, Dexedrine or DextroStat may be used.

The suggested initial dose for children between 6 and 12 years of age is 5 milligrams per day. The doctor may increase the daily dose in increments of 5 milligrams at weekly intervals until it becomes effective.

Children 12 years of age and older will be started with 10 milligrams daily. The daily dosage may be raised in increments of 10 milligrams at weekly intervals until effective. If side effects such as insomnia or loss of appetite appear, the dosage will probably be reduced.

ATTENTION DEFICIT HYPERACTIVITY DISORDER

This drug is not recommended for children under 3 years of age.

Children from 3 to 5 Years of Age: The usual starting dose is 2.5 milligrams daily, in tablet form. The doctor may raise the daily dosage by 2.5 milligrams at weekly intervals until the drug becomes effective.

Children 6 Years of Age and Older: The usual starting dose is 5 milligrams once or twice a day. The doctor may raise the dose by 5 milligrams at weekly intervals untilis satisfied with the response. Only in rare cases will the child take more than 40 milligrams per day.

The child should take the first dose upon awakening; the remaining 1 or 2 doses are taken at intervals of 4 to 6 hours. Alternatively, the doctor may prescribe Dexedrine "Spansule" capsules that are taken once a day. The doctor may interrupt the schedule occasionally to see if behavioral symptoms come back enough to require continued therapy.

Overdosage

An overdose of Dexedrine can be fatal. If an overdose is suspected, seek medical attention immediately.

- *Symptoms of an acute Dexedrine overdose may include:*
  Abdominal cramps, assaultiveness, coma, confusion, convulsions, depression, diarrhea, fatigue, hallucinations, high fever, heightened reflexes, high or low blood pressure, irregular heartbeat, nausea, panic, rapid breathing, restlessness, tremor, vomiting

- *Symptoms of an acute DextroStat overdose may include:*
  Abdominal cramps, assaultiveness, coma, confusion, convulsions, depression, diarrhea, elevated body temperature, fatigue, hallucinations, heightened reflexes, high or low blood pressure, irregular heartbeat, muscle aches and pains, nausea, panic, rapid breathing, restlessness, tremor, vomiting

Dexmethylphenidate *See Focalin, page 88*

Dextroamphetamine *See Dexedrine, page 66*

DextroStat *See Dexedrine, page 66*

Diazepam *See Valium, page 243*

Disulfiram *See Antabuse, page 23*

Divalproex *See Depakote, page 57*

Donepezil *See Aricept, page 26*

DORAL
Quazepam

Why is this drug prescribed?
Doral, a sleeping medication available in tablet form, is taken as short-term treatment for insomnia. Symptoms of insomnia may include difficulty falling asleep, frequent awakenings throughout the night, or very early morning awakening.

Most important fact about this drug
Doral is a chemical cousin of Valium and is potentially addictive. Over time, the body will get used to the prescribed dosage of Doral, and a patient will no longer derive any benefit from it. If the patient were to increase the dosage against medical advice, the drug would again work as a sleeping pill, but only until the body adjusted to the higher dosage. This is a vicious circle that can lead to addiction. To avoid this danger, Doral must be used only as prescribed.

How should this medication be taken?
Doral must be used exactly as prescribed: one dose per day, at bedtime. Patients should keep in touch with their doctor. If they respond very well, it may be possible to cut their dosage in half after the first few nights. The older or more run-down the patient is, the more desirable it is to try for this early dosage reduction.

After taking Doral regularly for 6 weeks or so, patients may experience withdrawal symptoms if they stop suddenly, or even if they reduce the dosage without specific instructions on how to do it. They should see their doctor for instructions on how to taper off Doral.

* *Missed dose...*
  This medication should be taken only if needed.

* *Storage instructions...*
  Doral should be stored at room temperature, away from moisture.

What side effects may occur?
Side effects cannot be predicted. If any develop or change in intensity, patients should inform their doctor as soon as possible.

* *Side effects may include:*
  Drowsiness during the day, headache

In rare instances, Doral produces agitation, sleep disturbances, hallucinations, or stimulation—exactly the opposite of the desired effect. If this should happen, the patient should see the doctor, who will stop the medication.

Why should this drug not be prescribed?

Doral cannot be used by anyone who is sensitive to it or has ever had an allergic reaction to it or to another Valium-type medication.

Doral should not be used by patients with known or suspected sleep apnea (short periods of interrupted breathing that occur during sleep).

Doral must not be taken during pregnancy.

Special warnings about this medication

Because Doral may decrease daytime alertness, patients should not drive, climb, or operate dangerous machinery until they find out how the drug affects them. In some cases, Doral's sedative effect may last for several days after the last dose.

Doral may aggravate depression in patients with depressive disorders.

Patients with a history of alcohol or drug abuse are at special risk for addiction to Doral. It is important for patients to avoid increasing the dosage of Doral on their own. They should tell the doctor right away if the medication no longer seems to be working.

Patients should avoid drinking alcohol while taking Doral; it can increase the drug's effects.

Possible food and drug interactions when taking this medication

See the entry for the generic name quazepam on page 393.

Special information about pregnancy and breastfeeding

Because Doral may cause harm to the unborn child, it should not be taken during pregnancy. Patients should discontinue Doral before getting pregnant.

Babies whose mothers are taking Doral at the time of birth may experience withdrawal symptoms from the drug. Such babies may be "floppy" (flaccid) instead of having normal muscle tone.

Since Doral does appear in breast milk, patients should not take this medication while nursing a baby.

Recommended dosage

ADULTS

The recommended initial dose is 15 milligrams daily. The doctor may later reduce this dosage to 7.5 milligrams.

CHILDREN

Safety and efficacy of Doral in children under 18 years old have not been established.

OLDER ADULTS

Older patients may be more sensitive to this drug, and the doctor may reduce the dosage after only 1 or 2 nights.

Overdosage
Any medication taken in excess can have serious consequences. If an overdose of Doral is suspected, seek medical attention immediately.

• *Symptoms of an overdose of Doral may include:*
  Coma, confusion, extreme sleepiness

Doxepin *See Sinequan, page 211*

Duloxetine *See Cymbalta, page 50*

EFFEXOR
Venlafaxine hydrochloride
Other brand name: Effexor XR

Why is this drug prescribed?
Effexor is prescribed for the treatment of depression. Effexor XR is also prescribed to relieve generalized anxiety disorder and social anxiety disorder. The drug is thought to work by boosting levels of serotonin and norepinephrine, two important chemical messengers in the brain.

Most important fact about this drug
Serious, sometimes fatal reactions have occurred when Effexor is used in combination with drugs classified as MAO inhibitors, including the antidepressants Nardil and Parnate. Effexor must never be taken with one of these drugs, or within 14 days of discontinuing treatment with one of them. It is also important to allow at least 7 days between the last dose of Effexor and the first dose of an MAO inhibitor.

How should this medication be taken?
Effexor should be taken with food, exactly as prescribed. It may take several weeks before an effect is seen.

Effexor must be taken 2 or 3 times daily. The extended-release form, Effexor XR, permits once-a-day dosing, which should be taken at the same time each day. The capsule should be swallowed whole with water. It must not be divided, crushed, or chewed. However, if the patient has trouble swallowing pills, he or she may take Effexor XR by carefully opening the capsule and sprinkling the entire contents on a spoonful of applesauce, followed by a glass of water.

• *Missed dose...*
  It is not necessary to make up a forgotten dose. Patients should skip the missed dose and continue with the next scheduled dose. They should never take 2 doses at once.

- *Storage instructions...*
  Effexor should be stored in a tightly closed container at room temperature and protected from excessive heat and moisture.

What side effects may occur?
Side effects cannot be predicted. If any develop or change in intensity, patients should inform their doctor as soon as possible.

- *Side effects of Effexor may include:*
  Abnormal ejaculation/orgasm, anxiety, blurred vision, constipation, dizziness, dry mouth, impotence, insomnia, nausea, nervousness, sleepiness, sweating, tremor, vomiting, weakness, weight loss

- *Side effects of Effexor XR may include:*
  Abnormal dreams, abnormal ejaculation, constipation, dizziness, dry mouth, headache, insomnia, nausea, nervousness, sleepiness, sweating, weakness, weight loss

Why should this drug not be prescribed?
Remember that Effexor must never be combined with an MAO inhibitor (See "Most important fact about this drug"). This drug should also be avoided by anyone who has had an allergic reaction to it.

Special warnings about this medication
In clinical studies, antidepressants increased the risk of suicidal thinking and behavior in children and adolescents with depression and other psychiatric disorders. Anyone considering the use of Effexor, or any other antidepressant in a child or adolescent, must balance the risk with the clinical need. Effexor has not been studied in children or adolescents and is not approved for treating anyone less than 18 years old.

Additionally, the progression of major depression is associated with a worsening of symptoms and/or the emergence of suicidal thinking or behavior in both adults and children, whether or not they are taking antidepressants. Patients and caregivers should watch for any change in symptoms or any new symptoms that appear suddenly—especially agitation, anxiety, hostility, panic, restlessness, extreme hyperactivity, and suicidal thinking or behavior—and report them to the doctor immediately. Be especially observant at the beginning of treatment or whenever there is a change in dose.

Like all antidepressants, Effexor could cause episodes of mania. If a patient experiences a major depressive episode, there's a slight chance that it could be the first signs of bipolar disorder. The patient should tell the doctor about all of their symptoms. Note that Effexor is not approved for treating bipolar depression.

Effexor should be used with caution in patients with high blood pressure; heart, liver, or kidney disease; or a history of seizures or mania. It's important for patients to discuss all of their medical problems with their doctor before taking Effexor.

Effexor sometimes causes an increase in blood pressure. If this happens, the doctor may need to reduce the dose or discontinue the drug.

Effexor also tends to increase the heart rate, especially at higher doses. Effexor must be used cautiously in patients who have recently had a heart attack, suffer from heart failure, or have an overactive thyroid gland.

Effexor may increase cholesterol levels if it's taken for 3 months or longer. This effect is more common among patients taking higher doses.

Antidepressants such as Effexor may cause fluid retention, especially in older adults.

Effexor may cause patients to feel drowsy or less alert and may affect their judgment. They should avoid driving or operating dangerous machinery, or participating in any hazardous activity that requires full mental alertness, until they know how this drug affects them.

The doctor should regularly check any patient who has glaucoma (high pressure in the eye), or is at risk of developing it.

This drug should be discontinued only under supervision of a doctor. If it is stopped suddenly, patients may have withdrawal symptoms, even though Effexor does not seem to be habit-forming. The doctor will have them taper off gradually. If they have ever been addicted to drugs, they should tell the doctor before starting Effexor.

Patients who develop a skin rash or hives while taking Effexor should notify their doctor immediately. Effexor may also cause bleeding or bruising of the skin.

Combining Effexor with MAO inhibitors could cause a fatal reaction (see "Most important fact about this drug").

Although Effexor does not interact with alcohol, the manufacturer recommends avoiding alcohol while taking this medication.

Patients should consult their doctor before combining Effexor with other drugs that affect the central nervous system, including lithium, migraine medications such as Imitrex, weight-loss products such as phentermine, narcotic painkillers, sleep aids, tranquilizers, antipsychotic medicines such as haloperidol, and other antidepressants such as Celexa, Prozac, Tofranil, and Zoloft.

Effexor has been found to reduce blood levels of the HIV drug Crixivan. It's best for patients to check with their doctor before combining Effexor with any other drug or herbal product.

Possible food and drug interactions when taking this medication
See the entry for the generic name venlafaxine on page 421.

Special information about pregnancy and breastfeeding
The effects of Effexor during pregnancy have not been adequately studied. Patients should consult their doctor immediately if they are pregnant or are planning to become pregnant. Effexor should be used during pregnancy only if clearly needed.

If Effexor is taken shortly before delivery, the baby may suffer withdrawal symptoms. Effexor appears in breast milk and could cause serious side effects in a nursing infant. Patients will need to choose between nursing their baby and continuing treatment with Effexor.

Recommended dosage

EFFEXOR

The usual starting dose is 75 milligrams a day, divided into 2 or 3 smaller doses, and taken with food. If needed, the doctor may gradually increase the daily dose in steps of no more than 75 milligrams at a time, up to a maximum of 375 milligrams per day.

If the patient has kidney or liver disease, or is taking other medications, the doctor will adjust the dosage accordingly.

EFFEXOR XR

For both depression and anxiety, the usual starting dose is 75 milligrams once daily taken with food, although some people begin with a dose of 37.5 milligrams for the first 4 to 7 days. The doctor may gradually increase the dose, in steps of no more than 75 milligrams, up to a maximum of 225 milligrams daily. As with regular Effexor, the doctor will make adjustments in the dosage for patients with kidney or liver disease.

Overdosage

An overdose of Effexor, combined with other drugs or alcohol, can be fatal. If an overdose is suspected, seek medical attention immediately.

- *Symptoms of Effexor overdose may include:*
  Sleepiness, vertigo, rapid or slow heartbeat, low blood pressure, seizures, coma

---

EMSAM
Selegiline transdermal system

Why is this drug prescribed?
Emsam is a skin patch (transdermal system) used to treat depression. The patch is applied once a day and provides continuous delivery of medication through the skin and into the bloodstream.

Most important fact about this drug
Emsam belongs to a class of drugs known as monoamine oxidase inhibitors (MAOIs). These drugs, including Emsam, can interact with certain foods that contain tyramine and cause a life-threatening surge in blood pressure (known as hypertensive crisis). Side effects that indicate a hypertensive crisis include sudden onset of severe headache, nausea, stiff neck, fast heartbeat or palpitations, severe sweating, and confusion.

Patients who develop these symptoms should seek emergency medical treatment immediately.

Foods high in tyramine include aged cheeses and meats, pickled herring, fermented foods such as sauerkraut and tofu, and tap beer. Patients should see their doctor or pharmacist for a complete list of foods to avoid.

Patients must not eat or drink foods containing tyramine while using the Emsam 9 milligrams/24 hour or 12 milligrams/24 hour patches and for 2 weeks after stopping treatment with these patches. However, no diet changes are required when using the 6 milligrams/24 hour patch.

How should this medication be taken?
The Emsam patch should be applied to dry, smooth skin on the upper chest or back (below the neck and above the waist), upper thigh, or outside of the upper arm. Patients should choose a new site each time they change the patch. They should not use the same site 2 days in a row. After the patch has been applied, patients should wash their hands well with soap and water. They should be careful not to touch their eyes until after their hands are washed.

The patch delivers medicine continuously for 24 hours. A new patch should be applied every day. Patients should wear only one patch at a time.

The Emsam patch should never be kept or stored outside of its sealed pouch. Also, the patch should never be cut into smaller pieces to use.

- *Missed dose...*
  If patients forget to change their patch after 24 hours, they should remove the old patch, put on a new patch in a different area, and continue to follow their regular schedule.

- *Storage instructions...*
  Store Emsam patches at room temperature in their original pouches.

What side effects may occur?
Side effects cannot be predicted. If any develop or change in intensity, patients should inform their doctor as soon as possible.

- *Side effects may include:*
  Diarrhea, dry mouth, headache, insomnia, rash, sinusitis, skin reaction at the site of application, sore throat, upset stomach

Why should this drug not be prescribed?
Patients cannot use Emsam if they are allergic to any of its ingredients, or if they are taking certain drugs that could interact with Emsam (see "Special warnings about this medication").

Special warnings about this medication
In clinical studies, antidepressants increased the risk of suicidal thinking and behavior in children and adolescents with depression and other psychiatric

disorders. Anyone considering the use of Emsam, or any other antidepressant in a child or adolescent, must balance the risk with the clinical need. Emsam is not approved for use in patients less than 18 years old.

Additionally, the progression of major depression is associated with a worsening of symptoms and/or the emergence of suicidal thinking or behavior in both adults and children, whether or not they are taking antidepressants. Patients and caregivers should watch for any change in symptoms or any new symptoms that appear suddenly—especially agitation, anxiety, hostility, panic, restlessness, extreme hyperactivity, and suicidal thinking or behavior—and report them to the doctor immediately. Be especially observant at the beginning of treatment or whenever there is a change in dose.

Before taking Emsam, patients should inform the doctor about all their medical conditions, especially if they have a history of heart problems, mania or hypomania, seizures, low blood pressure, or fainting.

Any psychoactive drug has the potential to impair coordination, judgment, and the ability to think. Patients should not drive or operate dangerous machinery until they know how Emsam affects them.

Emsam can cause serious and life-threatening reactions if combined with certain medications. Patients should not take other medicines while using Emsam or for 2 weeks after stopping treatment without checking with their doctor first. Drugs that should never be combined with Emsam include:

Other antidepressants
Other medications containing the active ingredient selegiline, such as Eldepryl
Amphetamines
BuSpar (buspirone)
Decongestants
Demerol and other narcotic pain medicine such as tramadol, methadone, and propoxyphene
Dextromethorphan (often found in cough and cold medicine)
Flexeril or other drugs containing cyclobenzaprine
Tegretol or other drugs containing carbamazepine
Trileptal or other drugs containing oxcarbazepine
Over-the-counter diet pills or herbal weight-loss supplements
St. John's wort

Possible food and drug interactions when taking this medication
See the entry for the generic name selegiline on page 396.

Special information about pregnancy and breastfeeding
The effects of Emsam during pregnancy and breastfeeding have not been adequately studied. The drug is recommended only if its benefits are

thought to outweigh the potential risk to the baby. If a patient is pregnant, planning to become pregnant, or is breastfeeding she should inform her doctor immediately.

Recommended dosage

ADULTS

Emsam comes in three patch strengths: 6 milligrams, 9 milligrams, and 12 milligrams. The recommended starting dose is one 6-milligram patch applied every 24 hours. Based on the patient's response, the doctor may increase the dose by 3 milligrams every 2 weeks, up to a maximum of 12 milligrams a day.

Overdosage

No information on Emsam overdose is available. However, any medication taken in excess can have serious consequences. If an overdose is suspected, seek medical attention immediately.

EQUETRO

Carbamazepine

Why is this drug prescribed?

Equetro is used to treat acute manic and mixed episodes of bipolar I disorder.

The generic ingredient of Equetro—carbamazepine—is also the generic ingredient of another drug called Tegretol. Tegretol is used in the treatment of seizure disorders, including certain types of epilepsy. It is also prescribed for trigeminal neuralgia (severe pain in the jaws) and pain in the tongue and throat.

Most important fact about this drug

Patients should not begin treatment with Equetro if they are already being treated with a drug containing carbamazepine. If stopped abruptly, Equetro may cause a seizure in people with epilepsy.

Carbamazepine may cause severe harm during pregnancy.

How should this medication be taken?

Equetro capsules may be swallowed whole, or opened and sprinkled over food such as applesauce. Capsules may be taken with or without food. Patients should not crush or chew the capsules.

- *Missed dose...*
  If a dose is missed, patients should just continue on their normal schedule. Doses should never be doubled.

- *Storage instructions...*
  Equetro should be stored at room temperature, away from light.

What side effects may occur?

Side effects cannot be predicted. If any develop or change in intensity, patients should inform their doctor as soon as possible.

* *Side effects may include:*
  Blurred vision, dizziness, dry mouth, itchiness, muscle problems, nausea, speech problems, vomiting

Why should this drug not be prescribed?

Patients should not use Equetro if they have had problems with their bone marrow, or if they are allergic to any of the drug's ingredients.

Special warnings about this medication

People taking Equetro should avoid potentially harmful activities, such as driving and operating machinery, until they see how it affects them, as this drug may cause dizziness and blurred vision.

Patients should tell their doctor about all prescription, over-the-counter, and herbal medications they are taking before beginning treatment with Equetro. Also, they should talk to their doctor about their complete medical history, especially if they have liver problems, a seizure disorder, or previous blood problems.

Possible food and drug interactions when taking this medication

See the entry for the generic name carbamazepine on page 291.

Special information about pregnancy and breastfeeding

Women who are pregnant, plan to become pregnant, or are nursing should not take Equetro. This drug may cause severe problems during pregnancy, such as spina bifida (an opening in the spinal cord). Also, this drug may pass into breast milk.

Recommended dosage

ADULTS

The usual dosage of Equetro is 400 milligrams per day. The dosage may be adjusted by 200-milligram increments. The maximum dosage of this drug is 1,600 milligrams per day.

Overdosage

Any medication taken in excess can have serious consequences. If an overdose is suspected, seek medical attention immediately.

Escitalopram *See Lexapro, page 109*

Eskalith *See Lithium carbonate, page 116*

Estazolam *See ProSom, page 174*

Eszopiclone *See Lunesta, page 119*

EXELON
Rivastigmine tartrate

Why is this drug prescribed?
Exelon is used in the treatment of mild to moderate Alzheimer's disease. This progressive, degenerative disorder causes physical changes in the brain that disrupt the flow of information and interfere with memory, thinking, and behavior. By boosting levels of the chemical messenger acetylcholine, Exelon can temporarily improve brain function in some Alzheimer's sufferers, though it does not halt the progress of the underlying disease. Like other drugs for Alzheimer's, Exelon may become less effective as the disease progresses.

Most important fact about this drug
Patience is in order when starting this drug. It can take up to 12 weeks before Exelon's full benefits appear.

How should this medication be taken?
Exelon should be taken with food in the morning and in the evening.

- *Missed dose...*
  Generally, the forgotten dose should be given as soon as remembered. However, if it is almost time for the next dose, caregivers should skip the missed dose and go back to the regular schedule. Doses should never be doubled.

- *Storage instructions...*
  Exelon should be stored at room temperature in a tightly closed container.

What side effects may occur?
Side effects cannot be predicted. If any develop or change in intensity, caregivers should inform the doctor as soon as possible.

- *Side effects may include:*
  Abdominal pain, accidental injury, anxiety, aggression, confusion, constipation, depression, diarrhea, dizziness, drowsiness, fainting, fatigue, flu-like symptoms, gas, hallucinations, headache, high blood pressure, increased sweating, indigestion, inflamed nasal passages, insomnia, loss of appetite, nausea, tremor, unwell feeling, urinary infection, vomiting, weakness, weight loss

Why should this drug not be prescribed?
Exelon cannot be used if it causes an allergic reaction.

Special warnings about this medication
Exelon often causes nausea and vomiting, especially at the beginning of treatment. The problem is more likely in women, but it can lead to

significant weight loss in both women and men. The doctor should be informed immediately if these side effects occur.

The chance of severe vomiting increases when Exelon is given after an interruption of several days. Caregivers should check with the doctor before starting to give the drug again. The dosage may need to be reduced to the lowest starting level.

Exelon may aggravate asthma and other breathing problems and can increase the risk of seizures. Other drugs of its type are also known to increase the chance of ulcers, stomach bleeding, and urinary obstruction, although these problems have not been noted with Exelon. Drugs in this category can also slow the heartbeat, possibly causing fainting in people who have a heart condition. The doctor should be alerted if any of these problems occur.

Exelon has not been tested in children.

Possible food and drug interactions when taking this medication

See the entry for the generic name rivastigmine on page 395.

Special information about pregnancy and breastfeeding

Exelon is not intended for women of childbearing age, and its effects during pregnancy and breastfeeding have not been studied.

Recommended dosage

ADULTS

The usual starting dose is 1.5 milligrams 2 times a day for at least 2 weeks. At 2-week intervals, the doctor may then increase the dose to 3 milligrams, 4.5 milligrams, and finally 6.0 milligrams 2 times a day. Higher doses tend to be more effective. The maximum dosage is 12 milligrams daily.

If side effects such as nausea and vomiting begin to develop, the doctor may recommend skipping a few doses, then starting again at the same or next lowest dosage.

Overdosage

Any medication taken in excess can have serious consequences. If an overdose is suspected, seek emergency medical attention immediately.

- *Symptoms of Exelon overdose may include:*
  Collapse, convulsions, breathing difficulty, extreme muscle weakness (possibly ending in death if breathing muscles are affected), low blood pressure, salivation, severe nausea, slow heartbeat, sweating, vomiting

FazaClo ODT *See Clozaril, page 43*

Fluoxetine *See Prozac, page 179*

FLUPHENAZINE HYDROCHLORIDE

Why is this drug prescribed?

Fluphenazine is used to reduce the symptoms of severe mental disturbances such as schizophrenia.

Most important fact about this drug

Fluphenazine may cause tardive dyskinesia, a condition marked by involuntary muscle spasms and twitches in the face and body. This condition may be permanent and appears to be most common among the elderly, especially women.

How should this medication be taken?

The elixir form of fluphenazine should be examined before it's taken. The flavoring oils may have separated from the solution, causing globs or a wispy appearance. If this happens, the bottle should be gently shaken. The oil should blend in, and the solution should look clear. If the solution is not clear, it should not be used.

Avoid the use of alcohol when taking fluphenazine.

Fluphenazine concentrate can be mixed with homogenized milk, non-caffeinated soft drinks, or fruit juice. It should not be mixed with caffeine-containing beverages, tea, or apple juice.

- *Missed dose...*
  Patients who take 1 dose a day should take the forgotten dose as soon as they remember, then go back to their regular schedule. If they do not remember until the next day, they should skip the dose they missed and go back to their regular schedule. If they take more than 1 dose a day, they should take the forgotten dose as soon as they remember if it is within an hour or so of their scheduled time. If they do not remember until later, they should skip the dose they missed and go back to their regular schedule. Doses should never be doubled.

- *Storage instructions...*
  Fluphenazine should be stored at room temperature in a tightly closed container, away from light. The liquid forms should not be frozen. The tablets should be protected from excessive heat.

What side effects may occur?

Side effects cannot be predicted. If any develop or change in intensity, patients should inform their doctor as soon as possible.

- *Side effects may include:*
  Abnormal muscle rigidity, abnormal secretion of milk, abnormalities of movements and posture, asthma, blood disorders, blurred vision, body rigidly arches backwards, breast development in males, changed mental state, chewing movements, complete or almost complete loss of movement, constipation, dizziness, drowsiness, dry mouth, excessive

or spontaneous flow of milk, excessive urine, excitement, eye problems, eyeball rotation or state of fixed gaze, fluid accumulation and swelling, fluid accumulation in the brain, glaucoma, headache, heart attack, high blood pressure, high fever, hives, impotence, inability to sit still, increased sex drive in women, intestinal blockage, irregular blood pressure pulse heartbeat, irregular menstrual periods, loss of appetite, mask-like face and rigidity, muscle spasms, nasal congestion, nausea, oily scalp, painful muscle spasms, protruding tongue, puckering of mouth, puffing of cheeks, purple or red spots on the skin, rapid heartbeat, red blood spots, restlessness, salivation, sensitivity to light, severe allergic reactions, skin inflammation and peeling, skin itching or rash, skin lesions or crusts, sluggishness, sore throat mouth gums, strange dreams, sweating, swelling of the throat, twitching in the body neck and shoulders, face, visual problems, weight change, yellowing of the skin and whites of eyes

Why should this drug not be prescribed?

Do not give fluphenazine to someone in a comatose state. This drug should not be taken by anyone who is also taking large doses of hypnotic drugs such as Seconal, Halcion, and phenobarbital; who is very depressed; who has had brain or liver damage; or who has an abnormal bone marrow or blood condition. It should also be avoided by anyone who has ever had an allergic reaction to it or similar major tranquilizers.

Special warnings about this medication

Fluphenazine should be used with caution by anyone who has ever had breast cancer convulsive disorders heart or kidney disease or certain tumors. Caution is warranted, too, if the patient is exposed to extreme heat or certain pesticides.

Stomach inflammation, dizziness, nausea, vomiting, and tremors can result if fluphenazine is suddenly stopped. Patients must follow their doctor's instructions closely when discontinuing it.

Fluphenazine can cause a collection of symptoms called neuroleptic malignant syndrome. If the patient develops high fever, rigid muscles, changed mental state, irregular pulse or blood pressure, rapid or abnormal heartbeat, or excessive perspiration, the doctor should be notified immediately.

The doctor will periodically check the patient's liver, kidneys, and blood during fluphenazine therapy.

This drug may impair the ability to drive a car or operate potentially dangerous machinery. Patients should not participate in any activities that require full alertness if they are unsure of their ability.

Fluphenazine 2.5-, 5-, and 10-milligram tablets contain a coloring agent that can cause an allergic reaction in some people, especially those who are also allergic to aspirin.

Fluphenazine should not be used with epinephrine (EpiPen). Extreme drowsiness and other potentially serious effects can result if fluphenazine is combined with alcohol, narcotic pain relievers such as Percocet, sleeping medications such as Seconal, antihistamines such as Benadryl, or tranquilizers such as Valium. Fluphenazine may also interact with Atropine.

Possible food and drug interactions when taking this medication
See the entry for fluphenazine on page 325.

Special information about pregnancy and breastfeeding
Pregnant women should use fluphenazine only if clearly needed. Patients who are pregnant or plan to become pregnant should inform their doctor immediately.

Fluphenazine may appear in breast milk and could affect a nursing infant. If this medication is essential to the patient's health, the doctor may advise her not to breastfeed while taking it.

Recommended dosage
ADULTS

The usual beginning total daily dose is 2.5 to 10 milligrams. This amount is divided into 3 or 4 equal doses and taken 6 or 8 hours apart.

If necessary, the doctor may increase the total dosage to 40 milligrams daily. When symptoms are under control, the doctor may decrease the dose. A daily maintenance dose may range from 1 to 5 milligrams, usually taken once daily.

CHILDREN

Safety and efficacy of fluphenazine in children have not been established.

OLDER ADULTS

Older people may start with a daily dose of 1 to 2.5 milligrams. In general, they will take dosages of fluphenazine in the lower ranges. Older people (especially older women) may be more susceptible to tardive dyskinesia—a possibly permanent condition characterized by involuntary muscle spasms and twitches in the face and body.

Overdosage
Any medication taken in excess can have serious consequences. If an overdose of fluphenazine is suspected, seek medical help immediately.

Flurazepam *See Dalmane, page 52*

FLUVOXAMINE MALEATE

Why is this drug prescribed?

Fluvoxamine is prescribed for obsessive-compulsive disorder. It belongs to the class of drugs known as selective serotonin reuptake inhibitors (SSRIs). Fluvoxamine is thought to work by increasing levels of serotonin, a brain chemical associated with mood and thinking.

Most important fact about this drug

Before starting therapy with fluvoxamine, patients should tell the doctor what medications they are taking, both prescription and over-the-counter, since combining fluvoxamine with certain drugs may cause serious or even life-threatening effects. Fluvoxamine should never be combined with thioridazine or Orap. In addition, it should not be used within 14 days of taking any antidepressant drug classified as an MAO inhibitor, including Nardil and Parnate.

How should this medication be taken?

This medication should be taken only as directed by the doctor. It may be taken with or without food.

- *Missed dose...*
  Patients who are taking 1 dose a day should skip the missed dose and go back to their regular schedule. Patients who are taking 2 doses a day should take the missed dose as soon as possible, and then go back to their regular schedule. Patients should never take 2 doses at the same time.

- *Storage instructions...*
  Fluvoxamine should be stored at room temperature and protected from humidity.

What side effects may occur?

Side effects cannot be predicted. If any develop or change in intensity, patients should tell the doctor immediately.

- *Side effects may include:*
  Abnormal ejaculation, agitation, anxiety, diarrhea, dizziness, dry mouth, headache, indigestion, insomnia, nausea, nervousness, sleepiness, sweating, tremor, vomiting, weakness, weight loss

Why should this drug not be prescribed?

Patients who are sensitive to or have ever had an allergic reaction to fluvoxamine or similar drugs, such as Prozac and Zoloft, should not take this medication.

Fluvoxamine should never be combined with thioridazine or Orap, or taken within 14 days of taking an MAO inhibitor such as Nardil or Parnate. (See "Most important fact about this drug.")

Special warnings about this medication

In clinical studies, SSRI antidepressants increased the risk of suicidal thinking and behavior in children and adolescents with depression and other psychiatric disorders. Anyone considering the use of fluvoxamine, or any other antidepressant in a child or adolescent, must balance the risk with the clinical need. Fluvoxamine must be used with caution in children with depression. It is only approved for treating obsessive-compulsive disorder in children 8 years and older.

Additionally, the progression of major depression is associated with a worsening of symptoms and/or the emergence of suicidal thinking or behavior in both adults and children, whether or not they are taking antidepressants. Patients and caregivers should watch for any change in symptoms or any new symptoms that appear suddenly—especially agitation, anxiety, hostility, panic, restlessness, extreme hyperactivity, and suicidal thinking or behavior—and report them to the doctor immediately. Be especially observant at the beginning of treatment or whenever there is a change in dose.

Patients should discuss all medical problems with their doctor before starting therapy with fluvoxamine, as certain physical conditions or diseases may affect their reaction to the drug.

This medication should be used cautiously by anyone with a history of seizures. Patients who experience a seizure while taking fluvoxamine should stop taking the drug and call the doctor immediately.

The dosage of fluvoxamine may need adjustment if the patient has ever had suicidal thoughts. The drug should be used with caution by patients who have a history of mania.

The doctor will need to adjust the dosage if the patient has liver disease.

Fluvoxamine may cause patients to become drowsy or less alert and may affect their judgment. They should avoid driving, operating dangerous machinery, or participating in any hazardous activity that requires full mental alertness until they know how this medication affects them.

Fluvoxamine can also deplete the body's supply of salt, especially in older adults and people who take diuretics or suffer from dehydration. Under these conditions, the doctor will check salt levels regularly.

Serotonin-boosting drugs could potentially cause stomach bleeding, especially in older patients or those taking nonsteroidal anti-inflammatory drugs (NSAIDs) such as aspirin, ibuprofen (Advil, Motrin), naproxen (Aleve), and ketoprofen. Advise patients to consult their doctor before combining fluvoxamine with NSAIDs or blood-thinning medications.

If the patient develops a rash or hives, or any other allergic-type reaction, the physician should be notified immediately.

Patients should not drink alcohol while taking this medication. If they smoke, they should tell the doctor before starting fluvoxamine therapy, as their dosage may need adjustment.

Possible food and drug interactions when taking this medication

See the entry for fluvoxamine on page 327.

Special information about pregnancy and breastfeeding

The effects of fluvoxamine in pregnancy have not been adequately studied. Patients who are pregnant or plan to become pregnant should consult their doctor immediately.

Fluvoxamine passes into breast milk and may cause serious reactions in a nursing baby. If this medication is essential to the mother's health, her doctor may advise her to discontinue breastfeeding until treatment with fluvoxamine is finished.

Recommended dosage

ADULTS

The usual starting dose is one 50-milligram tablet taken at bedtime. The doctor may increase the dose, depending on response. The maximum daily dose is 300 milligrams. If the patient takes more than 100 milligrams a day, the doctor will divide the total amount into 2 doses; if the doses are not equal, the larger dose is taken at bedtime.

CHILDREN

For children aged 8 to 17, the recommended starting dose is 25 milligrams taken at bedtime. The dose may be increased to a maximum of 200 milligrams daily for children under 11, and 300 milligrams for children aged 11 to 17. Larger daily dosages are divided in two, as for adults.

OLDER ADULTS

Older adults and people with liver problems may need a reduced dosage.

Overdosage

An overdose of fluvoxamine can be fatal. If an overdose is suspected, seek medical help immediately.

- *Symptoms of fluvoxamine overdose may include:*
  Coma, breathing difficulties, sleepiness, rapid heartbeat, nausea, vomiting

Other possible symptoms include convulsions, tremor, diarrhea, exaggerated reflexes, and slow or irregular heartbeat. After recovery, some overdose victims have been left with kidney complications, bowel damage, an unsteady gait, or dilated pupils.

FOCALIN
Dexmethylphenidate hydrochloride
Other brand name: Focalin XR

Why is this drug prescribed?
Focalin is a mild central nervous system stimulant used to treat attention deficit hyperactivity disorder (ADHD) in children. The drug is a modified version of Ritalin (a common medication for attention disorders) and contains only the most active component of Ritalin. Because of this special formulation, the usual dose of Focalin is half the amount of the Ritalin dose. Focalin should be given as part of a total treatment program that includes psychological, educational, and social measures. Focalin XR is the extended-release form of Focalin. Like Focalin, Focalin XR is used for the treatment of ADHD.

Most important fact about this drug
Excessive doses of Focalin over a long period of time can produce addiction. It is also possible to develop tolerance to the drug, so that larger doses are needed to produce the original effect. Because of these dangers, the doctor should be consulted before making any change in dosage, and the drug should be withdrawn only under a doctor's supervision.

There have been reports of sudden death in patients who have heart problems or heart defects, stroke and heart attack in adults, and increased blood pressure and heart rate with use of Focalin, Focalin XR, and other stimulant medicines. The doctor should be alerted right away if a child has any signs of heart problems such as chest pain, shortness of breath, or fainting while taking Focalin or Focalin XR.

Psychiatric problems have also been reported with the use of Focalin, Focalin XR, and other stimulant medicines. All patients should be watched for new or worse behavior or thought problems, new or worse bipolar illness, and new or worse aggressive behavior or hostility. Children and teenagers have been reported to sometimes develop new psychotic symptoms or new manic symptoms during treatment with Focalin, Focalin XR, and other stimulant medicines.

How should this medication be taken?
Focalin can be taken with or without food. The drug is usually taken twice a day, at least 4 hours apart, but the doctor may adjust the schedule depending on the child's response.

Focalin XR should be taken exactly as prescribed by the doctor. The medication should be taken once each day in the morning. Focalin XR can be taken with or without food, but taking the medicine with food slows the time it will take to start working. Focalin XR capsules should be swallowed whole with water or other liquids. The capsules or beads in the capsules should not be chewed, crushed, or divided. If a child cannot swallow the capsule, it can be opened and sprinkled over a spoonful of applesauce, which should then be swallowed right away without chewing.

• *Missed dose...*
  The dose should be given to the child as soon as it's remembered. If it is almost time for the next dose, the missed dose should be skipped and the child should return to the regular schedule. Doses should never be doubled.

• *Storage instructions...*
  Like all drugs, this one should be kept out of reach of children. It should be stored below 86 degrees Fahrenheit in a tightly closed, light-resistant container. It should not be stored in hot, damp, or humid places.

What side effects may occur?

Side effects cannot be predicted. If any develop or change in intensity, the caregiver should inform the child's doctor as soon as possible.

• *Side effects of Focalin may include:*
  Fever, insomnia, loss of appetite, nausea, nervousness, and stomach pain

• *Side effects of Focalin XR may include:*
  Anxiety, decreased appetite, dizziness, dry mouth, headache, nervousness, trouble sleeping, upset stomach

The most common side effects reported for drugs that are similar to Focalin (including Ritalin) are nervousness and the inability to fall asleep or stay asleep. In children, loss of appetite, stomach pain, weight loss during long-term treatment, inability to fall asleep or stay asleep, and abnormally fast heartbeat are the more common side effects.

Why should this drug not be prescribed?

Focalin should not be used by people who suffer from anxiety, tension, and agitation, since the drug may aggravate these symptoms.

If Focalin, or similar drugs such as Ritalin, cause an allergic reaction, the drug should be avoided. It should not be taken by anyone with the eye condition known as glaucoma. It should also be avoided by anyone who suffers from motion tics (repeated, uncontrollable twitches) or verbal tics (uncontrollable repetition of words or sounds), or someone who suffers from, or has a family history of, Tourette's syndrome (severe and multiple tics).

Focalin should not be taken with drugs classified as monoamine oxidase (MAO) inhibitors, such as the antidepressants Nardil and Parnate, or within 14 days of stopping this type of medication.

Special warnings about this medication

The doctor will do a complete history and evaluation before prescribing Focalin. It is important to remember that the drug is only part of the over-all management of ADHD, and that the doctor should also recommend counseling or other therapy.

There is no information about the safety and effectiveness of long-term Focalin treatment in children. However, suppression of growth has been seen with the long-term use of stimulants, so it's important to watch the child carefully while he or she is taking this drug. If the child is not growing or gaining weight as expected, the doctor may have to stop Focalin treatment. This drug should not be given to children under 6 years of age; safety and effectiveness in this age group have not been established.

Blood pressure should be monitored in anyone taking Focalin, especially those with high blood pressure or abnormal heart rate or rhythm. Caution is also advised in those with heart or thyroid problems.

The doctor should be alerted if the child develops blurred vision while taking Focalin; some people have reported visual disturbances while taking stimulants similar to this drug.

The use of Focalin by anyone with a seizure disorder or psychosis is not recommended. Caution is also advisable for anyone with a history of emotional instability or substance abuse, due to the danger of addiction. Focalin should not be used for the prevention or treatment of normal fatigue, nor should it be used for the treatment of severe depression.

Focalin should not be shared with anyone else, and the child should be given only the number of tablets prescribed by the doctor. Caregivers should keep track of the number of tablets in a bottle so they can tell if any are missing. Incorrect use of Focalin can lead to dependence. The doctor should be consulted immediately if the drug is being used in more than the prescribed amount.

The doctor should be alerted if the patient or child takes drugs classi-fied as monoamine oxidase (MAO) inhibitors, seizure medicines, blood thinner medicines, blood pressure medicines, antacids, or cold or allergy medicines that contain decongestants.

Possible food and drug interactions when taking this medication

See the entry for the generic name dexmethylphenidate on page 312.

Special information about pregnancy and breastfeeding

The effects of Focalin during pregnancy have not been adequately studied. Caregivers should tell the doctor immediately if the patient becomes preg-nant. Focalin should be used during pregnancy only if clearly needed.

It is not known whether Focalin appears in breast milk. Caution is advised if the patient is nursing a baby.

Recommended dosage

FOCALIN

For patients who are not currently taking Ritalin, the usual starting dose is 5 milligrams a day. For those who are switching from Ritalin, the starting Focalin dose is half the amount of the Ritalin dose. In either case, the total daily dose of Focalin should be divided into 2 doses taken at least 4 hours apart.

Depending on the response, the doctor may increase the dose by 2.5 to 5 milligrams a day, up to a maximum daily dose of 20 milligrams (10 milligrams twice a day). Increases are usually made at weekly intervals.

FOCALIN XR

For patients who are not currently taking Ritalin, the usual starting dose is 5 milligrams a day for pediatric patients and 10 milligrams a day for adult patients. For those who are switching from Ritalin, the starting Focalin dose is half the amount of the Ritalin dose. Patients currently using Focalin may be switched to the same daily dose of Focalin XR. The maximum recommended daily dose is 20 milligrams a day for pediatric and adult patients.

Depending on the response, the doctor may increase the dose in 5-milligram increments up to a maximum daily dose of 20 milligrams for pediatric patients, and in increments of 10 milligrams up to a maximum of 20 milligrams a day for adult patients. Increases are usually made at weekly intervals.

Overdosage

If an overdose is suspected, seek medical attention immediately.

- *Symptoms of Focalin overdose may include:*
  Abnormal reflexes, agitation, confusion, convulsions (may be followed by coma), delirium, dryness of mucous membranes, enlarged pupils, exaggerated feeling of elation, extremely elevated body temperature, flushing, hallucinations, headache, high blood pressure, irregular or rapid heartbeat, muscle twitching, palpitations, sweating, tremors, vomiting

Galantamine *See Razadyne, page 184*

GEODON
Ziprasidone hydrochloride

Why is this drug prescribed?

Geodon is used in the treatment of schizophrenia and the manic episodes of bipolar disorder. Researchers believe that it works by opposing the action of serotonin and dopamine, two of the brain's major chemical messengers. Because of its potentially serious side effects, Geodon is typically prescribed only after other medications have proved inadequate. An intramuscular injection is available for use in agitated patients.

Most important fact about this drug

In some people with heart problems or a slow heartbeat, Geodon can cause serious and potentially fatal heartbeat irregularities. The chance of a problem is greater if the patient is taking a water pill (diuretic) or a medication that prolongs a part of the heartbeat known as the QT interval. Many of the drugs prescribed for heartbeat irregularities prolong the QT interval and should never be combined with Geodon. Other drugs to avoid when taking Geodon include Anzemet, Avelox, chlorpromazine, halofantrine hydrochloride, Inapsine, Lariam, thioridazine, Nebupent, Orap, levomethadyl acetate hydrochloride, Pentam, probucol, Prograf, gatifloxacin, Trisenox, and sparfloxacin. Patients should check with their doctor before combining Geodon with any drug they're unsure of.

How should this medication be taken?

Geodon capsules should be taken twice a day with food.

- *Missed dose...*
  Generally, the forgotten dose should be taken as soon as remembered. However, if it is almost time for the next dose, patients should skip the dose they missed and go back to their regular schedule. Doses should never be doubled.

- *Storage instructions...*
  Geodon should be stored at room temperature.

What side effects may occur?

Side effects cannot be predicted. If any develop or change in intensity, patients should inform their doctor as soon as possible.

- *Side effects may include:*
  Accidental injury, anorexia, cold symptoms, constipation, cough, diarrhea, dizziness, drowsiness, dry mouth, energy loss, headache, indigestion, involuntary muscle contractions, muscle aches, muscle tightness, nausea, rapid heartbeat, rash, skin fungus, stuffy and runny nose, twitching, upper respiratory infection, vision problems, vomiting, weakness

Why should this drug not be prescribed?

Geodon cannot be taken by anyone who has the heartbeat irregularity known as QT prolongation, has had a recent heart attack, or suffers from heart failure. This drug should also be avoided if it causes an allergic reaction.

Special warnings about this medication

Remember that Geodon can cause dangerous—even fatal—heartbeat irregularities. Warning signs include dizziness, palpitations, and fainting. The doctor should be consulted immediately if any of these symptoms develop.

Particularly during the first few days of therapy, Geodon can cause low blood pressure, with accompanying dizziness, fainting, and rapid heartbeat. The doctor should be notified of any of these side effects. To minimize such problems, the doctor will increase the dose gradually. If a patient is prone to low blood pressure, takes blood pressure medicine, becomes dehydrated, or has heart disease or poor circulation in the brain, Geodon should be used with caution.

Geodon may cause drowsiness and can impair judgment, thinking, and motor skills. Patients should use caution while driving and should avoid operating potentially dangerous machinery until they know how this drug affects them.

Antipsychotic drugs such as Geodon are associated with an increased risk of developing high blood sugar, which on rare occasions has led to coma or death. Patients should see their doctor right away if they develop signs of high blood sugar, including dry mouth, thirst, increased urination, and tiredness. Patients who have diabetes or have a high risk of developing it should see their doctor regularly for blood sugar testing.

While taking Geodon, some patients with bipolar disorder reported having anxiety, restlessness, depression, dizziness, muscle twitching, rashes, and vomiting. The patient should contact their doctor immediately if they develop these symptoms.

Animal studies suggest that Geodon may increase the risk of breast cancer, although human studies have not confirmed such a risk. Advise patients with a history of breast cancer to see their doctor regularly for checkups.

Geodon poses a very slight risk of seizures, especially if a patient is over age 65, has a history of seizures, or has Alzheimer's disease.

Drugs such as Geodon sometimes cause a condition called neuroleptic malignant syndrome. Symptoms include high fever, muscle rigidity, irregular pulse or blood pressure, rapid heartbeat, excessive perspiration, and changes in heart rhythm. If these symptoms appear, the doctor should be informed immediately. The patient will need to stop taking Geodon while the condition is under treatment.

There also is the risk of developing tardive dyskinesia, a condition marked by slow, rhythmical, involuntary movements. This problem is more likely to occur in mature adults, especially older women. When it does, use of Geodon is usually stopped.

Geodon can suppress the cough reflex, making it difficult to clear the airway. Some people taking Geodon also develop a rash. If this happens, the doctor should be informed. If the rash doesn't clear up with treatment, the drug may have to be discontinued.

Other antipsychotic medications have been known to interfere with the body's temperature-regulating mechanism, causing the body to overheat. Although this problem has not occurred with Geodon, caution is still advisable. Patients should avoid exposure to extreme heat, strenuous exercise, and dehydration. There also is a remote chance that this medication may cause abnormal, prolonged, and painful erections.

Possible food and drug interactions when taking this medication
See the entry for the generic name ziprasidone on page 422.

Special information about pregnancy and breastfeeding
Geodon has caused fetal harm when tested in animals. It should be taken during pregnancy only if the benefits outweigh the potential risk. Patients should notify their doctor as soon as they become pregnant or plan to become pregnant.

Although it is not known whether Geodon appears in breast milk, breast-feeding is not recommended.

Recommended dosage
ADULTS

Schizophrenia
The usual starting dose is 20 milligrams twice a day. If needed, the dosage may be increased at several-week intervals up to a maximum of 80 milligrams twice a day.

Acute Manic Episodes Associated with Bipolar Disorder
The usual starting dose is 40 milligrams twice a day with food. On the second day of treatment, the doctor will increase the dose to 60 or 80 milligrams twice a day. For maintenance treatment, the dosage range is usually 40 to 80 milligrams twice a day.

Overdosage
Any medication taken in excess can have serious consequences. If an overdose is suspected, seek medical help immediately.

- *Symptoms of Geodon overdose may include:*
  Anxiety, drowsiness, high blood pressure, slurred speech, tremors

---

HALCION
Triazolam

Why is this drug prescribed?
Halcion is used for short-term treatment of insomnia. It is a member of the benzodiazepine class of drugs, many of which are used as tranquilizers.

Most important fact about this drug

Sleep problems are usually temporary, requiring treatment for only a short time, usually 1 or 2 days and no more than 1 to 2 weeks. Insomnia that lasts longer than this may be a sign of another medical problem. If patients find they need this medicine for more than 7 to 10 days, they should check with their doctor.

How should this medication be taken?

This medication must be taken exactly as directed. It is important to never take more than the doctor has prescribed.

- *Missed dose...*
  Halcion should be taken only as needed.

- *Storage instructions...*
  This medication should be kept in the container it came in, tightly closed, and out of reach of children. It should be stored at room temperature.

What side effects may occur?

Side effects cannot be predicted. If any develop or change in intensity, patients should inform their doctor as soon as possible.

- *Side effects may include:*
  Coordination problems, dizziness, drowsiness, headache, light-headedness, nausea/vomiting, nervousness

Why should this drug not be prescribed?

Halcion should not be taken during pregnancy. Patients should also avoid it if they have had an allergic reaction to it or to other benzodiazepine drugs such as Valium. It should never be combined with the antifungal medications Nizoral or Sporanox, or the antidepressant nefazodone hydrochloride.

Special warnings about this medication

When Halcion is used every night for more than a few weeks, it loses its effectiveness. This is known as tolerance. Also, it can cause dependence, especially when it is used regularly for longer than a few weeks or at high doses.

Abrupt discontinuation of Halcion should be avoided, since it has been associated with withdrawal symptoms (convulsions, cramps, tremor, vomiting, sweating, feeling ill, perceptual problems, and insomnia). A gradual dosage tapering schedule is usually recommended for patients taking more than the lowest dose of Halcion for longer than a few weeks. The usual treatment period is 7 to 10 days.

If patients develop unusual and disturbing thoughts or behavior—including increased anxiety or depression—during treatment with Halcion, they should discuss them with their doctor immediately.

Traveler's amnesia has been reported by patients who took Halcion to induce sleep while traveling. To avoid this condition, patients should not take Halcion on an overnight airplane flight of less than 7 to 8 hours.

Some people suffer increased anxiety during the daytime while taking Halcion.

Because Halcion could have a carryover effect the next day, patients first starting therapy should use extreme care while doing anything that requires complete alertness, such as driving a car or operating machinery.

After discontinuing the drug, patients may experience rebound insomnia for the first 2 nights.

They should be aware that anterograde amnesia (forgetting events after an injury) has been associated with benzodiazepine drugs such as Halcion.

Halcion should be used with caution by anyone who has liver or kidney problems, lung problems, or a tendency to temporarily stop breathing while asleep.

Patients should avoid alcoholic beverages and grapefruit juice while taking Halcion.

Possible food and drug interactions when taking this medication

See the entry for the generic name triazolam on page 412.

Special information about pregnancy and breastfeeding

Since benzodiazepines have been associated with damage to the developing baby, women should not take Halcion if they are pregnant, think they may be pregnant, or are planning to become pregnant. Halcion must also be avoided while breastfeeding.

Recommended dosage

ADULTS

The usual dose is 0.25 milligrams before bedtime. The dose should never be more than 0.5 milligrams.

CHILDREN

Safety and effectiveness for children under the age of 18 have not been established.

OLDER ADULTS

To decrease the possibility of oversedation, dizziness, or impaired coordination, the usual starting dose is 0.125 milligrams. This may be increased to 0.25 milligrams if necessary.

Overdosage

Any medication taken in excess can have serious consequences. Severe overdosage of Halcion can be fatal. If an overdose is suspected, seek medical help immediately.

- *Symptoms of Halcion overdose may include:*
  Apnea (temporary cessation of breathing), coma, confusion, excessive sleepiness, problems in coordination, seizures, shallow or difficult breathing, slurred speech

---

HALOPERIDOL

Why is this drug prescribed?

Haloperidol is used to reduce the symptoms of mental disorders such as schizophrenia. It is also prescribed to control tics (uncontrolled muscle contractions of face, arms, or shoulders) and the unintended utterances that mark Tourette's syndrome.

It is used in the short-term treatment of children with severe behavior problems such as combative, explosive hyperexcitability. It is also prescribed for the short-term treatment of hyperactive children with conduct disorders marked by some or all of the following symptoms: impulsivity, difficulty sustaining attention, aggressivity, mood lability, and poor frustration tolerance. Haloperidol should be reserved for these two groups of children only after failure to respond to psychotherapy or medications other than antipsychotics.

Some doctors also prescribe haloperidol to relieve severe nausea and vomiting caused by cancer drugs, to treat drug problems such as LSD flashback and PCP intoxication, and to control symptoms of hemiballismus, a condition that causes involuntary writhing of one side of the body.

Most important fact about this drug

Haloperidol may cause tardive dyskinesia, a condition characterized by involuntary muscle spasms and twitches in the face and body. This condition can be permanent, and appears to be most common among the elderly, especially women.

How should this medication be taken?

Haloperidol may be taken with food or after eating. If taking haloperidol in a liquid concentrate form, patients will need to dilute it with milk or water.

Haloperidol should not be taken with coffee, tea, or other caffeinated beverages, or with alcohol.

Haloperidol causes dry mouth. Sucking on a hard candy or ice chips may help alleviate the problem.

• *Missed dose...*
The forgotten dose should be taken as soon as remembered. The rest of the doses for that day should follow at equally spaced intervals. Doses should never be doubled.

• *Storage instructions...*
Haloperidol should be stored away from heat, light, and moisture, in a tightly closed container. The liquid should not be frozen.

What side effects may occur?
Side effects cannot be predicted. If any develop or change in intensity, patients should inform their doctor as soon as possible.

• *Side effects may include:*
Breast development in men, breathing problems, cataracts, constipation, drowsiness, dry mouth, insomnia, involuntary muscle contractions, skin reactions, tardive dyskinesia (see "Most important fact about this drug"), tightening of the throat muscles, weight loss

Why should this drug not be prescribed?
Haloperidol should be avoided by anyone who has Parkinson's disease or is sensitive to or allergic to the drug.

Special warnings about this medication
Haloperidol should be used with caution by patients who have had or currently have breast cancer, a severe heart or circulatory disorder, chest pain, the eye condition known as glaucoma, seizures, or any drug allergies.

Temporary muscle spasms and twitches may occur if haloperidol is stopped abruptly. Patients need to follow the doctor's instructions closely when discontinuing the drug.

This drug may impair the ability to drive a car or operate potentially dangerous machinery. Patients should avoid any activities that require full alertness if they are unsure of their reaction to haloperidol.

Haloperidol may make the skin more sensitive to sunlight. Patients should use a sunscreen or wear protective clothing when spending time in the sun.

Patients should avoid exposure to extreme heat or cold. Haloperidol interferes with the body's temperature-regulating mechanism, so they could become overheated or suffer severe chills.

Extreme drowsiness and other potentially serious effects can result if haloperidol is combined with alcohol, narcotics, painkillers, sleeping medications, or other drugs that slow down the central nervous system.

Possible food and drug interactions when taking this medication
See the entry for haloperidol on page 334.

Special information about pregnancy and breastfeeding

The effects of haloperidol during pregnancy have not been adequately studied. Pregnant women should use haloperidol only if clearly needed. Patients should inform their doctor immediately if they are pregnant or plan to become pregnant. Haloperidol should not be used by women who are breastfeeding.

Recommended dosage

ADULTS

Moderate Symptoms

The usual dosage is 1 to 6 milligrams daily. This amount should be divided into 2 or 3 smaller doses.

Severe Symptoms

The usual dosage is 6 to 15 milligrams daily, divided into 2 or 3 smaller doses.

CHILDREN

Children younger than 3 years old should not take haloperidol. For children between the ages of 3 and 12, weighing approximately 33 to 88 pounds, doses should start at 0.5 milligram per day. The doctor will increase the dose if needed.

For Psychotic Disorders

The daily dose may range from 0.05 milligram to 0.15 milligram for every 2.2 pounds of body weight.

For Non-Psychotic Behavior Disorders and Tourette's Syndrome

The daily dose may range from 0.05 milligram to 0.075 milligram for every 2.2 pounds of body weight.

OLDER ADULTS

In general, older people take dosages of haloperidol in the lower ranges. Older adults (especially older women) may be more susceptible to tardive dyskinesia. Doses may range from 1 to 6 milligrams daily.

Overdosage

Any medication taken in excess can have serious consequences. If an overdose is suspected, seek medical help immediately.

* *Symptoms of haloperidol overdose may include:*
  Catatonic (unresponsive) state, coma, decreased breathing, low blood pressure, rigid muscles, sedation, tremor, weakness

Hydroxyzine *See Vistaril, page 246*

Imipramine *See Tofranil, page 231*

INVEGA
Paliperidone

Why is this drug prescribed?
Invega is used to treat schizophrenia. It is thought to work by muting the impact of dopamine and serotonin, two of the brain's key chemical messengers.

Most important fact about this drug
Invega may cause tardive dyskinesia, a condition marked by involuntary muscle spasms and twitches in the face and body. This condition can become permanent and is most common among older people, especially women. Patients should see their doctor immediately if they begin to have any involuntary movements. They may need to discontinue Invega therapy.

In addition, elderly patients with dementia who are treated with antipsychotic drugs such as Invega have an increased risk of stroke and death. Invega is not approved to treat dementia-related psychosis.

How should this medication be taken?
Invega should be taken once a day in the morning. It can be taken with or without food.

Patients should swallow the tablets whole with water or other liquid. The tablets should not be chewed, divided, or crushed. Because the tablet shell passes through the body, patients may see it in their stool; this is normal and no cause for alarm.

- *Missed dose...*
  Generally, forgotten doses should be taken as soon as remembered. However, if it is almost time for the next dose, patients should skip the one they missed and return to their regular schedule. Doses should never be doubled.

- *Storage instructions...*
  Store at room temperature and protect from moisture.

What side effects may occur?
Side effects cannot be anticipated. If any develop or change in intensity, patients should inform their doctor as soon as possible.

- *Side effects may include:*
  Anxiety, dizziness, headache, involuntary movements, rapid heartbeat, restlessness, sleepiness, tremors and muscle stiffness, upset stomach and nausea

Why should this drug not be prescribed?
Invega cannot be taken by anyone who is sensitive to or has ever had an allergic reaction to it or to Risperdal (risperidone), a similar antipsychotic drug.

Special warnings about this medication

Invega should be used with caution in patients who have liver, kidney, or heart disease; seizures; diabetes or increased blood sugar; or problems with their esophagus, stomach, or small or large intestine.

Invega may cause a change in heart rhythm. Because this effect is potentially serious, patients should alert their doctors about any current or past heart problems.

Invega may cause neuroleptic malignant syndrome, a serious nervous system problem marked by muscle stiffness and rigidity, fast heartbeat or irregular pulse, increased sweating, high fever, and high or low blood pressure. Unchecked, this condition can prove fatal. Patients should call their doctor immediately if they notice any of these symptoms.

Be aware that Invega may mask signs and symptoms of drug overdose and of conditions such as intestinal obstruction, brain tumor, and Reye's syndrome (a dangerous neurological condition that may follow viral infections, usually occurring in children).

Certain antipsychotic drugs similar to Invega are associated with an increased risk of developing high blood sugar, which on rare occasions has led to coma or death. Patients should see their doctor right away if they develop signs of high blood sugar, including dry mouth, thirst, increased urination, and tiredness. Patients who have diabetes or have a high risk of developing it should see their doctor regularly for blood sugar testing.

Patients at high risk of suicide attempts should be prescribed the lowest dose possible to reduce the risk of intentional overdose.

This drug may impair the ability to drive a car or operate potentially dangerous machinery. Patients should avoid participating in any activities that require full alertness until they are sure of how this drug affects them.

Invega can interfere with the body's temperature regulation, leading to overheating and dehydration. Caution patients to be careful when exercising or doing activities in the heat.

Invega can cause orthostatic hypotension (low blood pressure when rising to a standing position) with dizziness, rapid heartbeat, and fainting, especially at the start of therapy. This problem should be reported to the doctor if it develops. The dosage can be adjusted to reduce the symptoms.

Invega has not been studied in children less than 18 years old.

Invega is chemically related to Risperdal (risperidone). Using the two drugs together could potentially increase the risk of side effects.

Patients should avoid alcohol while taking Invega.

Possible food and drug interactions when taking this medication

See the entry for the generic name paliperidone on page 366.

Special information about pregnancy and breastfeeding

The effects of Invega during pregnancy have not been adequately studied. The drug is recommended only if its benefits are thought to outweigh the potential risk to the baby. If a patient is pregnant or planning to become pregnant, she should inform her doctor immediately.

Women taking Invega should not breastfeed, since the drug can show up in breast milk.

Recommended dosage

ADULTS

The recommended dosage is 6 milligrams once a day in the morning. Depending on the patient's response, the doctor may adjust the dose up or down within the usual dosage range of 3 to 12 milligrams a day. Patients with kidney problems will need a reduced dosage (a maximum of 6 milligrams a day for mild impairment and 3 milligrams a day for moderate to severe impairment).

Overdosage

Any medication taken in excess can have serious consequences. If an overdose is suspected, seek medical attention immediately.

- *Symptoms of Invega overdose may include:*
  Drowsiness, low blood pressure, movement or muscle problems (such as tremors, trouble walking, or muscle stiffness), rapid heartbeat, sedation

---

KLONOPIN

Clonazepam

Why is this drug prescribed?

Klonopin has two major uses. In the mental health field it is prescribed for panic disorder. In neurology it is used, alone or along with other medications, to treat convulsive disorders such as epilepsy. Klonopin belongs to the class of drugs known as benzodiazepines.

Most important fact about this drug

Klonopin works best when there is a constant amount in the bloodstream. It is important for patients to take their doses at regularly spaced intervals and to avoid missing any if possible.

How should this medication be taken?

Klonopin should be taken exactly as prescribed. If patients are taking it for panic disorder and find it makes them sleepy, the doctor may recommend a single dose at bedtime.

- *Missed dose...*
  If it is within an hour after the scheduled time, the dose should be taken as soon as remembered. If the dose is not remembered until later, the

patient should skip it and go back to the regular schedule. Doses should never be doubled.

- *Storage instructions...*
Klonopin should be stored at room temperature away from heat, light, and moisture.

What side effects may occur?
Side effects cannot be predicted. If any develop or change in intensity, patients should inform their doctor as soon as possible.

- *Side effects in panic disorder may include:*
Allergic reaction, constipation, coordination problems, depression, dizziness, fatigue, inflamed sinuses or nasal passages, flu, memory problems, menstrual problems, nervousness, reduced thinking ability, respiratory infection, sleepiness, speech problems, vaginal inflammation

- *Side effects in seizure disorders may include:*
Behavior problems, drowsiness, lack of muscular coordination. Klonopin can also cause aggressive behavior, agitation, anxiety, excitability, hostility, irritability, nervousness, nightmares, sleep disturbances, and vivid dreams.

- *Side effects due to rapid decrease in dose or abrupt withdrawal from Klonopin may include:*
Abdominal and muscle cramps, behavior disorders, convulsions, depressed feeling, hallucinations, restlessness, sleeping difficulties, tremors

Why should this drug not be prescribed?
This medication should be avoided by anyone who is sensitive to or has ever had an allergic reaction to it or to similar drugs, such as Librium and Valium. Klonopin also cannot be used in patients with severe liver disease or the eye condition known as acute narrow-angle glaucoma.

Special warnings about this medication
Klonopin makes some people drowsy or less alert. Patients should avoid driving, operating dangerous machinery, or participating in any hazardous activity that requires full mental alertness until they know how this drug affects them.

If a patient suffers from several types of seizures, this drug may increase the possibility of grand mal seizures (epilepsy). Patients should inform their doctor immediately if this occurs. The doctor may wish to prescribe an additional anticonvulsant drug or increase the dose of Klonopin.

Klonopin can be habit-forming and can lose its effectiveness as patients build up a tolerance to it. They may experience withdrawal symptoms—such as convulsions, hallucinations, tremor, and abdominal and muscle cramps—if they stop using this drug abruptly. Patients should discontinue or change their dose only in consultation with their doctor.

Klonopin slows the nervous system, and its effects may be intensified by alcohol. Patients should avoid alcohol while taking this medication.

Possible food and drug interactions when taking this medication

See the entry for the generic name clonazepam on page 308.

Special information about pregnancy and breastfeeding

Klonopin should be avoided if at all possible during the first 3 months of pregnancy; there is a risk of birth defects. When taken later in pregnancy, the drug can cause other problems, such as withdrawal symptoms in the newborn. Patients who are pregnant or plan to become pregnant should inform their doctor immediately.

Klonopin appears in breast milk and could affect a nursing infant. Mothers taking this drug should not breastfeed.

Recommended dosage

PANIC DISORDER

Adults: The starting dose is 0.25 milligrams twice a day. After 3 days, the doctor may increase the dose to 1 milligram daily. Some people need as much as 4 milligrams a day.

Children: For panic disorder, safety and effectiveness have not been established in children under age 18.

Older Adults: Klonopin tends to build up in the body if the kidneys are weak—a common problem among older adults. Higher doses of the drug also tend to cause more drowsiness and confusion in older patients. People over age 65 are therefore started on low doses of Klonopin and watched with extra care.

SEIZURE DISORDERS

Adults: The starting dose should be no more than 1.5 milligrams per day, divided into 3 doses. The doctor may increase the daily dosage by 0.5 to 1 milligram every 3 days until the patient's seizures are controlled or the side effects become too bothersome. The maximum daily dosage is 20 milligrams.

Children: The starting dose for infants and children up to 10 years old or up to 66 pounds should be 0.01 to 0.03 milligrams—no more than 0.05 milligrams—per 2.2 pounds (1 kilogram) of body weight daily. The daily dosage should be given in 2 or 3 smaller doses. The doctor may increase the dose by 0.25 to 0.5 milligram every 3 days until seizures are controlled or side effects become too bad. If the dose cannot be divided into 3 equal

doses, the largest dose should be given at bedtime. The maximum maintenance dose is 0.1 to 0.2 milligrams per 2.2 pounds (1 kilogram) daily.

Overdosage
Any medication taken in excess can have serious consequences. If an
overdose is suspected, seek medical attention immediately.

- *Symptoms of Klonopin overdose may include:*
  Coma, confusion, sleepiness, slowed reaction time

LAMICTAL
Lamotrigine
Other brand name: Lamictal CD

Why is this drug prescribed?
Lamictal is used to help prevent the manic and/or depressive phases of
bipolar disorder.

This drug is also prescribed to control partial seizures in people with
epilepsy and the epileptic condition known as Lennox-Gastaut syndrome.
Lamictal is used in combination with other antiepileptic drugs or as a
replacement for another medication such as Tegretol, Dilantin, phenobarbital, or Mysoline.

Most important fact about this drug
Lamictal may cause a rash during the first 2 to 8 weeks of therapy, particularly if the patient is also taking Depakene or Depakote. If this happens, the doctor should be notified immediately. The rash could become
severe and even dangerous, particularly in children. Signs of a more serious reaction include hives, fever, swollen lymph glands, painful sores in
the mouth or around the eyes, or swelling of the lips or tongue. A slight
possibility of this problem remains for up to 6 months.

How should this medication be taken?
Instruct patients to take Lamictal exactly as instructed by their doctor.
Taking more than the prescribed amount can increase the risk of developing a serious rash. Patients should not stop taking this medication without first discussing it with their doctor. An abrupt halt could increase the
risk of seizures and other adverse effects.

Lamictal Chewable Dispersible (CD) tablets may be swallowed whole,
chewed, or dissolved in liquid. When chewing the tablets, patients should
drink a small amount of water or diluted fruit juice to aid in swallowing.
When dissolving the tablets, patients should add them to a small amount
of water or diluted fruit juice (about 1 teaspoonful), and wait 1 minute
until the tablets are completely dissolved. They should swirl and drink the
solution immediately. Patients should not try to cut the dose by drinking
only part of the solution.

- *Missed dose...*
  Patients should take the forgotten dose as soon as they remember. If it is almost time for their next dose, patients should skip the dose they missed and go back to their regular schedule. Patients should never double the dose.

- *Storage instructions...*
  Lamictal should be stored in a tightly closed container at room temperature. It should be kept dry and protected from light.

What side effects may occur?

Side effects cannot be predicted. If any develop or change in intensity, patients should inform their doctor as soon as possible.

- *Side effects may include:*
  Abdominal pain, back pain, blurred vision, constipation, dizziness, double vision, dry mouth, fatigue, headache, increased cough, insomnia, nausea, rash (sometimes serious), runny nose, sleepiness, sore throat, uncoordinated movements, vomiting

- *Additional side effects in children may include:*
  Bronchitis, convulsions, ear problems, eczema, facial swelling, hemorrhage, infection, indigestion, light sensitivity, lymph node problems, nervousness, penis disorder, sinus infection, swelling, tooth problems, urinary tract infection, vertigo, vision problems

Why should this drug not be prescribed?

This medication should be avoided by anyone who is sensitive to or has ever had an allergic reaction to Lamictal.

Special warnings about this medication

Remind patients to be alert for the development of any type of rash, especially during the first 2 to 8 weeks of treatment. They should contact their doctor immediately at the first sign of an allergic reaction, including fever, swollen lymph nodes, or rash.

Lamictal may cause some people to become drowsy, dizzy, or less alert. Patients should not drive or operate dangerous machinery or participate in any hazardous activity until they know how the drug affects them.

Before starting Lamictal therapy, patients should tell their doctor about any history of medical problems. Patients with heart problems or kidney or liver disease should use this drug with caution.

Lamictal may cause vision problems. If any develop, patients should notify their doctor immediately.

Patients with bipolar disorder should be aware that Lamictal should not be used to stop an episode of mania or depression once it has started. Patients who are taking Lamictal for seizure control should tell their doctor right away if their seizures get worse.

There are no clinical studies to prove the safety and effectiveness of Lamictal for treating bipolar disorder in children less than 18 years old.

Possible food and drug interactions when taking this medication

See the entry for the generic name lamotrigine on page 339.

Special information about pregnancy and breastfeeding

The effects of Lamictal during pregnancy have not been adequately studied. Patients who are pregnant or plan to become pregnant should tell their doctor immediately. Lamictal should be used during pregnancy only if clearly needed.

This medication appears in breast milk. Because the effects of Lamictal on an infant exposed to this medication are unknown, breastfeeding is not recommended during Lamictal therapy.

Recommended dosage

ADULTS

For Bipolar Disorder

Lamictal NOT combined with Depakene, Depakote, Tegretol, Dilantin, Phenobarbital, or Mysoline

One 25-milligram dose of Lamictal per day for weeks 1 and 2, then 50 milligrams per day for weeks 3 and 4, then 100 milligrams a day for week 5. After that, the doctor will have the patient take a total of 200 milligrams a day.

Lamictal combined with Depakene or Depakote

One 25-milligram dose of Lamictal every other day for weeks 1 and 2, then 25 milligrams once a day for weeks 3 and 4, then 50 milligrams a day for week 5. After that, the doctor will have the patient take a total of 100 milligrams a day.

Lamictal combined with Tegretol, Dilantin, Phenobarbital, or Mysoline

One 50-milligram dose of Lamictal per day for weeks 1 and 2, then 50 milligrams twice a day for weeks 3 and 4, then 100 milligrams twice a day for week 5. After that, the doctor will have the patient take a total of 300 to 400 milligrams a day, divided into 2 doses.

For Seizures

Lamictal combined with Tegretol, Dilantin, Phenobarbital, or Mysoline

One 50-milligram dose per day for 2 weeks, then two 50-milligram doses per day for 2 weeks. After that, the doctor may have the patient take a total of 300 to 500 milligrams a day, divided into 2 doses.

Lamictal combined with Depakene or Depakote, whether taken alone or with any of the previously mentioned medications
One 25-milligram dose every other day for 2 weeks, then 25 milligrams once a day for 2 weeks. After that, the doctor will prescribe a total of 100 to 400 milligrams a day, taken in 1 or 2 doses.

Lamictal as a replacement for Tegretol, Dilantin, Phenobarbital, or Mysoline, or Valproate
While patients continue to take the other drug, the doctor will add Lamictal, starting at a dose of 50 milligrams per day, then gradually increase the daily dose. Once the patient has reached a dosage of 500 milligrams per day divided into 2 doses, the doctor will then begin to gradually reduce the dosage of the other drug until, after 4 weeks, it has been completely eliminated. If the patient is switching from valproate, the doctor will follow a slightly different regimen.

The doctor will adjust the patient's dose accordingly when treatment with any of the medications is stopped, or when patients start or stop taking oral contraceptives or psychiatric drugs.

Due to the lack of clinical studies, Lamictal should be used cautiously in people with liver or kidney problems. The doctor may have these patients take less than the usual dose and raise it based on their body's response.

CHILDREN 2 YEARS OF AGE AND OLDER

For Bipolar Disorder
Due to the lack of clinical studies, Lamictal is not recommended for treating bipolar disorder in children under 18 years old.

For Seizures
Lamictal can be added to other epilepsy drugs prescribed for children under 16 who have partial seizures or a serious form of epilepsy known as Lennox-Gastaut syndrome. Doses for children under 12 are based on the child's weight. Children 12 and older receive the adult dose. Doses are increased gradually from a low starting level to limit the risk of severe rash. Lamictal is not used as a replacement drug for children under 16.

Overdosage
A massive overdose of Lamictal can be fatal. If an overdose is suspected, seek medical treatment immediately.

* *Symptoms of Lamictal overdose may include:*
  Coma, decreased level of consciousness, delayed heartbeat, increased seizures, lack of coordination, rolling eyeballs

Lamotrigine *See Lamictal, page 105*

LEXAPRO
Escitalopram oxalate

Why is this drug prescribed?
Lexapro is prescribed for major depression and generalized anxiety disorder. The drug is a close chemical cousin of the antidepressant medication Celexa.

Lexapro belongs to the class of drugs known as selective serotonin reuptake inhibitors (SSRIs). Serotonin is one of the chemical messengers believed to govern moods. Ordinarily, it is quickly reabsorbed after its release at the junctures between nerves. Reuptake inhibitors such as Lexapro slow this process, thereby boosting the levels of serotonin available in the brain.

Most important fact about this drug
Patients should be careful to avoid taking Lexapro for 2 weeks before or after taking any drug classified as an MAO inhibitor. Drugs in this category include the antidepressants Nardil and Parnate. Combining these drugs with Lexapro can cause serious and even fatal reactions marked by such symptoms as fever, rigidity, twitching, and agitation leading to delirium and coma.

How should this medication be taken?
Patients need to take Lexapro exactly as prescribed, even after they begin to feel better. Although improvement usually begins within 1 to 4 weeks, treatment typically continues for several months. Lexapro is available in tablet and liquid form and can be taken with or without food.

- *Missed dose...*
  The forgotten dose should be taken as soon as it's remembered. However, if it is almost time for the next dose, patients should skip the dose they missed and return to their regular schedule. Doses should never be doubled.

- *Storage instructions...*
  Lexapro should be stored at room temperature.

What side effects may occur?
Side effects cannot be anticipated. If any develop or change in intensity, patients should inform their doctor as soon as possible.

- *Side effects may include:*
  Constipation, decreased appetite, decreased sex drive, diarrhea, dizziness, dry mouth, ejaculation disorder, fatigue, flu-like symptoms, headache, impotence, indigestion, insomnia, nausea, runny nose, sinusitis, sleepiness, sweating

A variety of very rare side effects have also been reported. Patients should check with their doctor if they develop any new or unusual symptoms.

Why should this drug not be prescribed?

Patients should not use Lexapro if it causes an allergic reaction, or if they've ever had an allergic reaction to the related drug Celexa. Also remember that Lexapro, like all serotonin-boosting drugs, must never be combined with an MAO inhibitor such as Nardil or Parnate.

Special warnings about this medication

In clinical studies, antidepressants increased the risk of suicidal thinking and behavior in children and adolescents with depression and other psychiatric disorders. Anyone considering the use of Lexapro, or any other antidepressant in a child or adolescent, must balance the risk with the clinical need. Lexapro has not been studied in children or adolescents and is not approved for treating anyone less than 18 years old.

Additionally, the progression of major depression is associated with a worsening of symptoms and/or the emergence of suicidal thinking or behavior in both adults and children, whether or not they are taking antidepressants. Patients and caregivers should watch for any change in symptoms or any new symptoms that appear suddenly—especially agitation, anxiety, hostility, panic, restlessness, extreme hyperactivity, and suicidal thinking or behavior—and report them to the doctor immediately. Be especially observant at the beginning of treatment or whenever there is a change in dose.

Lexapro may cause patients to become drowsy, sleepy, or less alert. Until they know how the drug affects them, patients should use caution when driving a car or operating other hazardous machinery.

In rare cases, Lexapro can trigger mania (unreasonably high spirits and excess energy). If a patient has ever had this problem, it's important to make sure the doctor is aware of it.

It's also important to alert the doctor if a patient has liver problems or severe kidney disease. The dosage of Lexapro may need adjustment.

Convulsions have been reported during Lexapro treatment. Patients with a history of seizures should use this drug with caution.

Serotonin-boosting antidepressants could potentially cause stomach bleeding, especially in older patients or those taking nonsteroidal anti-inflammatory drugs (NSAIDs) such as aspirin, ibuprofen (Advil, Motrin), naproxen (Aleve), and ketoprofen. Advise patients to consult their doctor before combining Lexapro with NSAIDs or blood-thinning medications.

Patients should never stop taking Lexapro without consulting the doctor. An abrupt decrease in dose could cause withdrawal symptoms such as mood problems, lethargy, insomnia, and tingling sensations.

Patients should not use Lexapro if they are taking the related drug Celexa. In addition, Lexapro must never be combined with MAO inhibitors such as Nardil and Parnate.

Although Lexapro does not interact with alcohol, the manufacturer recommends avoiding alcoholic beverages.

Possible food and drug interactions when taking this medication

See the entry for the generic name escitalopram on page 319.

Special information about pregnancy and breastfeeding

There have been reports of newborns developing serious complications after exposure to Lexapro late in the third trimester. Patients who are pregnant or plan to become pregnant should inform their doctor immediately. Lexapro should be taken during pregnancy only if its benefits outweigh the potential risks.

Lexapro appears in breast milk and can affect a nursing infant. If a patient decides to breastfeed, Lexapro is not recommended.

Recommended dosage

ADULTS

The recommended dose of Lexapro tablets or oral solution is 10 milligrams once a day. If necessary, the doctor may increase the dose to 20 milligrams after a minimum of 1 week, but the higher dose is not recommended for most older adults and people with liver problems.

Overdosage

A massive overdose of Lexapro—especially when combined with alcohol or other drugs—can be fatal. If an overdose is suspected, seek emergency treatment immediately.

- *Symptoms of Lexapro overdose may include:*
  Dizziness, drowsiness, nausea, rapid heartbeat, seizures, sweating, tremors, vomiting

Rarely, an overdose may also cause memory loss, confusion, coma, breathing problems, muscle wasting, irregular heartbeat, and a bluish tinge to the skin.

LIBRIUM

Chlordiazepoxide

Why is this drug prescribed?

Librium is used in the treatment of anxiety disorders. It is also prescribed for short-term relief of the symptoms of anxiety, symptoms of withdrawal in acute alcoholism, and anxiety and apprehension before surgery. It belongs to a class of drugs known as benzodiazepines.

Most important fact about this drug

Librium is habit-forming and can lead to dependency. Warn patients that they could experience withdrawal symptoms if they stop taking the drug abruptly (see "What side effects may occur?"). They should discontinue or change their dose only on the advice of their doctor.

How should this medication be taken?
Instruct patients to take this medication exactly as prescribed.

* *Missed dose...*
  Patients should take the forgotten dose as soon as they remember if it is within an hour or so of the scheduled time. If they do not remember until later, they should skip the missed dose and go back to their regular schedule. Warn against taking 2 doses at once.

* *Storage instructions...*
  Librium should be stored away from heat, light, and moisture.

What side effects may occur?
Side effects cannot be predicted. If any develop or change in intensity, patients should inform their doctor as soon as possible.

* *Side effects may include:*
  Confusion, constipation, drowsiness, fainting, increased or decreased sex drive, liver problems, lack of muscle coordination, minor menstrual irregularities, nausea, skin rash or eruptions, swelling due to fluid retention, yellow eyes and skin

* *Side effects due to rapid decrease in dose or abrupt withdrawal from Librium may include:*
  Abdominal and muscle cramps, convulsions, exaggerated feeling of depression, sleeplessness, sweating, tremors, vomiting

Why should this drug not be prescribed?
This medication should be avoided by anyone who is sensitive to or has ever had an allergic reaction to Librium or similar tranquilizers.

Anxiety or tension related to everyday stress usually does not require treatment with Librium. Patients should discuss their symptoms thoroughly with the doctor.

Special warnings about this medication
Librium may cause patients to become drowsy or less alert. They should not drive or operate dangerous machinery or participate in any hazardous activity that requires full mental alertness until they know how they react to this drug.

Patients who are severely depressed or have suffered from severe depression should consult with their doctor before taking this medication. This drug may cause children to become less alert.

If Librium has been prescribed for a hyperactive, aggressive child, the doctor should be informed of contrary reactions such as excitement, stimulation, or acute rage.

Patients should check with their doctor before taking Librium if they are being treated for porphyria (a rare metabolic disorder) or kidney or liver disease.

Librium is a central nervous system depressant and may intensify the effects of alcohol or have an additive effect. Warn patients against drinking alcohol while taking this medication.

Possible food and drug interactions when taking this medication
See the entry for the generic name chlordiazepoxide on page 301.

Special information about pregnancy and breastfeeding
Women should not take Librium if they are pregnant or planning to become pregnant. There may be an increased risk of birth defects.

This drug may appear in breast milk and could affect a nursing infant. If Librium is essential to the patient's health, her doctor may advise her to discontinue breastfeeding until her treatment with the drug is finished.

Recommended dosage
ADULTS

Apprehension and Anxiety Before Surgery: On days preceding surgery, the usual dose is 5 to 10 milligrams, 3 or 4 times a day.

Mild or Moderate Anxiety: The usual dose is 5 or 10 milligrams, 3 or 4 times a day.

Severe Anxiety: The usual dose is 20 to 25 milligrams, 3 or 4 times a day.

Withdrawal Symptoms of Acute Alcoholism: The usual starting oral dose is 50 to 100 milligrams; the doctor will repeat this dose, up to a maximum of 300 milligrams per day, until agitation is controlled. The dose will then be reduced as much as possible.

CHILDREN

The usual dose for children 6 years of age and older is 5 milligrams, 2 to 4 times per day. Some children may need to take 10 milligrams, 2 or 3 times per day. The drug is not recommended for children under 6.

OLDER ADULTS

The doctor will limit the dose to the smallest effective amount in order to avoid oversedation or lack of coordination. The usual dose is 5 milligrams, 2 to 4 times per day.

Overdosage
Any medication taken in excess can cause symptoms of overdose. If an overdose is suspected, seek medical attention immediately.

• *Symptoms of Librium overdose may include:*
  Coma, confusion, sleepiness, slow reflexes

LIMBITROL
Amitriptyline hydrochloride with chlordiazepoxide
Other brand name: Limbitrol DS

Why is this drug prescribed?
Limbitrol is a combination of an antidepressant and an antianxiety drug. It is used in the treatment of moderate to severe depression associated with moderate to severe anxiety.

Most important fact about this drug
Limbitrol is habit-forming and can lead to dependency. Patients could experience withdrawal symptoms if they stop taking it abruptly (see "What side effects may occur?"). They should discontinue or change their dose only on the advice of their doctor.

How should this medication be taken?
It is important that this medication be taken exactly as prescribed.

- *Missed dose...*
  Patients should skip the missed dose and go back to their regular schedule. They should never take 2 doses at once.

- *Storage instructions...*
  Limbitrol should be stored away from heat, light, and moisture.

What side effects may occur?
Side effects cannot be predicted. If any develop or change in intensity, patients should inform their doctor as soon as possible.

- *Side effects may include:*
  Bloating, blurred vision, constipation, dizziness, drowsiness, dry mouth

- *Side effects due to rapid decrease in dose or abrupt withdrawal from Limbitrol may include:*
  Abdominal and muscle cramps, convulsions, exaggerated feeling of depression, headache, inability to fall asleep or stay asleep, nausea, restlessness, sweating, tremors, vague bodily discomfort, vomiting

Why should this drug not be prescribed?
Limbitrol should be avoided by anyone who is sensitive to or has ever had an allergic reaction to related drugs, such as benzodiazepine tranquilizers and tricyclic antidepressants.

Limbitrol should not be used by patients who have just had a heart attack.

Patients who are taking an antidepressant drug classified as an MAO inhibitor (Nardil, Parnate) should not take Limbitrol. MAO inhibitors are long-lasting. A minimum of 14 days should be allowed between stopping an MAO inhibitor and starting Limbitrol. Convulsions and death have occurred when the drugs were combined.

Special warnings about this medication

In clinical studies, antidepressants increased the risk of suicidal thinking and behavior in children and adolescents with depression and other psychiatric disorders. Anyone considering the use of Limbitrol, or any other antidepressant in a child or adolescent, must balance the risk with the clinical need. Limbitrol has not been studied in children less than 12 years old.

Additionally, the progression of major depression is associated with a worsening of symptoms and/or the emergence of suicidal thinking or behavior in both adults and children, whether or not they are taking antidepressants. Patients and caregivers should watch for any change in symptoms or any new symptoms that appear suddenly—especially agitation, anxiety, hostility, panic, restlessness, extreme hyperactivity, and suicidal thinking or behavior—and report them to the doctor immediately. Be especially observant at the beginning of treatment or whenever there is a change in dose.

Limbitrol may cause patients to become drowsy or less alert. They should not drive or participate in any hazardous activity that requires full mental alertness until they know how this drug affects them.

This drug, especially when given in high doses, can cause irregular heartbeat, an increase in heart rate, heart attack, or stroke. Patients who are being treated for a heart or circulatory disorder should consult their doctor before taking Limbitrol.

Patients who are severely depressed or have been treated for severe depression should check with their doctor before taking this medication.

They should also double check with the doctor before taking this medication if they are being treated for the eye condition known as angle-closure glaucoma or for inability to pass urine. The doctor should also be alerted if they have a thyroid condition or liver or kidney problems, or if they have ever had seizures.

Before elective surgery, the doctor will discontinue Limbitrol several days prior to the operation. Limbitrol should be used with caution in patients who are getting electroconvulsive therapy.

Limbitrol is a central nervous system depressant and may intensify the effects of alcohol. Patients should not drink alcohol while taking this medication.

Severe constipation may occur if Limbitrol is combined with spasm-quelling drugs such as Donnatal or Bentyl.

Possible food and drug interactions when taking this medication

See the entry for the generic names amitriptyline and chlordiazepoxide on pages 278 and 301.

Special information about pregnancy and breastfeeding
Women who are pregnant or plan to become pregnant should avoid Limbitrol. There is an increased risk of birth defects.

This drug may appear in breast milk and could affect a nursing infant. If this medication is essential to the patient's health, the doctor may advise her to discontinue breastfeeding until her treatment is finished.

Recommended dosage
ADULTS

Limbitrol Tablets
The usual starting dosage is a total of 3 or 4 tablets per day in several small doses. The larger portion of the daily dose may be taken at bedtime. A single bedtime dose may be sufficient.

Limbitrol DS (Double-strength)
The usual starting dosage is a total of 3 or 4 tablets per day divided into smaller doses. The doctor may increase the dose to 6 tablets per day or decrease it to 2 tablets per day, depending on response.

CHILDREN

Safety and effectiveness have not been established in children under 12 years old.

OLDER ADULTS

The doctor will prescribe the smallest amount possible in order to avoid side effects such as oversedation, confusion, and loss of muscle control.

Overdosage
Any medication taken in excess can have serious consequences. If an overdose is suspected, seek medical attention immediately.

- *Symptoms of Limbitrol overdose may include:*
  Abnormally fast heart rate, agitation, coma, confusion, congestive heart failure, convulsions, dilated pupils, disturbed concentration, drowsiness, exaggerated reflexes, hallucinations, high fever, irregular heartbeat, muscle rigidity, reduction of body temperature, severe low blood pressure, stupor, vomiting

Lisdexamfetamine *See Vyvanse, page 252*

LITHIUM CARBONATE
Brand names: Eskalith, Lithobid

Why is this drug prescribed?
Lithium is used to treat the manic episodes of bipolar disorder. Once the mania subsides, lithium treatment may be continued over the long term,

at a somewhat lower dosage, to prevent or reduce the intensity of future manic episodes.

Some doctors also prescribe lithium for premenstrual tension, eating disorders such as bulimia, certain movement disorders, and sexual addictions.

Most important fact about this drug

If the lithium dosage is too low, patients derive no benefit; if it is too high, they could suffer lithium poisoning. Patient and doctor must work together to find the correct dosage. Initially, this means frequent blood tests to find out how much of the drug is actually circulating in the patient's bloodstream. Later, the patient must stay alert for side effects.

Signs of lithium poisoning include vomiting, unsteady walking, diarrhea, drowsiness, tremor, and weakness. If any of these symptoms develop, the patient should stop taking the drug and call the doctor.

How should this medication be taken?

To avoid stomach upset, lithium should be taken immediately after meals or with food or milk.

It is unwise to change from one brand of lithium to another without consulting a doctor or pharmacist. The drug should be taken exactly as prescribed.

While taking lithium, patients should drink 10 to 12 glasses of water or fluid a day. To minimize the risk of harmful side effects, they should eat a balanced diet that includes some salt and lots of liquids. Patients who have been sweating a great deal or have had diarrhea should be sure to get extra liquids and salt.

Patients should keep in close touch with their doctor if they develop an infection with a fever. They may need to cut back on their Lithium dosage or even quit taking it temporarily.

Long-acting forms of lithium, such as Lithobid, should be swallowed whole. They should not be chewed, crushed, or broken.

- *Missed dose...*
  Patients need to check with the doctor; requirements vary for each individual. Doses should never be doubled.

- *Storage instructions...*
  Lithium should be stored at room temperature.

What side effects may occur?

The possibility of side effects varies with the level of lithium in the bloodstream. Patients should inform their doctor as soon as possible if they experience unfamiliar symptoms of any kind.

- *Side effects may include:*
  Discomfort, frequent urination, hand tremor, mild thirst, nausea

Why should this drug not be prescribed?

Although doctors are cautious under certain conditions, lithium may be prescribed for anyone.

Special warnings about this medication

Lithium may affect judgment or coordination. Patients should avoid driving, climbing, or performing hazardous tasks until they find out how this drug affects them.

Lithium should be used with extra caution in patients who have a heart or kidney problem, brain or spinal cord disease, or a weak, run-down, or dehydrated condition. It's important for patients to make sure the doctor is aware of any medical problems they may have, including diabetes, epilepsy, thyroid problems, Parkinson's disease, and difficulty urinating.

Patients should avoid activities that cause heavy sweating. They should also avoid drinking large amounts of coffee, tea, or cola, which can cause dehydration through increased urination. It is unwise for patients to make a major change in eating habits or to go on a weight loss diet without consulting the doctor. The loss of water and salt from the body could lead to lithium poisoning.

Possible food and drug interactions when taking this medication

See the entry for lithium on page 341.

Special information about pregnancy and breastfeeding

The use of lithium during pregnancy can harm the developing baby. Patients should inform the doctor immediately if they are pregnant or plan to become pregnant.

Lithium appears in breast milk and is considered potentially harmful to a nursing infant. If this medication is essential to the patient's health, the doctor may advise her to discontinue breastfeeding while she is taking it.

Recommended dosage

ADULTS

Acute Episodes

The usual dosage is a total of 1,800 milligrams per day. Immediate-release forms are taken in 3 or 4 doses per day; long-acting forms are taken twice a day.

Dosage is individualized according to the levels of the drug in the patient's blood. Blood levels will be checked at least twice a week when the drug is first prescribed and on a regular basis thereafter.

Long-term Control

Dosage will vary from one individual to another, but a total of 900 to 1,200 milligrams per day is typical. Immediate-release forms are taken in 3 or 4 doses per day; long-acting forms are taken twice a day. Blood levels in most cases should be checked every 2 months.

CHILDREN

Safety and effectiveness of lithium in children under 12 years of age have not been established.

OLDER ADULTS

Older people often need less lithium and may show signs of overdose at a dosage that younger people can handle well.

Overdosage

Any medication taken in excess can have serious consequences. If an overdose of lithium is suspected, seek medical attention immediately.

The harmful levels are close to those needed for treatment. Patients need to watch for early signs of overdose, such as diarrhea, drowsiness, lack of coordination, vomiting, and weakness. If they develop any of these signs, they should stop taking the drug and call the doctor.

Lithobid *See Lithium carbonate, page 116*

Lorazepam *See Ativan, page 28*

LUNESTA
Eszopiclone

Why is this drug prescribed?
Lunesta is prescribed for insomnia. It's used for adults who have trouble getting to sleep, wake frequently during the night, or wake up too early in the morning.

Most important fact about this drug
Rarely, Lunesta can cause changes in behavior or thinking. The patient or caregiver should contact the doctor immediately if they notice any of the following changes:

- More outgoing or aggressive behavior than normal
- Confusion
- Strange behavior
- Agitation
- Hallucinations
- Worsening of depression
- Suicidal thoughts

Sleep problems are usually temporary and require only short-term treatment with medication, typically 7 to 10 days. If the patient's insomnia continues or becomes worse, the doctor should be contacted.

How should this medication be taken?

Lunesta should be taken only when the patient is ready to get in bed or if they are already in bed and have trouble falling asleep. Patients should not take Lunesta unless they are able to get 8 or more hours of sleep before they have to be active again.

For Lunesta to work best, it should not be taken with or immediately after a high-fat, heavy meal. The tablet should be swallowed whole; it should not be split, crushed, or chewed.

Patients should not stop taking Lunesta suddenly or change the dose without the doctor's approval. The patient could experience signs of withdrawal such as abnormal dreams, anxiety, nausea, sleeplessness, or upset stomach.

- *Missed dose...*
  The prescribed dose of Lunesta should only be taken immediately before bedtime.

- *Storage instructions...*
  Lunesta should be stored at room temperature in a dry place.

What side effects may occur?

Side effects cannot be predicted. If any develop or change in intensity, patients should inform their doctor as soon as possible.

- *Side effects may include:*
  Difficulty with coordination, dizziness, drowsiness, light-headedness

Why should this drug not be prescribed?

At this time, there are no known contraindications for Lunesta.

Special warnings about this medication

Lunesta should be used with caution in patients who have problems with metabolism or blood circulation, breathing problems, or severe liver disease.

Patients must be ready for bed or already be in bed before taking Lunesta. If a patient stays awake after taking Lunesta, they may become dizzy or light-headed and may risk falling. To prevent injury to themselves and others, they should never attempt to drive a car, operate any machinery, or engage in hazardous activities after taking this drug. Also, patients could have memory problems while taking Lunesta, especially if they are 65 or older.

Sometimes drugs used for sleep can affect a patient the next day. Patients should be cautious when planning activities the day after taking Lunesta until they know its effects.

Drugs like Lunesta can lead to psychological or physical dependence, especially if the patient has a history of alcohol or drug abuse, or if they have mental and emotional problems. Be sure the doctor is aware of the complete medical history.

Depression can sometimes worsen when taking drugs like Lunesta. It is important to notify the doctor right away if the patient becomes more depressed or if they or their family notice unusual thoughts or behaviors, especially thoughts of suicide.

After stopping Lunesta, patients may have trouble falling asleep (known as rebound insomnia). This should go away after the first night or two.

Lunesta has not been studied in children.

Taking Lunesta after a high-fat, heavy meal could slow or reduce its effect.

Also, it's best to avoid drinking alcohol while taking Lunesta, since this may increase the drug's effects.

It is important to check with the doctor before combining Lunesta with drugs that relax the central nervous system, such as medicines used for allergies, anxiety, seizures, or sleep.

Possible food and drug interactions when taking this medication

See the entry for the generic name eszopiclone on page 321.

Special information about pregnancy and breastfeeding

The effects of taking Lunesta during pregnancy have not been studied. Patients who are pregnant or plan to become pregnant should contact their doctor immediately.

It is not known whether Lunesta appears in breast milk; patients should talk to their doctor if they plan to breastfeed.

Recommended dosage

ADULTS 18 YEARS AND OLDER

The usual starting dose is 2 milligrams taken immediately before bedtime. If the patient has trouble staying asleep, the doctor may increase the dosage. For patients with severe liver disease, the usual starting dose is 1 milligram, not to exceed 2 milligrams in one night.

OLDER ADULTS

For patients who are 65 years or older and have trouble falling asleep, the usual starting dose is 1 milligram taken immediately before bedtime. The doctor may increase the dose to 2 milligrams if the patient cannot stay asleep.

Overdosage

Any medication taken in excess can have serious consequences. If an overdose is suspected, seek emergency treatment immediately. There is little information on overdoses with Lunesta. Overdoses of similar drugs have been known to cause confusion, dizziness, and possibly loss of consciousness.

MAPROTILINE HYDROCHLORIDE

Why is this drug prescribed?

Maprotiline is used to treat depression and anxiety associated with depression. It is also used for depression in people with manic-depressive illness.

Maprotiline is classified as a tetracyclic antidepressant. It is thought to work by boosting sensitivity at nerve junctions in the brain.

Most important fact about this drug

Seizures have been associated with maprotiline, particularly when the drug was taken in amounts larger than prescribed, the dosage was increased too fast, or it was taken with certain other drugs such as chlorpromazine and trifluoperazine. To reduce the risk of seizures, patients should be sure to follow the doctor's instructions for taking this medication.

How should this medication be taken?

The doctor may prescribe a single daily dose or several smaller doses.

Improvement may not be evident for 2 to 3 weeks. Patients should not let this discourage them. They should continue maprotiline therapy until instructed otherwise by the doctor.

- *Missed dose...*
  Patients who take 1 dose at bedtime should check with their doctor. Taking it in the morning may cause side effects during the day.

  Patients who take more than 1 dose a day should take the forgotten dose as soon as they remember. If it is almost time for the next dose, they should skip the dose they missed and go back to their regular schedule. They should never try to "catch up" by doubling the dose.

- *Storage instructions...*
  Maprotiline should be stored at room temperature in a tightly closed container.

What side effects may occur?

Side effects cannot be predicted. If any develop or change in intensity, patients should inform the doctor as soon as possible.

- *Side effects may include:*
  Anxiety, blurred vision, constipation, dizziness, drowsiness, dry mouth, fatigue, headache, nervousness, tremors, weakness

Why should this drug not be prescribed?

Maprotiline should not be used by anyone who has had a recent heart attack. It should be avoided by patients who have taken one of the anti-depressant drugs known as MAO inhibitors, including Parnate and Nardil, within the preceding 14 days.

It should not be used by people who have had seizures. Maprotiline should not be taken by individuals known to be hypersensitive to it.

Special warnings about this medication

Maprotiline should be used cautiously if the patient has ever had glaucoma (excessive pressure in the eyes), heart disease, heart attacks, irregular heartbeats, strokes, thyroid disease, or difficulty urinating.

This drug may impair patients' ability to drive a car or operate potentially dangerous machinery. They should not participate in any activities that require full alertness if they are unsure of their response to the drug.

Maprotiline may cause sensitivity to light. Patients should avoid prolonged exposure to the sun; they should use sunscreens and wear protective clothing until they learn their tolerance.

Extreme drowsiness and other potentially serious effects can result if maprotiline is combined with alcohol, sleeping medications such as Seconal, and other drugs that depress the central nervous system.

Maprotiline should not be combined with MAO inhibitors such as Nardil.

Possible food and drug interactions when taking this medication

See the entry for maprotiline on page 349.

Special information about pregnancy or breastfeeding

The effects of maprotiline during pregnancy have not been adequately studied. Women who are pregnant or plan on becoming pregnant should inform their doctor immediately. Pregnant women should use maprotiline only if clearly needed.

Maprotiline appears in breast milk and could affect a nursing infant. Women who nurse infants should use the drug cautiously and only when the potential benefits clearly outweigh the potential risks.

Recommended dosage

ADULTS

For Mild to Moderate Depression

Dosages usually start at 75 milligrams a day, taken as a single daily dose or divided into smaller doses. The doctor may increase the dose gradually to a maximum of 150 milligrams daily.

For Moderate to Severe Depression

For those who are hospitalized, dosages as high as 225 milligrams daily may be prescribed.

CHILDREN

Safety and effectiveness for children under 18 years old have not been established.

OLDER ADULTS

For Mild to Moderate Depression
Dosages usually start at 25 milligrams a day and may range up to 50 to 75 milligrams daily.

Overdosage

Any medication taken in excess can have serious consequences. An overdose of maprotiline can be fatal. If an overdose is suspected, seek medical help immediately.

- *Symptoms of maprotiline overdose may include:*
  Agitation, bluish skin, coma, convulsions, dilated pupils, drowsiness, heart failure, high fever, irregular heart rate, lack of coordination, loss of consciousness, muscle rigidity, rapid heartbeat, restlessness, severely low blood pressure, shock, vomiting, writhing movement of the hands

---

MEBARAL
Mephobarbital sodium

Why is this drug prescribed?

Mebaral is a barbiturate used as a sedative for the relief of anxiety, tension, and apprehension. It also works as an anticonvulsant and is prescribed to treat certain types of epilepsy, including grand mal and petit mal seizures.

Most important fact about this drug

If taken for a long enough time, Mebaral can cause physical and psychological addiction. An overdose can be fatal. Mebaral should be used in the smallest possible amount, and it should always be stored in child-resistant containers.

How should this medication be taken?

Mebaral should be taken exactly as prescribed. Patients should never increase the dose or use the drug more often than the doctor has instructed.

Patients who are using Mebaral to control seizures should take it at bedtime if the attacks generally occur at night, and during the day if the attacks happen in the daytime.

- *Missed dose...*
  Patients should take the forgotten dose as soon as they remember. If it is almost time for their next dose, they should skip the one they missed and go back to their regular schedule. Patients should never take two doses at once.

- *Storage instructions...*
  Mebaral should be stored at room temperature.

What side effects may occur?

Side effects cannot be predicted. If any develop or change in intensity, patients should inform their doctor as soon as possible.

*   *Side effects may include:*
    Abnormal or increased muscle movement, agitation, confusion, fainting, headache, impaired coordination, low blood pressure, nausea, shallow or slowed breathing, slowed heartbeat, stoppage of breathing (apnea), sleepiness, vomiting

Why should this drug not be prescribed?

People with the rare blood disorder porphyria and those who are allergic or sensitive to barbiturates must avoid Mebaral.

Special warnings about this medication

Mebaral must not be stopped abruptly. Doing so can result in severe withdrawal symptoms and even death. To reduce any possible withdrawal symptoms, patients should follow their doctor's instructions closely when stopping this drug. Minor withdrawal symptoms may appear 8 to 12 hours after the last dose, and usually occur in the following order: anxiety, muscle twitching, tremors of hands and fingers, progressive weakness, dizziness, visual problems, nausea, vomiting, insomnia, and lightheadedness on standing up. Major withdrawal symptoms include convulsions and delirium, which may occur within 16 hours of abruptly stopping Mebaral and can last up to 5 days.

Barbiturates such as Mebaral should be used cautiously, if at all, in patients who have a history of depression, suicidal tendencies, or drug abuse.

In some people, Mebaral may cause excitement rather than sedation. Others experience depression and confusion. Such reactions are more likely in elderly or debilitated patients.

The doctor will prescribe this drug cautiously in patients with any of the following: liver damage, kidney impairment, heart problems, breathing difficulties, the muscle disorder myasthenia gravis, or myxedema (a type of skin swelling associated with poor thyroid function). Caution is also advised in patients with acute or chronic pain, since Mebaral treatment could induce paradoxical excitement or mask important pain symptoms.

Mebaral may impair the ability to drive a car or operate potentially dangerous machinery. Patients should not participate in any activities that require full alertness if they are unsure of the drug's effects.

Mebaral may cause vitamin D deficiency. Patients should ask their doctor about increasing their vitamin D intake.

Mebaral could lessen the effectiveness of oral contraceptives. Women who take this drug may need to consider another type of birth control.

Barbiturates such as Mebaral may lose their effect when taken regularly. If this happens, patients should contact the doctor. They should never increase the dose in an effort to get the drug to work again.

Warn patients not to drink alcohol while using Mebaral. Combining the two could cause serious effects due to central nervous system depression.

Possible food and drug interactions when taking this medication

See the entry for the generic name mephobarbital on page 350.

Special information about pregnancy and breastfeeding

Mebaral can cause damage to developing babies and withdrawal symptoms in newborns. Patients who are pregnant or plan to become pregnant should inform their doctor immediately.

This drug appears in breast milk and should be used with caution by nursing mothers.

Recommended dosage

SEDATION

Adults: The recommended optimum dose is 50 milligrams 3 to 4 times a day. The effective dosage can range from 32 to 100 milligrams 3 to 4 times a day.

Children: Dosages for children range from 16 to 32 milligrams 3 to 4 times a day.

EPILEPSY

Adults: The average dose is 400 to 600 milligrams a day.

Children 5 years of age and older: 32 to 64 milligrams 3 to 4 times a day.

Children under 5 years of age: 16 to 32 milligrams 3 to 4 times a day.

DOSAGE ADJUSTMENT

Patients who are taking Mebaral with other anticonvulsants, particularly phenobarbital, may be prescribed a reduced dosage. The doctor will also prescribe lower dosages for patients who are elderly, debilitated, or suffering from liver or kidney problems.

Overdosage

An overdose of Mebaral can be fatal. If an overdose is suspected, seek medical help immediately.

• *Symptoms or complications of Mebaral overdose may include:*
  Coma, constriction (or sometimes dilation) of pupils, difficulty breathing, fluid in the lungs, heart failure, kidney failure, lack of reflexes, low blood pressure, low body temperature, pneumonia, rapid or irregular heartbeat, reduced flow of urine

Memantine *See Namenda, page 131*

Mephobarbital *See Mebaral, page 124*

MEPROBAMATE

Why is this drug prescribed?

Meprobamate is a tranquilizer used in the treatment of anxiety disorders and for short-term relief of the symptoms of anxiety.

Most important fact about this drug

Meprobamate can be habit-forming. Patients can develop tolerance and dependence, and may experience withdrawal symptoms if they stop using this drug abruptly. They should discontinue this drug or change the dose only on their doctor's advice.

How should this medication be taken?

Meprobamate should be taken exactly as prescribed.

* *Missed dose...*
  The dose should be taken as soon as remembered if it is within an hour of the scheduled time. If it's not remembered until later, the patient should skip it and go back to the regular schedule. Doses should never be doubled.

* *Storage instructions...*
  Meprobamate should be stored at room temperature in a tightly closed container.

What side effects may occur?

Side effects cannot be predicted. If any develop or change in intensity, patients should inform their doctor as soon as possible.

* *Side effects may include:*
  Broken capillary blood vessels, diarrhea, drowsiness, impaired coordination, irregular or rapid heartbeat, low red blood cell count, nausea, rash, slurred speech, vertigo, vomiting, weakness

* *Side effects due to rapid decrease in dose or abrupt withdrawal from meprobamate:*
  Anxiety, confusion, convulsions, hallucinations, inability to fall asleep or stay asleep, loss of appetite, loss of coordination, muscle twitching, tremors, vomiting

Withdrawal symptoms usually become apparent within 12 to 48 hours after discontinuation of this medication and should disappear in another 12 to 48 hours.

Why should this drug not be prescribed?

Meprobamate should be avoided by anyone who is sensitive to or has ever had an allergic reaction to it or related drugs such as carisoprodol (Soma).

Meprobamate should not be taken by individuals with acute intermittent porphyria, an inherited disease of the body's metabolism. It can make the symptoms worse.

Anxiety or tension related to everyday stress usually does not require treatment with meprobamate.

Special warnings about this medication

Patients who develop a skin rash, sore throat, fever, or shortness of breath should contact their doctor immediately. They may be having an allergic reaction to the drug.

Meprobamate may cause patients to become drowsy or less alert. They should not drive, operate dangerous machinery, or participate in any hazardous activity that requires full mental alertness until they know how this drug affects them.

Long-term use of this drug should be evaluated by the doctor periodically for its usefulness. If the patient has liver or kidney disorders, the doctor should be made aware of these conditions before therapy begins.

Use of this drug may bring on seizures in people with epilepsy. They need to consult with their doctor before taking this medication.

Meprobamate may intensify the effects of alcohol. Patients should not drink alcohol while taking this medication.

Possible food and drug interactions when taking this medication

See the entry for meprobamate on page 356.

Special information about pregnancy and breastfeeding

Meprobamate should not be taken by patients who are pregnant or are planning to become pregnant. There is an increased risk of birth defects.

Meprobamate appears in breast milk and could affect a nursing infant. If this medication is essential to the mother's health, the doctor may advise her to discontinue breastfeeding until her treatment is finished.

Recommended dosage

ADULTS

The usual dosage is 1,200 to 1,600 milligrams per day divided into 3 or 4 doses. The maximum dosage is 2,400 milligrams a day.

CHILDREN

The usual dose for children 6 to 12 years of age is 200 to 600 milligrams per day divided into 2 or 3 doses.

Meprobamate is not recommended for children under age 6.

OLDER ADULTS

The doctor will limit the dose to the smallest effective amount to avoid oversedation.

Overdosage

Any medication taken in excess can have serious consequences. If an overdose is suspected, seek emergency medical attention immediately.

* *Symptoms of meprobamate overdose may include:*
  Coma, drowsiness, loss of muscle control, severely impaired breathing, shock, sluggishness, and unresponsiveness

Metadate *See Ritalin, page 199*

Methamphetamine *See Desoxyn, page 60*

Methylin *See Ritalin, page 199*

Methylphenidate, oral *See Ritalin, page 199*

Methylphenidate, patch *See Daytrana, page 54*

Mirtazapine *See Remeron, page 186*

MOBAN
Molindone hydrochloride

Why is this drug prescribed?
Moban is used in the treatment of schizophrenia.

Most important fact about this drug?
Moban can cause tardive dyskinesia, a condition marked by involuntary movements in the face and body, including chewing movements, puckering, puffing the cheeks, and sticking out the tongue. This condition may be permanent and appears to be most common among the elderly, especially women.

How should this medication be taken?
Moban should be taken exactly as prescribed. It should not be taken with alcohol.

* *Missed dose...*
  Generally, the forgotten dose should be taken as soon as remembered. However, if it is almost time for the next dose, the missed dose should be skipped and the patient should return to the regular schedule. Doses should never be doubled.

* *Storage instructions...*
  Moban should be stored at room temperature and protected from light.

What side effects may occur?

Side effects cannot be predicted. If any develop or change in intensity, patients should inform their doctor as soon as possible.

- *Side effects may include:*
  Blurred vision, depression, drowsiness (especially at the start of therapy), dry mouth, euphoria, hyperactivity, nausea, Parkinson's-like movements, restlessness

Why should this drug not be prescribed?

Moban should not be combined with alcohol, barbiturates (sleep aids), narcotics (painkillers), or other substances that slow down the nervous system, nor should it be given to anyone in a comatose state. Moban cannot be used by anyone who is hypersensitive to the drug. The concentrate form of Moban contains a sulfite that may cause life-threatening allergic reactions in some people, especially in those with asthma.

Special warnings about this medication

Drugs such as Moban can cause a potentially fatal condition called neuroleptic malignant syndrome. Symptoms include high fever, rigid muscles, irregular pulse or blood pressure, rapid heartbeat, excessive perspiration, and changes in heart rhythm. If patients develop these symptoms, they need to contact their doctor immediately. Moban should be discontinued.

Moban should be used with caution by anyone who has ever had breast cancer. The drug stimulates production of a hormone that promotes the growth of certain types of tumors.

Because this drug may cause drowsiness, patients should not participate in activities that require full alertness, such as driving or operating machinery, until they are sure how this medicine affects them.

Moban may mask signs of a brain tumor or intestinal blockage. It causes increased activity in some people. On rare occasions, it causes seizures.

Remember that Moban must never be combined with alcohol, barbiturates, or narcotics. In addition, Moban tablets contain calcium, which may interfere with the absorption of tetracycline antibiotics (Sumycin) and phenytoin (Dilantin).

Possible food and drug interactions when taking this medication

See the entry for the generic name molindone on page 360.

Special information about pregnancy and breastfeeding

The safety and effectiveness of Moban during pregnancy have not been adequately studied. Patients who are pregnant or planning to become pregnant should tell their doctor immediately. Moban should be used during pregnancy only if the benefits outweigh the potential risks.

It is not known whether Moban appears in breast milk. Patients should check with their doctor before deciding to breastfeed.

Recommended dosage

ADULTS

The usual starting dose is 50 to 75 milligrams a day. The doctor may increase the dose to 100 milligrams a day after 3 or 4 days of treatment.

The long-term maintenance dose depends on the patient's response to the medication. The usual maintenance dose for treatment of mild symptoms is 5 to 15 milligrams taken 3 or 4 times a day. For moderate symptoms it is 10 to 25 milligrams taken 3 or 4 times a day. For severe symptoms, up to 225 milligrams a day may be prescribed. Older adults generally take lower dosages of Moban.

CHILDREN

The safety and effectiveness of Moban in children under age 12 have not been established.

Overdosage

Any medication taken in excess can have serious consequences. If an overdose of Moban is suspected, seek medical help immediately.

Modafinil *See Provigil, page 177*

Molindone *See Moban, page 129*

Naltrexone, injection *See Vivitrol, page 251*

Naltrexone, tablets *See ReVia, page 193*

NAMENDA

Memantine

Why is this drug prescribed?

Namenda is used to treat moderate to severe Alzheimer's disease. While other Alzheimer's drugs work to prevent the breakdown of the brain chemical acetylcholine, Namenda works by targeting glutamate. Both chemicals are associated with memory and learning.

Studies show that Namenda can help improve the mental state and daily functioning of some—but not all—people with Alzheimer's disease. As with other Alzheimer's drugs, Namenda does not cure or slow the progression of the disease; it merely treats the symptoms.

Most important fact about this drug

Namenda should not be taken by anyone who has ever had an allergic reaction to this medication.

Namenda has not been evaluated for use in patients with seizure disorders. Conditions that raise urine pH, such as severe urinary tract infections, may increase levels of Namenda. Dosage should be reduced in patients with severe renal impairment.

Namenda treatment should not be stopped, or the dose changed, without consulting a doctor. Caregivers need to pay particular attention to the doctor's instructions on dose increases. It can take up to 4 weeks for any positive effects to appear.

How should this medication be taken?

Namenda is available in tablet and oral solution forms. Caregivers should give Namenda exactly as prescribed. The dose of Namenda is increased gradually at 1-week intervals. Using doses that are higher than recommended provides no additional benefit and could increase the risk of side effects. Namenda can be given with or without food.

* *Missed dose...*
  It should be given as soon as it's remembered. However, if it is almost time for the next dose, caregivers should skip the dose they missed and return to the regular schedule. Doses should never be doubled.

* *Storage instructions...*
  Namenda should be stored at room temperature.

What side effects may occur?

Side effects cannot be predicted. If any develop or change in intensity, the doctor should be informed as soon as possible.

* *Side effects may include:*
  Confusion, constipation, coughing, dizziness, hallucinations, headache, high blood pressure, pain, sleepiness, vomiting

Why should this drug not be prescribed?

People who have ever had an allergic reaction to Namenda should not take this medication.

Special warnings about this medication

Namenda is not recommended for patients with severe kidney impairment.

Certain conditions can alter the alkaline balance of the urine, which may cause a buildup of Namenda in the body. Caregivers should alert the doctor about any major dietary changes, kidney problems such as renal acidosis, or urinary tract infections.

The doctor should be told about any history of seizures. Namenda has not been formally studied in people with seizure disorders.

Possible food and drug interactions when taking this medication
See the entry for the generic name memantine on page 349.

Special information about pregnancy and breastfeeding
Namenda is not usually prescribed for women of childbearing age. There are no adequate and well-controlled studies in pregnant women. It should be used in pregnant women only if the potential benefit to the mother outweighs the risk to the fetus.

It is not known whether Namenda appears in human breast milk. If this drug is essential to the patient's health, the doctor may advise her to stop nursing until treatment is finished.

Recommended dosage
ADULTS

The recommended dosage is 10 milligrams twice a day. The doctor will start treatment at 5 milligrams once a day for 7 days, and gradually increase the dose by 5 milligrams every 7 days, up to a maximum total daily dose of 20 milligrams.

If Namenda causes side effects, the doctor may wait more than 1 week to increase the dose. People who have impaired kidney function may require lower doses.

Overdosage
Any medication taken in excess can have serious consequences. If an overdose is suspected, seek emergency treatment immediately.

- *Symptoms of Namenda overdose may include:*
  Loss of consciousness, hallucinations, psychosis, restlessness, sleepiness, stupor

---

NARDIL
Phenelzine sulfate

Why is this drug prescribed?
Nardil is a monoamine oxidase (MAO) inhibitor used to treat depression as well as anxiety or phobias mixed with depression. MAO is an enzyme responsible for breaking down certain neurotransmitters in the brain. By inhibiting MAO, Nardil boosts the levels of these neurotransmitters and helps restore more normal mood states. Unfortunately, MAO inhibitors such as Nardil also block MAO activity throughout the body, an action that can have serious, even fatal, side effects, especially if MAO inhibitors are combined with certain foods or drugs containing a substance called tyramine.

Most important fact about this drug
It is essential that patients avoid the following foods, beverages, and medications while taking Nardil and for 2 weeks after stopping Nardil treatment:

Anchovies
Avocado
Beer (including alcohol-free or reduced-alcohol beer)
Caffeine (in excessive amounts)
Caviar
Cheese (except for cottage cheese and cream cheese)
Chocolate (in excessive amounts)
Dry sausage (including Genoa salami, hard salami, pepperoni, and
  Lebanon bologna)
Fava bean pods
Liver
Meat extracts or meat prepared with tenderizers
Pickled herring
Pickled, fermented, aged, or smoked meat, fish, or dairy products
Sauerkraut
Sour cream
Soy sauce
Spoiled or improperly stored meat, fish, or dairy products
Wine (including alcohol-free or reduced-alcohol wine)
Yeast extract (including large amounts of brewer's yeast)
Yogurt

Also, patients should avoid taking Nardil with L-tryptophan-containing products.

Taking Nardil with any of the above foods, beverages, or medications can cause serious, potentially fatal, high blood pressure. When taking Nardil patients should immediately report the occurrence of a headache, heart palpitations, or any other unusual symptom. In addition, patients should be sure to inform any physician or dentist they see that they are currently taking Nardil or have taken Nardil within the last 2 weeks.

How should this medication be taken?
Nardil may be taken with or without food. It can take up to 4 weeks for the drug to begin working. Use of Nardil may complicate other medical treatment. Patients should carry a card that says they are taking Nardil, or wear a Medic Alert bracelet.

• *Missed dose...*
  Generally, the dose should be taken as soon as remembered. However, if it is within 2 hours of the next dose, the patient should skip the missed dose and go back to the regular schedule. Doses should never be doubled.

• *Storage instructions...*
  Nardil should be stored at room temperature.

What side effects may occur?

Side effects cannot be predicted. If any develop or change in intensity, patients should inform their doctor as soon as possible.

- *Side effects may include:*
  Constipation, dizziness, drowsiness, dry mouth, headache, liver problems, low blood pressure upon standing, sexual problems, sleep disturbances, stomach and intestinal problems, water retention, weight gain

Why should this drug not be prescribed?

This drug cannot be taken by anyone with pheochromocytoma (a tumor of the adrenal gland), congestive heart failure, a history of liver disease, or an allergy to the drug's ingredients.

Nardil should not be combined with medications that may increase blood pressure (such as amphetamines, cocaine, allergy and cold medications, or Ritalin), other MAO inhibitors, L-dopa, methyldopa, phenylalanine, L-tryptophan, L-tyrosine, flextime (Prozac), bastioned (Bus par), bupropion (Wellbutrin), guanethidine, meperidine (Demerol), dextromethorphan, or substances that slow the central nervous system such as alcohol and narcotics. It is also important to avoid foods, beverages, or medications listed in the "Most important fact about this drug" section.

Special warnings about this medication

In clinical studies, antidepressants increased the risk of suicidal thinking and behavior in children and adolescents with depression and other psychiatric disorders. Anyone considering the use of Nardil, or any other antidepressant in a child or adolescent, must balance the risk with the clinical need. Nardil is not approved for treating children.

Additionally, the progression of major depression is associated with a worsening of symptoms and/or the emergence of suicidal thinking or behavior in both adults and children, whether or not they are taking antidepressants. Patients and caregivers should watch for any change in symptoms or any new symptoms that appear suddenly—especially agitation, anxiety, hostility, panic, restlessness, extreme hyperactivity, and suicidal thinking or behavior—and report them to the doctor immediately. Be especially observant at the beginning of treatment or whenever there is a change in dose.

Patients must follow the food and drug limitations established by the physician; failure to do so may lead to potentially fatal side effects. While taking Nardil, they should promptly report the occurrence of a headache or any other unusual symptoms. Consult the "Most important fact about this drug" and "Why should this drug not be prescribed?" sections for lists of the foods, beverages, and medications that should be avoided while taking Nardil.

In addition, blood pressure medications (including water pills and beta blockers) should be used with caution by anyone taking Nardil, since excessively low blood pressure may result. Symptoms of low blood pressure include dizziness when rising from a lying or sitting position, fainting, and tingling in the hands or feet.

The doctor should prescribe Nardil with caution if the patient has diabetes, since it is not clear how MAO inhibitors affect blood sugar levels.

Patients need to tell the doctor that they are taking Nardil before deciding to have elective surgery.

Abrupt discontinuation of Nardil may trigger withdrawal symptoms. They may include nightmares, agitation, strange behavior, and convulsions.

Possible food and drug interactions when taking this medication

See the entry for the generic name phenelzine on page 374.

Special information about pregnancy and breastfeeding

The effects of Nardil during pregnancy have not been adequately studied. Nardil should be used during pregnancy only if the benefits of therapy clearly outweigh the potential risks to the fetus. If a patient is pregnant or plans to become pregnant, she should inform her doctor immediately.

Nursing mothers should use Nardil only after consulting their physician, since it is not known whether Nardil appears in breast milk.

Recommended dosage

ADULTS

The usual starting dose is 15 milligrams (1 tablet) 3 times a day. The doctor may increase the dosage to 90 milligrams per day.

It may be 4 weeks before the drug starts to work. Once the patient responds, the doctor may gradually reduce the dose, possibly to as low as 15 milligrams daily or every 2 days.

CHILDREN

Nardil is not recommended, since safety and efficacy for children have not been determined.

OLDER ADULTS

Because older people are more likely to have poor liver, kidney, or heart function, or other diseases that could increase the likelihood of side effects, a relatively low dose of Nardil is usually recommended at the start.

Overdosage

Any medication taken in excess can have serious consequences. An overdose of Nardil can be fatal. If an overdose is suspected, seek medical help immediately.

* *Symptoms of Nardil overdose may include:*
  Agitation, backward arching of the head neck back, cool and clammy skin, coma, convulsions, difficult breathing, dizziness, drowsiness,

fainting, hallucinations, high blood pressure, high fever, hyperactivity, irritability, jaw muscle spasms, low blood pressure, pain in the heart area, rapid and irregular pulse, rigidity, severe headache, sweating

NAVANE

Thiothixene

Why is this drug prescribed?

Navane is used to treat schizophrenia. Researchers theorize that this type of antipsychotic medication works by lowering levels of dopamine, a neurotransmitter in the brain. Excessive levels of dopamine are believed to be related to psychotic behavior.

Most important fact about this drug

Navane may cause tardive dyskinesia—a condition marked by involuntary muscle spasms and twitches in the face and body. This condition can be permanent and appears to be most common among the elderly, especially women.

How should this medication be taken?

Navane may be taken in liquid or capsule form. For the liquid form, a dropper is supplied.

- *Missed dose...*
  Generally, it should be taken as soon as remembered. However, if it is within 2 hours of the next dose, patients can skip the missed dose and go back to their regular schedule. Doses should never be doubled.

- *Storage instructions...*
  Navane should be stored at room temperature away from heat, light, and moisture. The liquid form should not be allowed to freeze.

What side effects may occur?

Side effects cannot be predicted. If any develop or change in intensity, patients should inform their doctor as soon as possible.

- *Side effects may include:*
  Agitation, blood disorders, blurred vision, drowsiness, dry mouth, exaggerated reflexes, fainting, high blood pressure, insomnia, lightheadedness, low blood pressure, Parkinson's-like movements, profuse sweating, rapid or irregular heartbeat, rash, sensitivity to sunlight, skin color changes

Why should this drug not be prescribed?

Navane should not be given to comatose individuals. It should be avoided by anyone known to be hypersensitive to it. Also, it should not be used when the activity of the central nervous system is slowed down by a sleeping medication, circulatory system collapse, or an abnormal bone marrow or blood condition.

Special warnings about this medication

Navane may hide symptoms of brain tumor and intestinal obstruction. The doctor will prescribe Navane cautiously if the patient has or has ever had a brain tumor, breast cancer, convulsive disorders, the eye condition called glaucoma, intestinal blockage, or heart disease. It should also be avoided by patients exposed to extreme heat and those recovering from alcohol addiction.

This drug may impair the ability to drive a car or operate potentially dangerous machinery. Patients should not participate in any activities that require full alertness if they are unsure of their ability.

Extreme drowsiness and other potentially serious effects can result if Navane is combined with alcohol or other central nervous system depressants such as painkillers, narcotics, or sleeping medications.

Possible food and drug interactions when taking this medication

See the entry for the generic name thiothixene on page 403.

Special information about pregnancy and breastfeeding

If a patient is pregnant or plans to become pregnant, she should inform her doctor immediately; pregnant women should use Navane only if clearly needed. The doctor may also advise her to avoid breastfeeding while she is taking Navane.

Recommended dosage

Dosages of Navane are tailored to the individual. Usually treatment begins with a small dose, which is increased if needed.

ADULTS

For Milder Conditions

The usual starting dosage is a daily total of 6 milligrams, divided into doses of 2 milligrams taken 3 times a day. The doctor may increase the dose to a total of 15 milligrams a day.

For More Severe Conditions

The usual starting dosage is a daily total of 10 milligrams, taken in 2 doses of 5 milligrams each. The doctor may increase this dose to a total of 60 milligrams a day.

Taking more than 60 milligrams a day rarely increases the benefits of Navane.

Some people are able to take Navane once a day. Patients should check with their doctor to see whether they can follow this schedule.

CHILDREN

Navane is not recommended for children younger than 12 years old.

OLDER ADULTS

In general, older adults are prescribed dosages of Navane in the lower ranges. Because older adults may develop low blood pressure while taking Navane, their doctors will monitor them closely. Older adults (especially women) may be more susceptible to such side effects as involuntary muscle spasms and twitches in the face and body.

Overdosage

Any medication taken in excess can have serious consequences. If an overdose is suspected, seek medical help immediately.

- *Symptoms of Navane overdose may include:*
  Central nervous system depression, coma, difficulty swallowing, dizziness, drowsiness, head tilted to the side, low blood pressure, muscle twitching, rigid muscles, salivation, tremors, walking disturbances, weakness

---

NEFAZODONE HYDROCHLORIDE

Why is this drug prescribed?

Nefazodone is prescribed for the treatment of major depression. Researchers believe it works by boosting levels of two of the brain's key chemical messengers, serotonin and norepinephrine. However, the drug is chemically unrelated to the family of serotonin-boosters that includes Prozac and Paxil.

Most important fact about this drug

Nefazodone has been known to produce very rare cases of potentially fatal liver failure. Ordinarily, the drug is not prescribed for people with active liver disease or with high enzyme levels on liver function tests, and the doctor may periodically test the patient's liver function. If a patient develops warning signs of liver problems—such as nausea, abdominal pain, loss of appetite that lasts several days or longer, unusually dark urine, or yellowing of the skin or eyes—the doctor should be alerted immediately. Treatment with nefazodone will probably have to be stopped.

How should this medication be taken?

Patients must take nefazodone exactly as prescribed, even if they no longer feel depressed.

- *Missed dose...*
  Generally, a missed dose should be taken as soon as remembered. However, if it is within 4 hours of the next dose, patients should skip the dose they missed and go back to their regular schedule. Doses should never be doubled.

- *Storage instructions...*
  Nefazodone should be stored at room temperature in a tightly closed
  container.

What side effects may occur?
Side effects cannot be predicted. If any develop or change in intensity,
patients should tell their doctor as soon as possible.

- *Side effects may include:*
  Blurred or abnormal vision, confusion, constipation, dizziness, dry
  mouth, light-headedness, nausea, sleepiness, weakness

Why should this drug not be prescribed?
This medication should be avoided by anyone who is sensitive to or has
ever had an allergic reaction to it or to similar drugs, such as Desyrel.
Likewise, patients should not take nefazodone if previous treatment had
to be stopped due to signs of liver injury.

Serious, sometimes fatal reactions have occurred when nefazodone is
used in combination with drugs known as MAO inhibitors, including the
antidepressants Nardil and Parnate. Nefazodone must never be taken with
one of these drugs or within 14 days of discontinuing treatment with one
of them. Also, patients should allow at least 7 days between the last dose
of nefazodone and the first dose of an MAO inhibitor.

Nefazodone should also be avoided by people taking terfenadine,
astemizole, cisapride, Halcion, or Tegretol, and should never be combined with Orap, as heart problems could result.

Special warnings about this medication
In clinical studies, antidepressants increased the risk of suicidal thinking
and behavior in children and adolescents with depression and other psychiatric disorders. Anyone considering the use of nefazodone, or any
other antidepressant in a child or adolescent, must balance the risk with
the clinical need. Nefazodone has not been studied in children or adolescents and is not approved for treating anyone less than 18 years old.

Additionally, the progression of major depression is associated with a
worsening of symptoms and/or the emergence of suicidal thinking or
behavior in both adults and children, whether or not they are taking antidepressants. Patients and caregivers should watch for any change in
symptoms or any new symptoms that appear suddenly—especially agitation, anxiety, hostility, panic, restlessness, extreme hyperactivity, and
suicidal thinking or behavior—and report them to the doctor immediately.
Be especially observant at the beginning of treatment or whenever there
is a change in dose.

The doctor will prescribe nefazodone with caution if the patient has a
history of suicide attempts, seizures, mania, or heart or liver disease.
Nefazodone should also be used with caution in patients who have had a
heart attack, stroke, or angina; take drugs for high blood pressure; or suffer

from dehydration. Under these circumstances, nefazodone could cause an unwanted drop in blood pressure. Patients should discuss all of their medical problems with the doctor before taking this drug.

Nefazodone may cause patients to become drowsy or less alert and may affect their judgment. They should not drive, operate dangerous machinery, or participate in any hazardous activity that requires full mental alertness until they know how the drug affects them.

Before having surgery, dental treatment, or any diagnostic procedure requiring anesthesia, patients should tell the doctor or dentist they are taking nefazodone. If they develop an allergic reaction such as a skin rash or hives while taking nefazodone, they should notify the doctor. Men who experience a prolonged or inappropriate erection while taking nefazodone should discontinue the drug and call their doctor.

Nefazodone should be used with caution in people who have been addicted to drugs.

Possible food and drug interactions when taking this medication
See the entry for nefazodone on page 361.

Special information about pregnancy and breastfeeding
The effects of nefazodone during pregnancy have not been adequately studied. Women who are pregnant or are planning to become pregnant should tell their doctor immediately. Nefazodone should be used during pregnancy only if clearly needed.

Nefazodone may appear in breast milk. If this medication is essential to the patient's health, the doctor may tell her to discontinue breastfeeding until treatment with nefazodone is finished.

Recommended dosage
ADULTS

The usual starting dose is 200 milligrams a day, divided into 2 doses. If needed, the doctor may increase the dose gradually to 300 to 600 milligrams a day. Remind patients that it may take several weeks before they feel the full antidepressant effects.

CHILDREN

The safety and effectiveness of nefazodone have not been established in children less than 18 years of age.

OLDER ADULTS

The usual starting dose for older people and those in a weakened condition is 100 milligrams a day, taken in 2 doses. The doctor will adjust the dose according to the patient's response.

Overdosage

Any medication taken in excess can have serious consequences. If an overdose is suspected, seek medical attention immediately.

* *Symptoms of nefazodone overdose may include:*
  Nausea, sleepiness, vomiting

NEMBUTAL

Pentobarbital sodium

Why is this drug prescribed?

Nembutal is used as a sedative. It is prescribed on a short-term basis to help people fall asleep. After 2 weeks, it appears to lose its effectiveness as a sleep aid.

Most important fact about this drug

If taken for a long enough time, Nembutal can cause physical and psychological addiction. An overdose can be fatal. Nembutal should be used in the smallest possible amount, and it should always be stored in child-resistant containers.

How should this medication be taken?

Nembutal should be taken at bedtime, only as prescribed.

* *Missed dose...*
  This drug is for use only at bedtime. The dose should never be doubled.

* *Storage instructions...*
  Nembutal may be stored at room temperature.

What side effects may occur?

Side effects cannot be predicted. If any develop or change in intensity, patients should inform their doctor as soon as possible.

* *More common side effects may include:*
  Extreme sleepiness

* *Less common or rare side effects may include:*
  Agitation, anemia, anxiety, central nervous system depression, confusion, constipation, difficulty breathing, disturbed thinking, dizziness, fainting, fever, hallucinations, headache, insomnia, lack of coordination, low blood pressure, nausea, nervousness, nightmares, overactivity, skin inflammation and flaking, skin rash, slow heartbeat, temporary failure to breathe, vomiting

Why should this drug not be prescribed?

People with the rare blood disorder porphyria and those who are allergic or sensitive to barbiturates must avoid Nembutal.

Special warnings about this medication

Nembutal must not be stopped abruptly. Doing so can result in withdrawal symptoms and even death. To reduce any possible withdrawal symptoms, patients should follow the doctor's instructions closely when stopping Nembutal.

Minor withdrawal symptoms may include increased dreams or nightmares. Other minor withdrawal symptoms usually occur in the following order: anxiety, muscle twitching, tremors of hands and fingers, progressive weakness, dizziness, visual problems, nausea, vomiting, insomnia, and light-headedness on standing up. Major withdrawal symptoms may include convulsions and delirium.

The doctor will prescribe Nembutal cautiously if the patient has had liver disease or has a history of depression or substance abuse.

Patients should tell the doctor if they suffer from pain. Nembutal may hide pain-causing symptoms that require treatment.

Older adults may become confused, depressed, or excited while taking Nembutal, and should be prescribed lower doses. People with kidney or liver problems should also use lower doses.

Nembutal may lessen the effectiveness of oral contraceptives. Women who take Nembutal may need to consider another type of birth control.

The 100-milligram strength of Nembutal contains a coloring agent that may cause allergic reactions in some people.

This drug may impair the ability to drive a car or operate potentially dangerous machinery. Patients should not participate in any activities that require full alertness if they are unsure of their ability.

Nembutal may lose its effect when taken regularly. Patients should not increase the dose in an effort to get the drug to work again. Instead, they should contact the doctor.

Extreme drowsiness and other potentially serious effects can result if Nembutal is combined with alcohol or drugs that slow down the central nervous system, such as Percocet and Demerol.

Possible food and drug interactions when taking this medication

See the entry for the generic name pentobarbital on page 372.

Special information about pregnancy and breastfeeding

Nembutal causes damage to developing babies and withdrawal symptoms in newborns. Patients who are pregnant or plan to become pregnant should inform their doctor immediately.

This drug appears in breast milk and should be used with caution by nursing mothers.

Recommended dosage

ADULTS

The usual dose is 100 milligrams at bedtime.

CHILDREN

Dosages for children should be based on the child's age and weight.

OLDER ADULTS

Because older adults may be more sensitive to Nembutal, it will be prescribed at lower dosages.

Overdosage

Any medication taken in excess can have serious consequences. An overdose of Nembutal can be fatal. If an overdose is suspected, seek medical help immediately.

- *Symptoms of Nembutal overdose may include:*
  Coma, constriction (or sometimes dilation) of pupils, difficulty breathing, fluid in the lungs, heart failure, kidney failure, lack of reflexes, low blood pressure, low body temperature, pneumonia, rapid or irregular heartbeat, reduced flow of urine

NIRAVAM

Alprazolam orally disintegrating tablets

Why is this drug prescribed?

Niravam is used to treat anxiety disorder, panic disorder (with or without a fear of crowds or being in small places), and to provide short-term relief of anxiety symptoms.

Most important fact about this drug

Niravam may cause dependence. If taken at certain dosages, dependence becomes more likely. Dependence on Niravam has a greater chance of occurrence if the patient has a history of drug or alcohol abuse.

How should this medication be taken?

With clean, dry hands, patients should place a Niravam tablet on their tongue. It will begin to dissolve within seconds. Niravam can be taken with or without water.

- *Missed dose...*
  Generally, forgotten doses should be taken as soon as remembered. However, if it is almost time for the next dose, patients should skip the one they missed and return to their regular schedule. Doses should never be doubled.

- *Storage instructions...*
  Niravam should be stored at room temperature, away from moisture.

What side effects may occur?

Side effects cannot be predicted. If any develop or change in intensity, patients should inform their doctor as soon as possible.

• *Side effects may include:*
Drowsiness, fatigue, headache, impaired coordination, insomnia, irritability, light-headedness, memory impairment

Why should this drug not be prescribed?
Niravam should not be taken by patients who have acute narrow-angle glaucoma (increased eye pressure), or are taking a potent antifungal medication such as ketoconazole or itraconazole.

Special warnings about this medication
Patients should not drive a car or operate heavy machinery until they know how Niravam affects them. Patients also should not change or stop taking the prescribed dose of Niravam without talking to the doctor first.

Patients should tell their doctor about all prescription, over-the-counter, and herbal medications they are taking before beginning treatment with Niravam. Also, they should talk to their doctor about their complete medical history, especially if they have kidney or liver problems, or if they are pregnant or plan to become pregnant.

Possible food and drug interactions when taking this medication
See the entry for the generic name alprazolam on page 277.

Special information about pregnancy and breastfeeding
It is not recommended to take Niravam while pregnant. Women who are pregnant, planning to become pregnant, or are breastfeeding, should talk to their doctor about the best therapy for them. Niravam may pass into breast milk.

Recommended dosage
ADULTS

Anxiety Disorder
The initial dose is usually 0.25 to 0.5 milligrams taken 3 times a day. The dosage may be increased every 3 to 4 days to a maximum of 4 milligrams per day. Elderly patients may need to take a lower dose.

Panic Disorder
The initial dose is usually is 0.5 milligrams taken 3 times a day. The dosage may be increased every 3 to 4 days to a maximum of 4 milligrams per day.

Overdosage
Any medication taken in excess can have serious consequences. If an overdose is suspected, seek medical attention immediately.

• *Symptoms of Niravam overdose may include:*
Coma, confusion, coordination problems, reflex problems, sleepiness

NORPRAMIN
Desipramine hydrochloride

Why is this drug prescribed?

Norpramin is used in the treatment of depression. It is one of a family of drugs called tricyclic antidepressants. Drugs in this class are thought to work by affecting the levels of neurotransmitters in the brain, and adjusting the brain's response to them.

Norpramin has also been used to treat bulimia and attention deficit disorders, and to help with cocaine withdrawal.

Most important fact about this drug

Serious—sometimes fatal—reactions have been known to occur when drugs such as Norpramin are taken with another type of antidepressant called an MAO inhibitor. Drugs in this category include Nardil and Parnate. Norpramin cannot be taken within two weeks of taking one of these drugs.

How should this medication be taken?

Norpramin should be taken exactly as prescribed. Patients should continue taking Norpramin even if they feel no immediate effect. It can take up to 2 or 3 weeks for improvement to begin. Norpramin can cause dry mouth. Sucking hard candy or chewing gum can help this problem.

* *Missed dose...*
  Patients who take several doses per day should take the forgotten dose as soon as they remember, then take any remaining doses for the day at evenly spaced intervals. If the patient takes Norpramin once a day at bedtime and doesn't remember until morning, the missed dose should be skipped. Doses should never be doubled in an effort to "catch up."

* *Storage instructions...*
  Norpramin can be stored at room temperature. It should be protected from excessive heat.

What side effects may occur?

Side effects cannot be predicted. If any develop or change in intensity, patients should inform their doctor as soon as possible.

* *Side effects may include:*
  Anxiety, confusion, dizziness, dry mouth, frequent urination or problems urinating, high blood pressure, hallucinations, hives, impaired coordination, irregular heartbeat, low blood pressure, numbness, rapid heartbeat, sensitivity to sunlight, sex drive changes, tingling, tremors

Why should this drug not be prescribed?

Norpramin should not be used by anyone known to be hypersensitive to it, or by someone who has had a recent heart attack.

People who take antidepressant drugs known as MAO inhibitors (including Nardil and Parnate) should not take Norpramin.

Special warnings about this medication

In clinical studies, antidepressants increased the risk of suicidal thinking and behavior in children and adolescents with depression and other psychiatric disorders. Anyone considering the use of Norpramin, or any other antidepressant in a child or adolescent, must balance the risk with the clinical need. Norpramin has not been studied in children.

Additionally, the progression of major depression is associated with a worsening of symptoms and/or the emergence of suicidal thinking or behavior in both adults and children, whether or not they are taking antidepressants. Patients and caregivers should watch for any change in symptoms or any new symptoms that appear suddenly—especially agitation, anxiety, hostility, panic, restlessness, extreme hyperactivity, and suicidal thinking or behavior—and report them to the doctor immediately. Be especially observant at the beginning of treatment or whenever there is a change in dose.

Norpramin should be used with caution in patients who have heart or thyroid disease, a seizure disorder, a history of being unable to urinate, or high pressure in the eyes (glaucoma).

Nausea, headache, and uneasiness can result if Norpramin is discontinued abruptly. Patients should consult their doctor and follow instructions closely when discontinuing Norpramin.

This drug may impair the ability to drive a car or operate potentially dangerous machinery. Patients should not participate in any activities that require full alertness if they are unsure about their ability.

Norpramin may increase the skin's sensitivity to sunlight. Overexposure could cause rash, itching, redness, or sunburn. Patients should avoid direct sunlight or wear protective clothing.

Patients planning to have elective surgery should make sure that the doctor is aware that they are taking Norpramin. It should be discontinued as soon as possible prior to surgery.

The doctor should be alerted if a fever and sore throat develop during Norpramin therapy. He may want to do some blood tests.

People who take antidepressant drugs known as MAO inhibitors (including Nardil and Parnate) should not take Norpramin.

Extreme drowsiness and other potentially serious side effects can result if Norpramin is combined with alcohol or other depressants, including narcotic painkillers such as Percocet and Demerol, sleeping medications such as Halcion and Nembutal, and tranquilizers such as Valium and Xanax.

Possible food and drug interactions when taking this medication

See the entry for the generic name desipramine on page 309.

Special information about pregnancy and breastfeeding

Pregnant women or mothers who are nursing an infant should use Norpramin only when the potential benefits clearly outweigh the potential risks. If a patient is pregnant or planning to become pregnant, she should inform her doctor immediately.

Recommended dosage

Doses are tailored to individual needs.

ADULTS

The usual dosage ranges from 100 to 200 milligrams per day, taken in 1 dose or divided into smaller doses. If needed, the dosage may gradually be increased to 300 milligrams a day. Dosages above 300 milligrams per day are not recommended.

CHILDREN

Norpramin is not recommended for children.

OLDER ADULTS AND ADOLESCENTS

The usual dose ranges from 25 to 100 milligrams per day. If needed, the dosage may gradually be increased to 150 milligrams a day. Dosages above 150 milligrams per day are not recommended.

Overdosage

Any medication taken in excess can have serious consequences. An overdose of Norpramin can be fatal. If an overdose is suspected, seek medical help immediately.

- *Symptoms of Norpramin overdose may include:*
  Agitation, coma, confusion, convulsions, dilated pupils, disturbed concentration, drowsiness, extremely low blood pressure, hallucinations, high fever, irregular heart rate, low body temperature, overactive reflexes, rigid muscles, stupor, vomiting

Nortriptyline *See Pamelor, page 151*

Olanzapine *See Zyprexa, page 270*

Olanzapine and fluoxetine *See Symbyax, page 224*

OXAZEPAM

Why is this drug prescribed?

Oxazepam is used in the treatment of anxiety disorders, including anxiety associated with depression.

This drug seems to be particularly effective for anxiety, tension, agitation, and irritability in older people. It is also prescribed to relieve symptoms of acute alcohol withdrawal.

Oxazepam belongs to a class of drugs known as benzodiazepines.

Most important fact about this drug

Oxazepam can be habit-forming or addicting and can lose its effectiveness over time as patients develop a tolerance for it. They may experience withdrawal symptoms if they stop using the drug abruptly. When discontinuing the drug, the doctor will reduce the dose gradually.

How should this medication be taken?

Oxazepam should be taken exactly as prescribed.

- *Missed dose...*
  If remembered within an hour or so, the dose should be taken immediately. If not remembered until later, the dose should be skipped and the patient should return to the regular schedule. Doses should never be doubled.

- *Storage instructions...*
  Oxazepam should be stored at room temperature in a tightly closed container.

What side effects may occur?

Side effects cannot be predicted. If any develop or change in intensity, patients should inform their doctor as soon as possible. The doctor should periodically reassess the need for this drug.

- *Side effects may include:*
  Dizziness, drowsiness, headache, memory impairment, paradoxical excitement, transient amnesia, vertigo

- *Side effects due to rapid decrease in dose or abrupt withdrawal from oxazepam:*
  Abdominal and muscle cramps, convulsions, depression, inability to fall asleep or stay asleep, sweating, tremors, vomiting

Why should this drug not be prescribed?

Anyone who is sensitive to or has ever had an allergic reaction to oxazepam or other tranquilizers such as Valium should not take this medication. Patients should make sure the doctor is aware of any drug reactions they have experienced.

Anxiety or tension related to everyday stress usually does not require treatment with oxazepam. Patients should discuss their symptoms thoroughly with their doctor.

Oxazepam should not be prescribed for people who are being treated for mental disorders more serious than anxiety.

Special warnings about this medication

Oxazepam may cause patients to become drowsy or less alert. They should not drive, operate dangerous machinery, or participate in any hazardous activity that requires full mental alertness until they know how this drug affects them.

Oxazepam may cause a drop in blood pressure. People with heart problems should check with their doctor before taking this medication.

Oxazepam may intensify the effects of alcohol. It may be best to avoid alcohol while taking this medication.

Possible food and drug interactions when taking this medication

See the entry for oxazepam on page 366.

Special information about pregnancy and breastfeeding

Patients should not take oxazepam if they are pregnant or planning to become pregnant. There is an increased risk of birth defects.

Oxazepam may appear in breast milk and could affect a nursing infant. If this drug is essential to the patient's health, the doctor may advise her to stop breastfeeding until her treatment with this medication is finished.

Recommended dosage

ADULTS

Mild to Moderate Anxiety with Tension, Irritability, or Agitation
The usual dose is 10 to 15 milligrams 3 or 4 times per day.

Severe Anxiety, Depression with Anxiety, or Alcohol Withdrawal
The usual dose is 15 to 30 milligrams 3 or 4 times per day.

CHILDREN

Safety and effectiveness have not been established for children less than 6 years of age, nor have dosage guidelines been established for children 6 to 12 years old. The doctor will adjust the dosage to fit the child's needs.

OLDER ADULTS

The usual starting dose is 10 milligrams 3 times a day. The doctor may increase the dose to 15 milligrams 3 or 4 times a day, if needed.

Overdosage

An overdose of oxazepam can be fatal. If an overdose is suspected, seek medical attention immediately.

* *Symptoms of mild oxazepam overdose may include:*
  Confusion, drowsiness, lethargy

- *Symptoms of more serious overdose may include:*
  Coma, hypnotic state, lack of coordination, limp muscles, low blood pressure

Paliperidone *See Invega, page 100*

PAMELOR
Nortriptyline hydrochloride
Other brand name: Aventyl

Why is this drug prescribed?
Pamelor is prescribed to relieve the symptoms of depression. It is one of the drugs known as tricyclic antidepressants.

Some doctors also prescribe Pamelor to treat chronic hives, premenstrual depression, attention deficit hyperactivity disorder in children, and bedwetting.

Most important fact about this drug
Pamelor must be taken regularly to be effective, and it may be several weeks before the patient begins to feel better. It's important to keep taking regular doses, even if they seem to make no difference.

How should this medication be taken?
Pamelor should be taken exactly as prescribed. This drug can make the mouth dry. Sucking on hard candy, chewing gum, or melting ice chips in the mouth can provide relief.

- *Missed dose...*
  A forgotten dose should be taken as soon as remembered, unless it is almost time for the next dose. If that's the case, the missed dose should be skipped and the patient should return to the regular schedule.

  Patients who take Pamelor once a day at bedtime and miss a dose should not take it in the morning, since disturbing side effects could occur. Doses should never be doubled.

- *Storage instructions...*
  Pamelor should be kept in the container it came in, tightly closed and away from light. It is especially important to keep this drug out of reach of children; an overdose is particularly dangerous in the young. Pamelor should be stored at room temperature.

What side effects may occur?
Side effects cannot be predicted. If any develop or change in intensity, patients should inform their doctor as soon as possible.

- *Side effects may include:*
  Anxiety, blurred vision, confusion, dry mouth, hallucinations, heart attack or vascular heart blockage, heartbeat irregularities, high blood pressure, insomnia, loss of muscle coordination, low blood pressure, rapid heartbeat, sensitivity to sunlight, skin rash, stroke, tremors, weight loss

- *Side effects due to rapid decrease in dose or abrupt withdrawal from Pamelor after prolonged treatment include:*
  Headache, nausea, vague feeling of bodily discomfort

These side effects do not indicate addiction to this drug.

Why should this drug not be prescribed?

Anyone who is sensitive to or has ever had an allergic reaction to Pamelor or similar drugs should not take this medication.

Pamelor must be avoided by people who are taking—or have taken within the past 14 days—a drug classified as an MAO inhibitor. Drugs in this category include the antidepressants Nardil and Parnate. Combining these drugs with Pamelor can cause fever and convulsions, and could even be fatal.

Unless directed to do so by a doctor, patients should not take this medication while recovering from a heart attack or taking any other antidepressant drugs.

Patients who have been taking Prozac typically have to wait at least 5 weeks before beginning therapy with Pamelor. Otherwise, a drug interaction could result.

Special warnings about this medication

In clinical studies, antidepressants increased the risk of suicidal thinking and behavior in children and adolescents with depression and other psychiatric disorders. Anyone considering the use of Pamelor, or any other antidepressant in a child or adolescent, must balance the risk with the clinical need. Pamelor is not approved for use in children.

Additionally, the progression of major depression is associated with a worsening of symptoms and/or the emergence of suicidal thinking or behavior in both adults and children, whether or not they are taking antidepressants. Patients and caregivers should watch for any change in symptoms or any new symptoms that appear suddenly—especially agitation, anxiety, hostility, panic, restlessness, extreme hyperactivity, and suicidal thinking or behavior—and report them to the doctor immediately. Be especially observant at the beginning of treatment or whenever there is a change in dose.

Pamelor may cause patients to become drowsy or less alert. They should not drive, operate dangerous machinery, or participate in any hazardous activity that requires full mental alertness until they know how this drug affects them.

Pamelor should be used with caution in people who have a history of seizures, difficulty urinating, diabetes, or chronic eye conditions such as glaucoma. Caution is also warranted with patients who have heart disease, high blood pressure, or an overactive thyroid, and with those who are receiving thyroid medication.

If a patient is being treated for a severe mental disorder (schizophrenia or manic depression), the doctor should be made aware of this before Pamelor therapy begins.

Pamelor may make the skin more sensitive to sunlight. Patients should stay out of the sun, wear protective clothing, and apply a sunblock.

Before any surgery, dental treatment, or diagnostic procedure is undertaken, the doctor should be informed that the patient is taking Pamelor. Certain drugs used during these procedures, such as anesthetics and muscle relaxants, may interact with Pamelor.

Pamelor may intensify the effects of alcohol. Patients should avoid alcohol while taking this medication.

Possible food and drug interactions when taking this medication

See the entry for the generic name nortriptyline on page 363.

Special information about pregnancy and breastfeeding

The effects of Pamelor during pregnancy have not been adequately studied. Patients who are pregnant or planning to become pregnant should inform their doctor immediately. The doctor should also be consulted about breastfeeding.

Recommended dosage

This medication is available in tablet and liquid form. Only tablet dosages are listed. For liquid dosages, check with the doctor.

ADULTS

Doctors monitor response to this medication carefully, and gradually increase or decrease the dose to suit the patient's needs. Some doctors use blood tests to help determine the ideal dose.

The usual starting dosage is 25 milligrams, 3 or 4 times per day. Alternatively, the doctor may instruct that the total daily dose be taken once a day. Doses above 150 milligrams per day are not recommended.

CHILDREN

The safety and effectiveness of Pamelor have not been established for children and its use is not recommended. However, adolescents may be given 30 to 50 milligrams per day, either in a single dose or divided into smaller doses, as determined by the doctor.

OLDER ADULTS

The usual dose is 30 to 50 milligrams taken in a single dose or divided into smaller doses, as determined by the doctor.

Overdosage

An overdose of this type of antidepressant can be fatal. If an overdose is suspected, seek medical help immediately.

- *Symptoms of Pamelor overdose may include:*
  Agitation, coma, confusion, congestive heart failure, convulsions, dilated pupils, disturbed concentration, drowsiness, excessive reflexes, extremely high fever, fluid in the lungs, hallucinations, irregular heartbeat, low body temperature, restlessness, rigid muscles, severely low blood pressure, shock, stupor, vomiting

---

PARNATE

Tranylcypromine sulfate

Why is this drug prescribed?

Parnate is prescribed for the treatment of major depression. A member of the class of drugs known as monoamine oxidase (MAO) inhibitors, it works by increasing concentrations of the brain chemicals epinephrine, norepinephrine, and serotonin.

Most important fact about this drug

Parnate is a potent drug with the capability of producing serious side effects. It is typically prescribed only if other antidepressants fail, and then only for adults who are under close medical supervision. It is considered especially risky because it can interact with a long list of drugs and foods to produce life-threatening side effects (see "Possible food and drug interactions when taking this medication").

How should this medication be taken?

Dosage is adjusted according to the patient's individual needs and response. The drug usually produces improvement within 48 hours to 3 weeks after starting therapy.

- *Missed dose...*
  Generally, the forgotten dose should be taken as soon as remembered. However, if it is within 2 hours of the next dose, the missed dose should be skipped and the patient should return to the regular schedule. Doses should never be doubled.

- *Storage instructions...*
  Parnate should be stored at room temperature.

What side effects may occur?
Side effects cannot be predicted. If any develop or change in intensity, patients should inform their doctor as soon as possible.

* *Side effects may include:*
Blood disorders, diarrhea, dizziness, drowsiness, dry mouth, insomnia, muscle spasm, nausea, overstimulation, rapid or irregular heartbeat, restlessness, ringing in the ears, water retention, weakness, weight loss

Why should this drug not be prescribed?
Parnate should be avoided by anyone in danger of a stroke; by those who have heart or liver disease, high blood pressure, or a history of headaches; by individuals who have a type of tumor known as pheochromocytoma; and by anyone who will be undergoing elective surgery requiring general anesthesia.

Special warnings about this medication
In clinical studies, antidepressants increased the risk of suicidal thinking and behavior in children and adolescents with depression and other psychiatric disorders. Anyone considering the use of Parnate, or any other antidepressant in a child or adolescent, must balance the risk with the clinical need. Parnate is not approved for use in children.

Additionally, the progression of major depression is associated with a worsening of symptoms and/or the emergence of suicidal thinking or behavior in both adults and children, whether or not they are taking antidepressants. Patients and caregivers should watch for any change in symptoms or any new symptoms that appear suddenly—especially agitation, anxiety, hostility, panic, restlessness, extreme hyperactivity, and suicidal thinking or behavior—and report them to the doctor immediately. Be especially observant at the beginning of treatment or whenever there is a change in dose.

The most dangerous reaction to Parnate is a surge in blood pressure, which has sometimes been fatal. For this reason, patients should report promptly to their doctor any of the following symptoms: constriction or pain in the throat or chest, dizziness, fever, headache, irregular heartbeat, light sensitivity, nausea, neck stiffness or soreness, palpitations, pupil dilation, sweating, or vomiting.

A number of people who take Parnate experience low blood pressure, faintness, or drowsiness. Great care should be exercised when performing potentially hazardous tasks, such as driving a car or operating machinery.

Some people become physically dependent on Parnate and experience withdrawal symptoms when the drug is stopped, including restlessness, anxiety, depression, confusion, hallucinations, headache, weakness, and diarrhea.

If the patient has kidney problems, the doctor should be made aware of it. The doctor may need to reduce the dosage of Parnate to avoid a buildup of the drug. Parnate should also be used with caution by people who have an overactive thyroid gland.

MAO inhibitors can suppress heart pain that would otherwise serve as a warning sign of a heart attack. For this reason and others, Parnate should be used with caution by older adults. Also, it should be used with caution by diabetics and people with epilepsy or other convulsive disorders because it can alter the level of drugs used to treat these conditions.

While taking Parnate, patients should also avoid foods that contain a high amount of a substance called tyramine, including:

Anchovies
Avocado
Beer (including alcohol-free or reduced-alcohol beer)
Caffeine (in excessive amounts)
Caviar
Cheese (except for cottage cheese and cream cheese)
Chocolate (in excessive amounts)
Dry sausage (including Genoa salami, hard salami, pepperoni, and
  Lebanon bologna)
Fava bean pods
Liver
Meat extracts or meat prepared with tenderizers
Pickled herring
Pickled, fermented, aged, or smoked meat, fish, or dairy products
Sauerkraut
Soy sauce
Sour cream
Spoiled or improperly stored meat, fish, or dairy products
Wine (including alcohol-free or reduced-alcohol wine)
Yeast extract (including large amounts of brewer's yeast)
Yogurt

Likewise, patients taking Parnate should avoid alcohol and large amounts of caffeine.

Possible food and drug interactions when taking this medication
See the entry for the generic name tranylcypromine on page 403.

Special information about pregnancy and breastfeeding
Patients who are pregnant or plan to become pregnant should inform their doctor immediately. Parnate should be used during pregnancy only if its benefits outweigh potential risks.

Parnate makes its way into breast milk. If the drug is essential to the patient's health, the doctor may advise her to stop nursing until her treatment is finished.

Recommended dosage

ADULTS

The usual dosage is 30 milligrams per day, divided into smaller doses. If ineffective, the dosage may be slowly increased under the doctor's supervision to a maximum of 60 milligrams per day.

Overdosage

Any medication taken in excess can have serious consequences. If an overdose of Parnate is suspected, seek medical help immediately.

- *Symptoms of Parnate overdose may include:*
  Agitation, confusion, coma, dizziness, drowsiness, high fever, incoherence, rigid muscles, severe headache, twitching, weakness

Paroxetine *See Paxil, page 157*

PAXIL

Paroxetine hydrochloride
Other brand names: Paxil CR, Pexeva (paroxetine mesylate)

Why is this drug prescribed?

Paxil and Pexeva relieve a variety of emotional problems. These medications can be prescribed for major depressive disorder, obsessive-compulsive disorder (OCD), panic disorder, and generalized anxiety disorder. Paxil is also prescribed for social anxiety disorder (also known as social phobia), and post-traumatic stress disorder.

Paxil CR, the controlled-release version, is indicated for major depressive disorder, panic disorder, social anxiety disorder, and severe premenstrual symptoms classified as premenstrual dysphoric disorder.

Paxil belongs to the class of drugs known as selective serotonin reuptake inhibitors (SSRIs). Serotonin is one of the chemical messengers believed to govern moods. Ordinarily, it is quickly reabsorbed after its release at the junctures between nerves. Reuptake inhibitors such as Paxil slow this process, thereby boosting the levels of serotonin available in the brain.

Most important fact about this drug

Improvement may be noted within 1 to 4 weeks after treatment begins. Patients should continue taking the medication even if they begin to feel better.

How should this medication be taken?

Paxil is taken once a day, with or without food, usually in the morning. The oral suspension must be thoroughly shaken before each use. Paxil CR and Pexeva should be swallowed whole; they should not be chewed or crushed.

Pexeva is taken as one single daily dose with or without food, usually in the morning.

• *Missed dose...*
Patients should skip the forgotten dose and go back to their regular schedule with the next dose. They should not take a double dose to make up for the one they missed.

• *Storage instructions...*
Paxil tablets and suspension can be stored at room temperature. Pexeva should also be stored at room temperature and protected from humidity.

What side effects may occur?
Side effects cannot be predicted. If any develop or change in intensity, patients should inform their doctor as soon as possible.

During the first 4 to 6 weeks, patients may find some side effects less troublesome (nausea and dizziness, for example) than others (dry mouth, drowsiness, and weakness).

• *Side effects of Paxil may include:*
Constipation, decreased appetite, decreased libido, diarrhea, dizziness, dry mouth, ejaculation problems, impotence, insomnia, nausea, sleepiness, sweating, tremors, vomiting, weakness, yawning

• *Side effects of Paxil CR may include:*
Dry mouth, impaired concentration, nausea, sleepiness, weakness

• *Side effects of Pexeva may include:*
Abnormal ejaculation or ejaculatory disturbance and other male genital disorders, constipation, decreased appetite or libido, dizziness, dry mouth, female genital disorders, impotence, infection, insomnia, nausea, nervousness, sleepiness, sweating, tremor, weakness

Why should this drug not be prescribed?
Dangerous and even fatal reactions are possible when Paxil or Pexeva are combined with thioridazine or drugs classified as monoamine oxidase (MAO) inhibitors, such as the antidepressants Nardil and Parnate. Paxil or Pexeva must not be taken with any of these medications, or within 2 weeks of starting or stopping use of an MAO inhibitor. Paxil and Pexeva must also be avoided if it causes an allergic reaction.

Pexeva and Paxil must not be taken by patients who are taking pimozide.

Special warnings about this medication
In clinical studies, antidepressants increased the risk of suicidal thinking and behavior in children and adolescents with depression and other psychiatric disorders. Anyone considering the use of Paxil, or any other antidepressant in a child or adolescent, must balance the risk with the clinical need. Paxil and Pexeva are not approved for use in pediatric patients.

Additionally, the progression of major depression is associated with a worsening of symptoms and/or the emergence of suicidal thinking or behavior in both adults and children, whether or not they are taking anti-depressants. Patients and caregivers should watch for any change in symptoms or any new symptoms that appear suddenly—especially agitation, anxiety, hostility, panic, restlessness, extreme hyperactivity, and suicidal thinking or behavior—and report them to the doctor immediately. Be especially observant at the beginning of treatment or whenever there is a change in dose.

SSRI antidepressants could potentially cause stomach bleeding, especially in older patients or those taking nonsteroidal anti-inflammatory drugs (NSAIDs) such as aspirin, ibuprofen (Advil, Motrin), naproxen (Aleve), and ketoprofen. Advise patients to consult their doctor before combining Paxil with NSAIDs or blood-thinning drugs.

Paxil should be used cautiously by people with a history of manic disorders and those with high pressure in the eyes (glaucoma). Caution is also warranted if the patient has a disease or condition that affects the metabolism or blood circulation.

If the patient has a history of seizures, the doctor should be informed about it. Paxil must be used with caution in this situation. If the patient develops seizures once therapy has begun, the drug should be discontinued.

Paxil may impair judgment, thinking, or motor skills. Patients should not drive, operate dangerous machinery, or participate in any hazardous activity that requires full mental alertness until they are sure the medication is not affecting them in this way.

It's best to avoid an abrupt discontinuation of Paxil therapy. It can lead to symptoms such as dizziness, abnormal dreams, and tingling sensations. To prevent such problems, the dosage is reduced gradually.

Remember that Paxil must never be combined with thioridazine, pimozide, or MAO inhibitors such as Nardil and Parnate, or taken within 2 weeks of starting or stopping an MAO inhibitor.

Because they have the same main ingredient, Pexeva should not be taken at the same time as Paxil or Paxil CR.

Possible food and drug interactions when taking this medication

See the entry for the generic name paroxetine on page 369.

Special information about pregnancy and breastfeeding

The effects of Paxil during pregnancy have not been adequately studied. There have been reports of serious complications in newborns who were exposed to Paxil late in the third trimester. Patients who are pregnant or plan to become pregnant should inform their doctor immediately.

Paxil and Pexeva appear in breast milk and could affect a nursing infant. If this medication is essential to the patient's health, the doctor may advise her to discontinue breastfeeding until her treatment with Paxil is finished.

Recommended dosage

The following indications and dosages are for adults. The safety and effectiveness of Paxil or Pexeva have not been established in children.

DEPRESSION

Paxil and Pexeva: The usual starting dose is 20 milligrams a day, taken as a single dose, usually in the morning. At intervals of at least 1 week, the dosage may be increased by 10 milligrams a day, up to a maximum of 50 milligrams a day.

Paxil CR: The recommended starting dose is 25 milligrams a day, usually taken in the morning. At intervals of at least 1 week, the dosage may be increased by 12.5 milligrams a day, up to a maximum of 62.5 milligrams a day.

OBSESSIVE-COMPULSIVE DISORDER

Paxil and Pexeva: The usual starting dose is 20 milligrams a day, typically taken in the morning. At intervals of at least 1 week, the dosage may be increased by 10 milligrams a day. The recommended long-term dosage is 40 milligrams daily. The maximum is 60 milligrams a day.

PANIC DISORDER

Paxil: The usual starting dose is 10 milligrams a day, taken in the morning. At intervals of 1 week or more, the dosage may be increased by 10 milligrams a day. The target dose is 40 milligrams daily; dosage should never exceed 60 milligrams.

Paxil CR: The recommended starting dose is 12.5 milligrams a day, usually taken in the morning. At intervals of at least 1 week, the dosage may be increased by 12.5 milligrams a day, up to a maximum of 75 milligrams a day.

GENERALIZED ANXIETY DISORDER

Paxil and Pexeva: The recommended dose is 20 milligrams taken once a day, usually in the morning.

SOCIAL ANXIETY DISORDER

Paxil: The recommended dose is 20 milligrams taken once a day, usually in the morning.

Paxil CR: The recommended starting dose is 12.5 milligrams a day, usually taken in the morning. At intervals of at least 1 week, the dosage may be increased by 12.5 milligrams a day, up to a maximum of 37.5 milligrams a day.

POST-TRAUMATIC STRESS DISORDER

Paxil: The recommended dose is 20 milligrams taken once a day, usually in the morning.

PREMENSTRUAL DYSPHORIC DISORDER

Paxil CR: The recommended starting dose is 12.5 milligrams a day, usually taken in the morning. The doctor will instruct the patient to take the dose either every day of the month or only during the 2 weeks before menstruation begins (the luteal phase of her cycle). If needed, the dose can be increased to 25 milligrams a day.

DOSAGE ADJUSTMENT

For older adults, the weak, and those with severe kidney or liver disease: Starting doses of Paxil and Pexeva are reduced to 10 milligrams daily, and later doses are limited to no more than 40 milligrams a day. Starting doses of Paxil CR are limited to 12.5 milligrams daily, and later doses are limited to no more than 50 milligrams a day.

Overdosage

Any medication taken in excess can have serious consequences. If an overdose is suspected, seek medical attention immediately.

- *Symptoms of Paxil overdose may include:*
  Coma, dizziness, drowsiness, facial flushing, nausea, sweating, tremor, vomiting

- *Symptoms of Pexeva overdose may include:*
  Coma, confusion, dizziness, nausea, rapid heartbeat, sleepiness, tremor, vomiting

PERPHENAZINE

Why is this drug prescribed?

Perphenazine is used to treat schizophrenia and to control severe nausea and vomiting in adults. It is a member of the phenothiazine family of antipsychotic medications, which includes such drugs as thioridazine, chlorpromazine, and trifluoperazine.

Most important fact about this drug

Perphenazine can cause tardive dyskinesia, a condition marked by involuntary muscle spasms and twitches in the face and body, including chewing movements, puckering, puffing the cheeks, and sticking out the tongue. This condition may be permanent and appears to be most common among older adults, especially women.

How should this medication be taken?

Perphenazine should be taken exactly according to physician instructions and for no longer than necessary.

• *Missed dose...*

If a patient takes one dose of perphenazine a day, they should take the missed dose as soon as they remember, then go back to the regular schedule the next day. If the patient does not remember until the next day, then they should skip the missed dose and take only the next regularly scheduled dose.

If a patient takes perphenazine on a regular schedule several times a day, they should take the missed dose within 1 hour of its regular time. If more than 1 hour has passed, they should skip the missed dose and take only the next regularly scheduled dose. Doses should never be doubled.

• *Storage instructions...*

This medication should be kept in the container it came in, tightly closed, and out of reach of children. Perphenazine should be stored at room temperature and away from excessive heat and moisture.

What side effects may occur?

Side effects cannot be predicted. If any develop or change in intensity, patients should inform their doctor as soon as possible.

• *Side effects may include:*

Aching or numbness of the limbs, brain swelling, breast milk production, diarrhea, drowsiness, dry mouth, low blood pressure upon standing, nausea, rapid or irregular heartbeat, restlessness, salivation, seizures, vomiting

Why should this drug not be prescribed?

People who are comatose or who are at reduced levels of consciousness or alertness should not take perphenazine. Nor should those who are taking large amounts of any substance that slows brain function, including barbiturates, alcohol, narcotics, pain killers, and antihistamines.

Perphenazine should also be avoided by people who have blood disorders, bone marrow problems, liver problems, or brain damage. It cannot be taken by anyone who is hypersensitive to its ingredients or to related drugs.

Special warnings about this medication

Drugs such as perphenazine are capable of triggering a potentially fatal condition known as neuroleptic malignant syndrome. Symptoms include high fever, muscle rigidity, altered mental status, unstable blood pressure, a rapid or irregular heartbeat, and excessive sweating. If any of these symptoms develop, patients should see their doctor immediately. Perphenazine therapy will need to be discontinued.

Any significant increase in body temperature should also be reported to the doctor. It could be an early warning that the drug cannot be tolerated.

Patients should alert their physician before taking perphenazine if they are going through alcohol withdrawal, suffer from convulsions or seizures, or have a depressive disorder. They will have to use the drug with caution. Patients taking an anticonvulsant agent as well as perphenazine may need to have their anticonvulsant dosage increased.

Perphenazine should also be used with caution by anyone who has a history of eye disorders such as glaucoma; difficulty urinating; breast cancer; breathing problems; or heart, liver, kidney, or thyroid disease. Caution is also advised if the patient is exposed to extreme heat or pesticides. Be aware that perphenazine may mask signs of brain tumor, intestinal blockage, and overdose of other drugs.

Perphenazine should be used cautiously in people who are severely depressed and may be at risk for suicide. Patients should be watched closely for signs of suicidal thoughts and behavior. The doctor will prescribe the lowest amount of drug possible to avoid the risk of overdose.

While taking this medication, patients may feel dizzy or light-headed or actually faint when getting up from a lying or sitting position. If getting up more slowly doesn't help or if the problem continues, patients should alert the doctor.

Perphenazine could make patients more sensitive to sunlight. Encourage them to stay out of the sun, wear protective clothing, and use sunblock.

Patients should tell the doctor or dentist they're taking perphenazine before having any surgery, dental work, or diagnostic procedure. Perphenazine could interact with anesthetics, muscle relaxants, and other drugs used during surgical procedures.

Perphenazine may impair the mental or physical abilities needed to drive a car or operate heavy machinery. Patients should not participate in any activities that require full alertness until they know how this drug affects them.

Stomach inflammation, dizziness, nausea, vomiting, and tremors may result if perphenazine is stopped suddenly. Therapy should be discontinued only under a doctor's supervision.

Perphenazine is not recommended for children under the age of 12 years.

Extreme drowsiness and other potentially serious effects can result if perphenazine is combined with alcohol or other central nervous system depressants such as narcotics, painkillers, and sleep medications. Perphenazine should also be used with caution in patients who are taking atropine or related drugs.

Caution should also be observed in giving perphenazine to patients who have had severe adverse reactions to other phenothiazines in the past.

Possible food and drug interactions when taking this medication
See the entry for perphenazine on page 372.

Special information about pregnancy and breastfeeding
Perphenazine may cause false-positive results on pregnancy tests. Patients who are pregnant or planning to become pregnant should tell their doctor immediately. The safe use of perphenazine during pregnancy has not been established. The possible benefits of using this medication must be weighed against the possible hazards to the mother and child.

Drugs similar to perphenazine appear in breast milk. If this medication is essential to the patient's health, the doctor may advise her to avoid breastfeeding until her treatment is finished.

Recommended dosage
The dosage of perphenazine is adjusted according to the severity of the condition and the drug's effect. Doctors aim for the lowest effective dose.

SCHIZOPHRENIA

The usual initial dosage of perphenazine tablets is 4 to 8 milligrams 3 times daily, up to a maximum daily dose of 24 milligrams. Hospitalized patients are usually given 8 to 16 milligrams 2 to 4 times daily, up to a maximum daily dose of 64 milligrams.

SEVERE NAUSEA AND VOMITING IN ADULTS

For this problem, the usual dosage of perphenazine tablets is 8 to 16 milligrams daily divided into smaller doses. Up to 24 milligrams daily is occasionally necessary.

Overdosage
Anyone suspected of having taken an overdose of perphenazine should be hospitalized immediately for emergency treatment.

• *Usual symptoms of perphenazine overdose include:*
  Stupor, coma, convulsions (in children)

Pexeva *See Paxil, page 157*

Phenelzine *See Nardil, page 133*

PHENERGAN
Promethazine hydrochloride

Why is this drug prescribed?
Phenergan is an antihistamine. Because antihistamines of this type cause drowsiness, the drug is used as a sedative and sleep aid for both children and adults.

Like other antihistamines, Phenergan is also prescribed to relieve the nasal stuffiness and red, inflamed eyes caused by hay fever and other allergies. It is used to treat itching, swelling, and redness from hives and other rashes; allergic reactions to blood transfusions; and, with other medications, anaphylactic shock (severe allergic reaction). It is prescribed to prevent and control nausea and vomiting before and after surgery, and to prevent and treat motion sickness. It is also used, with other medications, for pain after surgery.

Antihistamines work by decreasing the effects of histamine, a chemical the body releases in response to certain irritants. Histamine narrows air passages in the lungs and contributes to inflammation. Antihistamines reduce itching and swelling and dry up secretions from the nose, eyes, and throat.

Most important fact about this drug

Because Phenergan may cause considerable drowsiness, patients should not drive, operate dangerous machinery, or participate in any hazardous activity that requires full mental alertness until they know how they react to Phenergan. Children should be carefully supervised while they are bike-riding, roller-skating, or playing until the drug's effect on them is established.

How should this medication be taken?

Phenergan should be taken exactly as prescribed.

- *Missed dose...*
  If Phenergan is being taken on a regular schedule, the forgotten dose should be taken as soon as remembered. If it is almost time for the next dose, patients should skip the dose they missed and go back to their regular schedule. Doses should never be doubled.

- *Storage instructions...*
  Tablets should be stored at room temperature, away from light. Suppositories should be stored in the refrigerator, in a tightly closed container.

What side effects may occur?

Side effects cannot be predicted. If any develop or change in intensity, patients should inform their doctor as soon as possible.

- *Side effects may include:*
  Blurred vision, dizziness, drowsiness, dry mouth, increased or decreased blood pressure, nausea, rash, sedation, vomiting

Why should this drug not be prescribed?

Phenergan should be avoided by anyone who has ever had an allergic reaction to it or to related medications, such as Thorazine, thioridazine, Stelazine, or Prolixin. Phenergan is not for use in comatose patients, and should not be used to treat asthma or other breathing problems.

Special warnings about this medication

If the patient is taking other medications that cause sedation, the doctor may reduce the dosage of these medications or eliminate them during Phenergan therapy.

In people who have a seizure disorder, Phenergan may cause seizures to occur more often.

Phenergan can cause a serious—even fatal—decline in the breathing function. This medication should be avoided by people with chronic breathing problems such as emphysema, and those who suffer from sleep apnea (periods during sleep when breathing stops).

Phenergan can also cause a potentially fatal condition called neuroleptic malignant syndrome. Symptoms include high fever, rigid muscles, sweating, and a rapid or irregular heartbeat. Patients who develop these symptoms should stop taking Phenergan and see their doctor immediately.

Phenergan should be used with caution by anyone who has heart disease, high blood pressure or circulatory problems, liver problems, the eye condition called narrow-angle glaucoma, peptic ulcer or other abdominal obstructions, or urinary bladder obstruction due to an enlarged prostate.

Phenergan may affect the results of pregnancy tests and can raise blood sugar.

Some people have developed jaundice (yellow eyes and skin) while on this medication.

The doctor should be notified if the patient develops any uncontrolled movements or seems to be unusually sensitive to sunlight.

Remember that Phenergan can cause drowsiness.

Phenergan should not be given to children under 2 years of age, and should be used with caution in older children, due to the danger of impaired breathing. Large doses have been known to cause hallucinations, seizures, and sudden death, especially in children who are dehydrated. Drugs such as Phenergan are not recommended for the treatment of vomiting in children unless the problem is severe. Phenergan should also be avoided if the child has the serious neurological disease known as Reye's syndrome or any disease of the liver.

Phenergan may increase the effects of alcohol. Patients should avoid alcohol, or at least substantially reduce the amount they drink, while taking this medication.

Possible food and drug interactions when taking this medication

See the entry for the generic name promethazine on page 387.

Special information about pregnancy and breastfeeding

The effects of Phenergan during pregnancy have not been adequately studied. If the patient is pregnant or plans to become pregnant, she should inform her doctor immediately.

Although it is not known whether Phenergan appears in breast milk, there is a chance that it could cause a nursing infant serious harm. The use of Phenergan is not recommended during breastfeeding.

Recommended dosage

Phenergan is available in tablet, syrup, and suppository form. The suppositories are for rectal use only. Phenergan tablets and suppositories are not recommended for children under 2 years of age.

ALLERGY

Adults: The average oral dose is 25 milligrams taken before bed; however, your doctor may have you take 12.5 milligrams before meals and before bed.

Children: The usual dose is a single 25-milligram dose at bedtime or 6.25 to 12.5 milligrams 3 times daily.

INSOMNIA

Adults: The usual dose is 25 to 50 milligrams for nighttime sedation.

Children: The usual dose is 12.5 to 25 milligrams by tablets or rectal suppository at bedtime.

Older Adults: The dosage is usually reduced for people over 60.

MOTION SICKNESS

Adults: The average adult dose is 25 milligrams taken twice daily. The first dose should be taken one-half to 1 hour before the patient plans to travel, and the second dose 8 to 12 hours later, if necessary. On travel days after that, the recommended dose is 25 milligrams upon arising and again before the evening meal.

Children: The usual dose of Phenergan tablets, syrup, or rectal suppositories is 12.5 to 25 milligrams taken twice a day.

NAUSEA AND VOMITING

The average dose of Phenergan for nausea and vomiting in children or adults is 25 milligrams. When oral medication cannot be tolerated, use the rectal suppository. The doctor may prescribe 12.5 to 25 milligrams every 4 to 6 hours, if necessary.

For nausea and vomiting in children, the dose is usually calculated at 0.5 milligram per pound of body weight and will also be based on the age of the child and the severity of the condition being treated. Phenergan and other antivomiting drugs should not be given to children if the cause of the problem is unknown.

Overdosage
Any medication taken in excess can have serious consequences. An overdose of Phenergan can be fatal. If an overdose is suspected, seek medical treatment immediately.

* *Symptoms of Phenergan overdose may include:*
  Difficulty breathing, dry mouth, fixed and dilated pupils, flushing, heightened reflexes, loss of consciousness, muscle tension, poor coordination, seizures, slowdown in brain activity, slowed heartbeat, stomach and intestinal problems, very low blood pressure, writhing movements

Children may become overstimulated and have nightmares. Older adults may also become overstimulated.

PHENOBARBITAL

Why is this drug prescribed?
Phenobarbital, a barbiturate, is used as a sleep aid and to treat certain types of epilepsy, including generalized or grand mal seizures and partial seizures.

Most important fact about this drug
Phenobarbital can be habit-forming. One can become tolerant (needing more and more of the drug to achieve the same effect) and physically and psychologically dependent with continued use. Patients should never increase the amount of phenobarbital they take without first checking with their doctor.

How should this medication be taken?
It is important to take this medication exactly as prescribed.
  Patients taking phenobarbital for seizures should not discontinue it abruptly.

* *Missed dose...*
  Generally, a forgotten dose should be taken as soon as remembered. However, if it is almost time for the next dose, patients should skip the dose they missed and go back to their regular schedule. Doses should never be doubled.

* *Storage instructions...*
  Phenobarbital should be stored at room temperature in a tightly closed container.

What side effects may occur?
Side effects cannot be predicted. If any develop or change in intensity, patients should notify their doctor as soon as possible.

* *Side effects may include:*
  Allergic reaction, drowsiness, headache, lethargy, nausea, oversedation, sleepiness, slowed or delayed breathing, vertigo, vomiting

Why should this drug not be prescribed?

Phenobarbital should not be used by anyone suffering from porphyria (an inherited metabolic disorder), liver disease, or a lung disease that causes blockages or breathing difficulties, or by anyone who has ever had an allergic reaction to or is sensitive to phenobarbital or other barbiturates.

Special warnings about this medication

Remember that phenobarbital may be habit-forming. It must be taken exactly as prescribed.

Phenobarbital should be used with extreme caution, or not at all, by people who are depressed or have a history of drug abuse.

Patients should tell the doctor if they are in pain, or if they have constant pain, before they take phenobarbital.

Phenobarbital may cause excitement, depression, or confusion in elderly or weakened individuals, and excitement in children.

People with liver disease or poorly functioning adrenal glands should use phenobarbital with extra caution.

Barbiturates such as phenobarbital can cause people to become tired or less alert. Patients should be careful driving, operating machinery, or doing any activity that requires full mental alertness until they know how they react to this medication.

Phenobarbital may increase the effects of alcohol. Patients should avoid alcoholic beverages while taking phenobarbital.

Possible food and drug interactions when taking this medication

See the entry for phenobarbital on page 382.

Special information about pregnancy and breastfeeding

Barbiturates such as phenobarbital may cause damage to the developing baby during pregnancy. Withdrawal symptoms may occur in an infant whose mother took barbiturates during the last 3 months of pregnancy. Patients who are pregnant or plan to become pregnant should inform their doctor immediately.

Phenobarbital appears in breast milk and could affect a nursing infant. If phenobarbital is essential to the patient's health, the doctor may advise her to stop breastfeeding until her treatment is finished.

Recommended dosage

The following indications and dosages are for adults unless otherwise noted.

SEDATION

The usual initial dose of phenobarbital is a single dose of 30 to 120 milligrams. The doctor may repeat this dose at intervals, depending on the patient's response to this medication. The maximum amount allowable during a 24-hour period is 400 milligrams.

DAYTIME SEDATION

The usual dose is 30 to 120 milligrams a day, divided into 2 to 3 doses.

TO INDUCE SLEEP

The usual dose is 100 to 200 milligrams.

ANTICONVULSANT USE

Adults: Phenobarbital dosage must be individualized on the basis of specific laboratory tests. The usual dose is 60 to 200 milligrams daily.

Children: The phenobarbital dosage must be individualized on the basis of specific laboratory tests. The usual dose is 3 to 6 milligrams per 2.2 pounds (1 kilogram) of body weight per day.

DOSAGE ADJUSTMENT

For all indications, the doctor will need to prescribe a lower dosage for older adults, the weak, and those with liver or kidney disease.

Overdosage

Barbiturate overdose can be fatal. If an overdose is suspected, seek medical treatment immediately.

- *Symptoms of phenobarbital overdose may include:*
  Congestive heart failure, diminished breathing, extremely low body temperature, fluid in lungs, involuntary eyeball movements, irregular heartbeat, kidney failure, lack of muscle coordination, low blood pressure, poor reflexes, skin reddening or bloody blisters, slowdown of the central nervous system

---

PROCHLORPERAZINE

Why is this drug prescribed?

Prochlorperazine is used to treat symptoms of mental disorders such as schizophrenia, and is occasionally prescribed for anxiety. It is also used to control severe nausea and vomiting.

Most important fact about this drug

Prochlorperazine may cause tardive dyskinesia—involuntary muscle spasms and twitches in the face and body. This condition may be permanent. It appears to be most common among the elderly, especially women. Patients should see their doctor immediately at the first sign of this problem (spasms in the tongue may be an early warning). Antipsychotic medications usually must be discontinued if these symptoms appear.

How should this medication be taken?

Patients should never take more prochlorperazine than prescribed. Doing so can increase the risk of serious side effects.

If patients are using the suppository form of prochlorperazine and find it is too soft to insert, they can chill it in the refrigerator for about 30 minutes or run cold water over it before removing the wrapper.

To insert a suppository, patients should first remove the wrapper and moisten the suppository with cold water. They should then lie down on their side and use a finger to push the suppository well up into the rectum.

- *Missed dose...*
  Generally, the forgotten dose should be taken as soon as remembered. However, if it is almost time for the next dose, patients should skip the dose they missed and go back to their regular schedule. Doses should never be doubled.

- *Storage instructions...*
  Prochlorperazine should be stored at room temperature and protected from heat and light.

What side effects may occur?

Side effects cannot be predicted. If any develop or change in intensity, patients should inform their doctor as soon as possible.

- *Side effects may include:*
  Blurred vision, dizziness, drowsiness, jaundice, low blood pressure, menstrual irregularities, neuroleptic malignant syndrome (see "Special warnings about this medication"), skin reactions

Why should this drug not be prescribed?

Prochlorperazine must be avoided by anyone who is sensitive to or has ever had an allergic reaction to prochlorperazine or other phenothiazine drugs such as chlorpromazine, Prolixin, amitriptyline with perphenazine, thioridazine, or trifluoperazine.

Prochlorperazine should not be given to children who are undergoing surgery.

Special warnings about this medication

Patients should never take large amounts of alcohol, barbiturates, or narcotics when taking prochlorperazine. Serious problems can result.

If prochlorperazine is stopped suddenly, patients may experience a change in appetite, dizziness, nausea, vomiting, and tremors. Therapy should be discontinued only under a doctor's supervision.

Prochlorperazine should be used with caution if the patient is being treated for a brain tumor, intestinal blockage, heart disease, breast cancer, seizures, glaucoma, or an abnormal bone marrow or blood condition such as leukemia. Caution is also advised if the patient is exposed to pesticides or extreme heat.

Due to its ability to prevent vomiting, prochlorperazine can mask symptoms of an overdose of other drugs. It could also mask symptoms of brain tumor, intestinal blockage, and the neurological condition known as Reye's syndrome.

Prochlorperazine should be used cautiously in children suffering from dehydration or an acute illness such as chickenpox, measles, or other infection. The drug should be avoided altogether in children and adolescents who have symptoms that could indicate Reye's syndrome, including persistent or recurrent vomiting, listlessness, irritability, combativeness, and disorientation.

Prochlorperazine can cause a potentially fatal group of symptoms called neuroleptic malignant syndrome. Symptoms include extremely high body temperature, rigid muscles, mental changes, irregular pulse or blood pressure, rapid heartbeat, excessive sweating, and changes in heart rhythm. The doctor should be alerted immediately if these symptoms develop. Prochlorperazine therapy will need to be discontinued.

This drug may impair the ability to drive a car or operate potentially dangerous machinery. Patients should avoid any activities that require full alertness if they are unsure about their ability.

Patients should try to stay out of the sun while taking prochlorperazine. They should use sunblock and wear protective clothing. Their eyes may become more sensitive to sunlight, too, so they should keep sunglasses handy.

Prochlorperazine interferes with the body's ability to shed extra heat. Caution is warranted in hot weather.

Patients taking prochlorperazine for a prolonged period should see their doctor for regular evaluations, since side effects can get worse over time.

Prochlorperazine may cause false-positive phenylketonuria (PKU) tests.

Possible food and drug interactions when taking this medication

See the entry for prochlorperazine on page 385.

Special information about pregnancy and breastfeeding

Prochlorperazine is not usually recommended for pregnant women, although it is sometimes prescribed for severe nausea and vomiting if the potential benefits of the drug outweigh the potential risks.

Prochlorperazine appears in breast milk and may affect a nursing infant. If this drug is essential to a woman's health, her doctor may recommend that she stop breastfeeding until her treatment is finished.

Recommended dosage

The following dosages are for adults unless otherwise noted.

NONPSYCHOTIC ANXIETY

Tablets: The usual dose is 5 milligrams, taken 3 or 4 times a day.

Treatment should not continue for longer than 12 weeks, and daily doses should not exceed 20 milligrams.

SCHIZOPHRENIA

Relatively Mild Symptoms: The usual dose is 5 or 10 milligrams, taken 3 or 4 times daily.

Moderate to Severe Symptoms: Dosages usually start at 10 milligrams, taken 3 or 4 times a day. If needed, the dosage may be gradually increased; 50 to 75 milligrams daily has been helpful for some people.

Very Severe Symptoms: Dosages may range from 100 to 150 milligrams per day.

SEVERE NAUSEA AND VOMITING

Tablets: The usual dosage is one 5- or 10-milligram tablet 3 or 4 times a day.

The usual rectal dosage (suppository) is 25 milligrams, taken 2 times a day.

SCHIZOPHRENIA IN CHILDREN

Children 2 to 5 Years Old: The starting oral or rectal dose is 2.5 milligrams 2 or 3 times daily. Do not exceed 10 milligrams the first day and 20 milligrams thereafter.

Children 6 to 12 Years Old: The starting oral or rectal dose is 2.5 milligrams 2 or 3 times daily. Do not exceed 10 milligrams the first day and 25 milligrams thereafter.

SEVERE NAUSEA AND VOMITING IN CHILDREN

An oral or rectal dose of prochlorperazine is usually not needed for more than 1 day.

Children 20 to 29 Pounds: The usual dose is 2.5 milligrams 1 or 2 times daily. Total daily amount should not exceed 7.5 milligrams.

Children 30 to 39 Pounds: The usual dose is 2.5 milligrams 2 or 3 times daily. Total daily amount should not exceed 10 milligrams.

Children 40 to 85 Pounds: The usual dose is 2.5 milligrams 3 times daily, or 5 milligrams 2 times daily. Total daily amount should not exceed 15 milligrams.

NOTE: Children under 2 years of age or weighing less than 20 pounds should not be given prochlorperazine. If a child becomes restless or excited after taking prochlorperazine, the child should not get another dose.

DOSAGE ADJUSTMENT

In general, weak or older patients take lower dosages of prochlorperazine. Because they may develop low blood pressure while taking the drug, the doctor should monitor them closely. Older people (especially women) may be more susceptible to tardive dyskinesia.

Overdosage

An overdose of prochlorperazine can be fatal. If an overdose is suspected, seek medical help immediately.

- *Symptoms of prochlorperazine overdose may include:*
  Agitation, coma, convulsions, dry mouth, extreme sleepiness, fever, intestinal blockage, irregular heart rate, restlessness

Promethazine *See Phenergan, page 164*

PROSOM
Estazolam

Why is this drug prescribed?

ProSom, a sleeping pill, is given for the short-term treatment of insomnia. Insomnia may involve difficulty falling asleep, frequent awakenings during the night, or too-early awakening in the morning.

Most important fact about this drug

As a chemical cousin of Valium and similar tranquilizers, ProSom is potentially addictive. It should be used only as a temporary sleeping aid. Even after relatively short-term use of ProSom, withdrawal symptoms may occur when the medication is stopped.

How should this medication be taken?

ProSom must be taken exactly as prescribed. A typical schedule is 1 tablet at bedtime. For small, physically run-down, or older people, one-half a tablet may be a safer starting dose.

Patients should avoid drinking alcoholic beverages while taking ProSom.

• *Missed dose...*
ProSom should be taken at bedtime only as needed. It is not necessary to make up a missed dose.

• *Storage instructions...*
ProSom should be stored at room temperature.

What side effects may occur?

Side effects cannot be predicted. If any develop or change in intensity, patients should inform their doctor as soon as possible.

• *Side effects may include:*
Abnormal coordination, constipation, decreased movement or activity, dizziness, dry mouth, general feeling of illness, hangover, headache, leg and foot pain, memory problems, nausea, nervousness, sleepiness, weakness

Why should this drug not be prescribed?

ProSom should not be taken by anyone who is sensitive or allergic to it, or by anyone who has ever had an adverse reaction to another Valium-type medication.

ProSom should not be taken by women who are pregnant or plan on becoming pregnant. Drugs in this class may cause damage to the unborn child.

Special warnings about this medication

Since ProSom may cloud thinking, impair judgment, or interfere with normal physical coordination, patients should not drive, climb, or perform hazardous tasks until they know their reaction to this medication. It is important to remember that a tablet taken in the evening may continue to have effects well into the following day.

People who are older or physically run-down, and those who have liver or kidney damage or breathing problems, are particularly vulnerable to side effects from ProSom. They should use this medication with special caution.

Patients with a history of seizures should not abruptly stop taking ProSom, even if they are taking antiseizure medication. Instead, they should taper off from ProSom under their doctor's supervision.

Even if a patient has never had a seizure, it is better to taper off from ProSom than to stop taking the medication abruptly. Experience suggests that tapering off can help prevent drug withdrawal symptoms.

Typically, the only withdrawal symptoms caused by ProSom are mild and temporary insomnia or irritability. Occasionally, however, withdrawal can involve considerable discomfort or even danger, with symptoms such as abdominal and muscle cramps, convulsions, sweating, tremors, and vomiting.

Patients should not drink alcohol while taking ProSom; this combination could make them comatose or dangerously slow their breathing.

For the same reason, it is unwise to combine ProSom with any other medication that might calm or slow the functioning of the central nervous system.

Smokers tend to process and eliminate ProSom fairly quickly compared with nonsmokers.

Possible food and drug interactions when taking this medication

See the entry for the generic name estazolam on page 321.

Special information about pregnancy and breastfeeding

ProSom should not be used during pregnancy; it could cause birth defects in the developing baby.

When a pregnant woman takes ProSom or a similar medication shortly before giving birth, her baby is likely to have poor muscle tone (flaccidity) and/or experience drug withdrawal symptoms.

Because ProSom is thought to pass into breast milk, this medication should not be used while breastfeeding.

Recommended dosage

ADULTS

The recommended initial dose is 1 milligram at bedtime. Some people may need a 2-milligram dose.

CHILDREN

There is no information on the safety and effectiveness of ProSom in people under age 18.

OLDER ADULTS

The recommended usual dosage for older adults is 1 milligram. Some may require only 0.5 milligram.

Overdosage

Any medication taken in excess can have serious consequences. If an overdose is suspected, seek medical attention immediately.

* *Symptoms of a ProSom overdose may include:*
  Confusion, depressed breathing, drowsiness and eventually coma, lack of coordination, slurred speech

Protriptyline *See Vivactil, page 248*

PROVIGIL
Modafinil

Why is this drug prescribed?
Provigil is a stimulant drug used to treat unusually sleepy people who have been diagnosed with narcolepsy, obstructive sleep apnea/hypopnea syndrome, or shift work sleep disorder. The patient should be medically diagnosed with one of these sleep disorders before taking Provigil, since sleepiness can be a symptom of other medical conditions.

Most important fact about this drug
Provigil will not cure any sleep disorder; it merely treats the symptoms of sleepiness. This medication should not be used in place of getting enough sleep. The patient should follow the doctor's advice about maintaining good sleep habits.

Provigil, like other stimulants, has the potential for abuse. It can alter mood, perception, thinking, and feelings, providing an artificial "lift" and potentially leading to a certain degree of dependence (although discontinuation of the drug does not produce physical withdrawal symptoms). Patients should take only the prescribed dose; they should never increase the dose or take additional doses.

How should this medication be taken?
Food does not reduce the effectiveness of this medication. However, it will delay the onset of action by approximately 1 hour.

- *Missed dose...*
  The forgotten dose should be taken as soon as possible. If it's not remembered until the next day, patients should skip the forgotten dose and go back to their regular schedule. Doses should never be doubled.

- *Storage instructions...*
  Provigil should be stored at room temperature.

What side effects may occur?
Side effects cannot be predicted. If any develop or change in intensity, patients should inform their doctor as soon as possible.

- *Side effects may include:*
  Anxiety, depression, diarrhea, difficulty sleeping, dizziness, dry mouth, headache, infection, loss of appetite, loss of muscle strength, lung problems, nausea, nervousness, prickling or tingling feeling, runny nose, sore throat

Why should this drug not be prescribed?
Provigil should be avoided by anyone who has ever had an allergic reaction to it.

Special warnings about this medication

Provigil should be used with caution by patients with high blood pressure, liver or kidney problems, or a history of psychosis or drug abuse. The doctor should know the patient's complete medical history before prescribing this drug.

Provigil should be avoided by people with certain types of heart problems such as mitral valve prolapse. Patients should tell the doctor about any heart problems they have before taking this drug.

Provigil may cause serious skin reactions, such as Stevens-Johnson syndrome (blisters on the skin, mouth, and eyes) and erythema multiforme (a type of herpes that may cause bumps or blisters).

Leukopenia (low white-blood-cell count) has been reported in pediatric patients taking Provigil.

Provigil may impair judgment, thinking, or motor skills. Patients should not drive a car or operate hazardous machinery until they know how this drug affects them. Likewise, patients should be aware that Provigil may not restore complete wakefulness in certain people.

Provigil may interfere with the effectiveness of oral and implantable contraceptives. Patients should use an additional method of contraception while taking Provigil and for 1 month after discontinuing it.

The effect of combining Provigil with alcohol has not been studied. It's best to avoid alcohol while taking this drug.

Possible food and drug interactions when taking this medication

See the entry for the generic name modafinil on page 358.

Special information about pregnancy and breastfeeding

The possibility of harmful effects during pregnancy has not been ruled out. Patients who are pregnant or plan to become pregnant should inform their doctor immediately. Provigil is recommended during pregnancy only if the need for therapy outweighs the potential risk.

It is not known whether Provigil appears in breast milk. If the patient is breastfeeding an infant, she should tell her doctor. Nursing mothers should use Provigil with caution and only when clearly needed.

Recommended dosage

ADULTS

The usual dose of Provigil is 200 milligrams taken as a single dose in the morning. Patients with shift work sleep disorder should take Provigil about 1 hour before their shift starts.

CHILDREN

Children younger than 16 years old should not use Provigil.

OLDER ADULTS

People over 65 may need a lower dose if they have liver or kidney disease, which reduces the body's ability to metabolize this medication.

Overdosage

Any medication taken in excess can have serious consequences. If an overdose is suspected, seek medical treatment immediately.

* *Symptoms of Provigil overdose may include:*
  Aggressiveness, agitation, anxiety, confusion, diarrhea, fluttering heartbeat, insomnia, irritability, nausea, nervousness, sleep disturbances, slow blood clotting, tremor

---

PROZAC

Fluoxetine hydrochloride
Other brand names: Prozac Weekly, Sarafem

Why is this drug prescribed?

Prozac is prescribed for the treatment of major depression, panic disorder, and obsessive-compulsive disorder. The drug is also used in the treatment of bulimia and has been used to treat other eating disorders and obesity. Prozac Weekly is approved for treating major depression.

In children and adolescents, Prozac is approved to treat major depression and obsessive-compulsive disorder.

Under the brand name Sarafem, the active ingredient in Prozac is also prescribed for the treatment of premenstrual dysphoric disorder (PMDD), a severe form of premenstrual syndrome (PMS). Symptoms of PMDD include mood problems such as anxiety, depression, irritability or persistent anger, mood swings, and tension. Physical problems that accompany PMDD include bloating, breast tenderness, headache, and joint and muscle pain. Symptoms typically begin 1 to 2 weeks before a woman's menstrual period and are severe enough to interfere with day-to-day activities and relationships.

Prozac belongs to the class of drugs called selective serotonin reuptake inhibitors (SSRIs). Serotonin is one of the chemical messengers believed to govern moods. Ordinarily, it is quickly reabsorbed after its release at the junctures between nerves. Reuptake inhibitors such as Prozac slow this process, thereby boosting the levels of serotonin available in the brain.

Most important fact about this drug

Serious, sometimes fatal, reactions have been known to occur when Prozac is used in combination with drugs known as MAO inhibitors, including the antidepressants Nardil and Parnate, and when Prozac is discontinued and an MAO inhibitor is started. Prozac should never be taken with one of these drugs or within at least 14 days of discontinuing therapy with one of them; and 5 weeks or more should be allowed between stopping Prozac and starting an MAO inhibitor. Caution is especially warranted if the patient has been taking Prozac in high doses or for a long time.

In addition, Prozac should never be combined with thioridazine due to the risk of life-threatening drug interactions; and a minimum of 5 weeks should be allowed between stopping Prozac and starting thioridazine.

Patients who are taking any prescription or nonprescription drugs should notify their doctor before taking Prozac.

How should this medication be taken?

Prozac should be taken exactly as prescribed. It usually is taken once or twice a day. To be effective, it should be taken regularly. Patients should make a habit of taking it at the same time they do some other daily activity.

It may be 4 weeks before a patient feels any relief from depression, but the drug's effects should last about 9 months after a 3-month treatment regimen. For obsessive-compulsive disorder, the full effect may take 5 weeks to appear.

* *Missed dose...*
  The forgotten dose should be taken as soon as the patient remembers. If several hours have passed, the dose should be skipped. Patients should never try to "catch up" by doubling the dose.

* *Storage instructions...*
  Prozac should be stored at room temperature.

What side effects may occur?

Side effects cannot be predicted. If any develop or change in intensity, patients should inform their doctor as soon as possible.

* *Side effects may include:*
  Abnormal dreams, abnormal ejaculation, abnormal vision, anxiety, diarrhea, diminished sex drive, dizziness, dry mouth, flu-like symptoms, flushing, gas, headache, impotence, insomnia, itching, loss of appetite, nausea, nervousness, rash, sinusitis, sleepiness, sore throat, sweating, tremor, upset stomach, vomiting, weakness, yawning

A wide variety of other very rare reactions have been reported during Prozac therapy. Patients who develop any new or unexplained symptoms should tell their doctor without delay.

Why should this drug not be prescribed?

This drug should be avoided by anyone who is sensitive to or has ever had an allergic reaction to it or to similar drugs such as Paxil and Zoloft. Remember, too, that Prozac should never be combined with thioridazine or an MAO inhibitor (see "Most important fact about this drug"). Likewise, do not start taking thioridazine within 5 weeks of stopping Prozac.

Special warnings about this medication

In clinical studies, antidepressants increased the risk of suicidal thinking and behavior in children and adolescents with depression and other psychiatric disorders. Anyone considering the use of Prozac, or any other antidepressant in a child or adolescent, must balance the risk with the clinical need. Prozac is approved for treating major depression in children 8 years and older and for treating obsessive-compulsive disorder in children 7 years and older.

Additionally, the progression of major depression is associated with a worsening of symptoms and/or the emergence of suicidal thinking or behavior in both adults and children, whether or not they are taking antidepressants. Patients and caregivers should watch for any change in symptoms or any new symptoms that appear suddenly—especially agitation, anxiety, hostility, panic, restlessness, extreme hyperactivity, and suicidal thinking or behavior—and report them to the doctor immediately. Be especially observant at the beginning of treatment or whenever there is a change in dose.

Antidepressants such as Prozac could potentially cause stomach bleeding, especially in older patients or those taking nonsteroidal anti-inflammatory drugs (NSAIDs) such as aspirin, ibuprofen (Advil, Motrin), naproxen (Aleve), and ketoprofen. Advise patients to consult their doctor before combining Prozac with NSAIDs or blood-thinning medications.

Unless the doctor directs, this medication should not be taken by anyone who is recovering from a heart attack or has liver disease or diabetes.

Prozac may cause patients to become drowsy or less alert and may affect their judgment. Therefore, driving, operating dangerous machinery, or participating in any hazardous activity that requires full mental alertness is not recommended.

While taking this medication, some people may feel dizzy or light-headed or actually faint when getting up from a lying or sitting position. If getting up slowly doesn't help, or if this problem continues, the doctor should be notified.

Patients who develop a skin rash or hives while taking Prozac should discontinue use of the medication and notify the doctor immediately.

Prozac should be used with caution if the patient has a history of mania or seizures. All the patient's medical conditions should be discussed with the doctor before this medication is taken.

Prozac can occasionally cause decreased appetite and weight loss, especially in depressed people who are already underweight and in those with bulimia. The doctor should be alerted if the patient has a significant change in weight or appetite.

There have been rare reports of prolonged seizures in patients who received electroconvulsive therapy (ECT) while taking Prozac. To date, there are no clinical studies establishing the benefit of combined treatment with Prozac and ECT.

As with other SSRIs, Prozac therapy should be slowly tapered instead of abruptly stopped. If abruptly discontinued, drowsiness, irritability, agitation, anxiety, headache, and insomnia may occur.

Remember that combining Prozac with thioridazine or MAO inhibitors is dangerous. Alcohol should also be avoided by people on Prozac.

Possible food and drug interactions when taking this medication

See the entry for the generic name fluoxetine on page 322.

Special information about pregnancy and breastfeeding

The effects of Prozac during pregnancy have not been adequately studied. Patients who are pregnant or plan to become pregnant should inform their doctor immediately. There have been reports of newborns experiencing complications such as respiratory problems, bluish coloring of the skin, irregular breathing, muscular problems, vomiting, and constant crying after exposure to Prozac late in the third trimester.

This medication appears in breast milk, and breastfeeding is not recommended during Prozac therapy.

Recommended dosage

DEPRESSION

It may take 4 weeks before the full antidepressant effect of Prozac is seen.

Adults: The recommended starting dose is 20 milligrams a day, usually taken in the morning. If needed, the doctor may gradually increase the dose up to a maximum of 80 milligrams a day. The usual daily dose ranges from 20 to 60 milligrams. Daily doses above 20 milligrams should be taken in the morning or in two smaller doses taken in the morning and at noon.

Children 8 years and older: The usual starting dose is 10 or 20 milligrams a day. Children starting at 10 milligrams will have their dose increased to 20 milligrams a day after 1 week. Underweight children may need to remain at the 10-milligram dose.

Prozac Weekly: Patients need to wait at least 7 days after stopping their daily dose of Prozac before switching to the once-weekly formulation. One Prozac Weekly capsule contains 90 milligrams of medication.

OBSESSIVE-COMPULSIVE DISORDER

It may take 5 weeks before the full effects of Prozac are seen.

Adults: The recommended starting dose is 20 milligrams a day, usually taken in the morning. If needed, the doctor may gradually increase the dose up to a maximum of 80 milligrams a day. The usual daily dose ranges from 20 to 60 milligrams. Daily doses above 20 milligrams should be taken in the morning or in two smaller doses taken in the morning and at noon.

Children 7 years and older: The recommended starting dose is 10 milligrams a day. After 2 weeks, the doctor will increase the dose to 20 milligrams. If needed, the doctor may further increase the dose up to a maximum of 60 milligrams a day. The recommended dosage range for underweight children is 10 to 30 milligrams a day.

BULIMIA

Adults: The recommended dose is 60 milligrams a day taken in the morning. The doctor may start the patient at a lower dose and gradually increase it over a period of several days.

PANIC DISORDER

Adults: The recommended starting dose is 10 milligrams a day. After 1 week, the doctor will increase the dose to 20 milligrams. If no improvement is seen after several weeks, the doctor may increase the dose to a maximum of 60 milligrams a day.

PREMENSTRUAL DYSPHORIC DISORDER

Adults: The usual dose of Sarafem is 20 milligrams a day. The doctor will instruct the patient to take the dose either every day of the month or only during the 2 weeks before menstruation begins (the luteal phase of her cycle). If there's no improvement after several weeks, the dose can be increased, usually to 60 milligrams a day. The maximum dose is 80 milligrams daily.

DOSAGE ADJUSTMENT

For all indications, the doctor may need to prescribe a lower dose for patients who are elderly, have liver disease, or are taking other medications.

Overdosage
Any medication taken in excess can have serious consequences. An overdose of Prozac can be fatal. In addition, combining Prozac with certain other drugs can cause symptoms of overdose. If an overdose is suspected, seek medical attention immediately.

- *Common symptoms of Prozac overdose include:*
  Nausea, rapid heartbeat, seizures, sleepiness, vomiting

- *Other symptoms of Prozac overdose include:*
  Coma, delirium, fainting, high fever, irregular heartbeat, low blood pressure, mania, rigid muscles, sweating, stupor

Quazepam *See Doral, page 70*

Quetiapine *See Seroquel, page 207*

Ramelteon *See Rozerem, page 203*

RAZADYNE
Galantamine
Other brand name: Razadyne ER

Why is this drug prescribed?
Razadyne can delay or even reverse mental decline in some patients with mild to moderate Alzheimer's disease. It is thought to work by boosting levels of the chemical messenger acetylcholine in the brain. (In Alzheimer's disease, the cells that produce acetylcholine slowly deteriorate.)

Like other Alzheimer's drugs, Razadyne is a temporary remedy. It doesn't work for everyone, and it doesn't halt the underlying disease.

Most important fact about this drug
Razadyne therapy starts at a low dose and increases over several months. It is important to wait 4 weeks between dosage adjustments. If treatment with Razadyne is interrupted for several days or longer, the patient will need to start over again at the lowest dose, increasing the dose at 4-week intervals until the former dose is achieved.

How should this medication be taken?
Razadyne should be taken twice a day, preferably with the morning and evening meals. The drug is available in tablet form and as an oral solution. If the solution is used, the required amount should be drawn into the measuring pipette that comes with the bottle and emptied into 3 to 4 ounces of a non-alcoholic beverage. The mixture should be stirred well and administered immediately.

- *Missed dose...*
  Generally, it should be given as soon as remembered. However, if it is almost time for the next dose, the missed dose should be skipped and the next dose given on schedule. Doses should never be doubled.

- *Storage instructions...*
  Both the tablets and the oral solution may be stored at room temperature. The solution should be protected from freezing.

What side effects may occur?
Side effects cannot be predicted. If any develop or change in intensity, caregivers should inform the doctor as soon as possible.

- *Side effects may include:*
  Abdominal pain, anemia, blood in urine, depression, diarrhea, dizziness, fatigue, fever, headache, inability to sleep, indigestion, leg cramps, loss of appetite, nausea, rapid heartbeat, ringing in the ears, runny nose, sleepiness, tremor, urinary tract infection, vomiting, weakness, weight loss

Why should this drug not be prescribed?

Razadyne cannot be used if it gives the patient an allergic reaction. This drug is not recommended for patients with severe liver disease or kidney disease.

Special warnings about this medication

Razadyne should be used with caution if the patient has severe asthma, obstructive lung disease, liver or kidney problems, or a history of stomach ulcers.

Razadyne can slow the heart rate and cause fainting episodes. Caution is especially important if the patient has a heart irregularity.

Before surgery, the doctor should be made aware if the patient is using Razadyne.

Possible food and drug interactions when taking this medication

See the entry for the generic name galantamine on page 334.

Special information about pregnancy and breastfeeding

Razadyne is not usually prescribed for women of childbearing age. It should be used during pregnancy only if the potential benefit justifies the risk to the developing baby. Razadyne should not be used by nursing mothers.

Recommended dosage

ADULTS

Razadyne

The recommended starting dose of Razadyne is 4 milligrams twice a day. Four weeks later, the dose should be increased to 8 milligrams twice a day. After waiting an additional 4 weeks, the doctor may increase the dose to 12 milligrams twice a day if necessary.

For patients with moderate liver or kidney problems, the dosage should not exceed 16 milligrams per day. Razadyne is not recommended for patients with severe liver or kidney problems.

Razadyne ER

The recommended starting dose of Razadyne ER is 8 milligrams once a day. Four weeks later, the dose should be increased to 16 milligrams a day. After waiting another 4 weeks, the doctor may increase the dose to 24 milligrams a day if necessary.

For patients with moderate liver or kidney problems, the dosage should not exceed 16 milligrams per day. Razadyne ER is not recommended for patients with severe liver or kidney problems.

Overdosage

Any medication taken in excess can have serious consequences. A massive overdose of Razadyne could prove fatal. If an overdose is suspected, seek medical attention immediately.

* *Symptoms of Razadyne overdose may include:*
  Convulsions, drooling, fainting, hallucinations, incontinence, low blood pressure, muscle weakness, severe nausea, slow or irregular heartbeat, stomach cramps, sweating, teary eyes, twitching, weak breathing, vomiting

---

REMERON

Mirtazapine
Other brand name: Remeron SolTab

Why is this drug prescribed?

Remeron is prescribed for the treatment of major depression. It belongs to the class of drugs known as tetracyclics and is chemically unrelated to other antidepressants such as serotonin reuptake inhibitors and MAO inhibitors. Remeron is thought to work by adjusting the balance of the brain's natural chemical messengers, especially norepinephrine and serotonin.

Most important fact about this drug

Remeron makes some people drowsy or less alert, and may affect judgment and thinking. Patients should avoid driving or participating in any hazardous activity that requires full mental alertness until they know whether Remeron has this effect on them.

How should this medication be taken?

Remeron may be taken with or without food. It is preferable to take it in the evening before going to bed. Even though improvement may begin in 1 to 4 weeks, it is important for the patient to continue taking this medication exactly as prescribed. Regular daily doses are needed for the drug to work properly.

Patients using Remeron SolTab, an orally disintegrating form of the drug, should make sure their hands are dry before removing the tablet from the blister pack and should immediately place the tablet on their tongue. They should not attempt to split the tablet; it will fall apart rapidly and can be swallowed with saliva.

* *Missed dose...*
  If the forgotten dose is remembered within a few hours, it should be taken immediately. Otherwise, it should be skipped. Doses should never be doubled.

* *Storage instructions...*
  Remeron should be stored at room temperature in a tight, light-resistant container.

What side effects may occur?

Side effects cannot be predicted. If any develop or change in intensity, patients should tell their doctor as soon as possible.

* *Side effects may include:*
  Abnormal dreams and thinking, constipation, dizziness, dry mouth, flu-like symptoms, increased appetite, sleepiness, weakness, weight gain

Why should this drug not be prescribed?

Anyone who has ever had an allergic reaction to Remeron or similar drugs such as maprotiline and Desyrel should not take this medication. It is important for patients to tell the doctor about any drug reactions they have experienced.

Remeron must also be avoided by anyone taking the antidepressants Nardil or Parnate (see "Special warnings about this medication").

Special warnings about this medication

In clinical studies, antidepressants increased the risk of suicidal thinking and behavior in children and adolescents with depression and other psychiatric disorders. Anyone considering the use of Remeron, or any other antidepressant in a child or adolescent, must balance the risk with the clinical need. Remeron has not been studied in children or adolescents and is not approved for treating anyone less than 18 years old.

Additionally, the progression of major depression is associated with a worsening of symptoms and/or the emergence of suicidal thinking or behavior in both adults and children, whether or not they are taking antidepressants. Patients and caregivers should watch for any change in symptoms or any new symptoms that appear suddenly—especially agitation, anxiety, hostility, panic, restlessness, extreme hyperactivity, and suicidal thinking or behavior—and report them to the doctor immediately. Be especially observant at the beginning of treatment or whenever there is a change in dose.

Serious, sometimes fatal, reactions have been known to occur when drugs such as Remeron are taken in combination with other drugs known as MAO inhibitors, including the antidepressants Nardil and Parnate. Remeron should never be taken with one of these drugs or within 14 days of discontinuing therapy with one of them. Patients should also allow at least 14 days between stopping Remeron and starting an MAO inhibitor.

Patients who develop flu-like symptoms, a sore throat, chills or fever, mouth sores, or any other signs of infection should call their doctor; these symptoms may signal a serious underlying condition.

Remeron tends to raise cholesterol levels in some people. If the patient has a cholesterol problem, it should be mentioned to the doctor before Remeron therapy begins.

Remeron should be used with caution by people with active liver or kidney disease, or heart or blood pressure problems. The doctor should also be alerted if the patient has a history of seizures, mania, hypomania (mild excitability), drug use, or any other physical or emotional problems.

While first taking this medication, some people feel dizzy or lightheaded, especially when getting up from a lying or sitting position. If getting up slowly doesn't help, or if this problem continues, the doctor should be notified.

People who must avoid phenylalanine should not use the SolTab form of Remeron, which contains this substance.

Patients should not drink alcohol while taking this medication. It is especially important for patients to check with the doctor before combining Remeron with tranquilizers such as Valium, Xanax, and Ativan.

Possible food and drug interactions when taking this medication
See the entry for the generic name mirtazapine on page 358.

Special information about pregnancy and breastfeeding
The effects of Remeron during pregnancy have not been adequately studied. If the patient is pregnant or plans to become pregnant, she should tell her doctor immediately. It is not known whether Remeron appears in breast milk. However, because many drugs do make their way into breast milk, caution is advised.

Recommended dosage

ADULTS

The usual starting dose is 15 milligrams taken daily before going to sleep. Depending upon the patient's response, the dosage may be increased to as much as 45 milligrams a day.

CHILDREN

The safety and effectiveness of Remeron have not been established in children.

Overdosage
Any medication taken in excess can have serious consequences. If you suspect an overdose, seek medical attention immediately.

- *Symptoms of Remeron overdose may include:*
  Drowsiness, impaired memory, mental confusion, rapid heartbeat

RESERPINE

Why is this drug prescribed?
Reserpine is prescribed to treat high blood pressure. It is also used to treat severe agitation in people with psychotic disorders, especially those who

cannot tolerate other antipsychotic drugs or who also need blood pressure medication. Reserpine works by decreasing the heart rate and relaxing the blood vessels.

Most important fact about this drug

Because depression is a possible side effect of using reserpine, the drug should be used with extreme caution in patients with a history of depression. Reserpine should be stopped at the first signs of depression such as despondency, early morning insomnia, loss of appetite, impotence, or self-deprecation. Drug-induced depression may persist for several months after reserpine withdrawal, and may be severe enough to result in suicide.

How should this medication be taken?

Reserpine comes as a tablet. It is usually taken once a day, although patients should take it exactly as directed by their doctor.

- *Missed dose...*
  Generally, forgotten doses should be taken as soon as remembered. However, if it is almost time for the next dose, patients should skip the one they missed and return to their regular schedule. Doses should never be doubled.

- *Storage instructions...*
  Store at room temperature; protect from light and moisture.

What side effects may occur?

Side effects cannot be anticipated. If any develop or change in intensity, patients should inform their doctor as soon as possible.

- *Side effects may include:*
  Anxiety, breast tenderness or enlargement, depression, diarrhea, dizziness, drowsiness, dry mouth, fainting, headache, irregular heartbeat, impotence, increased saliva and stomach secretion, muscle aches, nasal congestion, rash, shortness of breath, swelling or water retention, upset stomach, vomiting, weight gain

Why should this drug not be prescribed?

Reserpine cannot be taken by anyone who is sensitive to or has ever had an allergic reaction to it. In addition, reserpine should not be used in patients with a history of depression (especially with suicidal tendencies), active peptic ulcer, ulcerative colitis, or in those receiving electroconvulsive therapy.

Special warnings about this medication

Reserpine should be used with caution in patients who have a history of gastrointestinal disease such as ulcers or gallstones. Caution is also advised in patients with kidney disease.

Patients who are scheduled to have surgery (including dental surgery) should let the doctor or dentist know they are taking reserpine.

Because reserpine can make some people sleepy, patients should be cautious about driving a car or operating potentially dangerous machinery until they are sure of how this drug affects them.

Animal studies suggest that extremely high doses of reserpine may increase the risk of tumors, including breast cancer. However, the risk in humans is unknown. Advise patients with a history of cancer to see their doctor regularly for checkups.

Reserpine is not recommended for use in children.

Possible food and drug interactions when taking this medication

See the entry for reserpine on page 393.

Special information about pregnancy and breastfeeding

The effects of reserpine during pregnancy have not been adequately studied. The drug is recommended only if its benefits are thought to outweigh the potential risk to the baby. If a patient is pregnant or planning to become pregnant, she should inform her doctor immediately.

Women taking reserpine should not breastfeed, since the drug can show up in breast milk and may cause adverse reactions in a nursing infant.

Recommended dosage

HIGH BLOOD PRESSURE

Adults: The usual initial dose is 0.5 milligram for 1 to 2 weeks, followed by a maintenance dose of 0.1 to 0.25 milligram daily. Higher dosages should be used cautiously due to the risk of severe depression and other side effects.

SEVERE AGITATION DUE TO MENTAL DISORDERS

Adults: The usual initial dose is 0.5 milligram a day. Depending on the patient's response, the doctor may adjust the dose up or down in the range of 0.1 to 1 milligram a day.

Overdosage

Any medication taken in excess can have serious consequences. If an overdose is suspected, seek medical attention immediately. A large overdose of reserpine could result in coma.

- *Symptoms of reserpine overdose may include:*
  Drowsiness, constricted pupils, diarrhea, flushing of the skin, increased saliva and stomach secretion, low blood pressure, low body temperature, slowed breathing, slowed heartbeat

RESTORIL

Temazepam

Why is this drug prescribed?

Restoril is used for the relief of insomnia (difficulty in falling asleep, waking up frequently at night, or waking up early in the morning). It belongs to a class of drugs known as benzodiazepines.

Most important fact about this drug

Sleep problems are usually temporary, requiring treatment for only a short time, usually 1 or 2 days and no more than 2 to 3 weeks. Insomnia that lasts longer than this may be a sign of another medical problem. Needing this medicine for more than 7 to 10 days is a signal to check with the doctor.

How should this medication be taken?

It is important to take this medication exactly as directed, and in no more than the prescribed amount.

- *Missed dose...*
  Restoril should be taken only as needed.

- *Storage instructions...*
  This medication should be kept in the container it came in, tightly closed, and out of the reach of children. It should be stored at room temperature.

What side effects may occur?

Side effects cannot be predicted. If any develop or change in intensity, patients should inform their doctor as soon as possible.

- *Side effects may include:*
  Dizziness, drowsiness, fatigue, headache, nausea, nervousness, sluggishness

- *Side effects due to rapid decrease in dose or abrupt withdrawal from Restoril:*
  Abdominal and muscle cramps, convulsions, feeling of discomfort, inability to fall asleep or stay asleep, sweating, tremors, vomiting

Why should this drug not be prescribed?

Women who are pregnant or plan to become pregnant should not take this medication. It poses a potential risk to the developing baby.

Special warnings about this medication

When Restoril is used every night for more than a few weeks, it loses its effectiveness to promote sleep. This is known as tolerance. Patients can also develop physical dependence on this drug, especially if they take it regularly for more than a few weeks, or take high doses.

When patients first start taking Restoril, the medication may have a carryover effect the next day. Therefore, they should use extreme care while doing anything that requires complete alertness such as driving a car or operating machinery.

Patients who are severely depressed, or have suffered from severe depression in the past, should double-check with their doctor before taking this medication. They should also make sure the doctor is aware of any kidney ailments, liver problems, or chronic lung disease they may have.

After stopping Restoril, patients may have more trouble sleeping than they had before they started taking it. This is called rebound insomnia and should clear up after 1 or 2 nights.

Restoril may intensify the effects of alcohol. Patients should avoid alcohol while taking this medication.

Possible food and drug interactions when taking this medication

See the entry for the generic name temazepam on page 399.

Special information about pregnancy and breastfeeding

Women who are pregnant or planning to become pregnant should not take Restoril. There is an increased risk of birth defects.

This drug may appear in breast milk and could affect a nursing infant. If this medication is considered essential to a woman's health, her doctor may advise her to discontinue breastfeeding until her treatment with this medication is finished.

Recommended dosage

ADULTS

The usual recommended dose is 15 milligrams at bedtime. However, 7.5 milligrams may be all that is necessary, while some people may need 30 milligrams. The doctor will tailor the dose to the patient's needs.

CHILDREN

The safety and effectiveness of Restoril have not been established in children under 18 years of age.

OLDER ADULTS

The doctor will prescribe the smallest effective amount in order to avoid side effects such as oversedation, dizziness, confusion, and lack of muscle coordination. The usual starting dose is 7.5 milligrams.

Overdosage

Any medication taken in excess can have serious consequences. If an overdose is suspected, seek medical attention immediately.

- *Symptoms of Restoril overdose may include:*
  Coma, confusion, diminished reflexes, low blood pressure, labored or difficult breathing, sleepiness

REVIA
Naltrexone hydrochloride

Why is this drug prescribed?
ReVia is prescribed to treat alcohol dependence and narcotic addiction. ReVia is not a cure. Patients must be ready to make a change and be willing to undertake a comprehensive treatment program that includes professional counseling, support groups, and close medical supervision.

Most important fact about this drug
Before taking ReVia for narcotic addiction, patients must be drug-free for at least 7 to 10 days. They must also be free of any drug withdrawal symptoms. Patients who think they are still in withdrawal should be sure to tell their doctor, since taking ReVia while narcotics are still in their system could cause serious physical problems. The doctor will perform tests to confirm a patient's drug-free condition.

How should this medication be taken?
It is important to take ReVia on schedule as directed by the doctor, and to follow through with counseling and support group therapy.

If a patient takes small doses of heroin or other narcotic drugs while taking ReVia, they will have no effect. Large doses combined with ReVia can be fatal.

- *Missed dose...*
  The missed dose should be taken as soon as possible. Patients who do not remember until the next day should skip the missed dose and go back to the regular dosing schedule. Doses should never be doubled.

- *Storage instructions...*
  No special measures are needed for storing ReVia.

What side effects may occur?
Side effects cannot be predicted. If any side effects develop or change in intensity, patients should inform their doctor immediately.

- *Side effects of treatment for alcoholism may include:*
  Dizziness, fatigue, headache, nausea, nervousness, sleeplessness, vomiting

- *Side effects of treatment for narcotic addiction may include:*
  Abdominal pain/cramps, anxiety, difficulty sleeping, headache, joint and muscle pain, low energy, nausea and/or vomiting, nervousness

Why should this drug not be prescribed?

Patients who are sensitive to ReVia, or have ever had an allergic reaction to it, should not take the drug. Also, people who have acute hepatitis (liver disease) or liver failure should not start therapy with ReVia. Remember, too, that patients must be narcotic-free before beginning ReVia therapy.

Special warnings about this medication

Since ReVia may cause liver damage when taken at high doses, a patient who develops symptoms that signal possible liver problems should stop taking ReVia immediately and see their doctor as soon as possible. These symptoms include abdominal pain lasting more than a few days, white bowel movements, dark urine, or yellowing of the eyes. The doctor may periodically test patients' liver function while they are on ReVia therapy. Caution is also advisable for patients who have kidney problems.

Patients who are narcotic-dependent and accidentally take ReVia may experience severe withdrawal symptoms lasting up to 48 hours, including confusion, sleepiness, hallucinations, vomiting, and diarrhea. If this occurs, seek help immediately.

Patients must not attempt to use narcotics while taking ReVia. Small doses will have no effect, and large doses could lead to coma or even death.

People who take ReVia should have a medication card to alert emergency medical personnel that they are taking the drug. They should carry this card with them at all times, and tell all of the doctors, dentists, and pharmacists who may assist them with medical treatment that they are taking ReVia.

The safety of ReVia in children under 18 years of age has not been established.

Since studies to evaluate the interaction of ReVia with drugs other than narcotics have not been performed, patients should not take any medications, either over-the-counter or prescription, without first notifying their doctor.

Patients should not use Antabuse while also taking ReVia; both drugs can damage the liver. Also, they should not take thioridazine (a drug used to treat depression and anxiety) while on ReVia therapy, as the combination may make them feel very sleepy and sluggish.

While taking ReVia, patients should avoid medicines that contain narcotics, including certain cough and cold preparations, certain antidiarrheal medications, and narcotic painkillers such as oxycodone.

Possible food and drug interactions when taking this medication

See the entry for the generic name naltrexone on page 360.

Special information about pregnancy and breastfeeding

The effects of ReVia during pregnancy have not been adequately studied. Patients who are pregnant or are planning to become pregnant should tell their doctor immediately. ReVia should be used during pregnancy only if clearly needed. ReVia may appear in breast milk. If this medication is essential to the patient's health, the doctor may tell her to discontinue breastfeeding until her treatment with ReVia is finished.

Recommended dosage

The following dosages and indications are for adults. The safety of ReVia in children under 18 years of age has not been established.

ALCOHOLISM

The usual starting dose is 50 milligrams once a day.

NARCOTIC DEPENDENCE

The usual starting dose is 25 milligrams once a day. If no withdrawal symptoms occur, the doctor may increase the dosage to 50 milligrams a day.

Overdosage

Any medication taken in excess can have serious consequences. If an overdose of ReVia is suspected, seek medical attention immediately.

RISPERDAL

Risperidone
Other brand name: Risperdal M-Tab, Risperdal Consta

Why is this drug prescribed?

Risperdal is prescribed for the treatment of schizophrenia and for the short-term treatment of mania associated with bipolar disorder. It is thought to work by muting the impact of dopamine and serotonin, two of the brain's key chemical messengers. Risperdal can also be used to treat irritability associated with autistic disorder in children and adolescents.

Risperdal M-Tab is the orally disintegrating tablet form of Risperdal and can be used for all of the same conditions for which Risperdal is prescribed.

Risperdal Consta is a deep intramuscular gluteal injection that is given by a healthcare professional every 2 weeks. It delivers the same medication as Risperdal and Risperdal M-Tabs, but is only used for the treatment of schizophrenia.

Most important fact about this drug

Risperdal may cause tardive dyskinesia, a condition that causes involuntary muscle spasms and twitches in the face and body. This condition can become permanent and is most common among older people, especially women. Patients should see their doctor immediately if they begin to have any involuntary movements. They may need to discontinue Risperdal therapy.

In addition, elderly patients with dementia who are treated with antipsychotic drugs such as Risperdal have an increased risk of stroke and death. Risperdal is not approved to treat dementia-related psychosis.

How should this medication be taken?
It is important for patients to take exactly the amount of Risperdal prescribed. Higher doses are more likely to cause unwanted side effects. Risperdal may be taken with or without food. Risperdal oral solution comes with a calibrated pipette to use for measuring. The oral solution can be taken with water, coffee, orange juice, and low-fat milk, but not with cola drinks or tea.

Risperdal M-Tabs are orally disintegrating tablets that come in blister packs. The tablets should not be removed from the package until patients are ready to take them. When it's time for their dose, patients should use dry fingers to peel back the foil of the blister pack to remove the tablet; they should not push the tablet through the foil because this could damage the tablet. Once removed, the tablet should be placed immediately on the tongue. The medication dissolves in the mouth quickly and can be swallowed with or without liquid. Risperdal M-Tabs should not be split or chewed.

Risperdal Consta is a deep intramuscular gluteal injection that is given by a healthcare professional every 2 weeks. Injections will be alternated between the two buttocks.

- *Missed dose...*
  Generally, the dose should be taken as soon as remembered. However, if it is almost time for the next dose, patients should skip the one they missed and go back to their regular schedule. Doses should never be doubled.

  Patients who miss their appointment to get their Risperdal Consta injection, should call their doctor right away to find out when they should come next for an injection.

- *Storage instructions...*
  Risperdal may be stored at room temperature. The tablets should be protected from light and moisture; the oral solution should be protected from light and freezing.

What side effects may occur?
Side effects cannot be predicted. If any develop or change in intensity, patients should inform their doctor as soon as possible.

- *Side effects of Risperdal may include:*
  Agitation, anxiety, constipation, dizziness, hallucination, headache, indigestion, insomnia, rapid or irregular heartbeat, restlessness, runny nose, sleepiness, vomiting, weight change

• *Side effects of Risperdal Consta may include:*
Constipation, dry mouth, feeling tired, restlessness, sleepiness, stomach upset, tremors and rigid muscles, weight increase

Why should this drug not be prescribed?

Risperdal cannot be taken by anyone who is sensitive to or has ever had an allergic reaction to it or to other antipsychotic medications.

Risperdal should not be used to treat elderly patients who have dementia because the drug could increase the risk of stroke.

Special warnings about this medication

Risperdal should be used with caution in patients who have kidney, liver, or heart disease; seizures; breast cancer; thyroid disorders; or any other diseases that affect the metabolism. Caution is also warranted in patients exposed to extremes of temperature.

Be aware that Risperdal may mask signs and symptoms of drug overdose and of conditions such as intestinal obstruction, brain tumor, and Reye's syndrome (a dangerous neurological condition that may follow viral infections, usually occurring in children).

Risperdal may cause neuroleptic malignant syndrome, a condition marked by muscle stiffness or rigidity, fast heartbeat or irregular pulse, increased sweating, high fever, and high or low blood pressure. Unchecked, this condition can prove fatal. Patients should call their doctor immediately if they notice any of these symptoms. Risperdal therapy should be discontinued.

Certain antipsychotic drugs, including Risperdal, are associated with an increased risk of developing high blood sugar, which on rare occasions has led to coma or death. Patients should see their doctor right away if they develop signs of high blood sugar, including dry mouth, thirst, increased urination, and tiredness. Patients who have diabetes or have a high risk of developing it should see their doctor regularly for blood sugar testing.

Patients at high risk of suicide attempts should be prescribed the lowest dose possible to reduce the risk of intentional overdose.

This drug may impair the ability to drive a car or operate potentially dangerous machinery. Patients should avoid participating in any activities that require full alertness if they are unsure of their ability.

Risperdal can cause orthostatic hypotension (low blood pressure when rising to a standing position), with dizziness, rapid heartbeat, and fainting, especially at the start of therapy. This problem should be reported to the doctor if it develops. The dosage can be adjusted to reduce the symptoms.

Risperdal is prescribed for the short-term treatment of rapid-onset bipolar mania; it is not approved for preventing future episodes. The effectiveness of the drug for treating mania for more than 3 weeks has not been studied.

People who have phenylketonuria and must avoid the amino acid phenylalanine should not use Risperdal M-Tabs, which contain this substance.

The safety and effectiveness of Risperdal have not been studied in children.

Risperdal tends to increase the effect of blood pressure medicines.

Patients may experience drowsiness and other potentially serious effects if Risperdal is combined with alcohol and other drugs that slow the central nervous system such as Valium, Percocet, Demerol, or haloperidol.

Patients should check with their doctor before taking any new medications.

Possible food and drug interactions when taking this medication

See the entry for the generic name risperidone on page 394.

Special information about pregnancy and breastfeeding

The safety and effectiveness of Risperdal during pregnancy have not been adequately studied. Patients who are pregnant or plan to become pregnant should tell their doctor immediately.

Risperdal makes its way into breast milk, so women taking Risperdal must avoid breastfeeding.

Recommended dosage

SCHIZOPHRENIA

Adults: Doses of Risperdal can be taken once a day, or divided in half and taken twice daily. The usual dose on the first day is 2 milligrams or 2 milliliters of oral solution. On the second day, the dose increases to 4 milligrams or milliliters, and on the third day rises to 6 milligrams or milliliters. Further dosage adjustments can be made at intervals of 1 week. Over the long term, typical daily doses range from 2 to 8 milligrams or milliliters.

Risperdal Consta is given after tolerability has already been established with oral Risperdal. Each Risperdal Consta dose should be administered by a healthcare professional every 2 weeks by deep intramuscular gluteal injection. Injections should alternate between the buttocks and should not be given intravenously. The usual dose is 25 milligrams every 2 weeks. Some patients may receive a higher dose, but the maximum dose should not exceed 50 milligrams every 2 weeks. The dosage should not be increased more frequently than every 4 weeks. For certain patients (such as those with liver or kidney impairment) an initial dose of 12.5 milligrams may be appropriate. Oral Risperdal, or another antipsychotic medication, should be given with the first injection of Risperdal Consta and continued for 3 weeks to ensure that the patient is receiving sufficient medication. Risperdal Consta has not been studied in children under 18 years of age.

BIPOLAR MANIA (SHORT-TERM TREATMENT OF ACUTE EPISODES)

Adults: The recommended starting dose is 2 to 3 milligrams (or milliliters of oral solution) per day, given as a single dose. If needed, the doctor will adjust the dose by 1 milligram at intervals of at least 24 hours. The effective dosage range is 1 to 6 milligrams a day.

IRRITABILITY ASSOCIATED WITH AUTISTIC DISORDER

The safety and effectiveness of Risperdal in pediatric patients with autistic disorder less than 5 years of age have not been established.

Children 5 to 16 years old: The doctor will adjust the dose based on the child's weight and response to the medication.

DOSAGE ADJUSTMENT

The doctor will prescribe lower doses for patients who are weak, elderly, have liver or kidney disease, or have a high risk for low blood pressure. The usual starting dose is 0.5 milligram (or 0.5 milliliter of oral solution) twice a day. The doctor may switch the patient to a once-a-day dosing schedule after the first 2 to 3 days of treatment.

If needed, each dose may be increased by increments of no more than 0.5 milligram. Increases to dosages above 1.5 milligrams twice a day should generally be made at intervals of at least 1 week.

Patients taking certain medications may also need their Risperdal dose adjusted. The list includes Dilantin, Paxil, phenobarbital, Prozac, Rifadin, and Tegretol.

Overdosage

Any medication taken in excess can have serious consequences. If an overdose of Risperdal is suspected, seek medical attention immediately.

- *Symptoms of Risperdal overdose may include:*
  Drowsiness, low blood pressure, rapid heartbeat, sedation

Risperidone *See Risperdal, page 195*

RITALIN
Methylphenidate hydrochloride
Other brand names: Concerta, Metadate CD, Metadate ER, Methylin, Methylin ER, Ritalin-SR, Ritalin LA

Why is this drug prescribed?
Ritalin and other brands of methylphenidate are mild central nervous system stimulants used in the treatment of attention deficit hyperactivity disorder (ADHD) in children. With the exception of Ritalin LA, Concerta, and Metadate CD, these products are also used in adults to treat narcolepsy.

When given for ADHD, this drug should be used as part of a broader treatment plan that includes psychological, educational, and social measures.

Most important fact about this drug

Excessive doses of this drug over a long period of time can produce addiction. It is also possible to develop tolerance to the drug, so that larger doses are needed to produce the original effect. Because of these dangers, dosage should be changed only as directed, and the drug should be withdrawn only under a doctor's supervision.

How should this medication be taken?

The doctor's directions should be followed carefully. It is recommended that methylphenidate be taken 30 to 45 minutes before meals. If the drug interferes with sleep, the child should receive the last dose before 6 p.m. Ritalin-SR, Ritalin LA, Metadate CD, Methylin ER, and Concerta are long-acting forms of the drug, taken less frequently. They should be swallowed whole, never crushed or chewed. (Ritalin LA and Metadate CD may also be given by sprinkling the contents of the capsule on a tablespoon of cool applesauce and administering immediately, followed by a drink of water.)

* *Missed dose...*
  It should be given as soon as remembered. The remaining doses for the day should then be administered at regularly spaced intervals. Doses should never be doubled.

* *Storage instructions...*
  This drug should be kept out of reach of children and stored below 86 degrees Fahrenheit in a tightly closed, light-resistant container. Ritalin-SR should be protected from moisture.

What side effects may occur?

Side effects cannot be predicted. If any develop or change in intensity, patients should inform their doctor as soon as possible.

* *Side effects may include:*
  Dizziness, headache, heart problems, inability to fall asleep or stay asleep, nausea, nervousness

These side effects can usually be controlled by reducing the dosage and omitting the drug in the afternoon or evening.

In children, loss of appetite, abdominal pain, weight loss during long-term therapy, inability to fall asleep or stay asleep, and abnormally fast heartbeat are more common side effects.

Why should this drug not be prescribed?

This drug should not be prescribed for anyone experiencing anxiety, tension, and agitation, since the drug may aggravate these symptoms.

Anyone sensitive or allergic to this drug should not take it.

This medication should not be taken by anyone with the eye condition known as glaucoma, anyone who suffers from tics (repeated, involuntary twitches), or someone with a family history of Tourette's syndrome (severe and multiple tics).

This drug is not intended for use in children whose symptoms may be caused by stress or a psychiatric disorder.

This medication should not be used for the prevention or treatment of normal fatigue, nor should it be used for the treatment of severe depression.

This drug should not be taken during treatment with drugs classified as monoamine oxidase inhibitors, such as the antidepressants Nardil and Parnate, nor for the 2 weeks following discontinuation of these drugs.

Special warnings about this medication

The doctor should do a complete history and evaluation before prescribing this drug. He or she will take into account the severity of the symptoms, as well as the child's age.

This drug should not be given to children under 6 years of age.

There is no information regarding the safety and effectiveness of long-term treatment in children. However, suppression of growth has been seen with the long-term use of stimulants, so the child should be monitored carefully while taking this drug.

Blood pressure should be monitored in anyone taking this drug, especially those with high blood pressure.

Some people have had visual disturbances such as blurred vision while being treated with this drug.

The use of this drug by anyone with a seizure disorder is not recommended. Make sure the doctor is aware of any problem in this area. Caution is also advisable for anyone with a history of emotional instability or substance abuse, due to the danger of addiction.

Possible food and drug interactions when taking this medication

See the entry for the generic name methylphenidate on page 357.

Special information about pregnancy and breastfeeding

The effects of this drug during pregnancy have not been adequately studied. Patients who are pregnant or plan to become pregnant should inform their doctor immediately.

It is not known if this drug appears in breast milk. If this medication is essential to a patient's health, the doctor may advise her to discontinue nursing until her treatment with this medication is finished.

Recommended dosage

ADULTS

Ritalin and Methylin Tablets

The average dosage is 20 to 30 milligrams a day, divided into 2 or 3 doses, preferably taken 30 to 45 minutes before meals. Some people may need 40 to 60 milligrams daily, others only 10 to 15 milligrams. The doctor will determine the best dose.

Ritalin-SR, Methylin ER, and Metadate ER Tablets

These tablets keep working for 8 hours. They may be used in place of the regular tablets if they deliver a comparable dose over an 8-hour period.

CHILDREN

This drug should not be given to children under 6 years of age.

Ritalin and Methylin Tablets

The usual starting dose is 5 milligrams taken twice a day, before breakfast and lunch. The doctor will increase the dose by 5 to 10 milligrams a week, up to a maximum of 60 milligrams a day. If improvement fails to appear after 1 month, the doctor may decide to discontinue the drug.

Ritalin-SR, Methylin ER, and Metadate ER Tablets

These tablets continue working for 8 hours. The doctor will decide if they should be used in place of the regular tablets.

Ritalin LA Capsules

The recommended starting dose is 10 to 20 milligrams once daily in the morning. At weekly intervals, the doctor may increase the dose by 10 milligrams, up to a maximum of 60 milligrams once a day.

Concerta Tablets

The recommended starting dose is 18 milligrams once daily in the morning. At weekly intervals, the doctor may increase the dose in 18-milligram steps. The maximum daily dose is 54 milligrams for children 6 to 12 year olds and 72 milligrams for adolescents 13 to 17 years old.

Metadate CD Capsules

The recommended starting dose is 20 milligrams once daily before breakfast. If necessary, the doctor may increase the dose in 20-milligram steps to a maximum of 60 milligrams once a day.

The doctor will periodically discontinue the ADHD drug in order to reassess the child's condition. Drug treatment should not, and need not, be indefinite, and usually can be discontinued after puberty.

Overdosage

If an overdose is suspected, seek medical attention immediately.

- *Symptoms of Ritalin overdose may include:*
Agitation, confusion, convulsions (may be followed by coma), delirium, dryness of mucous membranes, enlarging of the pupils, exaggerated feeling of elation, extremely elevated body temperature, flushing, hallucinations, headache, high blood pressure, irregular or rapid heartbeat, muscle twitching, sweating, tremors, vomiting

Rivastigmine *See Exelon, page 80*

ROZEREM
Ramelteon

Why is this drug prescribed?
Rozerem is prescribed for treatment of insomnia characterized by difficulty in falling asleep. (Other types of insomnia include awakening in the middle of the night or awakening too early in the morning.) Rozerem acts by activating some of the same pathways in the brain that are activated by melatonin, a chemical produced in the body that is believed to be involved in maintaining the daily sleep-wake cycle.

Most important fact about this drug
Sleep disturbance may be a symptom of a physical or psychiatric illness. Therefore, the doctor will need to evaluate the patient's overall health before prescribing Rozerem.

How should this medication be taken?
Rozerem is taken about 30 minutes before going to bed. After taking Rozerem, patients should only engage in activities related to preparing for bed. Any potentially hazardous activities, such as operating heavy machinery or driving a motor vehicle, should be avoided after taking Rozerem.

Rozerem should not be taken with or immediately after a high-fat meal.

- *Missed dose...*
Rozerem should be taken only when the patient is ready to sleep. The dose should never be doubled.

- *Storage instructions...*
Rozerem should be stored at room temperature.

What side effects may occur?
Side effects cannot be predicted. If any develop or change in intensity, patients should inform their doctor as soon as possible.

- *Side effects may include:*
Dizziness, tiredness

Why should this drug not be prescribed?

Rozerem should not be taken by anyone who has had an allergic reaction to any of its ingredients. Patients should not take Rozerem if they have severe liver damage or if they are taking the psychiatric drug fluvoxamine.

Special warnings about this medication

If the patient's insomnia does not improve after a reasonable treatment period, or if their insomnia worsens, the patient should notify the doctor. The doctor may further evaluate the patient to determine if there are any physical or psychiatric causes for insomnia.

Rozerem may cause cognitive or behavioral problems or worsening of insomnia. In depressed patients, sleep medications have been known to cause a worsening of depression, including suicidal thoughts.

Patients should not operate heavy machinery or drive a motor vehicle after taking Rozerem.

Alcohol consumption is not recommended in combination with Rozerem.

Rozerem is not recommended for patients with sleep apnea or chronic obstructive pulmonary disease.

Rozerem is not recommended for children under the age of 18.

Rozerem should not be taken with or immediately after a high-fat meal. Also, patients who are taking the psychiatric drug fluvoxamine, which is used to treat obsessive-compulsive disorder, should not take Rozerem.

Possible food and drug interactions when taking this medication

See the entry for the generic name ramelteon on page 393.

Special information if you are pregnant or breastfeeding

The effects of Rozerem during pregnancy have not been adequately studied. Women who are pregnant or plan to become pregnant should inform their doctor immediately. Rozerem is not recommended for nursing mothers.

Recommended dosage

Patients should take one 8-milligram tablet 30 minutes before going to bed.

Overdosage

Any medication taken in excess can have serious consequences. If an overdose is suspected, seek emergency treatment immediately.

Sarafem *See Prozac, page 179*

Secobarbital *See Seconal, page 205*

SECONAL
Secobarbital sodium

Why is this drug prescribed?
Seconal is a barbiturate used to treat insomnia on a short-term basis. After 2 weeks, Seconal appears to lose its effectiveness as a sleep aid. Seconal is also used as a sedative to relieve anxiety before surgery.

Most important fact about this drug
If taken for a long enough time, Seconal can cause physical addiction. Taken in a large enough amount, it can cause death.

How should this medication be taken?
Seconal should be taken only at bedtime, and only in the prescribed amount. It should not be taken with alcohol.

* *Missed dose...*
  Seconal is taken only as needed. It is not necessary to make up for a missed dose. Doses should never be doubled.

* *Storage instructions...*
  Seconal should be stored at room temperature in a tightly closed container.

What side effects may occur?
Side effects cannot be predicted. If any develop or change in intensity, patients should inform their doctor as soon as possible.

* *Side effects may include:*
  Agitation, anemia, anxiety, confusion, constipation, difficulty breathing, disturbed thinking, dizziness, fainting, fever, fluid retention, hallucinations, headache, insomnia, lack of coordination, low blood pressure, nausea, nervousness, nightmares, overactivity, slow heartbeat, skin rash, skin inflammation and/or peeling, temporary interruptions of breathing, vomiting

Why should this drug not be prescribed?
Seconal should be avoided by anyone who has the rare blood disorder porphyria, liver damage, or a lung disease that makes breathing difficult. The drug cannot be used by people who have ever had an allergic reaction to barbiturates.

Special warnings about this medication
Seconal should not be stopped suddenly, since this may result in severe withdrawal symptoms and even death. To reduce the possibility of withdrawal symptoms, patients should follow the doctor's instructions closely when discontinuing Seconal.

Minor withdrawal symptoms include (in order of occurrence): anxiety, muscle twitching, tremors of hands and fingers, progressive weakness, dizziness, visual problems, nausea, vomiting, insomnia, and light-headedness upon first standing up. Major withdrawal symptoms include convulsions and delirium.

Seconal should be used with caution by people who have had liver disease or have a history of depression or substance abuse.

Patients should inform the doctor if they have any pain. Seconal may hide pain-causing disorders that require treatment.

Children may become excited while taking Seconal. Elderly people may become confused, depressed, or excited.

Seconal may lessen the effectiveness of oral contraceptives. Women who take Seconal may need to consider another type of birth control.

This drug may impair the ability to drive a car or operate potentially dangerous machinery. Patients should not participate in any activities that require full alertness if they are unsure about their ability.

Extreme drowsiness and other potentially serious effects can result if Seconal is combined with alcohol and other drugs that slow the activity of the brain.

Possible food and drug interactions when taking this medication

See the entry for the generic name secobarbital on page 395.

Special information about pregnancy and breastfeeding

Studies have shown Seconal to have a potentially harmful effect on the unborn child. Patients who are pregnant or plan to become pregnant should inform their doctor immediately. This drug should be used during pregnancy only if clearly needed and only if potential benefits outweigh possible risks.

Small amounts of Seconal appear in breast milk. The doctor should be consulted before breastfeeding is undertaken.

Recommended dosage

ADULTS

For insomnia, the usual dose is 100 milligrams, taken at bedtime. To relieve anxiety before surgery, the usual dose is 200 to 300 milligrams, given 1 to 2 hours before the operation.

CHILDREN

Dosages for children, generally given to reduce anxiety before an operation, are based on the child's weight. The usual dose is 2 to 6 milligrams per 2.2 pounds (1 kilogram) of body weight, up to a maximum of 100 milligrams.

DOSAGE ADJUSTMENT

Because older people may be more sensitive to Seconal, they should take lower dosages; this is also true for people whose kidneys are not functioning properly and those who have liver disease.

Overdosage

Any medication taken in excess can have serious consequences. An overdose of Seconal can be fatal. If an overdose is suspected, seek medical help immediately.

- *Symptoms of Seconal overdose may be seen within 15 minutes and may include:*
  Blood blisters, difficulty breathing, extreme drowsiness, extreme low body temperature, fluid in the lungs, irregular heartbeat, low blood pressure

Selegiline *See Emsam, page 75*

SEROQUEL

Quetiapine fumarate
Other brand name: Seroquel XR

Why is this drug prescribed?

Seroquel is prescribed for the treatment of schizophrenia and for the treatment of mania and depressive episodes associated with bipolar disorder. Seroquel belongs to one of the newer classes of antipsychotic medications. Researchers believe that it works by diminishing the action of dopamine and serotonin, two of the brain's chief chemical messengers. Seroquel XR is the extended-release form of Seroquel, and is used for the treatment of schizophrenia.

Most important fact about this drug

Seroquel may cause tardive dyskinesia, a condition characterized by uncontrollable muscle spasms and twitches in the face and body. This problem can be permanent, and appears to be most common among older adults, especially women.

Seroquel is not approved for use in elderly patients with dementia (including Alzheimer's disease) due to the increased risk of sudden death, heart failure, and pneumonia.

How should this medication be taken?

Dosage is increased gradually until the drug takes effect. Patients who stop taking Seroquel for more than 1 week will need to build up to their ideal dosage once again.

Seroquel XR should be taken once a day, preferably in the evening. It should be taken without food or with a light meal (around 300 calories). In addition, Seroquel XR tablets should be swallowed whole, and not split, chewed, or crushed.

- *Missed dose...*
  Generally, a missed dose should be taken as soon as remembered. However, if it is almost time for the next dose, patients should skip the dose they missed and go back to their regular schedule. Doses should never be doubled.

- *Storage instructions...*
  Seroquel should be stored at room temperature.

What side effects may occur?
Side effects cannot be predicted. If any develop or change in intensity, patients should inform their doctor as soon as possible.

- *Side effects of Seroquel may include:*
  Abdominal pain, constipation, diminished movement, dizziness, drowsiness, dry mouth, excessive muscle tone, headache, indigestion, low blood pressure (especially upon standing), nasal inflammation, neck rigidity, rapid or irregular heartbeat, rash, sleepiness, tremor, uncontrollable movements, weakness

- *Side effects of Seroquel XR may include:*
  Constipation, dizziness, drowsiness or sleepiness, dry mouth, indigestion, low blood pressure (especially upon standing), sedation

Why should this drug not be prescribed?
If Seroquel causes an allergic reaction, the patient will not be able to use this drug.

Special warnings about this medication
In clinical studies, antidepressants increased the risk of suicidal thinking and behavior in children and adolescents with depression and other psychiatric disorders. Anyone considering the use of Seroquel, or any other antidepressant in a child or adolescent, must balance the risk with the clinical need. Seroquel and Seroquel XR are not approved for use in pediatric patients.

Additionally, the progression of major depression is associated with a worsening of symptoms and/or the emergence of suicidal thinking or behavior in both adults and children, whether or not they are taking antidepressants. Patients and caregivers should watch for any change in symptoms or any new symptoms that appear suddenly—especially agitation, anxiety, hostility, panic, restlessness, extreme hyperactivity, and suicidal thinking or behavior—and report them to the doctor immediately. Be especially observant at the beginning of treatment or whenever there is a change in dose.

Patients who develop muscle stiffness, confusion, irregular or rapid heartbeat, excessive sweating, and high fever should call their doctor immediately. These are signs of neuroleptic malignant syndrome, a serious—and potentially fatal—reaction to the drug. Patients should be especially wary if they have a history of heart attack, heart disease, heart failure, circulation problems, or irregular heartbeat.

Particularly during the first few days of therapy, Seroquel can cause low blood pressure, with accompanying dizziness, fainting, and rapid heartbeat. To minimize these effects, the doctor will increase the dose gradually. People who are prone to low blood pressure, take blood pressure medication, or become dehydrated should use Seroquel with caution.

Seroquel also tends to cause drowsiness, especially at the start of therapy, and can impair judgment, thinking, and motor skills. Until patients are certain of the drug's effect, they need to use caution when operating machinery or driving a car.

Certain antipsychotic drugs, including Seroquel, are associated with an increased risk of developing high blood sugar, which on rare occasions has led to coma or death. Patients should see their doctor right away if they develop signs of high blood sugar, including dry mouth, unusual thirst, increased urination, and tiredness. Patients who have diabetes or have a high risk of developing it should see their doctor regularly for blood sugar testing.

Patients at high risk of suicide attempts should be prescribed the lowest dose possible to reduce the risk of intentional overdose.

Seroquel should be used cautiously in older patients and those with Alzheimer's disease. Antipsychotic drug treatment has been associated with swallowing and breathing problems (aspiration).

Animal studies suggest that Seroquel may increase the risk of breast cancer, although human studies have not confirmed such a risk. Advise patients with a history of breast cancer to see their doctor regularly for checkups.

Patients should report any vision problems to the doctor. There is a chance that Seroquel may cause cataracts, and some people may be asked to see an eye doctor when they start Seroquel therapy, and every 6 months thereafter.

Seroquel poses a very slight risk of seizures, especially in people who are over 65 or have epilepsy or Alzheimer's disease. The drug can also suppress an underactive thyroid, and generally causes a minor increase in cholesterol levels. There is also a remote chance that it will trigger a prolonged and painful erection.

Other antipsychotic medications have been known to interfere with the body's temperature-regulating mechanism, causing patients to overheat. Although this problem has not occurred with Seroquel, caution is still advisable. Patients should avoid exposure to extreme heat, strenuous exercise, and dehydration.

Seroquel is prescribed for the short-term treatment of rapid-onset bipolar mania; it is not approved for preventing future episodes. The effectiveness of the drug for treating mania for more than 3 weeks has not been studied. The effectiveness of Seroquel XR in long-term use (more than 6 weeks) has not been evaluated in clinical trials. Therefore, doctors who prescribe Seroquel XR for extended use should periodically reevalute the long-term usefulness of the drug for the individual patient.

Seroquel increases the effects of alcohol. Patients should avoid alcoholic beverages while on Seroquel therapy.

Possible food and drug interactions when taking this medication
See the entry for the generic name quetiapine on page 393.

Special information about pregnancy and breastfeeding
The possibility of harm to a developing baby has not been ruled out. Women should take Seroquel during pregnancy only if the benefits outweigh this potential risk. They should notify their doctor as soon as they become pregnant or decide to become pregnant.

It is not known whether Seroquel appears in breast milk, and breastfeeding is not recommended.

Recommended dosage
SCHIZOPHRENIA

Seroquel
The usual dosage range is 300 to 400 milligrams a day, divided into 2 or 3 smaller doses. Doses as low as 150 milligrams a day sometimes prove effective, and the dose rarely exceeds 750 milligrams per day. Doses above 800 milligrams per day have not been tested for safety.

The dose is gradually increased over 4 days until the most effective dose is reached, using the following schedule:

Day 1: Patients take 25 milligrams twice a day.
Days 2, 3, and 4: Each daily dose is increased by 25 to 50 milligrams, taken either 2 or 3 times a day.
Day 5 and up: If needed, the doctor may increase each dose by 25 to 50 milligrams every 2 or more days.

Seroquel XR
The usual starting dose is 300 milligrams. Seroquel XR should be taken once a day, preferably in the evening. The dose range for Seroquel XR is 400 to 800 milligrams per day depending on the response and tolerance of the individual patient. Dose increases can be made at intervals as short as 1 day and in increments of up to 300 milligrams a day.

BIPOLAR MANIA (SHORT-TERM TREATMENT OF ACUTE EPISODES)

The usual dosage range is 400 to 800 milligrams a day. Doses above 800 milligrams a day have not been tested for safety. The dosage will be gradually increased over 4 to 6 days until the most effective dose is reached, using the following schedule:

Day 1: Patients take 50 milligrams twice a day.
Day 2: The dose is increased to 100 milligrams twice a day.
Day 3: The dose is increased to 150 milligrams twice a day.
Day 4: The dose is increased to 200 milligrams twice a day.
Days 5 and 6: If needed, the doctor may increase each dose by no more than 200-milligram increments to a total daily dose of 800 milligrams.

BIPOLAR DEPRESSION

The usual dose is 300 milligrams once a day at bedtime. The dosage will be gradually increased over 4 days, using the following schedule:

Day 1: Patients take 50 milligrams at bedtime.
Day 2: The dose is increased to 100 milligrams at bedtime.
Day 3: The dose is increased to 200 milligrams at bedtime.
Day 4: The dose is increased to 300 milligrams at bedtime.

DOSAGE ADJUSTMENT

Patients with liver problems will be started at 25 milligrams a day. The doctor will increase the dose as needed in increments of 25 to 50 milligrams a day based on the patient's tolerability.

The dosage may also need to be lowered for the weak, elderly, and those prone to low blood pressure reactions. Patients taking certain drugs, including Dilantin, Tegretol, and phenobarbital, may also need their dose adjusted.

Overdosage

Any medication taken in excess can have serious consequences. If an overdose is suspected, seek medical help immediately.

- *Symptoms of Seroquel overdose may include:*
  Dizziness, drowsiness, fainting, rapid heartbeat

Sertraline *See Zoloft, page 263*

SINEQUAN
Doxepin hydrochloride

Why is this drug prescribed?

Sinequan is used in the treatment of depression and anxiety. It helps relieve tension, improve sleep, elevate mood, increase energy, and generally ease feelings of fear, guilt, apprehension, and worry. It is effective in treating people whose depression and/or anxiety is psychological, associated with alcoholism, or a result of another disease (cancer, for example) or psychotic depressive disorders (severe mental illness). It is in the family of drugs called tricyclic antidepressants.

Most important fact about this drug

Serious, sometimes fatal, reactions have occurred when Sinequan has been used in combination with drugs known as MAO inhibitors, including the antidepressants Nardil and Parnate. Any drug of this type should be discontinued at least 2 weeks prior to starting treatment with Sinequan, and the patient should be carefully monitored by the doctor.

Patients should consult their doctor before combining Sinequan with any other prescription or nonprescription drugs.

How should this medication be taken?

This medication must be taken exactly as prescribed. It may take several weeks for its beneficial effects to appear.

- *Missed dose...*
  Patients taking several doses a day should take the missed dose as soon as they remember, then take any remaining doses for that day at evenly spaced intervals. If it is almost time for the next dose, they should skip the one they missed and go back to their regular schedule. Patients should never take 2 doses at the same time.

  Patients who take a single dose at bedtime and do not remember until the next morning should skip the dose. Doses should never be doubled.

- *Storage instructions...*
  Sinequan should be stored at room temperature.

What side effects may occur?

Side effects cannot be predicted. If any develop or change in intensity, patients should inform their doctor as soon as possible.

- *Side effects may include:*
  Blurred vision, constipation, dizziness, drowsiness, dry mouth, itchy or scaly skin (pruritus), light sensitivity, low blood pressure, nausea, rapid or irregular heartbeat, rash, trouble urinating, water retention

Why should this drug not be prescribed?

Anyone who is sensitive to or has ever had an allergic reaction to Sinequan or similar antidepressants should not take this medication. Sinequan should also be avoided by patients with the eye condition known as glaucoma and by those who have difficulty urinating.

Special warnings about this medication

In clinical studies, antidepressants increased the risk of suicidal thinking and behavior in children and adolescents with depression and other psychiatric disorders. Anyone considering the use of Sinequan, or any other antidepressant in a child or adolescent, must balance the risk with the clinical need. Sinequan is not approved for treating anyone less than 12 years old.

Additionally, the progression of major depression is associated with a worsening of symptoms and/or the emergence of suicidal thinking or behavior in both adults and children, whether or not they are taking antidepressants. Patients and caregivers should watch for any change in symptoms or any new symptoms that appear suddenly—especially agitation, anxiety, hostility, panic, restlessness, extreme hyperactivity, and suicidal thinking or behavior—and report them to the doctor immediately. Be especially observant at the beginning of treatment or whenever there is a change in dose.

Sinequan may cause the patient to become drowsy or less alert. Driving, operating dangerous machinery, or participating in any hazardous activity that requires full mental alertness is not recommended.

In a medical emergency, and before surgery or dental treatment, the doctor or dentist should be made aware that the patient is taking Sinequan.

Alcohol increases the danger in a Sinequan overdose. Patients should not drink alcohol while taking this medication.

Sinequan should never be combined with drugs known as MAO inhibitors. Medications in this category include the antidepressants Nardil and Parnate.

Patients switching from Prozac should wait at least 5 weeks after their last dose of Prozac before starting Sinequan.

Possible food and drug interactions when taking this medication

See the entry for the generic name doxepin on page 316.

Special information about pregnancy and breastfeeding

The effects of Sinequan during pregnancy have not been adequately studied. Women who are pregnant or are planning to become pregnant should inform their doctor immediately.

Sinequan may appear in breast milk and could affect a nursing infant. If this medication is essential to the patient's health, the doctor may advise her to discontinue breastfeeding until treatment is finished.

Recommended dosage

ADULTS

The starting dose for mild to moderate illness is usually 75 milligrams per day. This dose can be increased or decreased by the doctor according to individual need. The usual ideal dose ranges from 75 milligrams per day to 150 milligrams per day, although it can be as low as 25 to 50 milligrams per day. The total daily dose can be given once a day or divided into smaller doses. For people taking this drug once a day, the recommended dose is 150 milligrams at bedtime.

The 150-milligram capsule strength is intended for long-term therapy only and is not recommended as a starting dose.

For more severe illness, gradually increased doses of up to 300 milligrams may be required as determined by the doctor.

CHILDREN

Safety and effectiveness have not been established for use in children under 12 years of age.

OLDER ADULTS

Due to a greater risk of drowsiness and confusion, older people are usually started on a low dose.

Overdosage

An overdose of Sinequan can be fatal. The following symptoms signal the need for immediate medical attention.

- *Symptoms of Sinequan overdose may include:*
  Agitation, coma, confusion, convulsions, dilated pupils, disturbed concentration, drowsiness, hallucinations, high or low body temperature, irregular heartbeat, overactive reflexes, rigid muscles, severely low blood pressure, stupor, vomiting

---

SONATA
Zaleplon

Why is this drug prescribed?

Sonata is prescribed for people who have trouble falling asleep at bedtime. Because it has a short duration of action, it doesn't help those who suffer from frequent awakenings during the night or those who wake too early in the morning. It is intended only for short-term use (7 to 10 days).

Most important fact about this drug

Problems with sleep are usually temporary and require only short-term treatment with medication. Patients should call their doctor immediately if it seems the medication is making the problem worse, or if they notice any unusual changes in their thinking or behavior, such as hallucinations, amnesia, agitation, or a lack of inhibition. The emergence of new symptoms could be a sign of an undiagnosed medical or psychiatric condition.

How should this medication be taken?

Sonata is very fast-acting and should be taken only at bedtime.

* *Missed dose...*
Sonata should be taken only when the patient is ready to sleep. The dose should never be doubled.

* *Storage instructions...*
Sonata should be stored at room temperature in a light-resistant container.

What side effects may occur?
Side effects cannot be predicted. If any develop or change in intensity, patients should inform their doctor as soon as possible.

* *Side effects may include:*
Abdominal pain, amnesia, dizziness, drowsiness, eye pain, headache, memory loss, menstrual problems, nausea, sleepiness, tingling, weakness

A variety of other symptoms have been reported on very rare occasions. If Sonata is suspected of causing any sort of problem, it would be wise to check with the doctor.

Why should this drug not be prescribed?
Sonata is not recommended for people with severe liver disease and is best avoided during pregnancy.

Sonata contains FD&C Yellow No. 5 (tartrazine). Patients who are allergic to this dye, or any other ingredient in Sonata, should not take this drug. Tartrazine allergy is more likely in people with aspirin sensitivity.

Special warnings about this medication
Sonata should not be used unless the patient plans to be in bed for at least 4 hours after taking it. Those who need to be alert and active in less than 4 hours may find that their performance is impaired. No one should attempt to drive a car or operate other dangerous machinery right after taking Sonata.

Sonata should be used only for temporary relief of insomnia; sleep medicines tend to lose their effect when taken for more than a few weeks. Remember, too, that taking sleeping pills for extended periods or in high doses can lead to physical dependence and the danger of a withdrawal reaction when the drug is abruptly stopped. Special caution is warranted for patients who have had addiction problems with alcohol or other drugs.

Severe allergic reactions—including life-threatening ones that can cause severe breathing problems—have been reported. Patients who develop any of the following symptoms should seek medical attention immediately: agitation, difficulty breathing, sudden drop in blood pressure, fainting, tingling sensations, itchy and flushed skin, hives, or swelling. If a patient is allergic to FD&C Yellow No. 5 (tartrazine), they'll probably want to avoid Sonata, which contains this substance.

The safety and effectiveness of Sonata have not been established in children.

Patients should avoid alcoholic beverages when taking Sonata; the drug increases alcohol's effect. They should also forgo high-fat meals immediately before taking Sonata; they tend to slow or reduce the drug's effect.

Possible food and drug interactions when taking this medication

See the entry for the generic name zaleplon on page 422.

Special information about pregnancy and breastfeeding

Sonata can affect a developing baby, especially during the last weeks before delivery, and is therefore not recommended for use during pregnancy. This drug also appears in breast milk and should not be used by nursing mothers.

Recommended dosage

ADULTS

The usual dose is 10 milligrams taken once daily at bedtime. The doctor may adjust the dose according to individual need, especially for those who are in a weakened condition or have a low body weight. A dose of 5 milligrams is recommended if the patient has liver disease or uses the drug cimetidine.

OLDER ADULTS

The usual dose for older adults is 5 milligrams, as they may be more sensitive to the effects of Sonata.

Overdosage

An overdose of drugs such as Sonata can be fatal. If an overdose is suspected, seek medical attention immediately.

- *Symptoms of Sonata overdose may include:*
  Drowsiness, mental confusion, grogginess, lack of coordination, flaccid muscles, labored breathing, coma

---

STRATTERA

Atomoxetine hydrochloride

Why is this drug prescribed?

Strattera is used in the treatment of attention deficit hyperactivity disorder (ADHD). Medications such as Strattera should always be part of a comprehensive treatment program that includes psychological, educational, and social measures designed to remedy the problem.

Strattera is the first ADHD medication to avoid classification as a controlled substance (a drug with potential for abuse). It is thought to work by boosting levels of norepinephrine, one of the brain chemicals responsible for regulating activity. It is prescribed for children and adults.

Most important fact about this drug
During clinical trials, researchers found that Strattera slowed children's average rate of growth. It's not known whether final adult height and weight are affected, but the manufacturer recommends interrupting use of the drug if a child is not growing or gaining weight at the expected rate.

How should this medication be taken?
Strattera should be taken exactly as prescribed; higher-than-recommended doses provide no additional benefit. Strattera may be taken with or without food.

- *Missed dose...*
  The forgotten dose should be taken as soon as remembered. However, patients should take no more than the prescribed daily total during any 24-hour period.

- *Storage instructions...*
  Strattera should be stored at room temperature.

What side effects may occur?
Side effects cannot be anticipated. If any develop or change in intensity, patients should inform their doctor as soon as possible.

- *Side effects in children may include:*
  Appetite loss, constipation, cough, crying, diarrhea, dizziness, drowsiness, dry mouth, ear infection, fatigue, headache, indigestion, influenza, irritability, mood swings, nausea, runny nose, skin inflammation, stomach pain, vomiting, weight loss

- *Side effects in adults may include:*
  Abnormal dreams, abnormal orgasms, appetite loss, chills, constipation, diminished sex drive, dizziness, dry mouth, ejaculation disorders, erection problems, fatigue or sluggishness, fever, headache, hot flashes, impotence, indigestion, insomnia, gas, menstrual problems, muscle pain, nausea, palpitations, prostate inflammation, sinusitis, skin inflammation, sleep disorder, sweating, tingling, urinary problems, weight loss

Why should this drug not be prescribed?
Strattera must not be taken within 2 weeks of taking any drug classified as an MAO inhibitor, such as the antidepressants Nardil and Parnate. The combination can cause severe—even fatal—reactions, including symptoms such as high fever, rigid muscles, rapid changes in heart rate, delirium, and coma.

Patients should also avoid Strattera if they have narrow angle glaucoma (high pressure in the eye), or if the drug causes an allergic reaction.

Special warnings about this medication

Strattera can speed up the heart and boost blood pressure. It should be used with caution if the patient has high blood pressure, a rapid heart rate, heart disease, or any other circulation problem.

On the other hand, Strattera can also cause an attack of low blood pressure when the patient first stands up. Caution is warranted when the patient has a condition, such as severe dehydration, that can cause low blood pressure.

Strattera should be discontinued if a patient develops signs of liver damage, including jaundice (yellowing of the skin and eyes), dark urine, flu-like symptoms, and/or itchy spots. Patients should see their doctor at the first sign of these symptoms for testing and possible treatment options.

If a child with ADHD is becoming increasingly aggressive or hostile, this may be caused by Strattera. The doctor should be contacted immediately for proper evaluation.

Because Strattera sometimes causes sluggishness, patients should be careful when operating machinery or driving until they know how the drug affects them.

Remember that Strattera must never be combined with MAO inhibitors (see "Why should this drug not be prescribed?"). If patients are unsure about a particular medication possibly interacting with Strattera—whether prescription or over-the-counter—they should make a point of asking their doctor.

Possible food and drug interactions when taking this medication

See the entry for the generic name atomoxetine on page 285.

Special information about pregnancy and breastfeeding

Strattera has not been studied in pregnant women. If a woman is pregnant or plans to become pregnant she should notify her doctor immediately. Strattera should not be taken during pregnancy unless its benefits justify the potential risk to the baby.

It is not known whether Strattera makes its way into breast milk. Caution is warranted if the patient plans to nurse.

Recommended dosage

The daily dose of Strattera can be taken as a single dose in the morning, or divided into two equal doses taken in the morning and late afternoon or early evening.

ADULTS

For adults and teenagers weighing over 154 pounds, the usual starting dosage is 40 milligrams per day. After at least 3 days, the doctor may increase the daily total to a recommended level of 80 milligrams. After another 2 to 4 weeks, the dosage may be increased to a maximum of 100 milligrams daily. If the patient has liver problems, the dosage will be reduced.

CHILDREN

For children and teenagers weighing up to 154 pounds, the usual starting dosage is 0.5 milligram per 2.2 pounds (1 kilogram) of body weight per day. After at least 3 days, the doctor may increase the daily total to a recommended level of 1.2 milligrams per 2.2 pounds (1 kilogram). Daily doses should never exceed 1.4 milligrams per 2.2 pounds (1 kilogram) or a total of 100 milligrams, whichever is less. Strattera has not been tested in children under 6 years of age.

Overdosage

There is limited information on Strattera overdose. However, any medication taken in excess can have serious consequences. If an overdose is suspected, seek emergency treatment immediately.

- *Symptoms of a Strattera overdose may include:*
  Abnormal behavior, agitation, dilated pupils, dry mouth, hyperactivity, rapid heartbeat, sleepiness, stomach problems

---

SUBOXONE
Buprenorphine hydrochloride and naloxone hydrochloride dihydrate

Why is this drug prescribed?
Suboxone is prescribed to help treat opioid dependence, including an addiction to opioid drugs such as heroin, oxycodone, and other narcotic painkillers. It is used to help patients stay in treatment by suppressing symptoms of opioid withdrawal, decreasing cravings, reducing illicit opioid use, and blocking the effects of highly addictive opioids.

Suboxone is available as a sublingual tablet. The main active ingredient is buprenorphine. The other ingredient, naloxone, is included to discourage patients from dissolving the tablet and injecting it. When Suboxone is placed under the tongue, as directed, very little naloxone reaches the bloodstream, so the patient only feels the effects of buprenorphine. However, if naloxone is injected, it can cause the person to quickly go into withdrawal.

Most important fact about this drug
Suboxone sublingual tablets should never be misused by dissolving the medication and taking it as an injection. Severe reactions and even death can occur if Suboxone is injected, especially in combination with benzodiazepines and other nervous system depressants. Patients should be warned of the potential danger of misusing Suboxone or combining it with benzodiazepines and other depressants such as alcohol, sleeping pills, certain antidepressants, and other opioid medications.

How should this medication be taken?

Suboxone is taken once a day. The tablets should be placed under the tongue and allowed to dissolve completely. Patients should not swallow the medication, since this reduces its effectiveness.

• *Missed dose...*
Generally, forgotten doses should be taken as soon as remembered. However, if it is almost time for the next dose, patients should skip the one they missed and return to their regular schedule. Doses should never be doubled.

• *Storage instructions...*
Store at room temperature.

What side effects may occur?

Side effects cannot be anticipated. If any develop or change in intensity, patients should inform their doctor as soon as possible.

• *Side effects may include:*
Headache, insomnia, nausea, pain, sweating, withdrawal symptoms

In rare cases, Suboxone has caused serious allergic reactions. Patients should seek medical treatment immediately if any of the following occur: hives, swelling of the face, trouble breathing, wheezing, decreased blood pressure, and loss of consciousness (shock).

Why should this drug not be prescribed?

Suboxone should not be used by anyone who is allergic to the active ingredients buprenorphine or naloxone.

Special warnings about this medication

Because Suboxone is a partial opioid agonist, it has the potential for abuse and can cause dependence, although the withdrawal syndrome is milder than with full opioid agonists such as heroin and narcotic painkillers.

Before taking Suboxone, patients should inform the doctor about all their medical conditions, including a history of alcoholism, adrenal problems such as Addison's disease, benign prostatic hypertrophy (enlargement of the prostate gland), difficulty urinating, head injury, hallucinations, spinal problems that make it hard to breathe, gallbladder disease, stomach problems, kidney or liver disease, thyroid problems, and lung disease.

Family members should be made aware that if the patient needs emergency medical treatment, the attending doctor or emergency room staff should be alerted that the patient is physically dependent on narcotics and is being treated with Suboxone.

Liver problems have been reported in people receiving Suboxone. Patients should contact the doctor immediately if they develop any of the following: yellowing of the skin or whites of the eyes, dark-colored urine, light-colored stools, nausea, loss of appetite, and stomach pain.

Suboxone can cause drowsiness and slow reaction times. Patients should not drive or operate hazardous machinery until they know how this drug affects them.

Suboxone can also produce a sudden drop in blood pressure and cause dizziness when patients get up too quickly from a sitting or lying position. This is more common at the start of therapy. Advise patients to sit up slowly and rest their feet on the floor a few minutes before standing up.

Suboxone has not been studied in patients less than 16 years old.

Possible food and drug interactions when taking this medication

See the entries for the generic names buprenorphine and naloxone on pages 287 and 360.

Special information about pregnancy and breastfeeding

The effects of Suboxone during pregnancy have not been adequately studied. The drug is recommended only if its benefits are thought to outweigh the potential risk to the baby. If a patient is pregnant or planning to become pregnant, she should inform her doctor immediately.

Because Suboxone appears in breast milk and may harm a baby, women should not use it while breastfeeding.

Recommended dosage

ADULTS AND ADOLESCENTS 16 YEARS AND OLDER

The usual dose is 12 to 16 milligrams a day.

Overdosage

A large overdose of Suboxone can be fatal. If an overdose is suspected, seek emergency treatment immediately.

- *Symptoms of Suboxone overdose may include:*
  Confusion, constricted (pinpoint-sized) pupils, dizziness, feeling faint or losing consciousness, low blood pressure, slowed breathing

SURMONTIL

Trimipramine maleate

Why is this drug prescribed?

Surmontil is used to treat depression. It is a member of the family of drugs known as tricyclic antidepressants.

Most important fact about this drug

Serious—sometimes fatal—reactions have been known to occur when drugs such as Surmontil are taken with drugs classified as MAO inhibitors. Drugs in this category include the antidepressants Nardil and Parnate. Surmontil must not be used within 2 weeks of taking one of these drugs.

How should this medication be taken?

Surmontil may be taken in 1 dose at bedtime. Alternatively, the total daily dosage may be divided into smaller amounts taken during the day. The single bedtime dose is preferred for people on long-term therapy with Surmontil.

It is important to take Surmontil exactly as prescribed, even if the drug seems to have no effect. It may take up to 4 weeks for its benefits to appear.

Surmontil can make the mouth dry. Sucking hard candy or chewing gum can help this problem.

• *Missed dose...*
Generally, a missed dose should be taken as soon as remembered. However, if it is almost time for the next dose, patients should skip the dose they missed and go back to their regular schedule. Doses should never be doubled.

Patients who take Surmontil once a day at bedtime and miss a dose should not take it in the morning. It could cause disturbing side effects during the day.

• *Storage instructions...*
Surmontil should be stored at room temperature in a tightly closed container. Capsules in blister strips should be protected from moisture.

What side effects may occur?

Side effects cannot be predicted. If any develop or change in intensity, patients should inform their doctor as soon as possible.

• *Side effects may include:*
Allergic reactions, blood disorders, blurred vision, breast development in men, confusion, dry mouth, heartbeat irregularities, high blood pressure, insomnia, lack of coordination, low blood pressure, stomach and intestinal problems, urination problems

Why should this drug not be prescribed?

Surmontil should not be used by anyone recovering from a recent heart attack. It should not be taken by people who are sensitive to it or have ever had an allergic reaction to it or to similar drugs such as Tofranil.

Special warnings about this medication

In clinical studies, antidepressants increased the risk of suicidal thinking and behavior in children and adolescents with depression and other psychiatric disorders. Anyone considering the use of Surmontil, or any other antidepressant in a child or adolescent, must balance the risk with the clinical need. Surmontil has not been studied in children.

Additionally, the progression of major depression is associated with a worsening of symptoms and/or the emergence of suicidal thinking or behavior in both adults and children, whether or not they are taking antidepressants. Patients and caregivers should watch for any change in symptoms or any new symptoms that appear suddenly—especially agitation, anxiety, hostility, panic, restlessness, extreme hyperactivity, and suicidal thinking or behavior—and report them to the doctor immediately. Be especially observant at the beginning of treatment or whenever there is a change in dose.

Surmontil should be used with caution by patients who have a seizure disorder, the eye condition known as glaucoma, heart disease, or a liver disorder. Caution is also warranted if they have thyroid disease or are taking thyroid medication. People who have had problems urinating should also be careful about taking Surmontil.

Nausea, headache, and a general feeling of illness may result if Surmontil is stopped suddenly. This does not signify addiction, but the doctor's instructions should be followed closely when discontinuing the drug.

This drug may impair the ability to drive a car or operate potentially dangerous machinery. Patients should not participate in any activities that require full alertness if they are unsure of the drug's effect.

People who are taking antidepressants known as MAO inhibitors (Parnate and Nardil) should not take Surmontil. They need to wait 2 weeks after stopping an MAO inhibitor before starting Surmontil.

Extreme drowsiness and other potentially serious effects may result if the patient drinks alcoholic beverages while taking Surmontil.

Possible food and drug interactions when taking this medication

See the entry for the generic name trimipramine on page 417.

Special information about pregnancy and breastfeeding

The effects of Surmontil in pregnancy have not been adequately studied. Pregnant women should use Surmontil only when the potential benefits clearly outweigh the potential risks.

There is no information on whether Surmontil appears in breast milk. The doctor may tell the patient to stop nursing until her treatment is finished.

Recommended dosage

ADULTS

The usual starting dose is 75 milligrams per day, divided into equal smaller doses. The doctor may gradually increase the dose to 150 milligrams per day, divided into smaller doses. Doses over 200 milligrams a day are not recommended. Doses in long-term therapy may range from 50 to 150 milligrams daily. This total daily dosage can be taken at bedtime or spread out through the day.

CHILDREN

Safety and effectiveness of Surmontil in children have not been established.

OLDER ADULTS AND ADOLESCENTS

Dosages usually start at 50 milligrams per day. The doctor may increase the dose to 100 milligrams a day, if needed.

Overdosage

Any medication taken in excess can have serious consequences. An overdose of Surmontil can be fatal. If an overdose is suspected, seek medical help immediately.

- *Symptoms of Surmontil overdose may include:*
  Agitation, coma, confusion, convulsions, dilated pupils, disturbed concentration, drowsiness, hallucinations, high fever, irregular heart rate, low body temperature, muscle rigidity, overactive reflexes, severely low blood pressure, stupor, vomiting

Any of the symptoms listed under "What side effects may occur?" are also possible.

SYMBYAX

Olanzapine and fluoxetine hydrochloride

Why is this drug prescribed?

Symbyax is used to treat depressive episodes associated with bipolar disorder. The drug is a combination of the active ingredients in Prozac (fluoxetine), used to treat depression and other conditions, and Zyprexa (olanzapine), used to treat the manic phase of bipolar disorder as well as other conditions.

Most important fact about this drug

Serious, sometimes fatal, reactions have been known to occur when fluoxetine, one of the ingredients in Symbyax, is taken with other antidepressant drugs called MAO inhibitors, including Nardil and Parnate. Such reactions have also occurred when fluoxetine is discontinued and an MAO inhibitor is started. Patients should never take Symbyax with an MAO inhibitor, or within 14 days of discontinuing therapy with an MAO inhibitor. A minimum of 5 weeks should be allowed between stopping Symbyax and starting an MAO inhibitor. Caution is especially warranted if patients have been taking Symbyax in high doses or for a long time.

   In addition, Symbyax should never be combined with thioridazine due to the risk of life-threatening drug interactions, and a minimum of 5 weeks should be allowed between stopping Symbyax and starting thioridazine.

How should this medication be taken?

Symbyax can be taken with or without food. Symbyax should be taken exactly as prescribed. It is best to take in the evening. To be effective, Symbyax must be taken every day, even if the patient starts to feel better.

Patients should never change the dosage or stop taking the drug without consulting their doctor.

• *Missed dose...*
Patients should take the forgotten dose as soon as they remember. However, if it is almost time for their next dose, patients should skip the dose they missed and return to their regular schedule. They should never take two doses at once.

• *Storage instructions...*
Symbyax should be stored at room temperature in a tightly closed container. The drug should also be protected from moisture.

What side effects may occur?
Side effects cannot be predicted. If any develop or change in intensity, patients should inform their doctor as soon as possible.

• *Side effects may include:*
Abnormal thinking, increased appetite, lack of coordination, sleepiness, sore throat, tremor, water retention (especially in the arms and legs), weakness, weight gain

Why should this drug not be prescribed?
Symbyax should be avoided by anyone who has ever had an allergic reaction to any of the drug's ingredients or to the drugs Prozac or Zyprexa. Patients need to alert their doctor about any drug reaction they have experienced.

Remember, too, that Symbyax should never be combined with an MAO inhibitor or thioridazine (see "Most important fact about this drug").

Special warnings about this medication
In clinical studies, antidepressants increased the risk of suicidal thinking and behavior in children and adolescents with depression and other psychiatric disorders. Anyone considering the use of Symbyax, or any other antidepressant in a child or adolescent, must balance the risk with the clinical need. Symbyax is not approved for use in children.

Additionally, the progression of major depression is associated with a worsening of symptoms and/or the emergence of suicidal thinking or behavior in both adults and children, whether or not they are taking antidepressants. Patients and caregivers should watch for any change in symptoms or any new symptoms that appear suddenly—especially agitation, anxiety, hostility, panic, restlessness, extreme hyperactivity, and suicidal thinking or behavior—and report them to the doctor immediately. Be especially observant at the beginning of treatment or whenever there is a change in dose.

Certain antipsychotic drugs—including olanzapine, one of the ingredients in Symbyax—are associated with an increased risk of developing high blood sugar, which on rare occasions has led to coma or death. Patients should see their doctor right away if they develop signs of high blood sugar, including dry mouth, unusual thirst, increased urination, and tiredness. Patients who have diabetes or have a high risk of developing it should see their doctor regularly for blood sugar testing.

Symbyax should be used with caution in patients who have a history of heart disease, heart rhythm problems, stroke, seizures, or liver problems. Caution is also advised in patients who are at risk of developing low blood pressure or dehydration, and in those taking drugs to lower their blood pressure.

Serotonin-boosting antidepressants such as fluoxetine, one of the ingredients in Symbyax, could potentially cause stomach bleeding. This is especially likely in older adults or those taking nonsteroidal anti-inflammatory drugs (NSAIDs) such as aspirin, ibuprofen (Advil, Motrin), naproxen (Aleve), and ketoprofen. Advise patients to consult their doctor before combining Symbyax with NSAIDs or blood-thinning medications.

Symbyax has not been studied in people with certain diseases. However, the individual ingredients in this drug have been known to cause problems in people with specific illnesses. Patients should tell the doctor if they have a history of the following: heart attack, heart disease, an enlarged prostate, high or low blood pressure, abnormal bleeding, narrow-angle glaucoma, paralysis of the intestines, trouble swallowing, Alzheimer's disease, or dementia (in patients older than 65). Olanzapine, one of the ingredients in Symbyax, is not approved for treating elderly patients with dementia.

Animal studies suggest that olanzapine, one of the ingredients in Symbyax, may increase the risk of breast cancer, although human studies have not confirmed such a risk. Advise patients with a history of breast cancer to see their doctor regularly for checkups.

Symbyax can cause dizziness and even fainting when getting up from sitting or lying down (orthostatic hypotension). Patients who experience this should notify the doctor.

The ingredients in this drug could cause an allergic reaction. Patients should alert the doctor immediately if they develop a skin rash or hives.

Olanzapine and other antipsychotic drugs sometimes cause a condition called neuroleptic malignant syndrome. Symptoms include high fever, muscle rigidity, irregular pulse or blood pressure, rapid or irregular heartbeat, and excessive perspiration. If these symptoms appear, patients should alert the doctor immediately. The doctor will need to stop therapy with Symbyax while the condition is being treated.

Symbyax could increase the risk of developing tardive dyskinesia, a condition marked by slow, rhythmic, involuntary movements. This problem is more likely to surface in older adults, especially women. If it does, treatment with Symbyax will usually be stopped.

Symbyax could trigger a manic episode. The patient should be watched closely for symptoms of mania.

Medications such as Symbyax can interfere with regulation of body temperature. Patients should avoid getting overheated or becoming dehydrated while taking Symbyax. They should avoid extreme heat and drink plenty of fluids.

Symbyax sometimes causes drowsiness and can impair judgment, thinking, and motor skills. Patients should use caution while driving and shouldn't operate dangerous machinery until they know how the drug affects them.

Symbyax therapy should be slowly tapered instead of abruptly stopped. If abruptly discontinued, drowsiness, irritability, agitation, anxiety, headache, and insomnia may occur.

Prolonged seizures have occurred in people receiving electroconvulsive therapy (ECT) while taking fluoxetine, one of the ingredients in Symbyax. To date, there are no clinical studies establishing the benefit of combined treatment with fluoxetine and ECT.

Patients should avoid alcohol while taking Symbyax. The combination can cause a sudden drop in blood pressure.

Remember that Symbyax should never be combined with MAO inhibitors or thioridazine (see "Most important fact about this drug").

Symbyax should be used cautiously, if at all, with Zyprexa, Zyprexa Zydis, Prozac, Prozac Weekly, or Sarafem. Symbyax contains the same active ingredients as these medications.

Patients should let the doctor know if they smoke cigarettes, since this could affect how the body processes Symbyax.

Possible food and drug interactions when taking this medication

See the entries for the generic names olanzapine and fluoxetine on pages 322 and 366.

Special information about pregnancy and breastfeeding

Patients who are pregnant or planning to become pregnant should notify their doctor immediately. There have been reports of newborns experiencing complications such as respiratory problems, bluish coloring of the skin, irregular breathing, muscular problems, vomiting, and constant crying after exposure to fluoxetine (one of the ingredients in Symbyax) late in the third trimester. Symbyax should be used during pregnancy only if absolutely necessary.

Women should not breastfeed while taking Symbyax. The drug may pass into breast milk and harm the baby.

Recommended dosage

ADULTS

The usual starting dose is one capsule containing 6 milligrams of olanzapine and 25 milligrams of fluoxetine, taken once a day in the evening. If needed, the doctor may gradually increase the dose. The usual dosage range is 6 to 12 milligrams of olanzapine and 25 to 50 milligrams of fluoxetine.

CHILDREN

The safety and effectiveness of Symbyax have not been studied in children.

DOSAGE ADJUSTMENT

The doctor may adjust the dosage if patients have liver problems, a high risk of low blood pressure, or a combination of factors that may slow the body's processing of Symbyax (female, older age, nonsmoker).

Overdosage

Overdose with fluoxetine, one of the ingredients in Symbyax, can be fatal. There have been reports of patients dying after overdosing on fluoxetine and olanzapine taken as separate drugs at the same time. If an overdose is suspected, seek emergency treatment immediately.

- *Symptoms of Symbyax overdose may include:*
  Aggressive behavior, agitation, coma, confusion, convulsions, heart problems, irregular or fast heartbeat, loss of consciousness, problems with muscle coordination, problems with speech, sleepiness, sluggishness

Tacrine *See Cognex, page 47*

Temazepam *See Restoril, page 191*

THIORIDAZINE HYDROCHLORIDE

Why is this drug prescribed?

Thioridazine is used to treat schizophrenia. Because thioridazine has been known to cause dangerous heartbeat irregularities, it is usually prescribed only when at least two other medications have failed. Patients should receive an electrocardiogram before the drug is prescribed and periodically during thioridazine therapy.

Most important fact about this drug

The danger of potentially fatal cardiac irregularities increases when thioridazine is combined with any medication that prolongs a part of the heartbeat known as the QT interval. Many of the drugs prescribed for heartbeat irregularities (including Corduroyed, Internal, guanidine glaciate, guanidine sulfate, and Rhythmic) prolong the QT interval and should never be combined with thioridazine. Other drugs to be avoided during thioridazine therapy include fluvoxamine, Norvir, Paxil, pindolol, Prozac, Rescriptor, and Tagamet. Patients should make sure the doctor knows they are taking thioridazine whenever a new drug is prescribed.

How should this medication be taken?
Patients taking thioridazine in a liquid concentrate form can dilute it with distilled water, soft tap water, or juice just before taking it.

Patients should not change from one brand of thioridazine to another without consulting their doctor.

- *Missed dose...*
  Patients who take 1 dose a day and remember later in the day should take the dose immediately. If they don't remember until the next day, they should skip the dose and go back to their regular schedule. Patients who take more than 1 dose a day and remember the forgotten dose within an hour or so after its scheduled time should take it immediately. If they don't remember until later, they should skip the dose and go back to their regular schedule. Patients should never try to "catch up" by doubling a dose.

- *Storage instructions...*
  Thioridazine should be stored at room temperature, tightly closed, in the container the medication came in.

What side effects may occur?
Side effects cannot be predicted. If any develop or change in intensity, patients should inform the doctor as soon as possible.

- *Side effects may include:*
  Blurred vision, breast development in men, breast milk secretion, constipation, diarrhea, drowsiness, dry mouth, impotence, nausea, swelling in the arms and legs (edema), tardive dyskinesia (see "Special warnings about this medication"), vomiting

Why should this drug not be prescribed?
Due to the danger of cardiac irregularities, thioridazine must never be combined with drugs that increase its effects or prolong the part of the heartbeat known as the QT interval. (See "Most important fact about this drug.") It is also important to avoid combining thioridazine with excessive amounts of central nervous system depressants such as alcohol, barbiturates, or narcotics. It should not be used by anyone who has heart disease accompanied by severe high or low blood pressure.

Special warnings about this medication
Warning signs of the heartbeat irregularities that may be triggered by thioridazine include dizziness, palpitations, and fainting. Any patient who develops these symptoms should check with the doctor immediately.

Thioridazine may cause tardive dyskinesia—a condition marked by involuntary muscle spasms and twitches in the face and body. This condition may be permanent, and appears to be most common among the elderly, especially women.

Drugs such as thioridazine are also known to cause a potentially fatal condition known as neuroleptic malignant syndrome. Symptoms of this problem include high fever, rigid muscles, altered mental status, sweating, fast or irregular heartbeat, and changes in blood pressure. Patients who develop these symptoms should see their doctor immediately. Thioridazine therapy may have to be permanently discontinued.

Animal studies suggest that antipsychotics such as thioridazine may increase the risk of breast cancer, although human studies have not confirmed such a risk. Advise patients with a history of breast cancer to see their doctor regularly for checkups.

In rare cases, thioridazine has been known to trigger blood disorders and seizures. It can cause dizziness or faintness upon first standing up. High doses can also cause vision problems, including blurring, brownish coloring of vision, and poor night vision.

This drug may impair the ability to drive a car or operate potentially dangerous machinery. Patients should not participate in any activities that require full alertness until they are certain the drug will not interfere.

Extreme drowsiness and other potentially serious effects can result if thioridazine is combined with alcohol or other central nervous system depressants such as narcotics, painkillers, and sleeping medications. Patients should check with their doctor before adding any new drug to their regimen.

Possible food and drug interactions when taking this medication

See the entry for thioridazine on page 399.

Special information about pregnancy and breastfeeding

Pregnant women should use thioridazine only if clearly needed. Patients who are pregnant or plan to become pregnant should inform their doctor immediately.

There is no information on the effects of thioridazine during breastfeeding. The doctor may advise the patient to stop nursing until her treatment with this medication is finished.

Recommended dosage

The doctor will tailor the dose to the patient's needs, using the smallest effective amount.

ADULTS

The starting dose ranges from 50 to 100 milligrams 3 times a day. The doctor may gradually increase the dosage to as much as 800 milligrams a day, taken in 2 to 4 small doses. Once the symptoms improve, the doctor will decrease the dosage to the lowest effective amount.

CHILDREN

The usual starting dose for schizophrenic children is 0.5 milligram per 2.2 pounds (1 kilogram) of body weight per day, divided into smaller doses. The dose may be gradually increased to a maximum of 3 milligrams per 2.2 pounds (1 kilogram) per day.

Overdosage

Any medication taken in excess can have serious consequences. An overdose of thioridazine can be fatal. If an overdose is suspected, seek medical help immediately.

- *Symptoms of thioridazine overdose may include:*
Agitation, blurred vision, coma, confusion, constipation, difficulty breathing, dilated or constricted pupils, diminished flow of urine, dry mouth, dry skin, excessively high or low body temperature, extremely low blood pressure, fluid in the lungs, heart abnormalities, inability to urinate, intestinal blockage, nasal congestion, restlessness, sedation, seizures, shock

Thiothixene *See Navane, page 137*

Thorazine *See Chlorpromazine, page 39*

TOFRANIL

Imipramine hydrochloride
Other brand name: Tofranil-PM

Why is this drug prescribed?

Tofranil is used to treat major depression. It is a member of the family of drugs called tricyclic antidepressants.

Tofranil is also used on a short-term basis, along with behavioral therapies, to treat bed-wetting in children aged 6 and older. Its effectiveness may decrease with longer use.

Off-label uses of Tofranil include bulimia, attention deficit disorder in children, obsessive-compulsive disorder, and panic disorder.

Tofranil-PM, which is usually taken once daily at bedtime, is approved to treat major depression.

Most important fact about this drug

Serious, sometimes fatal, reactions have been known to occur when drugs such as Tofranil are taken with another type of antidepressant called an MAO inhibitor. Drugs in this category include Nardil and Parnate. Tofranil must not be taken within 2 weeks of taking one of these drugs.

How should this medication be taken?

Tofranil may be taken with or without food. It should not be combined with alcohol. Patients should keep taking Tofranil even if they feel no immediate effect. It can take from 1 to 3 weeks for improvement to begin. Tofranil can cause dry mouth. Sucking hard candy or chewing gum can help this problem.

- *Missed dose...*
  Patients who take 1 dose a day at bedtime should contact their doctor. They should not take the dose in the morning because of possible side effects. If a patient takes 2 or more doses a day, they should take the forgotten dose as soon as they remember. However, if it is almost time for the next dose, they should skip the dose they missed and go back to their regular schedule. Doses should never be doubled.

- *Storage instructions...*
  Tofranil should be stored at room temperature in a tightly closed container.

What side effects may occur?

Side effects cannot be predicted. If any develop or change in intensity, patients should inform their doctor as soon as possible.

- *Side effects may include:*
  Breast development in males, breast enlargement in females, breast milk production, confusion, diarrhea, dry mouth, hallucinations, hives, high blood pressure, low blood pressure upon standing, nausea, numbness, tremors, vomiting

- *The most common side effects in children being treated for bed-wetting are:*
  Nervousness, sleep disorders, stomach and intestinal problems, tiredness

- *Other side effects in children are:*
  Anxiety, collapse, constipation, convulsions, emotional instability, fainting

Why should this drug not be prescribed?

Tofranil should not be used by anyone recovering from a recent heart attack.

People who take drugs known as MAO inhibitors, such as the antidepressants Nardil and Parnate, should not take Tofranil. The drug should also be avoided by those who are sensitive or allergic to it.

Special warnings about this medication

In clinical studies, antidepressants increased the risk of suicidal thinking and behavior in children and adolescents with depression and other psychiatric disorders. Anyone considering the use of Tofranil, or any other antidepressant in a child or adolescent, must balance the risk with the clinical need. Tofranil has not been studied in children less than 6 years old. Tofranil-PM is not approved for use in children.

Additionally, the progression of major depression is associated with a worsening of symptoms and/or the emergence of suicidal thinking or behavior in both adults and children, whether or not they are taking antidepressants. Patients and caregivers should watch for any change in symptoms or any new symptoms that appear suddenly—especially agitation, anxiety, hostility, panic, restlessness, extreme hyperactivity, and suicidal thinking or behavior—and report them to the doctor immediately. Be especially observant at the beginning of treatment or whenever there is a change in dose.

Tofranil should be used with caution by people who have or have ever had narrow-angle glaucoma (increased pressure in the eye); difficulty urinating; heart, liver, kidney, or thyroid disease; or seizures. Caution is also warranted for people taking thyroid medication.

General feelings of illness, headache, and nausea can result if Tofranil is stopped abruptly. Patients need to follow the doctor's instructions closely when discontinuing Tofranil.

The doctor should be alerted if a sore throat or fever develops during Tofranil therapy.

This drug may impair the ability to drive a car or operate potentially dangerous machinery. Patients should avoid any activities that require full alertness if they are unsure about their ability.

Both increased and decreased blood sugar levels have been reported during Tofranil therapy. Patients with diabetes or low blood sugar (hypoglycemia) should be closely monitored by their doctors.

Tofranil could cause a manic episode in patients with bipolar disorder or a psychotic episode in those with schizophrenia. Such patients should be watched closely for signs of any problems during Tofranil therapy.

Unless it's absolutely essential, Tofranil is not recommended for patients undergoing electroconvulsive therapy (ECT).

This drug can make people sensitive to light. Patients should stay out of the sun as much as possible.

Tofranil should be discontinued before elective surgery.

Tofranil must never be combined with an MAO inhibitor (see "Most important fact about this drug").

Patients switching from Prozac should wait at least 5 weeks after the last dose of Prozac before starting Tofranil.

Extreme drowsiness and other potentially serious effects can result if Tofranil is combined with alcohol or other mental depressants, such as narcotic painkillers (Percocet), sleeping medications (Halcion), or tranquilizers (Valium).

Possible food and drug interactions when taking this medication

See the entry for the generic name imipramine on page 335.

Special information about pregnancy and breastfeeding

The effects of Tofranil during pregnancy have not been adequately studied. Pregnant women should use Tofranil only when the potential benefits clearly outweigh the potential risks. If a patient is pregnant or plans to become pregnant, she should inform her doctor immediately.

Tofranil may appear in breast milk and could affect a nursing infant. If this medication is essential to the patient's health, the doctor may advise her to stop breastfeeding until treatment is finished.

Recommended dosage

ADULTS

The usual starting dose is 75 milligrams a day. The doctor may increase this to 150 milligrams a day. The maximum daily dose is 200 milligrams. People who need to take 75 milligrams or more a day may use Tofranil-PM capsules instead of the regular tablets.

CHILDREN

Tofranil should be used in children only for the short-term treatment of bed-wetting. Safety and effectiveness in children under 6 years old have not been established. Tofranil-PM should not be used in children for any reason.

Total daily dosages for children should not exceed 2.5 milligrams for each 2.2 pounds of the child's weight. Doses usually begin at 25 milligrams per day, taken an hour before bedtime. If needed, this dose may be increased after 1 week to 50 milligrams (ages 6 through 11) or 75 milligrams (ages 12 and up), taken in one dose at bedtime or divided into 2 doses, 1 taken at mid-afternoon and 1 at bedtime.

OLDER ADULTS AND ADOLESCENTS

People in these two age groups should start with 30 to 40 milligrams per day of Tofranil tablets, since Tofranil-PM capsules are not available in these dosage strengths. The dose may be increased as necessary, but effective dosages usually do not exceed 100 milligrams a day.

Overdosage

Any medication taken in excess can have serious consequences. An overdose of Tofranil can be fatal. It has been reported that children are more sensitive than adults to overdoses of Tofranil. If an overdose is suspected, seek medical help immediately.

- *Symptoms of Tofranil overdose may include:*
  Agitation, bluish skin, coma, convulsions, difficulty breathing, dilated pupils, drowsiness, heart failure, high fever, involuntary writhing or jerky movements, irregular or rapid heartbeat, lack of coordination, low blood pressure, overactive reflexes, restlessness, rigid muscles, shock, stupor, sweating, vomiting

TRANXENE

Clorazepate dipotassium
Other brand names: Tranxene T-Tab, Tranxene-SD, Tranxene-SD Half Strength

Why is this drug prescribed?

Tranxene belongs to a class of drugs known as benzodiazepines. It is used to treat anxiety disorders and for short-term relief of anxiety symptoms.

It is also used to relieve the symptoms of acute alcohol withdrawal and to help in treating certain convulsive disorders such as epilepsy.

Most important fact about this drug

Tranxene can be habit-forming if taken regularly over a long period. Withdrawal symptoms may occur if this drug is stopped abruptly. Patients should consult the doctor before discontinuing Tranxene or making any change in their dose.

How should this medication be taken?

Tranxene should be taken exactly as prescribed.

- *Missed dose...*
  If it is within an hour or so of the scheduled time, the forgotten dose should be taken immediately. If it's not remembered until later, the patient should skip the dose and go back to the regular schedule. Doses should never be doubled.

- *Storage instructions...*
  Tranxene should be stored at room temperature and protected from excessive heat.

What side effects may occur?

Side effects cannot be predicted. If any develop or change in intensity, patients should inform their doctor as soon as possible.

- *Side effects may include:*
  Blurred vision, depression, difficulty in sleeping or falling asleep, dizziness, double vision, drowsiness, dry mouth, fatigue, genital and urinary tract disorders, headache, irritability, lack of muscle coordination, mental confusion, nervousness, skin rashes, slurred speech, stomach and intestinal problems, tremors

- *Side effects due to rapid decrease in dose or abrupt withdrawal from Tranxene may include:*
  Abdominal cramps, convulsions, diarrhea, difficulty in sleeping or falling asleep, hallucinations, impaired memory, irritability, muscle aches, nervousness, tremors, vomiting

Why should this drug not be prescribed?

Anyone who is sensitive to or has ever had an allergic reaction to Tranxene should not take this medication. It should also be avoided by people with the eye condition known as acute narrow-angle glaucoma.

Anxiety or tension related to everyday stress usually does not require treatment with such a strong drug. Patients should discuss their symptoms thoroughly with the doctor.

Tranxene is not recommended for use in more serious conditions such as depression or severe psychological disorders.

Special warnings about this medication

Tranxene may cause patients to become drowsy or less alert. They should not drive, operate dangerous machinery, or participate in any hazardous activity that requires full mental alertness until they know how this drug affects them.

Patients who are being treated for anxiety associated with depression will be prescribed the lowest dose possible to avoid the risk of overdose. They should not increase their dose without consulting the doctor.

Patients taking Tranxene for prolonged periods will need to have their blood counts and liver function checked periodically.

The elderly and people in a weakened condition are more apt to become unsteady or oversedated when taking Tranxene.

Tranxene slows down the central nervous system and may intensify the effects of alcohol. Patients should avoid alcohol while taking this medication.

Possible food and drug interactions when taking this medication

See the entry for the generic name clorazepate on page 308.

Special information about pregnancy and breastfeeding

The effects of Tranxene during pregnancy have not been adequately studied. However, because there is an increased risk of birth defects associated with this class of drug, its use during pregnancy should be avoided.

Tranxene may appear in breast milk and could affect a nursing infant. If this medication is essential to the patient's health, the doctor may advise her to discontinue breastfeeding until treatment with this medication is finished.

Recommended dosage

ANXIETY

Adults: The usual daily dosage is 30 milligrams divided into several smaller doses. A normal daily dose can be as little as 15 milligrams. The doctor may increase the dosage gradually to as much as 60 milligrams, according to the patient's individual needs.

Tranxene can also be taken in a single bedtime dose. The initial dose is 15 milligrams. The doctor may adjust the dose if necessary.

Tranxene-SD, a 22.5-milligram tablet, and Tranxene-SD Half Strength, an 11.25-milligram tablet, can be taken once every 24 hours. The doctor may switch patients to this form of the drug after they have been taking Tranxene for several weeks.

Older Adults: The usual starting dose is 7.5 to 15 milligrams a day.

ACUTE ALCOHOL WITHDRAWAL

Tranxene can be used in a multiday program for relief of the symptoms of acute alcohol withdrawal. Dosages are usually increased in the first 2 days from 30 to 90 milligrams and then reduced over the next 2 days to lower levels. The doctor will continue to lower the dose until the drug is no longer necessary.

WHEN USED WITH ANTIEPILEPTIC DRUGS

Tranxene can be used in conjunction with antiepileptic drugs. Recommended dosages must be followed carefully to avoid drowsiness.

Adults and Children over 12 Years Old: The starting dose is 7.5 milligrams 3 times a day. The doctor may increase the dosage by 7.5 milligrams per week to a maximum of 90 milligrams a day.

Children 9 to 12 Years Old: The starting dose is 7.5 milligrams twice a day. The doctor may increase the dosage by 7.5 milligrams a week to a maximum of 60 milligrams a day. Safety and effectiveness in children under 9 years of age have not been established.

Overdosage

Any medication taken in excess can have serious consequences. If an overdose is suspected, seek medical treatment immediately.

* *Symptoms of Tranxene overdose may include:*
  Coma, low blood pressure, sedation

Tranylcypromine *See Parnate, page 154*

Trazodone *See Desyrel, page 63*

Triazolam *See Halcion, page 94*

TRIFLUOPERAZINE HYDROCHLORIDE

Why is this drug prescribed?

Trifluoperazine is used to treat schizophrenia. It is also prescribed for anxiety that does not respond to ordinary tranquilizers.

Most important fact about this drug

Trifluoperazine may cause tardive dyskinesia, a condition marked by involuntary muscle spasms and twitches in the face and body. This condition may be permanent and appears to be most common among the elderly, especially women.

How should this medication be taken?

Patients taking trifluoperazine in a liquid concentrate form will need to dilute it with a carbonated beverage, coffee, fruit juice, milk, tea, tomato juice, or water. It can also be mixed with puddings, soups, and other semi-solid foods. It should not be mixed with alcohol.

Trifluoperazine should be diluted just before it's taken.

* *Missed dose...*
  Patients taking 1 dose a day should take the missed dose as soon as they remember, and then go back to their regular schedule. If they do not remember until the next day, they should skip the missed dose and go back to their regular schedule.

  Patients who take more than 1 dose a day should take the missed dose if it is within an hour or so of the scheduled time. If they do not remember until later, they should skip the missed dose and go back to their regular schedule. Doses should never be doubled.

* *Storage instructions...*
  Trifluoperazine should be stored at room temperature. The concentrate should be protected from light.

What side effects may occur?

Side effects cannot be predicted. If any develop or change in intensity, patients should inform their doctor as soon as possible.

* *Side effects may include:*
  Blood disorders, convulsions, dry mouth, headache, muscle stiffness or rigidity, nausea, restlessness, Parkinson's-like movements, tardive dyskinesia (see "Most important fact about this drug")

Why should this drug not be prescribed?

Trifluoperazine should be avoided by people with liver damage and those who are taking central nervous system depressants such as alcohol, barbiturates, or narcotic pain relievers. It is also contraindicated for people who have an abnormal bone marrow or blood condition.

Special warnings about this medication

Trifluoperazine should be used with caution by anyone who has ever had a brain tumor, breast cancer, intestinal blockage, the eye condition called glaucoma, heart or liver disease, or seizures. Caution is warranted, too, if the patient is exposed to certain pesticides or extreme heat.

Trifluoperazine may hide the signs of overdose of other drugs and may make it more difficult for the doctor to diagnose intestinal obstruction, brain tumor, and the dangerous neurological condition called Reye's syndrome.

Patients should inform the doctor if they have ever had an allergic reaction to any antipsychotic medication similar to trifluoperazine.

Dizziness, nausea, vomiting, and tremors can result if a patient suddenly stops taking trifluoperazine. The drug should be discontinued under a doctor's supervision.

The doctor should be alerted immediately if a patient experiences symptoms such as a fever or sore throat/mouth/or gums. These signs of infection may signal the need to stop trifluoperazine treatment. The doctor should be notified, too, of flu-like symptoms with fever.

This drug may impair the ability to drive a car or operate potentially dangerous machinery, especially during the first few days of treatment. Patients should not participate in any activities that require full mental alertness if they are unsure about their ability.

Any vision problems that develop should be reported to the doctor. Trifluoperazine has been known to cause vision problems.

Trifluoperazine concentrate contains a sulfite that may cause allergic reactions in some people, especially in those with asthma.

Trifluoperazine can cause a potentially fatal condition called neuroleptic malignant syndrome. Signs are high body temperature, rigid muscles, irregular pulse or blood pressure, rapid or abnormal heartbeat, excessive perspiration, and high fever. These symptoms should be reported to the doctor immediately. Antipsychotic therapy will have to be discontinued.

Extreme drowsiness and other potentially serious effects can result if trifluoperazine is combined with alcohol, tranquilizers such as Valium, narcotic painkillers such as Percocet, antihistamines such as Benadryl, and barbiturates such as phenobarbital.

Possible food and drug interactions when taking this medication

See the entry for trifluoperazine on page 414.

Special information about pregnancy and breastfeeding

Pregnant women should use trifluoperazine only if clearly needed. The effects of trifluoperazine during pregnancy have not been adequately studied. Women who are pregnant or plan to become pregnant should inform their doctor immediately.

Trifluoperazine appears in breast milk and may affect a nursing infant. If this medication is essential to the patient's health, the doctor may have her discontinue breastfeeding while she is taking it.

Recommended dosage

NONPSYCHOTIC ANXIETY

Adults: Doses usually range from 2 to 4 milligrams daily. This amount should be divided into 2 equal doses and taken twice a day. The maximum dose is 6 milligrams a day. Treatment should continue for no more than 12 weeks.

SCHIZOPHRENIA

Adults: The usual starting dose is 4 to 10 milligrams a day, divided into 2 equal doses; doses range from 15 to 40 milligrams daily.

Children 6 to 12 Years Old Who Are Closely Monitored or Hospitalized: Doses are based on the child's weight and the severity of his or her symptoms. The starting dose is 1 milligram a day, taken all at once or divided into 2 doses. The doctor will increase the dosage gradually, up to 15 milligrams a day.

DOSAGE ADJUSTMENT

Older people usually take trifluoperazine at lower doses. Because they may develop low blood pressure while taking this drug, the doctor will watch them closely. Older people (especially older women) may be more susceptible to tardive dyskinesia.

Overdosage

Any medication taken in excess can have serious consequences. If you suspect an overdose of trifluoperazine, seek medical help immediately.

• *Symptoms of trifluoperazine overdose may include:*
Agitation, coma, convulsions, difficulty breathing, difficulty swallowing, dry mouth, extreme sleepiness, fever, intestinal blockage, irregular heart rate, low blood pressure, restlessness

TRIHEXYPHENIDYL HYDROCHLORIDE

Why is this drug prescribed?

Trihexyphenidyl is used, in conjunction with other drugs, for the relief of certain symptoms of Parkinson's disease, a brain disorder that causes muscle tremor, stiffness, and weakness. It is also used to control certain side effects induced by antipsychotic drugs such as Thorazine and haloperidol. Trihexyphenidyl works by correcting the chemical imbalance that causes Parkinson's disease.

Most important fact about this drug

Trihexyphenidyl is not a cure for Parkinson's disease; it merely minimizes and reduces the frequency of symptoms such as tremors.

How should this medication be taken?

Trihexyphenidyl can be taken either before meals or after meals. The doctor will probably start the patient on a small amount and increase the dosage gradually. Trihexyphenidyl should be taken exactly as prescribed.

This drug can make the mouth dry. Sucking on hard candy, chewing gum, or simply sipping water can provide relief.

Trihexyphenidyl comes in tablet and liquid form, each of which is usually taken 3 or 4 times a day.

Once the best dosage has been reached, the doctor may switch the patient to sustained-release capsules ("Sequels") which are to be taken only once or twice a day. Sequels should be swallowed whole; patients should not open or crush them

- *Missed dose...*
  The missed dose should be taken as soon as it is remembered. If it is within 2 hours or the next dose, the patient should skip the missed dose and go back to the regular schedule. Doses should never be doubled.

- *Storage instructions...*
  Trihexyphenidyl should be stored at room temperature. The liquid should not be allowed to freeze.

What side effects may occur?

Side effects cannot be predicted. If any develop or change in intensity, the patient should inform their doctor as soon as possible.

- *Side effects may include:*
  Blurred vision, dry mouth, nausea, nervousness

These side effects, which appear in 30% to 50% of all people who take trihexyphenidyl, tend to be mild. They may disappear as the patient's body gets used to the drug; if they persist, the doctor may want to lower the dosage slightly.

Why should this drug not be prescribed?

Anyone who is known to be sensitive to trihexyphenidyl or who has ever had an allergic reaction to it or to other antiparkinson medications of this type should not take the drug.

Special warnings about this medication

The elderly are highly sensitive to drugs such as trihexyphenidyl and should use it with caution.

Trihexyphenidyl can reduce the body's ability to perspire, one of the key ways the body prevents overheating. Anyone taking trihexyphenidyl should avoid excess sun or exercise that can cause them to become overheated.

If a patient has any of the following conditions, the doctor should know about them, since trihexyphenidyl could make them worse:

Enlarged prostate
Glaucoma
Stomach/intestinal obstructive disease
Urinary tract obstructive disease

It is important to stick to the prescribed dosage; if a patient takes larger amounts than recommended, it could lead to an overdose.

Patients who have heart, liver, or kidney disease or high blood pressure should be carefully watched by their doctor. The doctor will also check their eyes frequently, and watch for the development of any allergic reactions.

Possible food and drug interactions when taking this medication
See the entry for trihexyphenidyl on page 415.

Special information about pregnancy and breastfeeding
No specific information is available concerning the use of trihexyphenidyl during pregnancy or breastfeeding. Women who are pregnant or plan to become pregnant while taking trihexyphenidyl should inform their doctor immediately.

Recommended dosage
The following indications and dosages are for adults. The doctor will individualize the dose to the patient's needs, starting with a low dose and then increasing it gradually, especially if the patient is over 60 years of age.

Patients will be able to handle the total daily intake of trihexyphenidyl tablets or liquid best if the medication is divided into 3 doses and taken at mealtimes. For patients who are taking high doses (more than 10 milligrams daily), the doctor may divide them into 4 parts, so that the patient takes 3 doses at mealtimes and the fourth at bedtime.

PARKINSON'S DISEASE

The usual starting dose, in tablet or liquid form, is 1 milligram on the first day.

After the first day, the doctor may increase the dose by 2 milligrams at intervals of 3 to 5 days, until the patient is taking a total of 6 to 10 milligrams a day.

The total daily dose will depend upon what is found to be the most effective level. For many people, 6 to 10 milligrams is most effective. Some, however, may require a total daily dose of 12 to 15 milligrams.

DRUG-INDUCED PARKINSONISM

The doctor will have to determine by trial and error the size and frequency of the dose of trihexyphenidyl needed to control the tremors and muscle rigidity that sometimes result from commonly used tranquilizers.

The total daily dosage usually ranges between 5 and 15 milligrams, although, in some cases, symptoms have been satisfactorily controlled on as little as 1 milligram daily.

The doctor may start the patient on 1 milligram of trihexyphenidyl a day. If symptoms are not controlled in a few hours, he or she may slowly increase the dose until satisfactory control is achieved.

USE OF TRIHEXYPHENIDYL WITH LEVODOPA

When trihexyphenidyl is used at the same time as levodopa, the usual dose of each may need to be reduced. The doctor will adjust the dosages carefully, depending on the side effects and the degree of symptom control. Trihexyphenidyl dosage of 3 to 6 milligrams daily, divided into equal doses, is usually adequate.

Overdosage
Overdosage with trihexyphenidyl may cause agitation, delirium, disorientation, hallucinations, or psychotic episodes.

* *Other symptoms may include:*
  Clumsiness or unsteadiness, fast heartbeat, flushing of skin, seizures, severe drowsiness, shortness of breath or troubled breathing, trouble sleeping, unusual warmth

If an overdose of trihexyphenidyl is suspected, seek medical attention immediately.

Trimipramine *See Surmontil, page 221*

VALIUM
Diazepam

Why is this drug prescribed?
Valium is used for treatment of anxiety disorders and for short-term relief of the symptoms of anxiety. It belongs to a class of drugs known as benzodiazepines.

Valium is also used to relieve the symptoms of acute alcohol withdrawal, to relax muscles, to relieve the uncontrolled muscle movements caused by disorders such as cerebral palsy and paralysis of the lower body and limbs, to control involuntary movement of the hands (athetosis), to relax tight and aching muscles, and, along with other medications, to treat convulsive disorders such as epilepsy.

The generic ingredient diazepam is also available as a rectal gel called Diastat, which is used to treat severe, uncontrollable seizures.

Most important fact about this drug

Valium can be habit-forming or addictive. Some patients may experience withdrawal symptoms if they stop using this drug abruptly. Patients should consult their doctor before discontinuing the drug or making any change in their dose.

How should this medication be taken?

This medication must be taken exactly as prescribed. People taking the drug for epilepsy should be sure to take it at the same times every day.

- *Missed dose...*
  If it is within an hour or so of the scheduled time, the forgotten dose should be taken as soon as remembered. Otherwise, it should be skipped and the patient should return to the regular schedule. Doses should never be doubled.

- *Storage instructions...*
  Valium should be stored away from heat, light, and moisture.

What side effects may occur?

Side effects cannot be predicted. If any develop or change in intensity, patients should inform their doctor as soon as possible.

- *Side effects may include:*
  Anxiety, drowsiness, fatigue, light-headedness, loss of muscle coordination

- *Side effects due to rapid decrease in dose or abrupt withdrawal from Valium:*
  Abdominal and muscle cramps, convulsions, sweating, tremors, vomiting

Why should this drug not be prescribed?

Anyone who is sensitive to or has ever had an allergic reaction to Valium should not take this medication. It should also be avoided by those with the eye condition known as acute narrow-angle glaucoma.

Anxiety or tension related to everyday stress usually does not require treatment with such a powerful drug as Valium. Patients should discuss their symptoms thoroughly with the doctor.

Valium should not be prescribed for patients who are being treated for mental disorders more serious than anxiety.

Special warnings about this medication

Valium causes some people to become drowsy or less alert. Patients should not drive, operate dangerous machinery, or participate in any hazardous activity that requires full mental alertness until they know how this drug affects them.

This medication should be used cautiously by people with liver or kidney problems.

Valium slows down the central nervous system and may intensify the effects of alcohol. Patients should avoid alcohol while taking this medication.

Possible food and drug interactions when taking this medication
See the entry for the generic name diazepam on page 314.

Special information about pregnancy and breastfeeding
Valium should not be taken during pregnancy. There is an increased risk of birth defects. If this medication is essential to the patient's health, the doctor may advise her to discontinue breastfeeding until her treatment with this drug is finished.

Recommended dosage
The following dosages are for adults unless otherwise noted.

ANXIETY DISORDERS AND SHORT-TERM RELIEF OF ANXIETY SYMPTOMS
The usual dose ranges from 2 to 10 milligrams 2 to 4 times daily, depending upon severity of symptoms.

ACUTE ALCOHOL WITHDRAWAL
The usual dose is 10 milligrams 3 or 4 times during the first 24 hours, then 5 milligrams 3 or 4 times daily as needed.

RELIEF OF MUSCLE SPASM
The usual dose is 2 to 10 milligrams 3 or 4 times daily.

CONVULSIVE DISORDERS
The usual dose is 2 to 10 milligrams 2 to 4 times daily.

DOSAGE ADJUSTMENT IN CHILDREN
Valium should not be given to children under 6 months of age.

The usual starting dose for children over 6 months is 1 to 2.5 milligrams 3 or 4 times a day. The doctor may increase the dosage gradually if needed.

DOSAGE ADJUSTMENT IN OLDER ADULTS
The usual starting dose is 2 to 2.5 milligrams once or twice a day. The doctor will increase the dose as needed, but will limit it to the smallest effective amount because older people are more apt to become oversedated or uncoordinated.

Overdosage

Any medication taken in excess can have serious consequences. If an overdose is suspected, seek medical attention immediately.

- *Symptoms of Valium overdose may include:*
  Coma, confusion, diminished reflexes, sleepiness

Varenicline *See Chantix, page 37*

Venlafaxine *See Effexor, page 72*

VISTARIL

Hydroxyzine pamoate

Why is this drug prescribed?

Vistaril is an antihistamine used to relieve the symptoms of common anxiety and tension and, in combination with other medications, to treat anxiety that results from physical illness. It also relieves itching from allergic reactions and can be used as a sedative before and after general anesthesia. Antihistamines work by decreasing the effects of histamine, a chemical the body releases that narrows air passages in the lungs and contributes to inflammation. Antihistamines reduce itching and swelling and dry up secretions from the nose, eyes, and throat.

Most important fact about this drug

Vistaril is not intended for long-term use (more than 4 months). The doctor should reevaluate the prescription periodically.

How should this medication be taken?

This medication should be taken exactly as prescribed. Vistaril oral suspension should be shaken vigorously until the product is completely resuspended.

- *Missed dose...*
  Generally, the dose should be taken as soon as remembered. However, if it is almost time for the next dose, the patient should skip the missed dose and go back to the regular schedule. Doses should never be doubled.

- *Storage instructions...*
  Tablets and syrup should be stored away from heat, light, and moisture. Syrup should be kept from freezing.

What side effects may occur?

Side effects cannot be predicted. If any develop or change in intensity, patients should inform their doctor as soon as possible.

Drowsiness, one of the most common side effects of Vistaril, is usually temporary and may disappear in a few days or when the dosage is reduced.

Other side effects include dry mouth, twitches, tremors, and convulsions. The last two usually occur with higher-than-recommended doses of Vistaril.

Why should this drug not be prescribed?

Vistaril should not be taken in early pregnancy. It should be avoided by anyone who is sensitive to or has ever had an allergic reaction to it.

Special warnings about this medication

Vistaril increases the effects of drugs that depress the activity of the central nervous system. If the patient is taking narcotics, non-narcotic analgesics, or barbiturates in combination with Vistaril, the dosage should be reduced.

This medication can cause drowsiness. Driving or operating dangerous machinery or participating in any hazardous activity that requires full mental alertness is not recommended until patients know how they react to Vistaril.

Vistaril may increase the effects of alcohol. Patients should avoid alcohol while taking this medication.

Possible food and drug interactions when taking this medication

See the entry for the generic name hydroxyzine on page 335.

Special information about pregnancy and breastfeeding

Although the effects of Vistaril during pregnancy have not been adequately studied in humans, birth defects have appeared in animal studies with this medication. Patients should avoid Vistaril in early pregnancy, and inform their doctor immediately if they are pregnant or plan to become pregnant.

Vistaril may appear in breast milk and could affect a nursing infant. If this medication is essential to the patient's health, the doctor may advise her to discontinue breastfeeding until her treatment is finished.

Recommended dosage

When treatment begins with injections, it can be continued with oral doses. The doctor will adjust the dosage based on the patient's response to the drug.

FOR ANXIETY AND TENSION

Adults: The usual dose is 50 to 100 milligrams 4 times per day.

Children under Age 6: The total dose is 50 milligrams daily, divided into several smaller doses.

Children over Age 6: The total dose is 50 to 100 milligrams daily, divided into several smaller doses.

FOR ITCHING DUE TO ALLERGIC CONDITIONS

Adults: The usual dose is 25 milligrams 3 or 4 times a day.

Children under Age 6: The total dose is 50 milligrams daily, divided into several smaller doses.

Children over Age 6: The total dose is 50 to 100 milligrams daily, divided into several smaller doses.

BEFORE AND AFTER GENERAL ANESTHESIA

Adults: The usual dose is 50 to 100 milligrams.

Children: The usual dose is 0.6 milligram per 2.2 pounds of body weight.

Overdosage
Any medication taken in excess can have serious consequences. If an overdose of Vistaril is suspected, seek medical attention immediately. The most common symptom of Vistaril overdose is excessive calm; blood pressure may drop, although it is not likely.

VIVACTIL
Protriptyline hydrochloride

Why is this drug prescribed?
Vivactil is used to treat the symptoms of mental depression in people who are under close medical supervision. It is particularly suitable for those who are inactive and withdrawn.

Vivactil is a member of the family of drugs called tricyclic antidepressants. Researchers don't know exactly how it works. Unlike the class of antidepressants known as monoamine oxidase (MAO) inhibitors, it does not act primarily through stimulation of the central nervous system. It tends to work more rapidly than some other tricyclic antidepressants. Improvement sometimes begins within a week.

Most important fact about this drug
For patients prone to anxiety or agitation, Vivactil can make the problem worse. It can also exaggerate the symptoms of bipolar disorder and schizophrenia. If this seems to be happening, the doctor should be alerted immediately. The dose of Vivactil may need to be reduced, or the doctor may need to add another drug to the patient's regimen.

How should this medication be taken?
Vivactil should be taken exactly as prescribed. It should not be taken with alcohol.

- *Missed dose...*
  Generally, the forgotten dose should be taken as soon as remembered. However, if it is almost time for the next dose, the missed dose should be skipped and the patient should return to the regular schedule. Doses should never be doubled.

- *Storage instructions...*
  Vivactil should be stored at room temperature in a tightly closed container.

What side effects may occur?
Side effects cannot be predicted. If any develop or change in intensity, patients should inform their doctor as soon as possible.

- *Side effects may include:*
  Anxiety, blood disorders, confusion, decreased libido, dizziness, flushing, headache, impotence, insomnia, low blood pressure, nightmares, rapid or irregular heartbeat, rash, seizures, sensitivity to sunlight, stomach and intestinal problems

Why should this drug not be prescribed?
Due to the possibility of life-threatening side effects, Vivactil must never be taken with drugs classified as MAO inhibitors, such as the antidepressants Nardil and Parnate. At least 14 days should be allowed between the last dose of one of these drugs and the first dose of Vivactil.

Vivactil should not be used during recovery from a heart attack. It also cannot be used by anyone who has had an allergic reaction to it.

Special warnings about this medication
In clinical studies, antidepressants increased the risk of suicidal thinking and behavior in children and adolescents with depression and other psychiatric disorders. Anyone considering the use of Vivactil, or any other antidepressant in a child or adolescent, must balance the risk with the clinical need. Vivactil is not approved for use in children.

Additionally, the progression of major depression is associated with a worsening of symptoms and/or the emergence of suicidal thinking or behavior in both adults and children, whether or not they are taking antidepressants. Patients and caregivers should watch for any change in symptoms or any new symptoms that appear suddenly—especially agitation, anxiety, hostility, panic, restlessness, extreme hyperactivity, and suicidal thinking or behavior—and report them to the doctor immediately. Be especially observant at the beginning of treatment or whenever there is a change in dose.

Drugs such as Vivactil sometimes cause heartbeat irregularities. Vivactil should be used with caution by people who have heart problems or a thyroid disorder. Caution is also advisable for those who have a history of seizures, difficulty urinating, glaucoma (high pressure in the eyes), or alcohol abuse.

This drug is not recommended during electroconvulsive therapy. Vivactil should be discontinued several days before any surgery. Vivactil may impair the physical and/or mental abilities required to drive a car or operate heavy machinery. Patients should not participate in any activities that require full alertness until they know how this drug affects them.

Remember that Vivactil must never be combined with MAO inhibitors such as Nardil and Parnate.

Possible food and drug interactions when taking this medication

See the entry for the generic name protriptyline on page 388.

Special information about pregnancy and breastfeeding

The effects of Vivactil during pregnancy have not been adequately studied. It should be used during pregnancy only if its benefits outweigh the potential risk. Patients who are pregnant or planning to become pregnant should inform their doctor immediately.

It is not known whether Vivactil makes its way into breast milk. Patients should consult with their doctor before deciding to breastfeed.

Recommended dosage

The doctor will start with a low dose and increase it gradually, watching for side effects and a positive response.

ADULTS

The usual adult dosage is 15 to 40 milligrams in 3 or 4 doses per day. The maximum dosage is 60 milligrams daily. Increases are made in the morning dose.

CHILDREN

The safety and efficacy of Vivactil have not been studied in children.

OLDER ADULTS AND ADOLESCENTS

Lower dosages are recommended for adolescents and older adults. Five milligrams 3 times a day may be given initially, followed by a gradual increase if necessary. Heart function must be monitored in older adults who are taking 20 or more milligrams per day.

Overdosage

An overdose of Vivactil can be fatal. If an overdose is suspected, seek medical help immediately.

- *Critical signs of Vivactil overdose may include:*
  Convulsions, irregular heartbeat, severely low blood pressure, reduced level of consciousness or even coma

• *Other signs of Vivactil overdose may include:*
Agitation, confusion, dilated pupils, disturbed concentration, drowsiness, fever, hyperactive reflexes, low body temperature, muscle rigidity, sporadic hallucinations, stupor, vomiting, or any of the other symptoms listed in "What side effects may occur?"

VIVITROL
Naltrexone

Why is this drug prescribed?
Vivitrol is used to treat alcohol dependence. Vivitrol is an opioid antagonist. It works by binding to opioid receptors in the brain.

Most important fact about this drug
Vivitrol may cause damage to the liver. If a patient already has liver problems, they should tell their doctor before beginning treatment with this drug.

Vivitrol may also cause depression and suicidal thoughts.

How should you take this medication?
Vivitrol should be injected into the buttocks, alternating sides with each injection, by the patient's doctor.

• *Missed dose...*
Patients who miss a dose of Vivitrol should see their doctor immediately for an injection.

What side effects may occur?
Side effects cannot be predicted. If any develop or change in intensity, patients should inform their doctor as soon as possible.

• *Side effects may include:*
Cramps, decreased appetite/anorexia, dizziness, dry mouth, fatigue, headache, injection-site reaction (redness/swelling at the injection), nausea, stomach pain, suicidal thoughts, vomiting

Why should this drug not be prescribed?
Patients who are taking an opioid (such as heroin), are dependent on opioids, are in opiate withdrawal, or have tested positive for opiates in their urine should not begin treatment with Vivitrol.

Also, if the patient is allergic to any of the ingredients in Vivitrol, or has liver problems, they should not begin therapy.

Special warnings about this medication
Vivitrol may cause dizziness. Patients should not drive a car, work with machines, or do other dangerous activities until they know how Vivitrol affects them.

Women should avoid nursing or becoming pregnant while taking Vivitrol. If a patient becomes pregnant while on Vivitrol, she should contact her doctor immediately.

Vivitrol should not be taken by people who are also taking an opioid such as heroin. This may cause serious injury, coma, or death. Patients should tell their doctor if they are dependent on an opiate. Vivitrol is not for the treatment of opiate-dependency.

Possible food and drug interactions when taking this medication

See the entry for the generic name naltrexone on page 360.

Special information about pregnancy and breastfeeding

Women should not take Vivitrol if they are pregnant, planning to become pregnant, or are breastfeeding. Vivitrol may cause harm to the unborn baby and may pass into breast milk.

Recommended dosage

ADULTS

The recommended dosage of Vivitrol is 380 milligrams injected every 4 weeks by a doctor.

Overdosage

Any medication taken in excess can have serious consequences. If an overdose is suspected, seek medical attention immediately.

VYVANSE

Lisdexamfetamine dimesylate

Why is this drug prescribed?

Vyvanse is a stimulant medication used to treat attention deficit hyperactivity disorder (ADHD). It belongs to the class of drugs known as amphetamines. When used appropriately, Vyvanse can help increase attention and decrease ADHD symptoms such as impulsiveness and hyperactivity. Vyvanse should be used as part of a broader treatment plan that includes psychological, educational, and social measures.

Most important fact about this drug

Stimulants such as Vyvanse have a high potential for abuse. Excessive doses of this drug over a long period of time can produce addiction. It is also possible to develop tolerance to the drug, so that larger doses are needed to produce the original effect. Because of these dangers, the dosage should be changed only as directed, and the drug should be withdrawn only under a doctor's supervision.

How should this medication be taken?

Vyvanse should be taken once a day in the morning. It may be taken with or without food. Vyvanse comes as a capsule that can be swallowed whole, or the capsule may be opened and the entire contents emptied into a glass of water. The dissolved medication should be taken immediately; it should never be stored for future use.

• *Missed dose...*
Generally, forgotten doses should be taken as soon as remembered. However, if it is almost time for the next dose, patients should skip the one they missed and return to their regular schedule. Doses should never be doubled.

• *Storage instructions...*
Store at room temperature in a tightly closed, light-resistant container.

What side effects may occur?

Side effects cannot be predicted. If any develop or change in intensity, patients should inform their doctor as soon as possible.

• *Side effects may include:*
Decreased appetite, dizziness, dry mouth, insomnia, irritability, nausea, upper stomach pain, vomiting, weight loss

• *Rare but serious side effects may include:*
Blurred vision or eyesight changes, heart-related problems, seizures (mainly in patients with a history of seizures), slowing of growth (height and weight) in children, thought and behavior changes

Why should this drug not be prescribed?

Vyvanse should never be prescribed for patients with any of the following:

Heart disease or hardening of the arteries
High blood pressure
High pressure in the eye (glaucoma)
Overactive thyroid gland
History of drug abuse

In addition, this drug should not be prescribed for anyone experiencing anxiety, tension, or agitation, since the drug may aggravate these symptoms.

Patients should never use Vyvanse while taking a drug classified as an MAO inhibitor, such as the antidepressants Nardil and Parnate, or within 14 days of stopping such a drug. A potentially life-threatening spike in blood pressure could result.

Vyvanse should not be used by anyone who is sensitive to or has had an allergic reaction to other stimulant drugs.

Special warnings about this medication

Amphetamines like Vyvanse may cause heart-related side effects such as increased blood pressure and heart rate. Amphetamines are also associated with life-threatening reactions, including stroke and heart attack in adults and sudden death in patients who have underlying heart problems or defects. Patients should contact their doctor immediately if they develop signs of heart problems such as chest pain, shortness of breath, or fainting while using Vyvanse.

The doctor should do a complete history and evaluation before prescribing this drug. Patients should inform the doctor about all their medical conditions, especially if they have a history of heart problems, heart defects, or high blood pressure; mental problems including psychosis, mania, or depression; tics or Tourette's syndrome; liver or kidney problems; thyroid problems; and seizures or an abnormal brain-wave test (EEG).

Vyvanse should be used cautiously with certain medications, especially antidepressants, antipsychotic drugs, lithium, blood pressure medication, anticonvulsants, and narcotic painkillers. Patients should not start taking any new medication without checking with their doctor first.

Vyvanse has not been studied in children less than 6 years old. The manufacturer does not recommend using this drug in children less than 3 years old.

There is no information regarding the safety and effectiveness of long-term treatment in children. However, suppression of growth has been seen with the long-term use of stimulants, so the child should be monitored carefully while taking this drug.

Blood pressure should be monitored in anyone taking this drug, especially those with high blood pressure.

The use of this drug by anyone with a seizure disorder is not recommended. Caution is also advisable for anyone with a history of emotional instability or substance abuse, due to the danger of addiction.

Patients should be aware that some people have had visual disturbances such as blurred vision while being treated with stimulant medication such as Vyvanse.

Possible food and drug interactions when taking this medication

See the entry for the generic name lisdexamfetamine on page 339.

Special information about pregnancy and breastfeeding

The effects of Vyvanse during pregnancy have not been adequately studied. The drug is recommended only if its benefits are thought to outweigh the potential risk to the baby. If a patient is pregnant or planning to become pregnant, she should inform her doctor immediately.

Patients taking Vyvanse should not breastfeed, since the drug can show up in breast milk.

Recommended dosage
CHILDREN 6 TO 12 YEARS OLD

The recommended dose is 30 milligrams once a day in the morning. Depending on the patient's response, the doctor may raise the dose in increments of 20 milligrams, up to a maximum of 70 milligrams a day.

Vyvanse has not been studied in children less than 6 or more than 12 years of age.

Overdosage
Fatal poisoning with amphetamines has occurred. If an overdose is suspected, seek medical attention immediately.

* *Symptoms of amphetamine overdose may include:*
  Abdominal cramps, agitation, confusion, convulsions (may be followed by coma), delirium, diarrhea, dryness of mucous membranes, enlarging of the pupils, exaggerated feeling of elation, extremely elevated body temperature, flushing, hallucinations, headache, high blood pressure, irregular or rapid heartbeat, muscle twitching, nausea, sweating, tremors, vomiting

WELLBUTRIN
Bupropion hydrochloride
Other brand name: Wellbutrin SR, Wellbutrin XL

Why is this drug prescribed?
Wellbutrin and Wellbutrin SR (the sustained-release form) are prescribed to help relieve major depression. They are thought to work by altering levels of the brain chemicals norepinephrine and dopamine. Wellbutrin is not chemically related to other antidepressants such as MAO inhibitors (Nardil, Parnate), tricyclics (amitriptyline), or serotonin inhibitors (Prozac). The extended-release version of the drug, Wellbutrin XL, is used to treat the symptoms of major depression and also to prevent seasonal depression that occurs from autumn to winter (also known as seasonal affective disorder).

Most important fact about this drug
Wellbutrin is associated with an increased risk of seizures. This risk is greater at higher doses (approximately 4 in 1,000 patients at dosages of 300 to 450 milligrams a day). Certain factors increase the risk of seizure, including:

A history of head trauma or previous seizure
Central nervous system tumor
Severe liver disease such as cirrhosis
A history of eating disorders, including anorexia and bulimia
Excessive use of alcohol, or abrupt withdrawal from alcohol or sedatives

Taking medications that lower the seizure threshold (see "Possible food and drug interactions when taking this medication")

To minimize the risk of seizures, dose increases should be done gradually, and the total daily dose of Wellbutrin should not exceed 450 milligrams. Additionally, patients need to inform their doctor about all medical conditions and not take any other medications (both prescription and over-the-counter) unless the doctor approves.

How should this medication be taken?
Wellbutrin should be taken exactly as prescribed. The usual dosing regimen is 3 equal doses spaced evenly throughout the day. At least 6 hours should elapse between doses. The doctor will probably start at a low dosage and gradually increase it; this helps minimize side effects.

Wellbutrin SR, the sustained-release form, should be taken in 2 doses at least 8 hours apart. Wellbutrin XL extended-release tablets should be taken once a day in the morning. Wellbutrin SR and Wellbutrin XL tablets must be swallowed whole; not chewed, divided, or crushed. If Wellbutrin proves effective, the doctor will probably continue therapy for at least several months. Wellbutrin XL may be taken with or without food.

- *Missed dose...*
  Generally, a forgotten dose should be taken as soon as remembered. However, if it is within 4 hours of the next dose, the missed dose should be skipped and the patient should go back to the regular schedule. Doses should never be doubled.

- *Storage instructions...*
  Wellbutrin should be stored at room temperature and should be protected from light and moisture.

What side effects may occur?
Side effects cannot be predicted. If any develop or change in intensity, patients should inform their doctor as soon as possible.

- *Side effects of Wellbutrin may include:*
  Agitation, constipation, dizziness, dry mouth, excessive sweating, headache, nausea, vomiting, skin rash, sleep disturbances, tremor

- *Side effects of Wellbutrin SR may include:*
  Agitation, constipation, dizziness, dry mouth, insomnia, nausea, rash, sweating, weight loss

- *Side effects of Wellbutrin XL may include:*
  Abdominal pain, agitation, anxiety, constipation, diarrhea, dizziness, dry mouth, heart palpitations, increased urination, insomnia, muscle soreness, nausea, rash, ringing in the ears, sore throat, sweating

Why should this drug not be prescribed?

Anyone who is sensitive to or has ever had an allergic reaction to Wellbutrin should avoid it.

Since Wellbutrin causes seizures in some people, it should not be taken by anyone who has any type of seizure disorder. It should also be avoided by people who are taking another medication containing bupropion, such as Zyban, the quit-smoking aid. Patients who have a seizure while taking Wellbutrin should stop taking the medication and never take it again.

Wellbutrin must be avoided by patients who currently have, or formerly had, an eating disorder. For some reason, people with a history of anorexia nervosa or bulimia seem to be more likely to experience Wellbutrin-related seizures.

Wellbutrin should not be used if, within the past 14 days, the patient has taken a monoamine oxidase inhibitor (MAO inhibitor) such as the antidepressants Nardil and Parnate. This particular drug combination could cause a sudden, dangerous rise in blood pressure.

Wellbutrin must also be avoided by patients undergoing abrupt discontinuation of alcohol or sedatives (including benzodiazepines such as Valium and Xanax). Rapid withdrawal increases the risk of seizures.

Patients who have had any kind of heart trouble or liver or kidney disease should be sure to tell their doctor before they start taking this medication. Wellbutrin should be used with extreme caution in patients who have severe cirrhosis of the liver. The doctor may need to reduce the dosage for patients with any sort of liver or kidney problem.

Special warnings about this medication

In clinical studies, antidepressants increased the risk of suicidal thinking and behavior in children and adolescents with depression and other psychiatric disorders. Anyone considering the use of Wellbutrin, or any other antidepressant in a child or adolescent, must balance the risk with the clinical need. Wellbutrin has not been studied in children or adolescents and is not approved for treating anyone less than 18 years old.

Additionally, the progression of major depression is associated with a worsening of symptoms and/or the emergence of suicidal thinking or behavior in both adults and children, whether or not they are taking antidepressants. Patients and caregivers should watch for any change in symptoms or any new symptoms that appear suddenly—especially agitation, anxiety, hostility, panic, restlessness, extreme hyperactivity, and suicidal thinking or behavior—and report them to the doctor immediately. Be especially observant at the beginning of treatment or whenever there is a change in dose.

Patients who have had any kind of heart trouble or liver or kidney disease should be sure to alert the doctor before they start taking this drug. It must be used with extreme caution by people with severe cirrhosis of the liver. A reduced dosage may be needed for those with any sort of liver or kidney problem.

Although Wellbutrin occasionally causes weight gain, a more common effect is weight loss. About a quarter of people who take this medication in clinical studies lost 5 pounds or more. If depression has already caused a decline in weight, and if further weight loss would be detrimental to the patient's health, Wellbutrin may not be the best choice.

Like all antidepressants, Wellbutrin could trigger a manic episode. Patients with bipolar disorder should be watched closely for symptoms of mania.

Patients should stop taking Wellbutrin and call the doctor immediately if they have difficulty breathing or swallowing; notice swelling in the face, lips, tongue, or throat; develop swollen arms and legs; or break out with itchy eruptions. These are warning signs of a potentially severe allergic reaction.

Wellbutrin may impair coordination or judgment. Patients should not drive or operate dangerous machinery and avoid activities that require full alertness until they know how the medication affects them.

Patients should avoid alcohol while taking Wellbutrin; an interaction between alcohol and Wellbutrin could increase the possibility of a seizure. Also, Wellbutrin should not be combined with drugs that lower the seizure threshold.

Before taking Wellbutrin XL, patients should be sure to tell their doctor if they are diabetic and are taking insulin or other medicines to control blood sugar.

Possible food and drug interactions when taking this medication
See the entry for the generic name bupropion on page 289.

Special information about pregnancy and breastfeeding
Patients who are pregnant or plan to become pregnant should notify their doctor immediately. Wellbutrin should be taken during pregnancy only if clearly needed.

Wellbutrin does pass into breast milk and may cause serious reactions in a nursing baby. New mothers may need to discontinue breastfeeding while they are taking this medication.

Recommended dosage
The safety and effectiveness of Wellbutrin, Wellbutrin XL, and Wellbutrin SR have not been established in pediatric patients.

No single dose of Wellbutrin should exceed 150 milligrams.

ADULTS

Wellbutrin
At the beginning, the dose will probably be 200 milligrams per day, taken as 100 milligrams 2 times a day. After at least 3 days at this dose, the doctor may increase the dosage to 300 milligrams per day, taken as 100 mil-

ligrams 3 times a day, with at least 6 hours between doses. This is the usual adult dose. The maximum recommended dosage is 450 milligrams per day taken in doses of no more than 150 milligrams each.

Wellbutrin SR

The usual starting dose is 150 milligrams in the morning. After 3 days, if the patient responds well, the doctor will prescribe another 150 milligrams at least 8 hours after the first dose. It may be 4 weeks before the patient feels the benefit, and therapy may continue for several months. The maximum recommended dose is 400 milligrams a day, taken in doses of 200 milligrams each.

For people with severe cirrhosis of the liver, the dosage should be no more than 75 milligrams once a day. With less serious liver and kidney problems, the dosage will be reduced as needed.

Wellbutrin XL

Patients with severe liver damage should use this drug with extreme caution. Their dose should not exceed 150 milligrams every other day. Patients with mild to moderate liver damage or kidney impairment will be prescribed a lower dose as well.

MAJOR DEPRESSION

The usual starting dose is 150 milligrams taken once a day in the morning. If this dose is well tolerated after a minimum of 3 days, the doctor may increase the dose to 300 milligrams, also taken once a day in the morning. If no improvement is seen after several weeks of treatment, the doctor may increase the dose to a maximum of 450 milligrams once a day.

SEASONAL AFFECTIVE DISORDER

Wellbutrin XL should generally be started in autumn before the first signs of depression appear. Treatment should continue through winter and the dose gradually decreased and then stopped in early spring. The usual starting dose is 150 milligrams taken once a day in the morning. If this dose is well tolerated, the doctor may increase the dose to 300 milligrams once a day after 1 week. Doses higher than 300 milligrams a day have not been studied for the prevention of seasonal depression.

Overdosage

There have been rare reports of death after an overdose of Wellbutrin. Any medication taken in excess can have serious consequences. If an overdose of Wellbutrin is suspected, seek medical attention immediately.

- *Symptoms of Wellbutrin overdose may include:*
  Hallucinations, heart failure, loss of consciousness, rapid heartbeat, seizures

- *Symptoms of Wellbutrin SR overdose may include:*
  Blurred vision, confusion, jitteriness, lethargy, light-headedness, nausea, seizures, vomiting

- *An overdose that involves other drugs in combination with Wellbutrin may also cause these symptoms:*
  Breathing difficulties, coma, fever, rigid muscles, stupor

XANAX

Alprazolam
Other brand name: Xanax XR

Why is this drug prescribed?

Xanax is a tranquilizer used for the treatment of anxiety disorders and the short-term relief of symptoms of anxiety. Xanax is also used in the treatment of panic disorder and anxiety associated with depression. Some doctors prescribe Xanax to treat alcohol withdrawal, fear of open spaces and strangers, depression, irritable bowel syndrome, and premenstrual syndrome.

Xanax XR is prescribed to treat panic disorder.

Most important fact about this drug

Tolerance and dependence can occur with the use of Xanax. Withdrawal symptoms may occur if the drug is stopped abruptly or the dosage is reduced. Patients should discontinue the drug or change the dose only under a doctor's supervision. Withdrawal symptoms are listed under "What side effects may occur?"

How should this medication be taken?

Xanax must be taken exactly as prescribed. It may be taken with or without food. Xanax XR tablets should be swallowed whole; they should not be broken in half, chewed, or crushed.

- *Missed dose...*
  If it is less than 1 hour late, the dose should be taken as soon as remembered. Otherwise it should be skipped and the patient should go back to the regular schedule. Doses should never be doubled.

- *Storage instructions...*
  Store Xanax at room temperature.

What side effects may occur?

Side effects cannot be predicted. If any develop or change in intensity, patients should inform their doctor as soon as possible.

Side effects of Xanax are usually seen at the beginning of treatment and disappear with continued medication. However, if the dosage is increased, side effects will be more likely.

- *Side effects of Xanax may include:*
  Decreased libido, drowsiness, fatigue, impaired coordination, memory impairment, speech difficulties, weight changes

- *Side effects of Xanax XR may include:*
  Constipation, decreased libido, depression, drowsiness, fatigue, impaired coordination, memory problems, mental impairment, nausea, sedation, sleepiness, speech difficulties, weight changes

- *Side effects due to decrease in dose or abrupt withdrawal from Xanax:*
  Blurred vision, decreased concentration, decreased mental clarity, diarrhea, heightened awareness of noise or bright lights, impaired sense of smell, loss of appetite, loss of weight, muscle cramps, seizures, tingling sensation, twitching

Why should this drug not be prescribed?

Anyone who is sensitive to or has ever had an allergic reaction to Xanax or other antianxiety agents should not take this medication. It should be avoided by people who have the eye condition called narrow-angle glaucoma. It must not be combined with the antifungal drugs Sporanox or Nizoral.

Anxiety or tension related to everyday stress usually does not require treatment with Xanax. Patients should discuss their symptoms thoroughly with the doctor. The doctor should periodically reassess the need for this drug.

Special warnings about this medication

Xanax may cause patients to become drowsy or less alert. Driving, operating dangerous machinery, or participating in any hazardous activity that requires full mental alertness is not recommended.

Individuals being treated for panic disorder may need a higher dose of Xanax than those being treated for anxiety alone. High doses—more than 4 milligrams a day—taken for long intervals may cause emotional and physical dependence. The doctor should monitor such patients carefully.

As with all antianxiety medication, there is a slight chance that Xanax could encourage suicidal thoughts or manic episodes. The doctor should be alerted immediately if any new or unusual symptoms appear.

Xanax should be used with caution in older or weak patients, and in those with lung disease, alcoholic liver disease, or any disorder that could hinder the elimination of the drug.

Xanax may intensify the effect of alcohol. Patients should avoid alcohol while taking this medication.

Xanax should never be combined with Sporanox or Nizoral. These drugs cause a buildup of Xanax in the body.

Possible food and drug interactions when taking this medication
See the entry for the generic name alprazolam on page 277.

Special information about pregnancy and breastfeeding
Xanax should be avoided by patients who are pregnant or plan to become pregnant. There is an increased risk of respiratory problems and muscular weakness in the baby. Infants may also experience withdrawal symptoms.

Xanax may appear in breast milk and could affect a nursing infant. If this medication is essential to the mother's health, the doctor may advise her to stop breastfeeding until treatment is finished.

Recommended dosage
The following dosages are for adults. The safety and effectiveness of Xanax have not been established in children less than 18 years old.

ANXIETY DISORDER

Xanax
The usual starting dose is 0.25 to 0.5 milligram taken 3 times a day. The dose may be increased every 3 to 4 days to a maximum daily dose of 4 milligrams, divided into smaller doses.

PANIC DISORDER

Xanax
The usual starting dose is 0.5 milligram 3 times a day. The dose may be increased by 1 milligram a day every 3 or 4 days. The daily dose ranges from 1 milligram up to a total of 10 milligrams, according to the patient's needs. A typical dose is 5 to 6 milligrams a day.

Xanax XR
The usual starting dose is 0.5 to 1 milligram taken once a day, preferably in the morning. If needed, the dose can be increased by no more than 1 milligram a day every 3 or 4 days. The usual effective dose ranges from 3 to 6 milligrams a day, but doses as high as 10 milligrams a day have occasionally been needed.

DOSAGE ADJUSTMENT

In patients who are older, weak, or have advanced liver disease, the usual starting dose of Xanax is 0.25 milligram, 2 or 3 times a day. For Xanax XR, the starting dose is 0.5 milligram taken once a day, preferably in the morning. If needed, the doctor will increase the dose gradually based on the patient's tolerance.

Overdosage
An overdose of Xanax, alone or after combining it with alcohol, can be fatal. If an overdose is suspected, seek medical attention immediately.

- *Symptoms of Xanax overdose may include:*
  Confusion, coma, impaired coordination, sleepiness, slowed reaction time

Zaleplon *See Sonata, page 214*

Ziprasidone *See Geodon, page 91*

ZOLOFT
Sertraline

Why is this drug prescribed?
Zoloft is prescribed for major depressive disorder and obsessive-compulsive disorder. It is also used for the treatment of panic disorder, social anxiety disorder, premenstrual dysphoric disorder (PMDD), and post-traumatic stress disorder.

Zoloft is a member of the family of drugs called selective serotonin re-uptake inhibitors (SSRIs). Serotonin is one of the chemical messengers believed to govern moods. Ordinarily, it is quickly reabsorbed after its release at the junctures between nerves. Reuptake inhibitors such as Zoloft slow this process, thereby boosting the levels of serotonin available in the brain.

Most important fact about this drug
Zoloft must not be used within 2 weeks of taking any drug classified as an MAO inhibitor, such as the antidepressants Nardil and Parnate. When serotonin boosters such as Zoloft are combined with MAO inhibitors, serious and sometimes fatal reactions can occur. In addition, patients should not combine Zoloft with the drug Orap.

How should this medication be taken?
Zoloft should be taken exactly as prescribed, once a day in either the morning or the evening.

Zoloft is available in tablet and oral concentrate forms. Zoloft oral concentrate should be prepared with the dropper provided. The amount of concentrate prescribed by the doctor should be mixed with 4 ounces of water, ginger ale, lemon/lime soda, lemonade, or orange juice. (No other type of beverage should be used.) The mixture must be taken immediately; it should not be prepared in advance for later use. At times, a slight haze may appear after mixing, but this is normal.

Improvement with Zoloft may not be seen for several days to a few weeks. Treatment typically lasts for at least several months. Zoloft may make the mouth dry. Sucking a hard candy, chewing gum, or melting bits of ice in the mouth can provide temporary relief.

- *Missed dose...*
  Generally, the forgotten dose should be taken as soon as remembered. However, if several hours have passed, it should be skipped and the patient should return to the regular schedule. Doses should never be doubled.

- *Storage instructions...*
  Zoloft should be stored at room temperature.

What side effects may occur?

Side effects cannot be predicted. If any develop or change in intensity, patients should inform their doctor as soon as possible.

- *Side effects may include:*
  Abdominal pain, agitation, anxiety, constipation, decreased appetite, decreased sex drive, diarrhea or loose stools, difficulty with ejaculation, dizziness, dry mouth, fatigue, gas, headache, increased sweating, indigestion, insomnia, nausea, nervousness, pain, rash, sleepiness, tingling or pins and needles, tremor, vision problems, vomiting

Many people lose a pound or two of body weight while taking Zoloft. This usually poses no problem but may be a concern if depression has already caused a great deal of weight loss.

In a few people, Zoloft may trigger the grandiose, inappropriate, out-of-control behavior called mania or the similar, but less dramatic, "hyper" state called hypomania.

Why should this drug not be prescribed?

Anyone who has ever had an allergic reaction to Zoloft should not take it.

This drug should never be combined with pimozide (Orap) or an MAO inhibitor (see "Most important fact about this drug"). Due to its alcohol content, Zoloft oral concentrate cannot be used with the anti-alcohol medication Antabuse.

Special warnings about this medication

In clinical studies, antidepressants increased the risk of suicidal thinking and behavior in children and adolescents with depression and other psychiatric disorders. Anyone considering the use of Zoloft, or any other antidepressant in a child or adolescent, must balance the risk with the clinical need. Zoloft is only approved for treating obsessive-compulsive disorder in children 6 years and older.

Additionally, the progression of major depression is associated with a worsening of symptoms and/or the emergence of suicidal thinking or behavior in both adults and children, whether or not they are taking antidepressants. Patients and caregivers should watch for any change in symptoms or any new symptoms that appear suddenly—especially agitation, anxiety, hostility, panic, restlessness, extreme hyperactivity, and suicidal thinking or behavior—and report them to the doctor immediately.

Be especially observant at the beginning of treatment or whenever there is a change in dose.

Patients with a kidney or liver disorder, and those with a history of heart disease, seizures, or bleeding problems, need to take Zoloft cautiously and under close medical supervision.

Zoloft could cause weight loss in children. The manufacturer recommends regular monitoring of weight and growth during long-term treatment in pediatric patients.

SSRI antidepressants could potentially cause stomach bleeding, especially in patients taking nonsteroidal anti-inflammatory drugs (NSAIDs) such as aspirin, ibuprofen (Advil, Motrin), naproxen (Aleve), and ketoprofen. Advise patients to consult their doctor before combining Zoloft with NSAIDs or blood-thinning medications.

Like all antidepressants, Zoloft could trigger a manic episode. Patients with bipolar disorder should be watched closely for symptoms of mania.

Zoloft has not been found to impair the ability to drive or operate machinery. Nevertheless, the manufacturer recommends caution until patients know how the drug affects them.

As with other SSRIs, Zoloft therapy should be slowly tapered instead of abruptly stopped. If abruptly discontinued, drowsiness, irritability, agitation, anxiety, headache, and insomnia may occur.

People who are sensitive to latex should use caution when handling the dropper provided with the oral concentrate.

Remember that Zoloft must never be combined with pimozide (Orap) or an MAO inhibitor (see "Most important fact about this drug").

Although alcohol does not appear to interact with Zoloft, the manufacturer recommends avoiding the combination. Likewise, over-the-counter remedies should be used with caution. Although none is known to interact with Zoloft, interactions remain a possibility.

Possible food and drug interactions when taking this medication

See the entry for the generic name sertraline on page 396.

Special information about pregnancy and breastfeeding

Patients who are pregnant or plan to become pregnant should inform their doctor immediately. There have been reports of newborns experiencing complications such as respiratory problems, bluish coloring of the skin, irregular breathing, muscular problems, vomiting, and constant crying after exposure to SSRI antidepressants late in the third trimester. Zoloft should be used during pregnancy only if absolutely necessary.

It is not known whether Zoloft appears in breast milk. Caution is advised when using Zoloft during breastfeeding.

Recommended dosage

The following indications and dosages are for adults only unless otherwise noted.

DEPRESSION OR OBSESSIVE-COMPULSIVE DISORDER

The usual starting dose is 50 milligrams once a day, taken either in the morning or in the evening. The doctor may increase the dose depending upon the patient's response. The maximum dose is 200 milligrams a day.

PREMENSTRUAL DYSPHORIC DISORDER

For patients with PMDD, the doctor will assess whether Zoloft should be taken throughout the menstrual cycle or only during the 2 weeks preceding menstruation. The starting dose is 50 milligrams a day. If this proves insufficient, the doctor will increase the dose in 50-milligram steps at the start of each new menstrual cycle up to a maximum of 100 milligrams per day in the 2-week regimen or 150 milligrams per day in the full-cycle regimen. (During the first 3 days of the 2-week regimen, doses are always limited to 50 milligrams.)

PANIC DISORDER, SOCIAL ANXIETY DISORDER, OR
POST-TRAUMATIC STRESS DISORDER

During the first week, the usual dose is 25 milligrams once a day. After that, the dose increases to 50 milligrams once a day. Depending on the response, the doctor may continue to increase the dose up to a maximum of 200 milligrams a day.

OBSESSIVE-COMPULSIVE DISORDER IN CHILDREN
6 TO 17 YEARS OLD

The starting dose for children 6 to 12 years old is 25 milligrams, and for adolescents 13 to 17 years old, the initial dose is 50 milligrams. The doctor will adjust the dose as necessary.

Safety and effectiveness have not been established for children under 6 years old.

DOSAGE ADJUSTMENT

The doctor will need to reduce the dosage for patients with liver disease.

Overdosage

Any medication taken in excess can have serious consequences. An overdose of Zoloft can be fatal. If an overdose is suspected, seek medical attention immediately.

- *Common symptoms of Zoloft overdose may include:*
  Agitation, dizziness, nausea, rapid heartbeat, sleepiness, tremor, vomiting

Other possible symptoms include coma, stupor, fainting, convulsions, delirium, hallucinations, mania, high or low blood pressure, and slow, rapid, or irregular heartbeat.

Zolpidem *See Ambien CR, page 7*

ZYBAN
Bupropion hydrochloride

Why is this drug prescribed?
Zyban is a nicotine-free smoking-cessation aid. Instead of nicotine, it contains the chemical buproprion, which is also the active ingredient in the antidepressant Wellbutrin.

Zyban is thought to work by boosting levels of the brain chemicals norepinephrine and dopamine. With more of these chemicals at work, patients experience a reduction in nicotine withdrawal symptoms and a weakening of the urge to smoke. More than a third of the people who take Zyban while participating in a support program are able to quit smoking for at least 1 month. Zyban can also prove helpful when people with conditions such as chronic bronchitis and emphysema decide it's time to quit. Zyban should be a part of a broader treatment plan that includes behavior modification, counseling, and other support programs.

Most important fact about this drug
About 1 person in 1,000 suffers a seizure while taking Zyban. For this reason, people with epilepsy or a history of seizures should never take the drug. In addition, a variety of conditions or medications can increase the risk of having a seizure while using Zyban, including:

Prior head injuries
Prior seizures
Central nervous system tumor
Cirrhosis of the liver
History of bulimia or anorexia
Too much alcohol
Abrupt withdrawal from alcohol, tranquilizers, or sedatives
Addiction to narcotics or cocaine
Over-the-counter stimulants or diet pills
Diabetes medications
Antidepressants, major tranquilizers, steroids, or theophylline

It's important that patients inform the doctor about their complete medical history. Also, patients should not take any other medicines while using Zyban unless their doctor approves.

How should this medication be taken?

Treatment with this drug begins while patients are still smoking. Zyban needs about a week to reach an effective level in the body; to improve the chance of success, patients should not attempt to quit until the second week of treatment. They should set a firm date for quitting. If patients are still smoking after that date, their odds of breaking the habit will be worse. Zyban should be used for 7 to 12 weeks.

Zyban tablets should be swallowed whole. They should not be chewed, divided, or crushed. Each dose of Zyban should be taken at about the same time every day, and doses should be separated by at least 8 hours.

Nicotine patches can be used along with Zyban. However, combining the two treatments can raise blood pressure, so it's important for patients to tell the doctor if they plan to use both. Patients should not smoke while using a patch, because too much nicotine can cause serious side effects.

Patients should be reminded that participating in a counseling or support program will make success more likely.

- *Missed dose...*
  If patients miss a dose, they should not take an extra tablet to make up for the dose they forgot. They should wait and take their next tablet at the regular time. This is very important, since taking too much Zyban at once could increase the chance of having a seizure.

- *Storage instructions...*
  Store at room temperature in a tightly closed container. Keep out of direct sunlight.

What side effects may occur?

Side effects cannot be predicted. If any develop or change in intensity, patients should inform their doctor as soon as possible.

- *Common side effects may include:*
  Dry mouth, sleeplessness

These are generally mild and usually disappear after a few weeks. If patients continue to have difficulty sleeping, they should avoid taking Zyban close to bedtime and ask their doctor about reducing the dosage.

- *Rare but serious side effects may include:*
  High blood pressure, seizure, severe allergic reaction, unusual thoughts or behaviors (including delusions, hallucinations, paranoia, and confusion)

Patients who have a serious side effect while taking Zyban should call their doctor immediately.

Why should this drug not be prescribed?

Zyban should not be prescribed for any patient who:

- Has ever had a seizure disorder or epilepsy
- Is taking any other drug that contains the ingredient bupropion, including Wellbutrin, Wellbutrin SR, and Wellbutrin XL
- Abruptly stops drinking alcohol or taking sedatives after excessive use
- Has taken a drug classified as an MAO inhibitor (such as the antidepressants Nardil or Parnate) within the last 14 days before starting Zyban
- Has a history of an eating disorder such as anorexia or bulimia
- Is allergic or sensitive to any of the ingredients in Zyban

Special warnings about this medication

Although Zyban is not a treatment for depression, it contains the same active ingredient as the antidepressant medications Wellbutrin, Wellbutrin SR, and Wellbutrin XL. Patients should be aware that antidepressants can increase the risk of suicidal thinking and behavior in children and teenagers. Adult and pediatric patients taking antidepressants should be watched closely for changes in moods or actions, especially when they first start therapy or when their dose is increased or decreased. Patients and family members are advised to contact the doctor immediately if new symptoms develop or seem to get worse. Signs to watch for include anxiety, hostility, insomnia, restlessness, impulsive or dangerous behavior, and thoughts about suicide or dying. Zyban is not approved for use in pediatric patients.

To lower the risk of seizure, patients should never take more than one 150-milligram tablet at a time, and the total daily dosage should be limited to 2 tablets (300 milligrams).

Patients should stop taking Zyban and call the doctor immediately if they have difficulty breathing or swallowing; notice swelling in their face, lips, tongue, or throat; develop swollen arms and legs; or break out in hives or a rash. These are warning signs of a potentially severe allergic reaction.

Before starting treatment with Zyban, patients should let the doctor know if they have liver or kidney problems, heart problems or high blood pressure, of if they drink a lot of alcohol. They may need a change in their dosage or treatment plan.

Zyban can interfere with driving ability. Patients should not drive or operate dangerous machinery until they know how this drug affects them.

Quitting smoking, with or without Zyban treatment, could change how certain drugs are metabolized; for example, theophylline and warfarin. Patients should make sure the doctor knows about all prescription and over-the-counter medicines, they are taking including herbs and dietary supplements.

Possible food and drug interactions when taking this medication

See the entry for the generic name bupropion on page 289.

Special information about pregnancy and breastfeeding

Zyban has not been tested in pregnant women. The drug is recommended only if its benefits are thought to outweigh the potential risk to the baby. Patients who are pregnant should be encouraged to quit smoking with the aid of counseling and support programs before turning to drug therapy. If a patient is pregnant or planning to become pregnant, she should inform her doctor immediately.

Zyban appears in breast milk and could affect a nursing infant. Patients should talk to their doctor about whether it's best to discontinue the medication or to stop breastfeeding.

Recommended dosage

ADULTS

The usual starting dose is one 150-milligram tablet in the morning for the first 3 days. After that, patients will be instructed to take one 150-milligram tablet in the morning and another in the early evening. Doses should be kept at least 8 hours apart. The maximum recommended dose is 300 milligrams daily. Zyban is usually taken for 7 to 12 weeks; however, the doctor may recommend continuing treatment for up to 6 months.

For patients with kidney or liver problems, the doctor may reduce the frequency of doses to avoid high blood levels of Zyban. Patients with severe cirrhosis of the liver should take no more than 150 milligrams every other day.

Overdosage

Information on Zyban overdose is limited. However, any medication taken in excess can have serious consequences. If an overdose is suspected, seek medical attention immediately.

* *Symptoms of Zyban overdose may include:*
  Blurred vision, confusion, grogginess, jitteriness, light-headedness, nausea, seizure, sluggishness, visual hallucinations

ZYPREXA

Olanzapine
Other brand names: Zyprexa IntraMuscular, Zyprexa Zydis

Why is this drug prescribed?

Zyprexa helps manage symptoms of schizophrenia, the manic phase of bipolar disorder, and other psychotic disorders. It is thought to work by opposing the action of serotonin and dopamine, two of the brain's major chemical messengers. The drug is available as Zyprexa tablets, Zyprexa

IntraMuscular injection, and Zyprexa Zydis, which dissolves rapidly with or without liquid. Zyprexa IntraMuscular is used to treat the agitation associated with schizophrenia and bipolar I mania.

Most important fact about this drug

Elderly patients with dementia who are treated with antipsychotic drugs such as Zyprexa have an increased risk of stroke and death. Zyprexa is not approved to treat dementia-related psychosis.

At the start of Zyprexa therapy, the drug can cause extreme low blood pressure, increased heart rate, dizziness, and, in rare cases, a tendency to faint when first standing up. These problems are more likely if the patient is dehydrated, has heart disease, or takes blood pressure medicine. To avoid such problems, the doctor may start with a low dose of Zyprexa and increase the dosage gradually.

How should this medication be taken?

Zyprexa should be taken once a day with or without food. To use Zyprexa Zydis, patients should open the sachet, peel back the foil on the blister pack, remove the tablet, and place the entire tablet in their mouth. The tablet should not be pushed through the foil. The medication can be taken with or without water; saliva will cause the tablet to dissolve. Zyprexa IntraMuscular is an injection given by healthcare professionals.

- *Missed dose...*
  Generally, a forgotten dose should be taken as soon as remembered. However, if it is almost time for the next dose, the missed dose should be skipped and the patient should go back to the regular schedule. Doses should never be doubled.

- *Storage instructions...*
  Zyprexa should be stored at room temperature away from light and moisture. Zyprexa IntraMuscular should be protected from light and should not be frozen.

What side effects may occur?

Side effects cannot be predicted. If any develop or change in intensity, patients should inform their doctor as soon as possible.

- *Side effects of Zyprexa may include:*
  Agitation, change in personality, constipation, dizziness, dry mouth, increased appetite, indigestion, low blood pressure upon standing, sleepiness, tremor, weakness, weight gain

- *Side effects of Zyprexa IntraMuscular may include:*
  Dizziness, low blood pressure, sleepiness, weakness

Why should this drug not be prescribed?

Anyone who is allergic to Zyprexa cannot use this drug.

Special warnings about this drug

Certain antipsychotic drugs, including Zyprexa, are associated with an increased risk of developing high blood sugar, which on rare occasions has led to coma or death. Patients should see their doctor right away if they develop signs of high blood sugar, including dry mouth, thirst, increased urination, and tiredness. Patients who have diabetes or have a high risk of developing it should see their doctor regularly for blood sugar testing.

Zyprexa should not be used to treat elderly patients who have dementia because the drug could increase the risk of stroke.

Animal studies suggest that Zyprexa may increase the risk of breast cancer, although human studies have not confirmed such a risk. Advise patients with a history of breast cancer to see their doctor regularly for checkups.

Patients at high risk of suicide attempts should be prescribed the lowest dose possible to reduce the risk of intentional overdose.

Zyprexa sometimes causes drowsiness and can impair judgment, thinking, and motor skills. Patients should use caution while driving and shouldn't operate dangerous machinery until they know how the drug affects them.

Medicines such as Zyprexa can interfere with regulation of the body's temperature. Patients should avoid getting overheated or becoming dehydrated while taking Zyprexa. They need to stay away from extreme heat and drink plenty of fluids.

People with the following conditions should use Zyprexa with caution: Alzheimer's disease, trouble swallowing, narrow angle glaucoma (high pressure in the eye), an enlarged prostate, heart irregularities, heart disease, heart failure, liver disease, or a history of heart attack, seizures, or intestinal blockage.

Drugs such as Zyprexa sometimes cause a condition called neuroleptic malignant syndrome. Symptoms include high fever, muscle rigidity, irregular pulse or blood pressure, rapid heartbeat, excessive perspiration, and changes in heart rhythm. If these symptoms appear, the doctor will discontinue Zyprexa while the condition is under treatment.

There is also a risk of developing tardive dyskinesia, a condition marked by slow, rhythmical, involuntary movements. This problem is more likely to surface in older adults, especially elderly women. When it does, use of Zyprexa is usually stopped.

Zyprexa can cause low blood pressure upon standing, resulting in dizziness, rapid heartbeat, and fainting, especially at the start of therapy. Patients who experience this should alert the doctor; the dosage can be adjusted to reduce the symptoms.

Patients who have phenylketonuria and must avoid the amino acid phenylalanine should not take the rapidly disintegrating form of this drug, Zyprexa Zydis, which contains this substance.

The safety and effectiveness of Zyprexa have not been studied in children.

Patients should avoid alcohol while taking Zyprexa. The combination can cause a sudden drop in blood pressure.

When patients are receiving a dose of Zyprexa IntraMuscular, they should be lying down if they feel dizzy or drowsy after the injection until the healthcare professional can check that they are not experiencing a slow heartbeat, a sudden drop in blood pressure, or hypoventilation.

Possible food and drug interactions when taking this medication

See the entry for the generic name olanzapine on page 366.

Special information about pregnancy and breastfeeding

Patients who are pregnant or plan to become pregnant should inform their doctor immediately. Zyprexa should be used during pregnancy only if absolutely necessary.

This drug appears in breast milk; women on Zyprexa therapy should not breastfeed.

Recommended dosage

SCHIZOPHRENIA

Adults: The usual starting dose is 5 to 10 milligrams once a day. If the patient starts at the lower dose, after a few days the doctor will increase it to 10 milligrams. After that, the dosage will be increased no more than once a week, 5 milligrams at a time, up to a maximum of 20 milligrams a day.

MANIC EPISODES IN BIPOLAR DISORDER

Adults: The usual starting dose is 10 to 15 milligrams once a day. If needed, the dose can be increased every 24 hours by 5 milligrams a day, up to a maximum daily dose of 20 milligrams. After the patient is stabilized, the doctor may continue maintenance therapy at a dosage range of 5 to 20 milligrams a day. If Zyprexa is being combined with lithium or valproate (Depakene, Depakote), the usual starting dose is 10 milligrams a day.

AGITATION ASSOCIATED WITH SCHIZOPHRENIA AND

BIPOLAR I MANIA

Adults: The usual starting dose is 10 milligrams. A lower dose of 5 or 7.5 milligrams may be considered for some patients. If additional doses are necessary, they may be given in subsequent doses up to 10 milligrams. However, the safety of total daily doses greater than 30 milligrams has not been evaluated.

DOSAGE ADJUSTMENT

The doctor will need to lower the dosage in debilitated patients, those prone to low blood pressure, and nonsmoking women over 65 (because they tend to have a slower metabolism). The recommended starting dose is 5 milligrams a day. Any dose increases should be done cautiously.

Overdosage

An overdose of Zyprexa is usually not life-threatening, but fatalities have been reported. If an overdose is suspected, seek medical attention immediately.

- *Symptoms of Zyprexa overdose may include:*
  Agitation, drowsiness, rapid or irregular heartbeat, slurred or disrupted speech, stupor

Overdoses of Zyprexa have also led to breathing difficulties, changes in blood pressure, excessive perspiration, fever, muscle rigidity, cardiac arrest, coma, and convulsions.

Interactions with Psychotropic Drugs

Listed in this section are over 1,600 possible interactions with the psychotropic medications profiled in Section 1. Entries are organized alphabetically, first by the generic name of the psychotropic drug, then by the generic name of the potentially interactive medication. Each entry includes a brief description of the possible results of concurrent use, plus ratings of the interaction's rapidity of onset, degree of severity, and level of supporting documentation. A key to these ratings follows.

Onset

0 = **Unspecified**
1 = **Rapid:** Develops within 24 hours
2 = **Delayed:** Will not occur during the first 24 hours

Severity

1 = **Contraindicated:** The interaction may be life-threatening. Concomitant use of the interacting agents is contraindicated.
2 = **Major:** The interaction may be life-threatening and/or require medical intervention to minimize or prevent serious adverse effects.
3 = **Moderate:** The interaction may result in an exacerbation of the patient's condition and/or require an alteration in therapy.
4 = **Minor:** The interaction would have limited clinical effects. Manifestations may include an increase in the frequency or severity of side effects but generally would not require a major alteration in therapy.

Evidence

1 = **Excellent:** Controlled studies have clearly established the existence of the interaction.
2 = **Good:** Documentation strongly suggests the interaction exists, but well-controlled studies are lacking.
3 = **Fair:** Available documentation is fair, but pharmacologic considerations lead clinicians to suspect the interaction exists; or, documentation is good for a pharmacologically similar drug.
4 = **Poor:** Documentation is poor (such as limited case reports), but the interaction is theoretically possible.

The information in this section is extracted from the DRUG-REAX System, a drug therapy screening program produced by *Physicians' Desk Reference*® affiliate Thomson Micromedex, a world leader in specialized information on pharmaceuticals. The entries are based on an independent review of the medical literature by a staff of more than 100 clinicians.

Acamprosate (Campral)

No drug interactions have been reported by the manufacturer.

Alprazolam (Niravam, Xanax, Xanax XR)

INTERACTION	ONSET	SEVERITY	EVIDENCE
CIMETIDINE Concurrent use may result in an increased risk of alprazolam toxicity (central nervous system depression).	1	3	3
CLARITHROMYCIN Concurrent use may result in increased alprazolam toxicity (central nervous system depression, ataxia, lethargy).	2	3	3
ERYTHROMYCIN Concurrent use may result in increased alprazolam toxicity (central nervous system depression, ataxia, lethargy).	2	3	3
ETHANOL Concurrent use may result in increased sedation.	1	3	2
FLUCONAZOLE Concurrent use may result in increased alprazolam serum concentrations and potential alprazolam toxicity (sedation, slurred speech, central nervous system depression).	2	1	3
FLUOXETINE Concurrent use may result in an increased risk of alprazolam toxicity (somnolence, dizziness, ataxia, slurred speech, hypotension, psychomotor impairment).	1	3	2
FLUVOXAMINE Concurrent use may result in elevated plasma alprazolam levels and an increased risk of side effects (central nervous system depression).	2	3	2
ITRACONAZOLE Concurrent use may result in increased alprazolam serum concentrations and potential alprazolam toxicity (sedation, slurred speech, central nervous system depression).	2	1	3
JOSAMYCIN Concurrent use may result in increased alprazolam toxicity (central nervous system depression, ataxia, lethargy).	2	3	3
KETOCONAZOLE Concurrent use may result in increased alprazolam serum concentrations and potential alprazolam toxicity (sedation, slurred speech, central nervous system depression).	2	1	3
NEFAZODONE Concurrent use may result in psychomotor impairment and sedation.	1	3	2
OMEPRAZOLE Concurrent use may result in alprazolam toxicity (central nervous system depression, ataxia, lethargy).	2	3	3

Onset: 0=Unspecified 1=Rapid 2=Delayed
Severity: 1=Contraindicated 2=Major 3=Moderate 4=Minor
Evidence: 1=Excellent 2=Good 3=Fair 4=Poor

INTERACTION	ONSET	SEVERITY	EVIDENCE
ORAL CONTRACEPTIVE Concurrent use may result in an increased risk of alprazolam toxicity (central nervous system depression, hypotension).	2	3	3
PROPOXYPHENE Concomitant administration may result in additive respiratory depression.	0	2	3
RITONAVIR Concurrent use may result in increased plasma concentrations of alprazolam and enhanced alprazolam effects.	2	3	3
ROXITHROMYCIN Concurrent use may result in increased alprazolam toxicity (central nervous system depression, ataxia, lethargy).	2	3	3
THEOPHYLLINE Concurrent use result in decreased alprazolam effectiveness.	1	3	2
TROLEANDOMYCIN Concurrent use may result in increased alprazolam toxicity (central nervous system depression, ataxia, lethargy).	2	3	3

Amitriptyline (Limbitrol)

INTERACTION	ONSET	SEVERITY	EVIDENCE
ACENOCOUMAROL Concurrent use may result in an increased risk of bleeding.	2	3	3
AMPRENAVIR Concurrent use may result in increased amitriptyline serum concentrations and potential toxicity (anticholinergic effects, sedation, confusion, cardiac arrhythmias).	2	2	3
ANISINDIONE Concurrent use may result in an increased risk of bleeding.	2	3	3
BEPRIDIL Concurrent use may result in an increased risk of cardiotoxicity (QT prolongation, torsade de pointes, cardiac arrest).	1	1	3
BETHANIDINE Concurrent use may result in decreased antihypertensive effectiveness.	1	3	2
CARBAMAZEPINE Concurrent use may result in decreased amitriptyline effectiveness.	2	3	3
CIMETIDINE Concurrent use may result in amitriptyline toxicity (dry mouth, blurred vision, urinary retention).	2	3	2
CISAPRIDE Concurrent use may result in cardiotoxicity (QT prolongation, torsade de pointes, cardiac arrest).	1	1	3
CLONIDINE Concurrent use may result in decreased antihypertensive effectiveness.	2	2	3

INTERACTION	ONSET	SEVERITY	EVIDENCE
CLORGYLINE Concurrent use may result in neurotoxicity, seizures, or serotonin syndrome (hypertension, hyperthermia, myoclonus, mental status changes).	2	1	3
DICUMAROL Concurrent use may result in an increased risk of bleeding.	2	3	3
DROPERIDOL Concurrent use may result in an increased risk of cardiotoxicity (QT prolongation, torsade de pointes, cardiac arrest).	0	2	3
EPINEPHRINE Concurrent use may result in hypertension, cardiac arrhythmias, and tachycardia.	1	2	2
ETHANOL Concurrent use may result in enhanced central nervous system depression and impairment of motor skills.	1	3	1
ETILEFRINE Concurrent use may result in hypertension, cardiac arrhythmias, and tachycardia.	1	2	2
FLUCONAZOLE Concurrent use result in an increased risk of amitriptyline toxicity and an increased risk of cardiotoxicity (QT prolongation, torsade de pointes, cardiac arrest).	2	2	3
FLUOXETINE Concurrent use may result in amitriptyline toxicity (dry mouth, urinary retention, sedation) and an increased risk of cardiotoxicity (QT prolongation, torsade de pointes, cardiac arrest).	0	2	3
FLUVOXAMINE Concurrent use may result in amitriptyline toxicity (dry mouth, urinary retention, sedation).	2	3	3
FURAZOLIDONE Concurrent use may result in neurotoxicity, seizures, or serotonin syndrome (hypertension, hyperthermia, myoclonus, mental status changes).	2	1	3
GREPAFLOXACIN Concurrent use may result in an increased risk of cardiotoxicity (QT prolongation, torsade de pointes, cardiac arrest).	2	1	3
GUANADREL Concurrent use may result in decreased antihypertensive effectiveness.	2	3	3
GUANETHIDINE Concurrent use may result in decreased antihypertensive effectiveness.	2	3	2

Onset: **0**=Unspecified **1**=Rapid **2**=Delayed
Severity: **1**=Contraindicated **2**=Major **3**=Moderate **4**=Minor
Evidence: **1**=Excellent **2**=Good **3**=Fair **4**=Poor

INTERACTION	ONSET	SEVERITY	EVIDENCE
GUANFACINE Concurrent use may result in decreased antihypertensive effectiveness.	2	3	3
HALOFANTRINE Concurrent use may result in an increased risk of cardiotoxicity (QT prolongation, torsade de pointes, cardiac arrest).	2	2	3
IPRONIAZID Concurrent use may result in neurotoxicity, seizures, or serotonin syndrome (hypertension, hyperthermia, myoclonus, mental status changes).	2	1	3
ISOCARBOXAZID Concurrent use may result in neurotoxicity, seizures, or serotonin syndrome (hypertension, hyperthermia, myoclonus, mental status changes).	2	1	3
LEVOMETHADYL Concurrent use may result in an increased risk of cardiotoxicity (QT prolongation, torsade de pointes, cardiac arrest).	2	1	3
METHOXAMINE Concurrent use may result in hypertension, cardiac arrhythmias, and tachycardia.	1	2	2
MIDODRINE Concurrent use may result in hypertension, cardiac arrhythmias, and tachycardia.	1	2	2
MOCLOBEMIDE Concurrent use may result in neurotoxicity, seizures, or serotonin syndrome (hypertension, hyperthermia, myoclonus, mental status changes).	2	1	3
NEFAZODONE Concurrent use may result in increased risk of serotonin syndrome (hypertension, hyperthermia, myoclonus, mental status changes).	1	2	3
NIALAMIDE Concurrent use may result in neurotoxicity, seizures, or serotonin syndrome (hypertension, hyperthermia, myoclonus, mental status changes).	2	1	3
NOREPINEPHRINE Concurrent use may result in hypertension, cardiac arrhythmias, and tachycardia.	1	2	2
OXILOFRINE Concurrent use may result in hypertension, cardiac arrhythmias, and tachycardia.	1	2	2
PARGYLINE Concurrent use may result in neurotoxicity, seizures, or serotonin syndrome (hypertension, hyperthermia, myoclonus, mental status changes).	2	1	3

INTERACTION	ONSET	SEVERITY	EVIDENCE
PHENELZINE Concurrent use may result in neurotoxicity, seizures, or serotonin syndrome (hypertension, hyperthermia, myoclonus, mental status changes).	2	1	3
PHENINDIONE Concurrent use may result in an increased risk of bleeding.	2	3	3
PHENPROCOUMON Concurrent use may result in an increased risk of bleeding.	2	3	3
PHENYLEPHRINE Concurrent use may result in hypertension, cardiac arrhythmias, and tachycardia.	1	2	2
PIMOZIDE Concurrent use may result in an increased risk of cardiotoxicity (QT prolongation, torsade de pointes, cardiac arrest).	0	1	3
PROCARBAZINE Concurrent use may result in neurotoxicity, seizures.	2	1	3
SELEGILINE Concurrent use may result in neurotoxicity, seizures, or serotonin syndrome (hypertension, hyperthermia, myoclonus, mental status changes).	2	1	3
SERTRALINE Concurrent use may result in elevated amitriptyline serum levels or possible serotonin syndrome (hypertension, hyperthermia, myoclonus, mental status changes).	2	2	3
SPARFLOXACIN Concurrent use may result in prolongation of the QTc interval and/or torsade de pointes.	2	1	3
TOLOXATONE Concurrent use may result in neurotoxicity, seizures, or serotonin syndrome (hypertension, hyperthermia, myoclonus, mental status changes).	2	1	3
TRAMADOL Concurrent use may result in an increased risk of seizures.	1	2	3
TRANYLCYPROMINE Concurrent use may result in neurotoxicity, seizures, or serotonin syndrome (hypertension, hyperthermia, myoclonus, mental status changes).	2	1	3
WARFARIN Concurrent use may result in an increased risk of bleeding.	2	3	3

Onset: 0=Unspecified 1=Rapid 2=Delayed
Severity: 1=Contraindicated 2=Major 3=Moderate 4=Minor
Evidence: 1=Excellent 2=Good 3=Fair 4=Poor

Amoxapine

INTERACTION	ONSET	SEVERITY	EVIDENCE
ACENOCOUMAROL Concurrent use may result in increased risk of bleeding.	2	3	3
AMPRENAVIR Concurrent use may result in increased amoxapine serum concentrations and potential toxicity (anticholinergic effects, sedation, confusion, cardiac arrhythmias).	2	2	3
ANISINDIONE Concurrent use may result in increased risk of bleeding.	2	3	3
BEPRIDIL Concurrent use may result in an increased risk of cardiotoxicity (QT prolongation, torsade de pointes, cardiac arrest).	1	1	3
CIMETIDINE Concurrent use result in amoxapine toxicity (dry mouth, urinary retention, blurred vision).	2	3	3
CISAPRIDE Concurrent use may result in cardiotoxicity (QT prolongation, torsade de pointes, cardiac arrest).	1	1	3
CLONIDINE Concurrent use may result in decreased antihypertensive effectiveness.	2	2	3
CLORGYLINE Concurrent use may result in neurotoxicity, seizures, or serotonin syndrome (hypertension, hyperthermia, myoclonus, mental status changes).	2	2	3
DICUMAROL Concurrent use may result in increased risk of bleeding.	2	3	3
DROPERIDOL Concurrent use may result in an increased risk of cardiotoxicity (QT prolongation, torsade de pointes, cardiac arrest).	0	2	3
EPINEPHRINE Concurrent use may result in hypertension, cardiac arrhythmias, and tachycardia.	1	2	2
ETILEFRINE Concurrent use may result in hypertension, cardiac arrhythmias, and tachycardia.	1	2	2
FLUOXETINE Concurrent use may result in amoxapine antidepressant toxicity (dry mouth, urinary retention, sedation) and an increased risk of cardiotoxicity (QT prolongation, torsade de pointes, cardiac arrest).	0	2	3
GREPAFLOXACIN Concurrent use may result in an increased risk of cardiotoxicity (QT prolongation, torsade de pointes, cardiac arrest).	2	1	3

INTERACTION	ONSET	SEVERITY	EVIDENCE
GUANADREL Concurrent use may result in decreased antihypertensive effectiveness.	2	3	3
HALOFANTRINE Concurrent use may result in an increased risk of cardiotoxicity (QT prolongation, torsade de pointes, cardiac arrest).	2	2	3
ISOCARBOXAZID Concurrent use may result in neurotoxicity, seizures, or serotonin syndrome (hypertension, hyperthermia, myoclonus, mental status changes).	2	1	3
LEVOMETHADYL Concurrent use may result in an increased risk of cardiotoxicity (QT prolongation, torsade de pointes, cardiac arrest).	2	1	3
METHOXAMINE Concurrent use may result in hypertension, cardiac arrhythmias, and tachycardia.	1	2	2
MIDODRINE Concurrent use may result in hypertension, cardiac arrhythmias, and tachycardia.	1	2	2
MOCLOBEMIDE Concurrent use may result in neurotoxicity, seizures, or serotonin syndrome (hypertension, hyperthermia, myoclonus, mental status changes).	2	2	3
NOREPINEPHRINE Concurrent use may result in hypertension, cardiac arrhythmias, and tachycardia.	1	2	2
OXILOFRINE Concurrent use may result in hypertension, cardiac arrhythmias, and tachycardia.	1	2	2
PHENELZINE Concurrent use may result in neurotoxicity, seizures, or serotonin syndrome (hypertension, hyperthermia, myoclonus, mental status changes).	2	2	3
PHENINDIONE Concurrent use may result in increased risk of bleeding.	2	3	3
PHENPROCOUMON Concurrent use may result in increased risk of bleeding.	2	3	3
PHENYLEPHRINE Concurrent use may result in hypertension, cardiac arrhythmias, and tachycardia.	1	2	2
PIMOZIDE Concurrent use may result in an increased risk of cardiotoxicity (QT prolongation, torsade de pointes, cardiac arrest).	0	1	3

Onset: 0=Unspecified 1=Rapid 2=Delayed
Severity: 1=Contraindicated 2=Major 3=Moderate 4=Minor
Evidence: 1=Excellent 2=Good 3=Fair 4=Poor

INTERACTION	ONSET	SEVERITY	EVIDENCE
PROCARBAZINE Concurrent use may result in neurotoxicity, seizures.	2	2	3
SELEGILINE Concurrent use may result in neurotoxicity, seizures, or serotonin syndrome (hypertension, hyperthermia, myoclonus, mental status changes).	2	2	3
TRAMADOL Concurrent use may result in an increased risk of seizures.	1	2	3
TRANYLCYPROMINE Concurrent use may result in neurotoxicity, seizures, or serotonin syndrome (hypertension, hyperthermia, myoclonus, mental status changes).	2	2	3
WARFARIN Concurrent use may result in an increased risk of bleeding.	2	3	3

Amphetamines (Adderall, Adderall XR)

INTERACTION	ONSET	SEVERITY	EVIDENCE
ACETAZOLAMIDE Concurrent use may result in amphetamine toxicity (hypertension, hyperpyrexia, seizures).	2	4	3
CLORGYLINE Concurrent use may result in hypertensive crisis (headache, hyperpyrexia, hypertension).	1	1	3
GUANETHIDINE Concurrent use may result in decreased guanethidine effectiveness.	1	3	2
IPRONIAZID Concurrent use may result in hypertensive crisis (headache, hyperpyrexia, hypertension).	1	1	3
ISOCARBOXAZID Concurrent use may result in hypertensive crisis (headache, hyperpyrexia, hypertension).	1	1	3
MOCLOBEMIDE Concurrent use may result in hypertensive crisis (headache, hyperpyrexia, hypertension).	1	1	3
NIALAMIDE Concurrent use may result in hypertensive crisis (headache, hyperpyrexia, hypertension).	1	1	3
PARGYLINE Concurrent use may result in hypertensive crisis (headache, hyperpyrexia, hypertension).	1	1	3
PHENELZINE Concurrent use may result in hypertensive crisis (headache, hyperpyrexia, hypertension).	1	1	2
PROCARBAZINE Concurrent use may result in hypertensive crisis (headache, hyperpyrexia, hypertension).	1	1	3

INTERACTION	ONSET	SEVERITY	EVIDENCE
SELEGILINE Concurrent use may result in hypertensive crisis (headache, hyperpyrexia, hypertension).	1	1	2
SIBUTRAMINE Concurrent use may result in an increased risk of hypertension and tachycardia.	1	1	3
SODIUM BICARBONATE Concurrent use may result in amphetamine toxicity (hypertension, hyperpyrexia, seizures).	2	3	3
TOLOXATONE Concurrent use may result in hypertensive crisis (headache, hyperpyrexia, hypertension).	1	1	3
TRANYLCYPROMINE Concurrent use may result in hypertensive crisis (headache, hyperpyrexia, hypertension).	1	1	2

Aripiprazole (Abilify, Abilify Discmelt)

INTERACTION	ONSET	SEVERITY	EVIDENCE
CARBAMAZEPINE Concurrent use may result in decreased aripiprazole concentrations.	2	2	3
FLUOXETINE Concurrent use may cause increased aripiprazole plasma levels.	2	2	3
KETOCONAZOLE Concurrent use may result in increased aripiprazole concentrations.	2	2	3
PAROXETINE Concurrent use may cause increased aripiprazole plasma levels.	2	2	3
QUINIDINE Concurrent use may result in increased aripiprazole plasma levels.	2	2	3

Atomoxetine (Strattera)

INTERACTION	ONSET	SEVERITY	EVIDENCE
ALBUTEROL Concurrent use may result in an increase in heart rate and blood pressure.	0	2	3
AMITRIPTYLINE Concurrent use may result in an increase in atomoxetine steady-state plasma concentrations.	0	3	3

Onset: 0=Unspecified 1=Rapid 2=Delayed
Severity: 1=Contraindicated 2=Major 3=Moderate 4=Minor
Evidence: 1=Excellent 2=Good 3=Fair 4=Poor

INTERACTION	ONSET	SEVERITY	EVIDENCE
AMOXAPINE Concurrent use may result in an increase in atomoxetine steady-state plasma concentrations.	0	3	3
CLOMIPRAMINE Concurrent use may result in an increase in atomoxetine steady-state plasma concentrations.	0	3	3
CLORGYLINE Concurrent use may result in an increased risk of serotonin syndrome (hypertension, hyperthermia, myoclonus, mental status changes).	0	1	3
DESIPRAMINE Concurrent use may result in an increase in atomoxetine steady-state plasma concentrations.	0	3	3
DIBENZEPIN Concurrent use may result in an increase in atomoxetine steady-state plasma concentrations.	0	3	3
DOTHIEPIN Concurrent use may result in an increase in atomoxetine steady-state plasma concentrations.	0	3	3
DOXEPIN Concurrent use may result in an increase in atomoxetine steady-state plasma concentrations.	0	3	3
FLUOXETINE Concurrent use may result in an increase in atomoxetine steady-state plasma concentrations.	0	3	3
IMIPRAMINE Concurrent use may result in an increase in atomoxetine steady-state plasma concentrations.	0	3	3
ISOCARBOXAZID Concurrent use may result in an increased risk of serotonin syndrome (hypertension, hyperthermia, myoclonus, mental status changes).	0	1	3
LAZABEMIDE Concurrent use may result in an increased risk of serotonin syndrome (hypertension, hyperthermia, myoclonus, mental status changes).	0	1	3
LOFEPRAMINE Concurrent use may result in an increase in atomoxetine steady-state plasma concentrations.	0	3	3
MOCLOBEMIDE Concurrent use may result in an increased risk of serotonin syndrome (hypertension, hyperthermia, myoclonus, mental status changes).	0	1	3
NORTRIPTYLINE Concurrent use may result in an increase in atomoxetine steady-state plasma concentrations.	0	3	3

INTERACTION	ONSET	SEVERITY	EVIDENCE
OPIPRAMOL Concurrent use may result in an increase in atomoxetine steady-state plasma concentrations.	0	3	3
PAROXETINE Concurrent use may result in an increase in atomoxetine steady-state plasma concentrations.	0	3	3
PHENELZINE Concurrent use may result in an increased risk of serotonin syndrome (hypertension, hyperthermia, myoclonus, mental status changes).	0	1	3
PROTRIPTYLINE Concurrent use may result in an increase in atomoxetine steady-state plasma concentrations.	0	3	3
QUINIDINE Concurrent use may result in an increase in atomoxetine steady-state plasma concentrations.	0	3	3
SELEGILINE Concurrent use may result in an increased risk of serotonin syndrome (hypertension, hyperthermia, myoclonus, mental status changes).	0	1	3
TRANYLCYPROMINE Concurrent use may result in an increased risk of serotonin syndrome (hypertension, hyperthermia, myoclonus, mental status changes).	0	1	3

Buprenorphine (Suboxone)

INTERACTION	ONSET	SEVERITY	EVIDENCE
ALFENTANIL Concurrent use may result in precipitation of withdrawal symptoms (abdominal cramps, nausea, vomiting, lacrimation, rhinorrhea, anxiety, restlessness, elevation of temperature or piloerection).	2	2	2
ALPHAPRODINE Concurrent use may result in precipitation of withdrawal symptoms (abdominal cramps, nausea, vomiting, lacrimation, rhinorrhea, anxiety, restlessness, elevation of temperature or piloerection).	2	2	2
CODEINE Concurrent use may result in precipitation of withdrawal symptoms (abdominal cramps, nausea, vomiting, lacrimation, rhinorrhea, anxiety, restlessness, elevation of temperature or piloerection).	2	2	2
DIAZEPAM Concurrent use may result in respiratory and cardiovascular collapse.	1	2	2

Onset: 0=Unspecified   1=Rapid   2=Delayed
Severity: 1=Contraindicated   2=Major   3=Moderate   4=Minor
Evidence: 1=Excellent   2=Good   3=Fair   4=Poor

INTERACTION	ONSET	SEVERITY	EVIDENCE
DIHYDROCODEINE Concurrent use may result in precipitation of withdrawal symptoms (abdominal cramps, nausea, vomiting, lacrimation, rhinorrhea, anxiety, restlessness, elevation of temperature or piloerection).	2	2	2
FENTANYL Concurrent use may result in precipitation of withdrawal symptoms (abdominal cramps, nausea, vomiting, lacrimation, rhinorrhea, anxiety, restlessness, elevation of temperature or piloerection).	2	2	2
HYDROCODONE Concurrent use may result in precipitation of withdrawal symptoms (abdominal cramps, nausea, vomiting, lacrimation, rhinorrhea, anxiety, restlessness, elevation of temperature or piloerection).	2	2	2
HYDROMORPHONE Concurrent use may result in precipitation of withdrawal symptoms (abdominal cramps, nausea, vomiting, lacrimation, rhinorrhea, anxiety, restlessness, elevation of temperature or piloerection).	2	2	2
LEVORPHANOL Concurrent use may result in precipitation of withdrawal symptoms (abdominal cramps, nausea, vomiting, lacrimation, rhinorrhea, anxiety, restlessness, elevation of temperature or piloerection).	2	2	2
MEPERIDINE Concurrent use may result in precipitation of withdrawal symptoms (abdominal cramps, nausea, vomiting, lacrimation, rhinorrhea, anxiety, restlessness, elevation of temperature or piloerection).	2	2	2
METHADONE Concurrent use may result in precipitation of withdrawal symptoms (abdominal cramps, nausea, vomiting, lacrimation, rhinorrhea, anxiety, restlessness, elevation of temperature or piloerection).	2	2	2
MORPHINE SULFATE LIPOSOME Concurrent use may result in precipitation of withdrawal symptoms (abdominal cramps, nausea, vomiting, lacrimation, rhinorrhea, anxiety, restlessness, elevation of temperature or piloerection).	2	2	2
MORPHINE Concurrent use may result in precipitation of withdrawal symptoms (abdominal cramps, nausea, vomiting, lacrimation, rhinorrhea, anxiety, restlessness, elevation of temperature or piloerection).	2	2	2
OXYCODONE Concurrent use may result in precipitation of withdrawal symptoms (abdominal cramps, nausea, vomiting, lacrimation, rhinorrhea, anxiety, restlessness, elevation of temperature or piloerection).	2	2	2

INTERACTION	ONSET	SEVERITY	EVIDENCE
OXYMORPHONE Concurrent use may result in precipitation of withdrawal symptoms (abdominal cramps, nausea, vomiting, lacrimation, rhinorrhea, anxiety, restlessness, elevation of temperature or piloerection).	2	2	2
PROPOXYPHENE Concurrent use may result in precipitation of withdrawal symptoms (abdominal cramps, nausea, vomiting, lacrimation, rhinorrhea, anxiety, restlessness, elevation of temperature or piloerection).	2	2	2
SUFENTANIL Concurrent use may result in precipitation of withdrawal symptoms (abdominal cramps, nausea, vomiting, lacrimation, rhinorrhea, anxiety, restlessness, elevation of temperature or piloerection).	2	2	2

Bupropion (Wellbutrin, Wellbutrin SR, Wellbutrin XL, Zyban)

INTERACTION	ONSET	SEVERITY	EVIDENCE
CLORGYLINE Concurrent use may result in bupropion toxicity.	1	1	3
DROPERIDOL Concurrent use may result in an increased risk of cardiotoxicity (QT prolongation, torsade de pointes, cardiac arrest).	1	2	3
ETHANOL Concurrent use may result in an increased risk of seizures.	2	2	3
IPRONIAZID Concurrent use may result in bupropion toxicity (seizures, agitation, psychotic changes).	1	1	3
ISOCARBOXAZID Concurrent use may result in bupropion toxicity (seizures, agitation, psychotic changes).	1	1	3
MOCLOBEMIDE Concurrent use may result in bupropion toxicity (seizures, agitation, psychotic changes).	1	1	3
NIALAMIDE Concurrent use may result in bupropion toxicity (seizures, agitation, psychotic changes).	1	1	3
PARGYLINE Concurrent use may result in bupropion toxicity (seizures, agitation, psychotic changes).	1	1	3
PHENELZINE Concurrent use may result in bupropion toxicity (seizures, agitation, psychotic changes).	1	1	3

Onset: 0=Unspecified 1=Rapid 2=Delayed
Severity: 1=Contraindicated 2=Major 3=Moderate 4=Minor
Evidence: 1=Excellent 2=Good 3=Fair 4=Poor

INTERACTION	ONSET	SEVERITY	EVIDENCE
PROCARBAZINE Concurrent use may result in bupropion toxicity (seizures, agitation, psychotic changes).	1	1	3
SELEGILINE Concurrent use may result in bupropion toxicity (seizures, agitation, psychotic changes).	1	1	3
TOLOXATONE Concurrent use may result in bupropion toxicity (seizures, agitation, psychotic changes).	1	1	3
TRANYLCYPROMINE Concurrent use may result in bupropion toxicity (seizures, agitation, psychotic changes).	1	1	3

Buspirone (BuSpar)

INTERACTION	ONSET	SEVERITY	EVIDENCE
CLORGYLINE Concurrent use may result in hypertensive crisis.	1	2	3
DILTIAZEM Concurrent use may result in an increased risk of enhanced buspirone effects.	1	3	3
ERYTHROMYCIN Concurrent use may result in increased buspirone plasma concentrations; increased buspirone side effects (impaired psychomotor performance, sedation).	1	3	3
GRAPEFRUIT JUICE Concurrent use may result in an increased risk of buspirone toxicity (dizziness, sedation).	1	3	3
IPRONIAZID Concurrent use may result in hypertensive crisis.	1	2	3
ISOCARBOXAZID Concurrent use may result in hypertensive crisis.	1	1	3
ITRACONAZOLE Concurrent use may result in increased buspirone plasma concentrations; increased buspirone side effects (impaired psychomotor performance, sedation).	1	3	3
MOCLOBEMIDE Concurrent use may result in hypertensive crisis.	1	2	3
NIALAMIDE Concurrent use may result in hypertensive crisis.	1	2	3
PARGYLINE Concurrent use may result in hypertensive crisis.	1	2	3
PHENELZINE Concurrent use may result in hypertensive crisis.	1	1	3
PROCARBAZINE Concurrent use may result in hypertensive crisis.	1	2	3

INTERACTION	ONSET	SEVERITY	EVIDENCE
RIFAMPIN Concurrent use may result in reduced anxiolytic effects of buspirone.	1	3	3
SELEGILINE Concurrent use may result in hypertensive crisis.	1	2	3
TOLOXATONE Concurrent use may result in hypertensive crisis.	1	2	3
TRANYLCYPROMINE Concurrent use may result in hypertensive crisis.	1	1	3
VERAPAMIL Concurrent use may result in an increased risk of enhanced buspirone effects.	1	3	3

Carbamazepine (Equetro)

INTERACTION	ONSET	SEVERITY	EVIDENCE
ACETAMINOPHEN Concurrent use may result in an increased risk of acetaminophen hepatotoxicity.	2	3	2
ACETYLCYSTEINE Concurrent use may result in subtherapeutic carbamazepine levels.	2	3	2
ACTIVATED CHARCOAL Concurrent use may result in decreased carbamazepine exposure.	1	3	3
ADENOSINE Concurrent use may result in a higher degree of heart block.	1	2	2
ALPRAZOLAM Concurrent use may result in decreased alprazolam effectiveness.	2	3	2
AMITRIPTYLINE Concurrent use may result in decreased amitriptyline effectiveness.	2	3	2
AMOXAPINE Concurrent use may result in decreased amoxapine concentration.	2	3	2
AMPRENAVIR Concurrent use may result in reduced amprenavir efficacy due to reduced amprenavir serum concentrations.	2	3	3
ANISINDIONE Concurrent use may result in decreased anticoagulant effectiveness.	2	3	2

Onset: 0=Unspecified 1=Rapid 2=Delayed
Severity: 1=Contraindicated 2=Major 3=Moderate 4=Minor
Evidence: 1=Excellent 2=Good 3=Fair 4=Poor

INTERACTION	ONSET	SEVERITY	EVIDENCE
APREPITANT Concurrent use may result in reduced plasma aprepitant concentrations and decreased aprepitant efficacy.	2	3	2
ARIPIPRAZOLE Concurrent use may result in decreased aripiprazole concentrations.	2	3	2
ATRACURIUM Concurrent use may result in decreased atracurium duration of action.	1	3	3
AZITHROMYCIN Concurrent use may result in increased serum carbamazepine levels.	0	4	3
BETAMETHASONE Concurrent use may result in decreased betamethasone effectiveness.	2	3	3
BROMPERIDOL Concurrent use may result in decreased bromperidol efficacy.	2	4	1
BUPROPION Concurrent use may result in decreased bupropion effectiveness.	2	4	2
CASPOFUNGIN Concurrent use may result in reduced caspofungin plasma levels.	2	3	2
CIMETIDINE Concurrent use may result in carbamazepine toxicity (ataxia, nystagmus, diplopia, headache, vomiting, apnea, seizures, coma).	2	3	3
CISATRACURIUM Concurrent use may result in resistance to neuromuscular blocking action.	1	4	3
CISPLATIN Concurrent use may result in decreased carbamazepine plasma concentrations.	2	3	3
CLARITHROMYCIN Concurrent use may result in an increased risk of carbamazepine toxicity (ataxia, nystagmus, diplopia, headache, vomiting, apnea, seizures, coma).	2	3	2
CLOBAZAM Concurrent use may result in decreased carbamazepine parent drug and/or increased active metabolite concentrations.	2	4	2
CLOMIPRAMINE Concurrent use may result in decreased clomipramine effectiveness.	2	3	3
CLONAZEPAM Concurrent use may result in reduced plasma levels of clonazepam.	2	3	2

INTERACTION	ONSET	SEVERITY	EVIDENCE
CLORGYLINE Concurrent use may result in hypertensive urgency, hyperpyrexia, and seizures.	1	1	3
CLOZAPINE Concurrent use may result in an increased risk of bone marrow suppression, asterixis, or decreased serum clozapine levels.	2	2	2
CORTISONE Concurrent use may result in decreased cortisone effectiveness.	2	3	3
CYCLOSPORINE Concurrent use may result in reduced cyclosporine serum levels and potentially increased risk for organ rejection.	2	3	3
DALFOPRISTIN Concurrent use may result in an increased risk of carbamazepine toxicity (ataxia, nystagmus, diplopia, headache, vomiting, apnea, seizures, coma).	2	3	2
DANAZOL Concurrent use may result in carbamazepine toxicity (ataxia, nystagmus, diplopia, headache, vomiting, apnea, seizures, coma).	2	3	2
DARUNAVIR Concurrent use may result in decreased darunavir plasma concentrations and potential loss of darunavir efficacy.	0	2	3
DEHYDROEPIANDROSTERONE Concurrent use may result in reduced effectiveness of carbamazepine.	2	3	3
DELAVIRDINE Concurrent use may result in decreased trough plasma delavirdine concentrations.	2	2	2
DESIPRAMINE Concurrent use may result in increased carbamazepine toxicity, decreased desipramine effectiveness.	2	3	2
DEXAMETHASONE Concurrent use may result in decreased dexamethasone effectiveness.	2	3	3
DICUMAROL Concurrent use may result in decreased anticoagulant effectiveness.	2	3	2
DILTIAZEM Concurrent use may result in carbamazepine toxicity (ataxia, nystagmus, diplopia, headache, vomiting, apnea, seizures, coma).	2	3	2

Onset: 0=Unspecified 1=Rapid 2=Delayed
Severity: 1=Contraindicated 2=Major 3=Moderate 4=Minor
Evidence: 1=Excellent 2=Good 3=Fair 4=Poor

INTERACTION	ONSET	SEVERITY	EVIDENCE
DOTHIEPIN Concurrent use may result in decreased dothiepin effectiveness.	2	3	3
DOXACURIUM Concurrent use may result in decreased doxacurium duration of action.	1	3	3
DOXEPIN Concurrent use may result in decreased doxepin effectiveness and possibly increased carbamazepine toxicity (diplopia, blurred vision, dizziness, tremor).	2	3	2
DOXORUBICIN HYDROCHLORIDE Concurrent use may result in decreased carbamazepine plasma concentrations.	2	3	3
DOXORUBICIN HYDROCHLORIDE LIPOSOME Concurrent use may result in decreased carbamazepine plasma concentrations.	2	3	3
DOXYCYCLINE Concurrent use may result in decreased doxycycline effectiveness.	2	3	3
EFAVIRENZ Concurrent use may result in decreased efavirenz plasma concentration and/or carbamazepine plasma concentration.	0	3	3
ERLOTINIB Concurrent use may result in increased erlotinib clearance and reduced erlotinib exposure.	0	2	3
ERYTHROMYCIN Concurrent use may result in carbamazepine toxicity (ataxia, nystagmus, diplopia, headache, vomiting, apnea, seizures, coma).	2	3	1
ETHOSUXIMIDE Concurrent use may result in decreased ethosuximide serum concentrations.	2	3	2
ETONOGESTREL Concurrent use may result in a decrease in plasma concentrations of estrogens and in estrogen effectiveness.	2	3	2
ETRETINATE Concurrent use may result in decreased etretinate effectiveness.	1	3	2
EVENING PRIMROSE Concurrent use may result in reduced anticonvulsant effectiveness.	2	3	3
FELODIPINE Concurrent use may result in decreased felodipine effectiveness.	2	4	2
FENTANYL Concurrent use may result in decreased plasma concentrations of fentanyl.	2	3	2

INTERACTION	ONSET	SEVERITY	EVIDENCE
FLUCONAZOLE Concurrent use may result in an increased risk of carbamazepine toxicity (ataxia, nystagmus, diplopia, headache, vomiting, apnea, seizures, coma).	1	3	2
FLUNARIZINE Concurrent use may result in increased carbamazepine serum levels and possible toxicity (ataxia, nystagmus, diplopia, headache, vomiting, apnea, seizures, coma).	2	3	2
FLUOXETINE Concurrent use may result in carbamazepine toxicity (ataxia, nystagmus, diplopia, headache, vomiting, apnea, seizures, coma).	2	3	2
FLUVOXAMINE Concurrent use may result in carbamazepine toxicity (ataxia, nystagmus, diplopia, headache, vomiting, apnea, seizures, coma).	2	3	3
FOSAMPRENAVIR Concurrent use may result in reduced effectiveness of fosamprenavir due to reduced serum concentrations.	2	3	2
GINKGO Concurrent use may result in decreased anticonvulsant effectiveness.	2	3	2
GRAPEFRUIT JUICE Concurrent use may result in increased carbamazepine bioavailability.	1	3	2
HALOPERIDOL Concurrent use may result in decreased haloperidol effectiveness.	2	3	2
HYDROCHLOROTHIAZIDE Concurrent use may result in hyponatremia.	2	3	2
HYDROCORTISONE Concurrent use may result in decreased hydrocortisone effectiveness.	2	3	3
IMATINIB Concurrent use may result in decreased plasma levels of imatinib.	2	2	3
IMIPRAMINE Concurrent use may result in decreased imipramine effectiveness.	2	3	2
INDINAVIR Concurrent use may result in decreased indinavir plasma concentrations and an increased risk of antiretroviral therapy failure.	2	3	2
INFLUENZA VIRUS VACCINE Concurrent use may result in increased carbamazepine serum concentrations.	2	3	2

Onset: 0=Unspecified 1=Rapid 2=Delayed
Severity: 1=Contraindicated 2=Major 3=Moderate 4=Minor
Evidence: 1=Excellent 2=Good 3=Fair 4=Poor

INTERACTION	ONSET	SEVERITY	EVIDENCE
ISOCARBOXAZID Concurrent use may result in hypertensive urgency, hyperpyrexia, and seizures.	2	1	3
ISONIAZID Concurrent use may result in elevated carbamazepine levels and toxicity (ataxia, nystagmus, diplopia, headache, vomiting, apnea, seizures, coma).	1	3	2
KETOCONAZOLE Concurrent use may result in increased carbamazepine serum levels.	2	3	3
LAPATINIB Concurrent use may result in decreased lapatinib exposure or plasma concentrations.	0	2	2
LEVETIRACETAM Concurrent use may result in symptoms of carbamazepine toxicity (nystagmus, ataxia, dizziness, double vision).	2	3	2
LEVONORGESTREL Concurrent use may result in a decrease in plasma concentrations of estrogens and in estrogen effectiveness.	2	3	2
LITHIUM Concurrent use may result in additive neurotoxicity (weakness, tremor, nystagmus, asterixis).	2	3	2
LOPINAVIR Concurrent use may result in decreased lopinavir exposure; increased serum carbamazepine levels and toxicity.	2	2	2
LOXAPINE Concurrent use may result in an increased risk of carbamazepine toxicity (ataxia, nystagmus, diplopia, headache, vomiting, apnea, seizures, coma).	2	3	2
MEBENDAZOLE Concurrent use may result in decreased mebendazole effectiveness.	2	3	3
MEFLOQUINE Concurrent use may result in loss of seizure control.	0	3	3
METHADONE Concurrent use may result in decreased methadone effectiveness.	2	4	3
METHYLPHENIDATE Concurrent use may result in loss of methylphenidate efficacy.	2	3	2
METHYLPREDNISOLONE Concurrent use may result in decreased methylprednisolone effectiveness.	2	3	2
METRONIDAZOLE Concurrent use may result in increased carbamazepine serum concentrations and potential carbamazepine toxicity.	2	3	2

INTERACTION	ONSET	SEVERITY	EVIDENCE
MIANSERIN Concurrent use may result in decreased mianserin serum concentrations.	2	3	2
MIDAZOLAM Concurrent use may result in decreased efficacy of midazolam.	1	3	2
MIFEPRISTONE Concurrent use may result in decreased serum levels of mifepristone and potentially decreased efficacy.	0	3	3
MILNACIPRAN Concurrent use may result in slight reductions in milnacipran plasma levels.	2	4	2
MIOKAMYCIN Concurrent use may result in an increase in carbamazepine plasma levels.	2	3	2
NEFAZODONE Concurrent use may result in an increased risk of carbamazepine toxicity (ataxia, nystagmus, diplopia, headache, vomiting, apnea, seizures, coma).	2	3	2
NELFINAVIR Concurrent use may result in decreased nelfinavir plasma concentrations; increased serum carbamazepine levels and toxicity.	2	2	3
NEVIRAPINE Concurrent use may result in decreased plasma concentrations of carbamazepine.	0	3	2
NIFEDIPINE Concurrent use may result in decreased nifedipine exposure and may decrease nifedipine efficacy.	2	3	3
NIMODIPINE Concurrent use may result in decreased nimodipine effectiveness.	2	4	2
NORELGESTROMIN Concurrent use may result in a decrease in plasma concentrations of estrogens and in estrogen effectiveness.	2	3	2
NORTRIPTYLINE Concurrent use may result in decreased nortriptyline effectiveness.	2	3	2
OLANZAPINE Concurrent use may result in reduced olanzapine efficacy.	1	3	2
OMEPRAZOLE Concurrent use may result in an increased risk of carbamazepine toxicity.	2	3	2

Onset: 0=Unspecified 1=Rapid 2=Delayed
Severity: 1=Contraindicated 2=Major 3=Moderate 4=Minor
Evidence: 1=Excellent 2=Good 3=Fair 4=Poor

INTERACTION	ONSET	SEVERITY	EVIDENCE
OXCARBAZEPINE Concurrent use may result in decreased plasma concentration of the active 10-monohydroxy metabolite of oxcarbazepine.	2	3	1
PANCURONIUM Concurrent use may result in decreased pancuronium duration of action.	1	3	3
PENTOBARBITAL Concurrent use may result in decreased carbamazepine effectiveness with loss of seizure control.	2	3	3
PHENELZINE Concurrent use may result in hypertensive urgency, hyperpyrexia, and seizures.	1	1	3
PHENOBARBITAL Concurrent use may result in decreased carbamazepine effectiveness with loss of seizure control.	2	3	3
PHENPROCOUMON Concurrent use may result in decreased anticoagulant effectiveness.	2	3	2
PHENYTOIN Concurrent use may result in increased phenytoin concentrations and decreased carbamazepine concentrations.	2	3	2
PIPECURONIUM Concurrent use may result in resistance to neuromuscular blockade.	1	3	2
PRAZIQUANTEL Concurrent use may result in decreased praziquantel effectiveness.	2	3	2
PREDNISOLONE Concurrent use may result in decreased prednisolone effectiveness.	2	3	3
PREDNISONE Concurrent use may result in decreased prednisone effectiveness.	2	3	3
PRIMIDONE Concurrent use may result in decreased carbamazepine effectiveness with loss of seizure control.	2	3	2
PROCARBAZINE Concurrent use may result in hypertensive urgency, hyperpyrexia, and seizures.	1	1	3
PROPOXYPHENE Concurrent use may result in an increased risk of carbamazepine toxicity (ataxia, nystagmus, diplopia, headache, vomiting, apnea, seizures, coma).	2	2	2

INTERACTION	ONSET	SEVERITY	EVIDENCE
PROTRIPTYLINE Concurrent use may result in decreased protriptyline plasma concentrations and increased carbamazepine plasma concentrations and possible toxicity (ataxia, nystagmus, apnea, seizures, coma).	2	3	2
PSYLLIUM Concurrent use may result in decreased absorption and effectiveness of carbamazepine.	1	3	2
QUETIAPINE Concurrent use may result in decreased serum quetiapine concentrations.	0	3	3
QUINUPRISTIN Concurrent use may result in an increased risk of carbamazepine toxicity (ataxia, nystagmus, diplopia, headache, vomiting, apnea, seizures, coma).	2	3	2
RAPACURONIUM Concurrent use may result in resistance to neuromuscular blocking action.	1	4	3
REMACEMIDE Concurrent use may result in reduced remacemide exposure and increased carbamazepine exposure.	2	3	2
REPAGLINIDE Concurrent use may result in decreased repaglinide plasma concentrations.	0	3	3
RIFAMPIN Concurrent use may result in elevated carbamazepine levels and toxicity (ataxia, nystagmus, diplopia, headache, vomiting, apnea, seizures, coma).	1	3	2
RIFAPENTINE Concurrent use may result in decreased anticonvulsant effectiveness.	2	3	2
RITONAVIR Concurrent use may result in increased carbamazepine serum concentrations and potential toxicity.	2	3	2
SABELUZOLE Concurrent use may result in reduced sabeluzole efficacy.	2	3	2
SAQUINAVIR Concurrent use may result in reduced saquinavir effectiveness.	1	3	2
SELEGILINE Concurrent use may result in an increase in selegiline concentrations.	1	1	3
SERTRALINE Concurrent use may result in an increased risk of carbamazepine toxicity (ataxia, nystagmus, diplopia, headache, vomiting, apnea, seizures, coma).	2	3	2

Onset: 0=Unspecified 1=Rapid 2=Delayed
Severity: 1=Contraindicated 2=Major 3=Moderate 4=Minor
Evidence: 1=Excellent 2=Good 3=Fair 4=Poor

INTERACTION	ONSET	SEVERITY	EVIDENCE
SIMVASTATIN Concurrent use may result in reduced simvastatin exposure.	2	3	2
SIROLIMUS Concurrent use may result in decreased plasma sirolimus concentration.	0	2	3
SORAFENIB Concurrent use may result in decreased sorafenib concentrations.	2	3	3
ST JOHN'S WORT Concurrent use may result in altered carbamazepine blood concentrations.	2	3	2
SUNITINIB Concurrent use may result in decreased plasma concentrations of sunitinib and its active metabolite.	2	2	3
TELITHROMYCIN Concurrent use may result in subtherapeutic telithromycin concentrations and/or elevated serum levels of carbamazepine.	0	3	2
TERFENADINE Concurrent use may result in carbamazepine toxicity (ataxia, nystagmus, diplopia, headache, vomiting, apnea, seizures, coma).	1	3	2
TIAGABINE Concurrent use may result in decreased tiagabine efficacy.	2	3	2
TICLOPIDINE Concurrent use may result in an increased risk of carbamazepine toxicity (ataxia, nystagmus, diplopia, headache, vomiting, apnea, seizures, coma).	2	3	2
TOPIRAMATE Concurrent use may result in decreased topiramate concentrations.	2	3	2
TRANYLCYPROMINE Concurrent use may result in hypertensive urgency, hyperpyrexia, and seizures.	1	1	3
TRAZODONE Concurrent use may result in decreased trazodone plasma concentrations.	2	3	2
TRIMIPRAMINE Concurrent use may result in decreased trimipramine effectiveness.	2	3	3
TROLEANDOMYCIN Concurrent use may result in carbamazepine toxicity (ataxia, nystagmus, diplopia, headache, vomiting, apnea, seizures, coma).	2	3	1
VALPROIC ACID Concurrent use may result in carbamazepine toxicity (ataxia, nystagmus, diplopia, headache, vomiting, apnea, seizures, coma) and/or decreased valproic acid effectiveness.	2	3	2

INTERACTION	ONSET	SEVERITY	EVIDENCE
VECURONIUM Concurrent use may result in decreased vecuronium duration of action.	1	3	1
VERAPAMIL Concurrent use may result in increased carbamazepine plasma concentrations and risk of toxicity (ataxia, nystagmus, diplopia, headache, vomiting, apnea, seizures, coma).	2	3	2
VIGABATRIN Concurrent use may result in carbamazepine toxicity (ataxia, nystagmus, diplopia, headache, vomiting, apnea, seizures, coma).	2	2	2
VILOXAZINE Concurrent use may result in carbamazepine toxicity (ataxia, nystagmus, diplopia, headache, vomiting, apnea, seizures, coma).	2	3	2
VORICONAZOLE Concurrent use may result in reduced systemic exposure to voriconazole.	0	1	3
WARFARIN Concurrent use may result in decreased anticoagulant effectiveness.	2	3	2

Chlordiazepoxide (Librium, Limbitrol)

INTERACTION	ONSET	SEVERITY	EVIDENCE
CIMETIDINE Concurrent use may result in chlordiazepoxide toxicity (central nervous system depression).	1	4	3
DISULFIRAM Concurrent use may result in an increased risk of chlordiazepoxide toxicity (central nervous system depression).	2	4	3
ETHANOL Concurrent use may result in increased sedation.	1	3	1
KETOCONAZOLE Concurrent use may result in increased chlordiazepoxide serum concentrations and potential chlordiazepoxide toxicity (sedation, slurred speech, central nervous system depression).	2	1	3
THEOPHYLLINE Concurrent use may result in decreased chlordiazepoxide effectiveness.	1	3	2

Onset: 0=Unspecified 1=Rapid 2=Delayed
Severity: 1=Contraindicated 2=Major 3=Moderate 4=Minor
Evidence: 1=Excellent 2=Good 3=Fair 4=Poor

Chlorpromazine

INTERACTION	ONSET	SEVERITY	EVIDENCE
ANTACIDS Concurrent use may result in decreased chlorpromazine effectiveness.	2	4	3
ATENOLOL Concurrent use may result in hypotension and/or chlorpromazine toxicity.	1	3	2
BELLADONNA Concurrent use may result in increased manic, agitated reactions, or enhanced anticholinergic effects resulting in cardiorespiratory failure, especially in cases of belladonna overdose.	1	3	2
BENZTROPINE Concurrent use may result in decreased chlorpromazine serum concentrations, decreased chlorpromazine effectiveness, enhanced anticholinergic effects (ileus, hyperpyrexia, sedation, dry mouth).	2	3	3
CABERGOLINE Concurrent use may result in the decreased therapeutic effect of both drugs.	1	3	3
CISAPRIDE Concurrent use may result in cardiotoxicity (QT prolongation, torsade de pointes, cardiac arrest).	1	1	3
DROPERIDOL Concurrent use may result in an increased risk of cardiotoxicity (QT prolongation, torsade de pointes, cardiac arrest).	0	2	3
EPINEPHRINE Concurrent use may result in hypotension and tachycardia.	1	3	3
ETHANOL Concurrent use may result in increased sedation.	1	3	2
FOSPHENYTOIN Concurrent use may result in increased or decreased phenytoin levels and possibly reduced chlorpromazine levels.	2	4	3
GREPAFLOXACIN Concurrent use may result in an increased risk of cardiotoxicity (QT prolongation, torsade de pointes, cardiac arrest).	2	1	3
GUANETHIDINE Concurrent use may result in decreased guanethidine effectiveness.	1	3	2
HALOFANTRINE Concurrent use may result in an increased risk of cardiotoxicity (QT prolongation, torsade de pointes, cardiac arrest).	0	2	3

INTERACTION	ONSET	SEVERITY	EVIDENCE
LEVODOPA Concurrent use may result in loss of levodopa efficacy.	1	3	2
LEVOMETHADYL Concurrent use may result in an increased risk of cardiotoxicity (QT prolongation, torsade de pointes, cardiac arrest).	2	1	3
LITHIUM Concurrent use may result in weakness, dyskinesias, increased extrapyramidal symptoms, encephalopathy, and brain damage.	2	2	1
MEPERIDINE Concurrent use may result in an increase in central nervous system and respiratory depression.	1	3	2
METOPROLOL Concurrent use may result in hypotension and/or chlorpromazine toxicity.	1	3	2
NOREPINEPHRINE Concurrent use may result in decreased norepinephrine effectiveness.	1	3	3
ORPHENADRINE Concurrent use may result in decreased chlorpromazine serum concentrations, decreased chlorpromazine effectiveness, enhanced anticholinergic effects (ileus, hyperpyrexia, sedation, dry mouth).	2	3	3
PHENMETRAZINE Concurrent use may result in decreased phenmetrazine effectiveness.	1	3	2
PHENOBARBITAL Concurrent use may result in decreased chlorpromazine effectiveness.	1	3	3
PHENYTOIN Concurrent use may result in increased or decreased phenytoin levels and possibly reduced chlorpromazine levels.	2	4	3
PORFIMER Concurrent use may result in excessive intracellular damage in photosensitized tissues.	2	3	3
PROCYCLIDINE Concurrent use may result in decreased chlorpromazine serum concentrations, decreased chlorpromazine effectiveness, enhanced anticholinergic effects (ileus, hyperpyrexia, sedation, dry mouth).	2	3	3
PROPRANOLOL Concurrent use may result in chlorpromazine toxicity (sedation, extrapyramidal effects, delirium), seizures.	2	3	3

Onset: 0=Unspecified 1=Rapid 2=Delayed
Severity: 1=Contraindicated 2=Major 3=Moderate 4=Minor
Evidence: 1=Excellent 2=Good 3=Fair 4=Poor

INTERACTION	ONSET	SEVERITY	EVIDENCE
SPARFLOXACIN Concurrent use may result in prolongation of the QTc interval and/or torsade de pointes.	2	1	3
TRAMADOL Concurrent use may result in an increased risk of seizures.	1	2	3
TRIHEXYPHENIDYL Concurrent use may result in decreased chlorpromazine serum concentrations, decreased chlorpromazine effectiveness, enhanced anticholinergic effects (ileus, hyperpyrexia, sedation, dry mouth).	2	3	3
ZIPRASIDONE Concurrent use may result in an increased risk of cardiotoxicity (QT prolongation, torsade de pointes, cardiac arrest).	0	1	3

Citalopram (Celexa)

INTERACTION	ONSET	SEVERITY	EVIDENCE
ALMOTRIPTAN Concurrent use may result in weakness, hyperreflexia, and/or incoordination.	0	3	3
CLORGYLINE Concurrent use may result in central nervous system toxicity or serotonin syndrome (hypertension, hyperthermia, myoclonus, mental status changes).	1	1	3
DEXFENFLURAMINE Concurrent use may result in serotonin syndrome (hypertension, hyperthermia, myoclonus, mental status changes).	1	2	3
DROPERIDOL Concurrent use may result in an increased risk of cardiotoxicity (QT prolongation, torsade de pointes, cardiac arrest).	1	2	3
FENFLURAMINE Concurrent use may result in serotonin syndrome (hypertension, hyperthermia, myoclonus, mental status changes).	1	2	3
FURAZOLIDONE Concurrent use may result in weakness, hyperreflexia, and incoordination.	2	1	3
HYDROXYTRYPTOPHAN Concurrent use may result in an increased risk of serotonin syndrome (hypertension, hyperthermia, myoclonus, mental status changes).	1	3	3
IPRONIAZID Concurrent use may result in central nervous system toxicity or serotonin syndrome (hypertension, hyperthermia, myoclonus, mental status changes).	1	1	3

INTERACTION	ONSET	SEVERITY	EVIDENCE
ISOCARBOXAZID Concurrent use may result in central nervous system toxicity or serotonin syndrome (hypertension, hyperthermia, myoclonus, mental status changes).	1	1	3
LEVOMETHADYL Concurrent use may result in an increased risk of cardiotoxicity (QT prolongation, torsade de pointes, cardiac arrest).	2	1	3
MOCLOBEMIDE Concurrent use may result in serotonin syndrome (hypertension, hyperthermia, myoclonus, mental status changes).	1	1	3
NIALAMIDE Concurrent use may result in central nervous system toxicity or serotonin syndrome (hypertension, hyperthermia, myoclonus, mental status changes).	1	1	3
PARGYLINE Concurrent use may result in central nervous system toxicity or serotonin syndrome (hypertension, hyperthermia, myoclonus, mental status changes).	1	1	3
PHENELZINE Concurrent use may result in central nervous system toxicity or serotonin syndrome (hypertension, hyperthermia, myoclonus, mental status changes).	1	1	3
PROCARBAZINE Concurrent use may result in central nervous system toxicity or serotonin syndrome (hypertension, hyperthermia, myoclonus, mental status changes).	1	1	3
SELEGILINE Concurrent use may result in central nervous system toxicity or serotonin syndrome (hypertension, hyperthermia, myoclonus, mental status changes).	1	1	3
SIBUTRAMINE Concurrent use may result in an increased risk of serotonin syndrome (hypertension, hypothermia, myoclonus, mental status changes).	1	2	3
TOLOXATONE Concurrent use may result in central nervous system toxicity or serotonin syndrome (hypertension, hyperthermia, myoclonus, mental status changes).	1	1	3
TRAMADOL Concurrent use may result in an increased risk of seizures and serotonin syndrome (hypertension, hyperthermia, myoclonus, mental status changes).	1	2	2

Onset: 0=Unspecified 1=Rapid 2=Delayed
Severity: 1=Contraindicated 2=Major 3=Moderate 4=Minor
Evidence: 1=Excellent 2=Good 3=Fair 4=Poor

INTERACTION	ONSET	SEVERITY	EVIDENCE
TRANYLCYPROMINE Concurrent use may result in central nervous system toxicity or serotonin syndrome (hypertension, hyperthermia, myoclonus, mental status changes).	1	1	3

Clomipramine (Anafranil)

INTERACTION	ONSET	SEVERITY	EVIDENCE
ACENOCOUMAROL Concurrent use may result in increased risk of bleeding.	2	3	3
AMPRENAVIR Concurrent use may result in increased clomipramine serum concentrations and potential toxicity (anticholinergic effects, sedation, confusion, cardiac arrhythmias).	2	2	3
ANISINDIONE Concurrent use may result in increased risk of bleeding.	2	3	3
BEPRIDIL Concurrent use may result in an increased risk of cardiotoxicity (QT prolongation, torsade de pointes, cardiac arrest).	1	1	3
BETHANIDINE Concurrent use may result in decreased antihypertensive effectiveness.	1	3	3
CIMETIDINE Concurrent use may result in clomipramine toxicity (dry mouth, blurred vision, urinary retention).	2	3	3
CISAPRIDE Concurrent use may result in cardiotoxicity (QT prolongation, torsade de pointes, cardiac arrest).	1	1	3
CLONIDINE Concurrent use may result in decreased antihypertensive effectiveness.	2	2	3
CLORGYLINE Concurrent use may result in neurotoxicity, seizures, or serotonin syndrome (hypertension, hyperthermia, myoclonus, mental status changes).	2	2	3
DICUMAROL Concurrent use may result in increased risk of bleeding.	2	3	3
EPINEPHRINE Concurrent use may result in hypertension, cardiac arrhythmias, and tachycardia.	1	2	2
ETILEFRINE Concurrent use may result in hypertension, cardiac arrhythmias, and tachycardia.	1	2	2
FLUVOXAMINE Concurrent use may result in clomipramine toxicity (dry mouth, urinary retention, sedation).	2	3	3

INTERACTION	ONSET	SEVERITY	EVIDENCE
GREPAFLOXACIN Concurrent use may result in an increased risk of cardiotoxicity (QT prolongation, torsade de pointes, cardiac arrest).	2	1	3
GUANADREL Concurrent use may result in decreased antihypertensive effectiveness.	2	3	3
HALOFANTRINE Concurrent use may result in an increased risk of cardiotoxicity (QT prolongation, torsade de pointes, cardiac arrest).	2	2	3
ISOCARBOXAZID Concurrent use may result in neurotoxicity, seizures, or serotonin syndrome (hypertension, hyperthermia, myoclonus, mental status changes).	2	1	3
METHOXAMINE Concurrent use may result in hypertension, cardiac arrhythmias, and tachycardia.	1	2	2
MIDODRINE Concurrent use may result in hypertension, cardiac arrhythmias, and tachycardia.	1	2	2
MOCLOBEMIDE Concurrent use may result in neurotoxicity, seizures, or serotonin syndrome (hypertension, hyperthermia, myoclonus, mental status changes).	1	2	3
NOREPINEPHRINE Concurrent use may result in hypertension, cardiac arrhythmias, and tachycardia.	1	2	2
OLANZAPINE Concurrent use may result in an increased risk of seizures.	2	2	2
OXILOFRINE Concurrent use may result in hypertension, cardiac arrhythmias, and tachycardia.	1	2	2
PHENELZINE Concurrent use may result in neurotoxicity, seizures, or serotonin syndrome (hypertension, hyperthermia, myoclonus, mental status changes).	2	2	3
PHENINDIONE Concurrent use may result in increased risk of bleeding.	2	3	3
PHENPROCOUMON Concurrent use may result in increased risk of bleeding.	2	3	3
PHENYLEPHRINE Concurrent use may result in hypertension, cardiac arrhythmias, and tachycardia.	1	2	2
PROCARBAZINE Concurrent use may result in neurotoxicity, seizures.	2	2	3

Onset: 0=Unspecified 1=Rapid 2=Delayed
Severity: 1=Contraindicated 2=Major 3=Moderate 4=Minor
Evidence: 1=Excellent 2=Good 3=Fair 4=Poor

INTERACTION	ONSET	SEVERITY	EVIDENCE
SELEGILINE Concurrent use may result in neurotoxicity, seizures, or serotonin syndrome (hypertension, hyperthermia, myoclonus, mental status changes).	2	2	3
TRAMADOL Concurrent use may result in an increased risk of seizures.	1	2	3
TRANYLCYPROMINE Concurrent use may result in neurotoxicity, seizures, or serotonin syndrome (hypertension, hyperthermia, myoclonus, mental status changes).	2	2	3
WARFARIN Concurrent use may result in an increased risk of bleeding.	2	3	3

Clonazepam (Klonopin)

INTERACTION	ONSET	SEVERITY	EVIDENCE
CARBAMAZEPINE Concurrent use may result in reduced plasma levels of clonazepam.	2	3	3
CIMETIDINE Concurrent use may result in clonazepam toxicity (central nervous system depression).	1	4	3
THEOPHYLLINE Concurrent use may result in decreased clonazepam effectiveness.	1	3	2

Clorazepate (Tranxene, Tranxene T-Tab, Tranxene-SD, Tranxene-SD Half Strength)

INTERACTION	ONSET	SEVERITY	EVIDENCE
CIMETIDINE Concurrent use may result in clorazepate toxicity (central nervous system depression).	1	4	3
ETHANOL Concurrent use may result in increased sedation.	1	3	2
THEOPHYLLINE Concurrent use may result in decreased clorazepate effectiveness.	1	3	2

Clozapine (Clozaril, FazaClo ODT)

INTERACTION	ONSET	SEVERITY	EVIDENCE
CARBAMAZEPINE Concurrent use may result in an increased risk of bone marrow suppression, asterixis, or decreased serum clozapine levels.	2	2	3
DROPERIDOL Concurrent use may result in an increased risk of cardiotoxicity (QT prolongation, torsade de pointes, cardiac arrest).	1	1	3

INTERACTION	ONSET	SEVERITY	EVIDENCE
ERYTHROMYCIN Concurrent use may result in increased clozapine serum concentrations and risk of side effects (sedation, incoordination, slurred speech, seizures, hematologic abnormalities).	2	3	3
FLUOXETINE Concurrent use may result in an increased risk of clozapine toxicity (sedation, seizures, hypotension).	2	3	3
FOSPHENYTOIN Concurrent use may result in decreased clozapine plasma levels associated with marked worsening of psychosis.	2	3	3
GUARANA Concomitant administration may lead to increased clozapine levels, (leukopenia, agranulocytosis, seizures) or increased guarana levels, (headache, insomnia, restlessness, diuresis, tachycardia).	2	3	3
LITHIUM Concurrent use may result in weakness, dyskinesias, increased extrapyramidal symptoms, encephalopathy, and brain damage.	2	2	1
LORAZEPAM Concurrent use may result in central nervous system depression.	1	4	3
PHENOBARBITAL Concurrent use may result in decreased clozapine plasma levels associated with marked worsening of psychosis.	2	3	3
PHENYTOIN Concurrent administration may result in decreased clozapine plasma levels associated with marked worsening of psychosis.	2	3	3
SERTRALINE Concurrent use may result in an increased risk of clozapine toxicity (sedation, seizures, hypotension).	2	3	3
TRAMADOL Concurrent use may result in an increased risk of seizures.	1	2	3

Desipramine (Norpramin)

INTERACTION	ONSET	SEVERITY	EVIDENCE
ACENOCOUMAROL Concurrent use may result in increased risk of bleeding.	2	3	3
AMPRENAVIR Concurrent use may result in increased desipramine serum concentrations and potential toxicity (anticholinergic effects, sedation, confusion, cardiac arrhythmias).	2	2	3
ANISINDIONE Concurrent use of may result in increased risk of bleeding.	2	3	3

Onset: 0=Unspecified 1=Rapid 2=Delayed
Severity: 1=Contraindicated 2=Major 3=Moderate 4=Minor
Evidence: 1=Excellent 2=Good 3=Fair 4=Poor

INTERACTION	ONSET	SEVERITY	EVIDENCE
BEPRIDIL Concurrent use may result in an increased risk of cardiotoxicity (QT prolongation, torsade de pointes, cardiac arrest).	1	1	3
BETHANIDINE Concurrent use may result in decreased antihypertensive effectiveness.	1	3	2
CIMETIDINE Concurrent use may result in desipramine toxicity (dry mouth, blurred vision, urinary retention).	2	3	2
CISAPRIDE Concurrent use may result in cardiotoxicity (QT prolongation, torsade de pointes, cardiac arrest).	1	1	3
CLONIDINE Concurrent use may result in decreased antihypertensive effectiveness.	2	2	2
CLORGYLINE Concurrent use may result in neurotoxicity, seizures, or serotonin syndrome (hypertension, hyperthermia, myoclonus, mental status changes).	2	2	3
DICUMAROL Concurrent use may result in increased risk of bleeding.	2	3	3
DROPERIDOL Concurrent use may result in an increased risk of cardiotoxicity (QT prolongation, torsade de pointes, cardiac arrest).	0	2	3
EPINEPHRINE Concurrent use may result in hypertension, cardiac arrhythmias, and tachycardia.	1	2	2
ETILEFRINE Concurrent use may result in hypertension, cardiac arrhythmias, and tachycardia.	1	2	2
FLUOXETINE Concurrent use may result in desipramine toxicity (dry mouth, urinary retention, sedation) and an increased risk of cardiotoxicity (QT prolongation, torsade de pointes, cardiac arrest).	0	2	3
GREPAFLOXACIN Concurrent use may result in an increased risk of cardiotoxicity (QT prolongation, torsade de pointes, cardiac arrest).	2	1	3
GUANADREL Concurrent use may result in decreased antihypertensive effectiveness.	2	3	3
GUANETHIDINE Concurrent use may result in decreased antihypertensive effectiveness.	2	3	1

INTERACTION	ONSET	SEVERITY	EVIDENCE
HALOFANTRINE Concurrent use may result in an increased risk of cardiotoxicity (QT prolongation, torsade de pointes, cardiac arrest).	2	2	3
ISOCARBOXAZID Concurrent use may result in neurotoxicity, seizures, or serotonin syndrome.	2	1	3
LEVOMETHADYL Concurrent use may result in an increased risk of cardiotoxicity (QT prolongation, torsade de pointes, cardiac arrest).	2	1	3
METHOXAMINE Concurrent use may result in hypertension, cardiac arrhythmias, and tachycardia.	1	2	2
MIDODRINE Concurrent use may result in hypertension, cardiac arrhythmias, and tachycardia.	1	2	2
MOCLOBEMIDE Concurrent use may result in neurotoxicity, seizures, or serotonin syndrome (hypertension, hyperthermia, myoclonus, mental status changes).	2	2	3
NOREPINEPHRINE Concurrent use may result in hypertension, cardiac arrhythmias, and tachycardia.	1	2	2
OXILOFRINE Concurrent use may result in hypertension, cardiac arrhythmias, and tachycardia.	1	2	2
PHENELZINE Concurrent use may result in neurotoxicity, seizures, or serotonin syndrome (hypertension, hyperthermia, myoclonus, mental status changes).	2	2	3
PHENINDIONE Concurrent use may result in increased risk of bleeding.	2	3	3
PHENPROCOUMON Concurrent use may result in increased risk of bleeding.	2	3	3
PHENYLEPHRINE Concurrent use may result in hypertension, cardiac arrhythmias, and tachycardia.	1	2	2
PIMOZIDE Concurrent use may result in an increased risk of cardiotoxicity (QT prolongation, torsade de pointes, cardiac arrest).	0	1	3
PROCARBAZINE Concurrent use may result in neurotoxicity, seizures.	2	2	3

Onset: 0=Unspecified 1=Rapid 2=Delayed
Severity: 1=Contraindicated 2=Major 3=Moderate 4=Minor
Evidence: 1=Excellent 2=Good 3=Fair 4=Poor

INTERACTION	ONSET	SEVERITY	EVIDENCE
QUINIDINE Concurrent use may result in an increased risk of cardiotoxicity (QT prolongation, torsade de pointes, cardiac arrest).	0	2	3
RITONAVIR Concurrent use may result in increased desipramine plasma concentrations and potential desipramine toxicity (dry mouth, urinary retention, sedation, blurred vision).	2	3	3
SELEGILINE Concurrent use may result in neurotoxicity, seizures, or serotonin syndrome (hypertension, hyperthermia, myoclonus, mental status changes).	2	2	3
SPARFLOXACIN Concurrent use may result in prolongation of the QTc interval and/or torsade de pointes.	2	1	3
TRAMADOL Concurrent use may result in an increased risk of seizures.	1	2	3
TRANYLCYPROMINE Concurrent use may result in neurotoxicity, seizures, or serotonin syndrome (hypertension, hyperthermia, myoclonus, mental status changes).	2	2	3
WARFARIN Concurrent use may result in an increased risk of bleeding.	2	3	3

Dexmethylphenidate (Focalin, Focalin XR)

INTERACTION	ONSET	SEVERITY	EVIDENCE
CLORGYLINE Concurrent use may result in hypertensive crisis (headache, palpitation, neck stiffness).	1	1	3
COUMARIN Concurrent use may result in an increased risk of bleeding.	1	3	3
IPRONIAZID Concurrent use may result in hypertensive crisis (headache, palpitation, neck stiffness).	1	1	3
ISOCARBOXAZID Concurrent use may result in hypertensive crisis (headache, palpitation, neck stiffness).	1	1	3
LAZABEMIDE Concurrent use may result in hypertensive crisis (headache, palpitation, neck stiffness).	1	1	3
MOCLOBEMIDE Concurrent use may result in hypertensive crisis (headache, palpitation, neck stiffness).	1	1	3
NIALAMIDE Concurrent use may result in hypertensive crisis (headache, palpitation, neck stiffness).	1	1	3

INTERACTION	ONSET	SEVERITY	EVIDENCE
PARGYLINE Concurrent use may result in hypertensive crisis (headache, palpitation, neck stiffness).	1	1	3
PHENELZINE Concurrent use may result in hypertensive crisis (headache, palpitation, neck stiffness).	1	1	3
PHENOBARBITAL Concurrent use may result in an increase in phenobarbital plasma concentrations.	1	3	3
PHENYTOIN Concurrent use may result in an increase in phenytoin plasma concentrations.	1	3	3
PRIMIDONE Concurrent use may result in an increase in primidone plasma concentrations.	1	3	3
PROCARBAZINE Concurrent use may result in hypertensive crisis (headache, palpitation, neck stiffness).	1	1	3
SELEGILINE Concurrent use may result in hypertensive crisis (headache, palpitation, neck stiffness).	1	1	3
TOLOXATONE Concurrent use may result in hypertensive crisis (headache, palpitation, neck stiffness).	1	1	3
TRANYLCYPROMINE Concurrent use may result in hypertensive crisis (headache, palpitation, neck stiffness).	1	1	3

Dextroamphetamine (Dexedrine, Dexedrine Spansules, DextroStat)

INTERACTION	ONSET	SEVERITY	EVIDENCE
ACETAZOLAMIDE Concurrent use may result in amphetamine toxicity (hypertension, hyperpyrexia, seizures).	1	3	2
ACIDIC FOODS Concurrent use may result in altered serum concentrations.	1	4	2
CLORGYLINE Concurrent use may result in a hypertensive crisis (headache, hyperpyrexia, hypertension).	1	1	3
FURAZOLIDONE Concurrent use may result in a hypertensive crisis (headache, hyperpyrexia, hypertension).	1	1	3
IPRONIAZID Concurrent use may result in a hypertensive crisis (headache, hyperpyrexia, hypertension).	1	1	3

Onset: 0=Unspecified 1=Rapid 2=Delayed
Severity: 1=Contraindicated 2=Major 3=Moderate 4=Minor
Evidence: 1=Excellent 2=Good 3=Fair 4=Poor

INTERACTION	ONSET	SEVERITY	EVIDENCE
ISOCARBOXAZID Concurrent use may result in a hypertensive crisis (headache, hyperpyrexia, hypertension).	1	1	3
MOCLOBEMIDE Concurrent use may result in a hypertensive crisis (headache, hyperpyrexia, hypertension).	1	1	3
NIALAMIDE Concurrent use may result in a hypertensive crisis (headache, hyperpyrexia, hypertension).	1	1	3
PARGYLINE Concurrent use may result in a hypertensive crisis (headache, hyperpyrexia, hypertension).	1	1	1
PHENELZINE Concurrent use may result in a hypertensive crisis (headache, hyperpyrexia, hypertension).	1	1	3
PROCARBAZINE Concurrent use may result in a hypertensive crisis (headache, hyperpyrexia, hypertension).	1	1	3
SELEGILINE Concurrent use may result in a hypertensive crisis (headache, hyperpyrexia, hypertension).	1	1	3
SIBUTRAMINE Concurrent use may result in an increased risk of hypertension and tachycardia.	1	1	3
SODIUM BICARBONATE Concurrent use may result in amphetamine toxicity (hypertension, hyperpyrexia, seizures).	2	3	3
TOLOXATONE Concurrent use may result in a hypertensive crisis (headache, hyperpyrexia, hypertension).	1	1	3
TRANYLCYPROMINE Concurrent use may result in a hypertensive crisis (headache, hyperpyrexia, hypertension).	1	1	3

Diazepam (Valium)

INTERACTION	ONSET	SEVERITY	EVIDENCE
CIMETIDINE Concurrent use may result in diazepam toxicity (central nervous system depression).	1	4	2
CLARITHROMYCIN Concurrent use may result in increased diazepam toxicity (central nervous system depression, ataxia, lethargy).	2	3	3
DISULFIRAM Concurrent use may result in an increased risk of central nervous system depression.	2	3	3

INTERACTION	ONSET	SEVERITY	EVIDENCE
ERYTHROMYCIN Concurrent use may result in increased diazepam toxicity (central nervous system depression, ataxia, lethargy).	2	3	3
ETHANOL Concurrent use may result in increased sedation.	1	3	1
FLUOXETINE Concurrent use may result in higher serum concentrations of diazepam.	2	4	3
FLUVOXAMINE Concurrent use may result in diazepam and N-desmethyldiazepam accumulation.	2	3	2
ITRACONAZOLE Concurrent use may result in increased diazepam serum concentrations and potential diazepam toxicity (sedation, slurred speech, central nervous system depression).	2	1	3
JOSAMYCIN Concurrent use may result in increased diazepam toxicity (central nervous system depression, ataxia, lethargy).	2	3	3
RIFAMPIN Concurrent use may result in decreased diazepam effectiveness.	2	3	3
ROXITHROMYCIN Concurrent use may result in increased diazepam toxicity (central nervous system depression, ataxia, lethargy).	2	3	3
THEOPHYLLINE Concurrent use may result in decreased diazepam effectiveness.	1	3	2
TROLEANDOMYCIN Concurrent use may result in increased diazepam toxicity (central nervous system depression, ataxia, lethargy).	2	3	3

Disulfiram (Antabuse)

INTERACTION	ONSET	SEVERITY	EVIDENCE
AMPRENAVIR Concurrent use may result in an increased risk of propylene glycol toxicity (seizures, tachycardia, lactic acidosis, renal toxicity, hemolysis).	2	1	2
ETHANOL Concurrent use may result in ethanol intolerance.	1	1	2
METRONIDAZOLE Concurrent use may result in CNS toxicity (psychotic symptoms, confusion).	1	1	2

Onset: 0=Unspecified 1=Rapid 2=Delayed
Severity: 1=Contraindicated 2=Major 3=Moderate 4=Minor
Evidence: 1=Excellent 2=Good 3=Fair 4=Poor

Donepezil (Aricept, Aricept ODT)

INTERACTION	ONSET	SEVERITY	EVIDENCE
SUCCINYLCHOLINE Concurrent use may result in prolonged neuromuscular blockade.	1	2	3

Doxepin (Sinequan)

INTERACTION	ONSET	SEVERITY	EVIDENCE
ACENOCOUMAROL Concurrent use may result in increased risk of bleeding.	2	3	3
AMPRENAVIR Concurrent use may result in increased doxepin serum concentrations and potential toxicity (anticholinergic effects, sedation, confusion, cardiac arrhythmias).	2	2	3
ANISINDIONE Concurrent use may result in increased risk of bleeding.	2	3	3
BEPRIDIL Concurrent use may result in an increased risk of cardiotoxicity (QT prolongation, torsade de pointes, cardiac arrest).	1	1	3
BETHANIDINE Concurrent use may result in decreased antihypertensive effectiveness.	1	3	2
CIMETIDINE Concurrent use may result in doxepin toxicity (dry mouth, blurred vision, urinary retention).	2	3	2
CISAPRIDE Concurrent use may result in cardiotoxicity (QT prolongation, torsade de pointes, cardiac arrest).	1	1	3
CLONIDINE Concurrent use may result in decreased antihypertensive effectiveness.	2	2	3
CLORGYLINE Concurrent use may result in neurotoxicity, seizures, or serotonin syndrome (hypertension, hyperthermia, myoclonus, mental status changes).	2	2	3
DICUMAROL Concurrent use may result in increased risk of bleeding.	2	3	3
DROPERIDOL Concurrent use may result in an increased risk of cardiotoxicity (QT prolongation, torsade de pointes, cardiac arrest).	0	2	3
EPINEPHRINE Concurrent use may result in hypertension, cardiac arrhythmias, and tachycardia.	1	2	2

INTERACTION	ONSET	SEVERITY	EVIDENCE
ETILEFRINE Concurrent use may result in hypertension, cardiac arrhythmias, and tachycardia.	1	2	2
FLUOXETINE Concurrent use may result in doxepin toxicity (dry mouth, urinary retention, sedation) and an increased risk of cardiotoxicity (QT prolongation, torsade de pointes, cardiac arrest).	0	2	3
GREPAFLOXACIN Concurrent use may result in an increased risk of cardiotoxicity (QT prolongation, torsade de pointes, cardiac arrest).	2	1	3
GUANADREL Concurrent use may result in decreased antihypertensive effectiveness.	2	3	3
GUANETHIDINE Concurrent use may result in decreased antihypertensive effectiveness.	2	3	3
HALOFANTRINE Concurrent use may result in an increased risk of cardiotoxicity (QT prolongation, torsade de pointes, cardiac arrest).	2	2	3
ISOCARBOXAZID Concurrent use may result in neurotoxicity, seizures, or serotonin syndrome (hypertension, hyperthermia, myoclonus, mental status changes).	2	1	3
METHOXAMINE Concurrent use may result in hypertension, cardiac arrhythmias, and tachycardia.	1	2	2
MIDODRINE Concurrent use may result in hypertension, cardiac arrhythmias, and tachycardia.	1	2	2
MOCLOBEMIDE Concurrent use may result in neurotoxicity, seizures, or serotonin syndrome (hypertension, hyperthermia, myoclonus, mental status changes).	2	2	3
NOREPINEPHRINE Concurrent use may result in hypertension, cardiac arrhythmias, and tachycardia.	1	2	2
OXILOFRINE Concurrent use may result in hypertension, cardiac arrhythmias, and tachycardia.	1	2	2
PHENELZINE Concurrent use may result in neurotoxicity, seizures, or serotonin syndrome (hypertension, hyperthermia, myoclonus, mental status changes).	2	2	3

Onset: 0=Unspecified 1=Rapid 2=Delayed
Severity: 1=Contraindicated 2=Major 3=Moderate 4=Minor
Evidence: 1=Excellent 2=Good 3=Fair 4=Poor

INTERACTION	ONSET	SEVERITY	EVIDENCE
PHENINDIONE Concurrent use may result in increased risk of bleeding.	2	3	3
PHENPROCOUMON Concurrent use may result in increased risk of bleeding.	2	3	3
PHENYLEPHRINE Concurrent use may result in hypertension, cardiac arrhythmias, and tachycardia.	1	2	2
PIMOZIDE Concurrent use may result in an increased risk of cardiotoxicity (QT prolongation, torsade de pointes, cardiac arrest).	0	1	3
PROCARBAZINE Concurrent use may result in neurotoxicity, seizures.	2	2	3
SELEGILINE Concurrent use may result in neurotoxicity, seizures, or serotonin syndrome (hypertension, hyperthermia, myoclonus, mental status changes).	2	2	3
TRAMADOL Concurrent use may result in an increased risk of seizures.	1	2	3
TRANYLCYPROMINE Concurrent use may result in neurotoxicity, seizures, or serotonin syndrome (hypertension, hyperthermia, myoclonus, mental status changes).	2	2	3
WARFARIN Concurrent use may result in an increased risk of bleeding.	2	3	3

Duloxetine (Cymbalta)

INTERACTION	ONSET	SEVERITY	EVIDENCE
CLORGYLINE Concurrent use may result in central nervous system toxicity or serotonin syndrome (hypertension, hyperthermia, myoclonus, mental status changes).	1	1	2
ISOCARBOXAZID Concurrent use may result in central nervous system toxicity or serotonin syndrome (hypertension, hyperthermia, myoclonus, mental status changes).	1	1	2
LAZABEMIDE Concurrent use may result in central nervous system toxicity or serotonin syndrome (hypertension, hyperthermia, myoclonus, mental status changes).	1	1	2
MOCLOBEMIDE Concurrent use may result in central nervous system toxicity or serotonin syndrome (hypertension, hyperthermia, myoclonus, mental status changes).	1	1	2
PHENELZINE Concurrent use may result in central nervous system toxicity or serotonin syndrome (hypertension, hyperthermia, myoclonus, mental status changes).	1	1	2

INTERACTION	ONSET	SEVERITY	EVIDENCE
SELEGILINE Concurrent use may result in central nervous system toxicity or serotonin syndrome (hypertension, hyperthermia, myoclonus, mental status changes).	1	1	2
RASAGILINE Concurrent use may result in central nervous system toxicity or serotonin syndrome (hypertension, hyperthermia, myoclonus, mental status changes).	1	1	2
THIORIDAZINE Concurrent use may result in increased thioridazine serum concentrations and risk of cardiac arrhythmia.	0	1	2
TRANYLCYPROMINE Concurrent use may result in central nervous system toxicity or serotonin syndrome (hypertension, hyperthermia, myoclonus, mental status changes).	1	1	2

Escitalopram (Lexapro)

INTERACTION	ONSET	SEVERITY	EVIDENCE
ALMOTRIPTAN Concurrent use may result in weakness, hyperreflexia, and/or incoordination.	0	3	3
CLORGYLINE Concurrent use may result in central nervous system toxicity or serotonin syndrome (hypertension, hyperthermia, myoclonus, mental status changes).	1	1	3
ENTACAPONE Concurrent use may result in decreased catecholamine metabolism.	1	2	3
ETHANOL Concurrent use may result in the potentiation of the cognitive and motor effects of alcohol.	0	3	3
FURAZOLIDONE Concurrent use may result in weakness, hyperreflexia, and incoordination.	2	1	3
HYDROXYTRYPTOPHAN Concurrent use may result in an increased risk of serotonin syndrome (hypertension, hyperthermia, myoclonus, mental status changes).	1	3	3
ISOCARBOXAZID Concurrent use may result in central nervous system toxicity or serotonin syndrome (hypertension, hyperthermia, myoclonus, mental status changes).	1	1	3
LAZABEMIDE Concurrent use may result in central nervous system toxicity or serotonin syndrome (hypertension, hyperthermia, myoclonus, mental status changes).	1	1	3

Onset: 0=Unspecified 1=Rapid 2=Delayed
Severity: 1=Contraindicated 2=Major 3=Moderate 4=Minor
Evidence: 1=Excellent 2=Good 3=Fair 4=Poor

INTERACTION	ONSET	SEVERITY	EVIDENCE
LINEZOLID Concurrent use may result in central nervous system toxicity or serotonin syndrome (hypertension, hyperthermia, myoclonus, mental status changes).	1	2	3
LITHIUM Concurrent use may result in possible lithium toxicity (weakness, tremor, excessive thirst, confusion, dizziness).	2	3	3
MOCLOBEMIDE Concurrent use may result in central nervous system toxicity or serotonin syndrome (hypertension, hyperthermia, myoclonus, mental status changes).	1	1	3
PHENELZINE Concurrent use may result in central nervous system toxicity or serotonin syndrome (hypertension, hyperthermia, myoclonus, mental status changes).	1	1	3
SELEGILINE Concurrent use may result in central nervous system toxicity or serotonin syndrome (hypertension, hyperthermia, myoclonus, mental status changes).	1	1	3
SIBUTRAMINE Concurrent use may result in an increased risk of serotonin syndrome (hypertension, hypothermia, myoclonus, mental status changes).	1	2	3
ST. JOHN'S WORT Concurrent use may result in an increased risk of serotonin syndrome (hypertension, hyperthermia, myoclonus, mental status changes).	1	2	3
SUMATRIPTAN Concurrent use may result in an increased risk of weakness, hyperreflexia, incoordination.	0	3	3
TOLCAPONE Concurrent use may result in decreased catecholamine metabolism.	1	2	3
TRAMADOL Concurrent use may result in an increased risk of seizures and serotonin syndrome (hypertension, hyperthermia, myoclonus, mental status changes).	1	2	3
TRANYLCYPROMINE Concurrent use may result in central nervous system toxicity or serotonin syndrome (hypertension, hyperthermia, myoclonus, mental status changes).	1	1	3
ZOLMITRIPTAN Concurrent use may result in weakness, hyperreflexia, and incoordination.	1	3	3

Estazolam (ProSom)

INTERACTION	ONSET	SEVERITY	EVIDENCE
CIMETIDINE Concurrent use may result in estazolam toxicity (central nervous system depression).	1	4	3
THEOPHYLLINE Concurrent use may result in decreased estazolam effectiveness.	1	3	2

Eszopiclone (Lunesta)

INTERACTION	ONSET	SEVERITY	EVIDENCE
CLARITHROMYCIN Concurrent use may result in increased plasma concentrations of eszopiclone.	0	3	3
ETHANOL Concurrent use may result in impaired psychomotor functions and risk of increased sedation.	1	3	2
HIGH FAT FOOD Concurrent use may result in decreased effect of eszopiclone on sleep onset.	1	4	2
ITRACONAZOLE Concurrent use may result in increased plasma concentrations of eszopiclone.	0	3	3
KETOCONAZOLE Concurrent use may result in increased plasma concentrations of eszopiclone.	0	3	2
NEFAZODONE Concurrent use may result in increased plasma concentrations of eszopiclone.	0	3	3
NELFINAVIR Concurrent use may result in increased plasma concentrations of eszopiclone.	0	3	3
OLANZAPINE Concurrent use may result in decreased psychomotor function.	0	4	3
RIFAMPIN Concurrent use may result in decreased plasma concentrations and decreased efficacy of eszopiclone.	0	3	3
RITONAVIR Concurrent use may result in increased plasma concentrations of eszopiclone.	0	3	3
TROLEANDOMYCIN Concurrent use may result in increased plasma concentrations of eszopiclone.	0	3	3

Onset: 0=Unspecified 1=Rapid 2=Delayed
Severity: 1=Contraindicated 2=Major 3=Moderate 4=Minor
Evidence: 1=Excellent 2=Good 3=Fair 4=Poor

Fluoxetine (Prozac, Prozac Weekly, Sarafem, Symbyax)

INTERACTION	ONSET	SEVERITY	EVIDENCE
ALMOTRIPTAN Concurrent use may result in weakness, hyperreflexia, and/or incoordination.	0	3	3
ALPRAZOLAM Concurrent use may result in an increased risk of alprazolam toxicity (somnolence, dizziness, ataxia, slurred speech, hypotension, psychomotor impairment).	1	3	2
AMITRIPTYLINE Concurrent use may result in amitriptyline toxicity (dry mouth, urinary retention, sedation) and an increased risk of cardiotoxicity (QT prolongation, torsade de pointes, cardiac arrest).	0	2	3
AMOXAPINE Concurrent use may result in amoxapine toxicity (dry mouth, urinary retention, sedation) and an increased risk of cardiotoxicity (QT prolongation, torsade de pointes, cardiac arrest).	0	2	3
ASTEMIZOLE Concurrent use may result in cardiotoxicity (QT interval prolongation, torsade de pointes, cardiac arrest).	1	2	3
CLORGYLINE Concurrent use may result in central nervous system toxicity or serotonin syndrome (hypertension, hyperthermia, myoclonus, mental status changes).	1	1	2
CLOZAPINE Concurrent use may result in an increased risk of clozapine toxicity (sedation, seizures, hypotension).	2	3	3
DESIPRAMINE Concurrent use may result in desipramine toxicity (dry mouth, urinary retention, sedation) and an increased risk of cardiotoxicity (QT prolongation, torsade de pointes, cardiac arrest).	0	2	3
DEXFENFLURAMINE Concurrent use may result in serotonin syndrome (hypertension, hyperthermia, myoclonus, mental status changes).	1	2	3
DEXTROMETHORPHAN Concurrent use may result in possible dextromethorphan toxicity (nausea, vomiting, blurred vision, hallucinations) or serotonin syndrome (hypertension, hyperthermia, myoclonus, mental status changes).	1	2	3
DIAZEPAM Concurrent use may result in higher serum concentrations of diazepam.	2	4	3
DIHYDROERGOTAMINE Concurrent use may result in an increased risk of ergotism (nausea, vomiting, vasospastic ischemia).	0	1	2

INTERACTION	ONSET	SEVERITY	EVIDENCE
DOXEPIN Concurrent use may result in doxepin toxicity (dry mouth, urinary retention, sedation) and an increased risk of cardiotoxicity (QT prolongation, torsade de pointes, cardiac arrest).	0	2	3
DROPERIDOL Concurrent use may result in an increased risk of cardiotoxicity (QT prolongation, torsade de pointes, cardiac arrest).	0	2	3
ERGOLOID MESYLATES Concurrent use may result in an increased risk of ergotism (nausea, vomiting, vasospastic ischemia).	0	1	2
ERGONOVINE Concurrent use may result in an increased risk of ergotism (nausea, vomiting, vasospastic ischemia).	0	1	2
ERGOTAMINE Concurrent use may result in an increased risk of ergotism (nausea, vomiting, vasospastic ischemia).	0	1	2
FENFLURAMINE Concurrent use may result in serotonin syndrome (hypertension, hyperthermia, myoclonus, mental status changes).	1	2	3
FOSPHENYTOIN Concurrent use may result in an increased risk of phenytoin toxicity (ataxia, hyperreflexia, nystagmus, tremor).	2	3	3
FURAZOLIDONE Concurrent use may result in weakness, hyperreflexia, and incoordination.	2	1	3
HYDROXYTRYPTOPHAN Concurrent use may result in an increased risk of serotonin syndrome (hypertension, hyperthermia, myoclonus, mental status changes).	1	3	3
IMIPRAMINE Concurrent use may result in imipramine toxicity (dry mouth, urinary retention, sedation) and an increased risk of cardiotoxicity (QT prolongation, torsade de pointes, cardiac arrest).	0	2	3
IPRONIAZID Concurrent use may result in central nervous system toxicity or serotonin syndrome (hypertension, hyperthermia, myoclonus, mental status changes).	1	1	2
ISOCARBOXAZID Concurrent use may result in central nervous system toxicity or serotonin syndrome (hypertension, hyperthermia, myoclonus, mental status changes).	1	1	2

Onset: 0=Unspecified 1=Rapid 2=Delayed
Severity: 1=Contraindicated 2=Major 3=Moderate 4=Minor
Evidence: 1=Excellent 2=Good 3=Fair 4=Poor

INTERACTION	ONSET	SEVERITY	EVIDENCE
LEVOMETHADYL Concurrent use may result in an increased risk of cardiotoxicity (QT prolongation, torsade de pointes, cardiac arrest).	2	1	3
METHYSERGIDE Concurrent use may result in an increased risk of ergotism (nausea, vomiting, vasospastic ischemia).	0	1	2
METHYLERGONOVINE Concurrent use may result in an increased risk of ergotism (nausea, vomiting, vasospastic ischemia).	0	1	2
MOCLOBEMIDE Concurrent use may result in central nervous system toxicity or serotonin syndrome (hypertension, hyperthermia, myoclonus, mental status changes).	1	1	3
NIALAMIDE Concurrent use may result in central nervous system toxicity or serotonin syndrome (hypertension, hyperthermia, myoclonus, mental status changes).	1	1	2
NORTRIPTYLINE Concurrent use may result in nortriptyline toxicity (dry mouth, urinary retention, sedation) and an increased risk of cardiotoxicity (QT prolongation, torsade de pointes, cardiac arrest).	0	2	3
PARGYLINE Concurrent use may result in central nervous system toxicity or serotonin syndrome (hypertension, hyperthermia, myoclonus, mental status changes).	1	1	2
PHENELZINE Concurrent use may result in central nervous system toxicity or serotonin syndrome (hypertension, hyperthermia, myoclonus, mental status changes).	1	1	2
PHENYTOIN Concurrent use may result in an increased risk of phenytoin toxicity (ataxia, hyperreflexia, nystagmus, tremor).	2	3	3
PIMOZIDE Concurrent use may result in bradycardia, somnolence, and potentially increased risk of cardiotoxicity (QT prolongation, torsades de pointes, cardiac arrest).	0	1	2
PROCARBAZINE Concurrent use may result in central nervous system toxicity or serotonin syndrome (hypertension, hyperthermia, myoclonus, mental status changes).	1	1	2
SELEGILINE Concurrent use may result in central nervous system toxicity or serotonin syndrome (hypertension, hyperthermia, myoclonus, mental status changes).	1	1	2

INTERACTION	ONSET	SEVERITY	EVIDENCE
SIBUTRAMINE Concurrent use may result in an increased risk of serotonin syndrome (hypertension, hypothermia, myoclonus, mental status changes).	1	2	3
TERFENADINE Concurrent use may result in cardiotoxicity (QT prolongation, torsades de pointes, cardiac arrest).	2	1	2
THIORIDAZINE Concurrent use may result in an increased risk of cardiotoxicity (QT prolongation, torsade de pointes, cardiac arrest).	1	1	3
TOLOXATONE Concurrent use may result in central nervous system toxicity or serotonin syndrome (hypertension, hyperthermia, myoclonus, mental status changes).	1	1	2
TRAMADOL Concurrent use may result in an increased risk of seizures and serotonin syndrome (hypertension, hyperthermia, myoclonus, mental status changes).	1	2	2
TRANYLCYPROMINE Concurrent use may result in central nervous system toxicity or serotonin syndrome (hypertension, hyperthermia, myoclonus, mental status changes).	1	1	2
TRAZODONE Concurrent use may result in trazodone toxicity (sedation, dry mouth, urinary retention) or serotonin syndrome (hypertension, hyperthermia, myoclonus, mental status changes).	2	2	3
TRIMIPRAMINE Concurrent use may result in trimipramine toxicity (dry mouth, urinary retention, sedation) and an increased risk of cardiotoxicity (QT prolongation, torsade de pointes, cardiac arrest).	0	2	3
TRYPTOPHAN Concurrent use may result in serotonin syndrome (hypertension, hyperthermia, myoclonus, mental status changes).	2	2	3
WARFARIN Concurrent use may result in an increased risk of bleeding.	2	3	3

Fluphenazine

INTERACTION	ONSET	SEVERITY	EVIDENCE
BELLADONNA Concurrent use may result in increased manic, agitated reactions, or enhanced anticholinergic effects resulting in cardiorespiratory failure, especially in cases of belladonna overdose.	1	3	2

Onset: 0=Unspecified 1=Rapid 2=Delayed
Severity: 1=Contraindicated 2=Major 3=Moderate 4=Minor
Evidence: 1=Excellent 2=Good 3=Fair 4=Poor

INTERACTION	ONSET	SEVERITY	EVIDENCE
BENZTROPINE Concurrent use may result in decreased fluphenazine serum concentrations, decreased fluphenazine effectiveness, enhanced anticholinergic effects (ileus, hyperpyrexia, sedation, dry mouth).	2	3	3
CABERGOLINE Concurrent use may result in the decreased therapeutic effect of both drugs.	1	3	3
CISAPRIDE Concurrent use may result in cardiotoxicity (QT prolongation, torsade de pointes, cardiac arrest).	1	1	3
ETHANOL Concurrent use may result in increased central nervous system depression and an increased risk of extrapyramidal reactions.	1	3	2
FOSPHENYTOIN Concurrent use may result in increased or decreased phenytoin levels and possibly reduced fluphenazine levels.	2	4	3
GREPAFLOXACIN Concurrent use may result in an increased risk of cardiotoxicity (QT prolongation, torsade de pointes, cardiac arrest).	2	1	3
LEVODOPA Concurrent use may result in loss of levodopa efficacy.	1	3	2
LITHIUM Concurrent use may result in weakness, dyskinesias, increased extrapyramidal symptoms, encephalopathy, and brain damage.	2	2	1
MEPERIDINE Concurrent use may result in an increase in central nervous system and respiratory depression.	1	3	2
ORPHENADRINE Concurrent use may result in decreased fluphenazine serum concentrations, decreased fluphenazine effectiveness, enhanced anticholinergic effects (ileus, hyperpyrexia, sedation, dry mouth).	2	3	3
PHENYTOIN Concurrent use may result in increased or decreased phenytoin levels and possibly reduced fluphenazine levels.	2	4	3
PORFIMER Concurrent use may result in excessive intracellular damage in photosensitized tissues.	2	3	3
PROCYCLIDINE Concurrent use may result in decreased fluphenazine serum concentrations, decreased fluphenazine effectiveness, enhanced anticholinergic effects (ileus, hyperpyrexia, sedation, dry mouth).	2	3	3

INTERACTION	ONSET	SEVERITY	EVIDENCE
TRAMADOL Concurrent use may result in an increased risk of seizures.	1	2	3
TRIHEXYPHENIDYL Concurrent use may result in decreased fluphenazine serum concentrations, decreased fluphenazine effectiveness, enhanced anticholinergic effects (ileus, hyperpyrexia, sedation, dry mouth).	2	3	3

Flurazepam (Dalmane)

INTERACTION	ONSET	SEVERITY	EVIDENCE
CIMETIDINE Concurrent use may result in flurazepam toxicity (central nervous system depression).	2	4	3
THEOPHYLLINE Concurrent use may result in decreased flurazepam. effectiveness.	1	3	2

Fluvoxamine

INTERACTION	ONSET	SEVERITY	EVIDENCE
ACECLOFENAC Concurrent use may result in an increased risk of bleeding.	0	3	2
ACEMETACIN Concurrent use may result in an increased risk of bleeding.	0	3	2
ALCLOFENAC Concurrent use may result in an increased risk of bleeding.	0	3	2
ALMOTRIPTAN Concurrent use may result in weakness, hyperreflexia, and/or incoordination.	0	3	3
ALOSETRON Concurrent use may result in increased alosetron exposure and increased side effects.	0	1	1
ALPRAZOLAM Concurrent use may result in elevated plasma alprazolam levels and an increased risk of side effects (central nervous system depression).	2	3	2
AMITRIPTYLINE Concurrent use may result in amitriptyline toxicity (dry mouth, urinary retention, sedation).	2	3	3
ASPIRIN Concurrent use may result in an increased risk of bleeding.	0	3	2
ASTEMIZOLE Concurrent use may result in cardiotoxicity (QT prolongation, torsade de pointes, cardiac arrest).	1	1	3
BENOXAPROFEN Concurrent use may result in an increased risk of bleeding.	0	3	2

Onset: **0**=Unspecified **1**=Rapid **2**=Delayed
Severity: **1**=Contraindicated **2**=Major **3**=Moderate **4**=Minor
Evidence: **1**=Excellent **2**=Good **3**=Fair **4**=Poor

INTERACTION	ONSET	SEVERITY	EVIDENCE
BROMFENAC Concurrent use may result in an increased risk of bleeding.	0	3	2
BUFEXAMAC Concurrent use may result in an increased risk of bleeding.	0	3	2
CARPROFEN Concurrent use may result in an increased risk of bleeding.	0	3	2
CELECOXIB Concurrent use may result in an increased risk of bleeding.	0	3	2
CISAPRIDE Concurrent use may result in cardiotoxicity (QT prolongation, torsade de pointes, cardiac arrest).	1	1	3
CLOMIPRAMINE Concurrent use may result in clomipramine toxicity (dry mouth, urinary retention, sedation).	2	3	3
CLONIXIN Concurrent use may result in an increased risk of bleeding.	0	3	2
CLORGYLINE Concurrent use may result in central nervous system toxicity or serotonin syndrome (hypertension, hyperthermia, myoclonus, mental status changes).	1	2	2
CLOZAPINE Concurrent use may result in increased serum clozapine concentrations.	2	3	3
DEXFENFLURAMINE Concurrent use may result in serotonin syndrome (hypertension, hyperthermia, myoclonus, mental status changes).	1	2	3
DEXKETOPROFEN Concurrent use may result in an increased risk of bleeding.	0	3	2
DIAZEPAM Concurrent use may result in diazepam and N-desmethyldiazepam accumulation.	2	3	2
DICLOFENAC Concurrent use may result in an increased risk of bleeding.	0	3	2
DIFLUNISAL Concurrent use may result in an increased risk of bleeding.	0	3	2
DIHYDROERGOTAMINE Concurrent use may result in an increased risk of ergotism (nausea, vomiting, vasospastic ischemia).	1	1	3
DIPYRONE Concurrent use may result in an increased risk of bleeding.	0	3	2
DROPERIDOL Concurrent use may result in an increased risk of cardiotoxicity (QT prolongation, torsade de pointes, cardiac arrest).	1	2	3

INTERACTION	ONSET	SEVERITY	EVIDENCE
DROXICAM Concurrent use may result in an increased risk of bleeding.	0	3	2
ERGOLOID MESYLATES Concurrent use may result in an increased risk of ergotism (nausea, vomiting, vasospastic ischemia).	1	1	3
ERGONOVINE Concurrent use may result in an increased risk of ergotism (nausea, vomiting, vasospastic ischemia).	1	1	3
ERGOTAMINE Concurrent use may result in an increased risk of ergotism (nausea, vomiting, vasospastic ischemia).	1	1	3
ETODOLAC Concurrent use may result in an increased risk of bleeding.	0	3	2
ETOFENAMATE Concurrent use may result in an increased risk of bleeding.	0	3	2
ETORICOXIB Concurrent use may result in an increased risk of bleeding.	0	3	2
FELBINAC Concurrent use may result in an increased risk of bleeding.	0	3	2
FENBUFEN Concurrent use may result in an increased risk of bleeding.	0	3	2
FENFLURAMINE Concurrent use may result in serotonin syndrome (hypertension, hyperthermia, myoclonus, mental status changes).	1	2	3
FENOPROFEN Concurrent use may result in an increased risk of bleeding.	0	3	2
FENTIAZAC Concurrent use may result in an increased risk of bleeding.	0	3	2
FLOCTAFENINE Concurrent use may result in an increased risk of bleeding.	0	3	2
FLUFENAMIC ACID Concurrent use may result in an increased risk of bleeding.	0	3	2
FLURBIPROFEN Concurrent use may result in an increased risk of bleeding.	0	3	2
FOSPHENYTOIN Concurrent use may result in an increased risk of phenytoin toxicity (ataxia, hyperreflexia, nystagmus, tremors).	2	3	3
FURAZOLIDONE Concurrent use may result in weakness, hyperreflexia, and incoordination.	2	1	3

Onset: 0=Unspecified 1=Rapid 2=Delayed
Severity: 1=Contraindicated 2=Major 3=Moderate 4=Minor
Evidence: 1=Excellent 2=Good 3=Fair 4=Poor

INTERACTION	ONSET	SEVERITY	EVIDENCE
GRAPEFRUIT JUICE Concurrent use may result in increased fluvoxamine exposure.	1	4	2
GUARANA Concomitant administration may result in symptoms of excessive caffeine (insomnia, headache, restlessness, nervousness, palpitations, and arrhythmias).	1	3	3
HYDROXYTRYPTOPHAN Concurrent use may result in an increased risk of serotonin syndrome (hypertension, hyperthermia, myoclonus, mental status changes).	1	3	3
IBUPROFEN Concurrent use may result in an increased risk of bleeding.	0	3	2
IMIPRAMINE Concurrent use may result in imipramine toxicity (dry mouth, urinary retention, sedation).	2	3	3
INDOMETHACIN Concurrent use may result in an increased risk of bleeding.	0	3	2
INDOPROFEN Concurrent use may result in an increased risk of bleeding.	0	3	2
IPRONIAZID Concurrent use may result in central nervous system toxicity or serotonin syndrome (hypertension, hyperthermia, myoclonus, mental status changes).	1	2	2
ISOCARBOXAZID Concurrent use may result in central nervous system toxicity or serotonin syndrome (hypertension, hyperthermia, myoclonus, mental status changes).	1	1	2
ISOXICAM Concurrent use may result in an increased risk of bleeding.	0	3	2
KETOPROFEN Concurrent use may result in an increased risk of bleeding.	0	3	2
KETOROLAC Concurrent use may result in an increased risk of bleeding.	0	3	2
LEVOMETHADYL Concurrent use may result in an increased risk of cardiotoxicity (QT prolongation, torsade de pointes, cardiac arrest).	2	1	3
LINEZOLID Concurrent use may result in central nervous system toxicity or serotonin syndrome (hypertension, hyperthermia, myoclonus, mental status changes).	1	1	2
LITHIUM Concurrent use may result in possible lithium toxicity (weakness, tremor, excessive thirst, confusion, dizziness).	2	3	3
LORNOXICAM Concurrent use may result in an increased risk of bleeding.	0	3	2

INTERACTION	ONSET	SEVERITY	EVIDENCE
MECLOFENAMATE Concurrent use may result in an increased risk of bleeding.	0	3	2
MEFENAMIC ACID Concurrent use may result in an increased risk of bleeding.	0	3	2
MELATONIN Concurrent use may result in increased central nervous system depression.	1	4	3
MELOXICAM Concurrent use may result in an increased risk of bleeding.	0	3	2
METHADONE Concurrent use may result in increased plasma methadone levels.	2	3	3
METHYLERGONOVINE Concurrent use may result in an increased risk of ergotism (nausea, vomiting, vasospastic ischemia).	1	1	3
MIDAZOLAM Concurrent use may result in elevated serum midazolam concentrations.	2	3	3
MOCLOBEMIDE Concurrent use may result in central nervous system toxicity or serotonin syndrome (hypertension, hyperthermia, myoclonus, mental status changes).	1	2	2
MORNIFLUMATE Concurrent use may result in an increased risk of bleeding.	0	3	2
NABUMETONE Concurrent use may result in an increased risk of bleeding.	0	3	2
NAPROXEN Concurrent use may result in an increased risk of bleeding.	0	3	2
NIALAMIDE Concurrent use may result in central nervous system toxicity or serotonin syndrome (hypertension, hyperthermia, myoclonus, mental status changes).	1	2	2
NIFLUMIC ACID Concurrent use may result in an increased risk of bleeding.	0	3	2
NIMESULIDE Concurrent use may result in an increased risk of bleeding.	0	3	2
OLANZAPINE Concurrent use may result in an increased risk of olanzapine adverse effects.	2	3	3
OXAPROZIN Concurrent use may result in an increased risk of bleeding.	0	3	2
PARECOXIB Concurrent use may result in an increased risk of bleeding.	0	3	2

Onset: 0=Unspecified 1=Rapid 2=Delayed
Severity: 1=Contraindicated 2=Major 3=Moderate 4=Minor
Evidence: 1=Excellent 2=Good 3=Fair 4=Poor

INTERACTION	ONSET	SEVERITY	EVIDENCE
PARGYLINE Concurrent use may result in central nervous system toxicity or serotonin syndrome (hypertension, hyperthermia, myoclonus, mental status changes).	1	2	2
PHENELZINE Concurrent use may result in central nervous system toxicity or serotonin syndrome (hypertension, hyperthermia, myoclonus, mental status changes).	1	1	2
PHENYLBUTAZONE Concurrent use may result in an increased risk of bleeding.	0	3	2
PHENYTOIN Concurrent use may result in an increased risk of phenytoin toxicity (ataxia, hyperreflexia, nystagmus, tremors).	2	3	3
PIRAZOLAC Concurrent use may result in an increased risk of bleeding.	0	3	2
PIROXICAM Concurrent use may result in an increased risk of bleeding.	0	3	2
PIRPROFEN Concurrent use may result in an increased risk of bleeding.	0	3	2
PROCARBAZINE Concurrent use may result in central nervous system toxicity or serotonin syndrome (hypertension, hyperthermia, myoclonus, mental status changes).	1	2	2
PROPRANOLOL Concurrent use may result in bradycardia and hypotension.	2	3	3
PROPYPHENAZONE Concurrent use may result in an increased risk of bleeding.	0	3	2
PROQUAZONE Concurrent use may result in an increased risk of bleeding.	0	3	2
RASAGILINE Concurrent use may result in CNS toxicity or serotonin syndrome (hypertension, hyperthermia, myoclonus, mental status changes).	0	1	2
ROFECOXIB Concurrent use may result in an increased risk of bleeding.	0	3	2
ROPIVACAINE Concurrent use may result in increased plasma levels of ropivacaine.	1	3	3
SELEGILINE Concurrent use may result in central nervous system toxicity or serotonin syndrome (hypertension, hyperthermia, myoclonus, mental status changes).	1	2	2
SIBUTRAMINE Concurrent use may result in an increased risk of serotonin syndrome (hypertension, hypothermia, myoclonus, mental status changes).	1	2	3

INTERACTION	ONSET	SEVERITY	EVIDENCE
ST. JOHN'S WORT Concurrent use may result in an increased risk of serotonin syndrome (hypertension, hyperthermia, myoclonus, mental status changes).	1	2	3
SULINDAC Concurrent use may result in an increased risk of bleeding.	0	3	2
SUMATRIPTAN Concurrent use may result in an increased risk of weakness, hyperreflexia, and incoordination.	2	2	3
SUPROFEN Concurrent use may result in an increased risk of bleeding.	0	3	2
TACRINE Concurrent use may result in an increase in the plasma concentration of tacrine.	1	3	3
TENIDAP Concurrent use may result in an increased risk of bleeding.	0	3	2
TENOXICAM Concurrent use may result in an increased risk of bleeding.	0	3	2
TERFENADINE Concurrent use may result in cardiotoxicity (QT prolongation, torsade de pointes, cardiac arrest).	1	1	3
THEOPHYLLINE Concurrent use may result in theophylline toxicity (nausea, vomiting, palpitations, seizures).	2	2	3
THIORIDAZINE Concurrent use may result in an increased risk of thioridazine toxicity, cardiotoxicity (QT prolongation, torsade de pointes, cardiac arrest).	1	1	3
TIAPROFENIC ACID Concurrent use may result in an increased risk of bleeding.	0	3	2
TIZANIDINE Concurrent use may result in increased tizanidine bioavailability and an increased risk of tizanidine adverse effects (profound hypotension, bradycardia, excessive drowsiness).	1	1	1
TOBACCO Concurrent use may result in increased fluvoxamine metabolism.	2	4	3
TOLMETIN Concurrent use may result in an increased risk of bleeding.	0	3	2
TOLOXATONE Concurrent use may result in central nervous system toxicity or serotonin syndrome (hypertension, hyperthermia, myoclonus, mental status changes).	1	2	2

Onset: 0=Unspecified 1=Rapid 2=Delayed
Severity: 1=Contraindicated 2=Major 3=Moderate 4=Minor
Evidence: 1=Excellent 2=Good 3=Fair 4=Poor

INTERACTION	ONSET	SEVERITY	EVIDENCE
TRAMADOL Concurrent use may result in an increased risk of seizures and serotonin syndrome (hypertension, hyperthermia, myoclonus, mental status changes).	1	2	2
TRANYLCYPROMINE Concurrent use may result in central nervous system toxicity or serotonin syndrome (hypertension, hyperthermia, myoclonus, mental status changes).	1	2	2
TRIAZOLAM Concurrent use may result in elevated serum triazolam concentrations.	2	3	3
VALDECOXIB Concurrent use may result in an increased risk of bleeding.	0	3	2
WARFARIN Concurrent use may result in an increased risk of bleeding.	2	3	3
ZOLMITRIPTAN Concurrent use may result in weakness, hyperreflexia, and incoordination.	1	3	3
ZOMEPIRAC Concurrent use may result in an increased risk of bleeding.	0	3	2

Galantamine (Razadyne, Razadyne ER)

INTERACTION	ONSET	SEVERITY	EVIDENCE
AMITRIPTYLINE Concurrent use may result in increased galantamine plasma concentrations.	0	3	2
FLUOXETINE Concurrent use may result in increased galantamine plasma concentrations.	0	3	2
FLUVOXAMINE Concurrent use may result in increased galantamine plasma concentrations.	0	3	2
KETOCONAZOLE Concurrent use may result in increased galantamine plasma concentrations.	0	3	2
PAROXETINE Concurrent use may result in increased galantamine plasma concentrations.	0	3	2
QUINIDINE Concurrent use may result in increased galantamine plasma concentrations.	0	3	2

Haloperidol

INTERACTION	ONSET	SEVERITY	EVIDENCE
BENZTROPINE Concurrent use may result in excessive anticholinergic effects (sedation, constipation, dry mouth).	2	3	2

INTERACTION	ONSET	SEVERITY	EVIDENCE
CABERGOLINE Concurrent use may result in the decreased therapeutic effect of both drugs.	1	3	3
CARBAMAZEPINE Concurrent use may result in decreased haloperidol effectiveness.	2	3	2
CISAPRIDE Concurrent use may result in worsening of psychotic symptoms and/or an increased risk of cardiotoxicity (QT prolongation, torsades de pointes, cardiac arrest).	2	1	1
DROPERIDOL Concurrent use may result in an increased risk of cardiotoxicity (QT prolongation, torsade de pointes, cardiac arrest).	0	2	3
LITHIUM Concurrent use may result in weakness, dyskinesias, increased extrapyramidal symptoms, encephalopathy, and brain damage.	2	2	1
RIFAMPIN Concurrent use may result in decreased haloperidol effectiveness.	2	3	3
SPARFLOXACIN Concurrent use may result in prolongation of the QTc interval and/or torsade de pointes.	2	1	3
TRAMADOL Concurrent use may result in an increased risk of seizures.	1	2	3

Hydroxyzine (Vistaril)

INTERACTION	ONSET	SEVERITY	EVIDENCE
PROCARBAZINE Concurrent use may result in CNS depression.	0	3	3

Imipramine (Tofranil, Tofranil-PM)

INTERACTION	ONSET	SEVERITY	EVIDENCE
ACENOCOUMAROL Concurrent use may result in increased risk of bleeding.	2	3	3
AMPRENAVIR Concurrent use may result in increased imipramine serum concentrations and potential toxicity (anticholinergic effects, sedation, confusion, cardiac arrhythmias).	2	2	3
ANISINDIONE Concurrent use may result in increased risk of bleeding.	2	3	3
BEPRIDIL Concurrent use may result in an increased risk of cardiotoxicity (QT prolongation, torsade de pointes, cardiac arrest).	1	1	3

Onset: 0=Unspecified 1=Rapid 2=Delayed
Severity: 1=Contraindicated 2=Major 3=Moderate 4=Minor
Evidence: 1=Excellent 2=Good 3=Fair 4=Poor

INTERACTION	ONSET	SEVERITY	EVIDENCE
BETHANIDINE Concurrent use may result in decreased antihypertensive effectiveness.	1	3	2
CARBAMAZEPINE Concurrent use may result in decreased imipramine effectiveness.	2	3	3
CIMETIDINE Concurrent use may result in imipramine toxicity (dry mouth, urinary retention, blurred vision).	2	3	2
CISAPRIDE Concurrent use may result in cardiotoxicity (QT prolongation, torsade de pointes, cardiac arrest).	1	1	3
CLONIDINE Concurrent use may result in decreased antihypertensive effectiveness.	2	2	3
CLORGYLINE Concurrent use may result in neurotoxicity, seizures, or serotonin syndrome (hypertension, hyperthermia, myoclonus, mental status changes).	2	2	3
DICUMAROL Concurrent use may result in increased risk of bleeding.	2	3	3
DILTIAZEM Concurrent use may result in imipramine toxicity (dry mouth, sedation).	2	4	3
DROPERIDOL Concurrent use may result in an increased risk of cardiotoxicity (QT prolongation, torsade de pointes, cardiac arrest).	0	2	3
EPINEPHRINE Concurrent use may result in hypertension, cardiac arrhythmias, and tachycardia.	1	2	2
ETILEFRINE Concurrent use may result in hypertension, cardiac arrhythmias, and tachycardia.	1	2	2
FLUOXETINE Concurrent use may result in imipramine antidepressant toxicity (dry mouth, urinary retention, sedation) and an increased risk of cardiotoxicity (QT prolongation, torsade de pointes, cardiac arrest).	0	2	3
FLUVOXAMINE Concurrent use may result in imipramine toxicity (dry mouth, urinary retention, sedation).	2	3	3
GREPAFLOXACIN Concurrent use may result in an increased risk of cardiotoxicity (QT prolongation, torsade de pointes, cardiac arrest).	2	1	3

INTERACTION	ONSET	SEVERITY	EVIDENCE
GUANADREL Concurrent use may result in decreased antihypertensive effectiveness.	2	3	3
GUANETHIDINE Concurrent use may result in decreased antihypertensive effectiveness.	2	3	2
GUANFACINE Concurrent use may result in decreased antihypertensive effectiveness.	2	3	3
HALOFANTRINE Concurrent use may result in an increased risk of cardiotoxicity (QT prolongation, torsade de pointes, cardiac arrest).	2	2	3
ISOCARBOXAZID Concurrent use may result in neurotoxicity, seizures, or serotonin syndrome (hypertension, hyperthermia, myoclonus, mental status changes).	2	1	3
LABETALOL Concurrent use may result in imipramine toxicity (dry mouth, urinary retention, sedation).	2	3	3
LEVOMETHADYL Concurrent use may result in an increased risk of cardiotoxicity (QT prolongation, torsade de pointes, cardiac arrest).	2	1	3
METHOXAMINE Concurrent use may result in hypertension, cardiac arrhythmias, and tachycardia.	1	2	2
MIDODRINE Concurrent use may result in hypertension, cardiac arrhythmias, and tachycardia.	1	2	2
MOCLOBEMIDE Concurrent use may result in neurotoxicity, seizures, or serotonin syndrome (hypertension, hyperthermia, myoclonus, mental status changes).	2	2	3
NOREPINEPHRINE Concurrent use may result in hypertension, cardiac arrhythmias, and tachycardia.	1	2	2
OXILOFRINE Concurrent use may result in hypertension, cardiac arrhythmias, and tachycardia.	1	2	2
PHENELZINE Concurrent use may result in neurotoxicity, seizures, or serotonin syndrome (hypertension, hyperthermia, myoclonus, mental status changes).	2	2	3

Onset: 0=Unspecified 1=Rapid 2=Delayed
Severity: 1=Contraindicated 2=Major 3=Moderate 4=Minor
Evidence: 1=Excellent 2=Good 3=Fair 4=Poor

INTERACTION	ONSET	SEVERITY	EVIDENCE
PHENINDIONE Concurrent use may result in increased risk of bleeding.	2	3	3
PHENPROCOUMON Concurrent use may result in increased risk of bleeding.	2	3	3
PHENYLEPHRINE Concurrent use may result in hypertension, cardiac arrhythmias, and tachycardia.	1	2	2
PHENYTOIN Concurrent use may result in an increased risk of phenytoin toxicity (ataxia, hyperreflexia, nystagmus, tremors).	2	3	3
PIMOZIDE Concurrent use may result in an increased risk of cardiotoxicity (QT prolongation, torsade de pointes, cardiac arrest).	0	1	3
PROCARBAZINE Concurrent use may result in neurotoxicity, seizures.	2	2	3
QUINIDINE Concurrent use may result in an increased risk of cardiotoxicity (QT prolongation, torsade de pointes, cardiac arrest).	0	2	3
QUINIDINE Concurrent use may result in imipramine toxicity (dry mouth, sedation) and an increased risk of cardiotoxicity QT prolongation, torsade de pointes, cardiac arrest).	2	3	3
SELEGILINE Concurrent use may result in neurotoxicity, seizures, or serotonin syndrome (hypertension, hyperthermia, myoclonus, mental status changes).	2	2	3
SPARFLOXACIN Concurrent use may result in prolongation of the QTc interval and/or torsade de pointes.	2	1	3
TOBACCO Concurrent use may result in decreased imipramine concentrations.	2	3	3
TRAMADOL Concurrent use may result in an increased risk of seizures.	1	2	3
TRANYLCYPROMINE Concurrent use may result in neurotoxicity, seizures, or serotonin syndrome (hypertension, hyperthermia, myoclonus, mental status changes).	2	2	3
VERAPAMIL Concurrent use may result in imipramine toxicity (dry mouth, sedation, urinary retention).	2	4	2
WARFARIN Concurrent use may result in an increased risk of bleeding.	2	3	3

Lamotrigine (Lamictal)

INTERACTION	ONSET	SEVERITY	EVIDENCE
CARBAMAZEPINE Concurrent use may result in reduced lamotrigine efficacy, loss of seizure control, and a potential risk of neurotoxicity (nausea, vertigo, nystagmus, ataxia).	2	3	3
EVENING PRIMROSE Concurrent use may result in reduced lamotrigine effectiveness.	2	3	3
FOSPHENYTOIN Concurrent use may result in reduced lamotrigine efficacy.	2	3	3
GINKGO Concurrent use may result in decreased lamotrigine effectiveness.	2	3	3
METHSUXIMIDE Concurrent use may result in reduced lamotrigine concentrations and possible loss of seizure control.	2	3	3
ORAL CONTRACEPTIVE Concurrent use may result in altered (increased or decreased) plasma lamotrigine concentrations.	2	3	2
OXCARBAZEPINE Concurrent use may result in reduced lamotrigine concentrations and possible loss of seizure control.	2	3	3
PHENOBARBITAL Concurrent use may result in reduced lamotrigine efficacy, loss of seizure control.	2	3	2
PHENYTOIN Concurrent use may result in reduced lamotrigine efficacy.	2	3	3
PRIMIDONE Concurrent use may result in decreased lamotrigine efficacy.	2	3	1
RITONAVIR Concurrent use may result in decreased lamotrigine serum concentrations.	2	3	3
VALPROIC ACID Concurrent use may result in increased elimination half-life of lamotrigine leading to lamotrigine toxicity (fatigue, drowsiness, ataxia) and an increased risk of life-threatening rashes.	2	2	3

Lisdexamfetamine (Vyvanse)

INTERACTION	ONSET	SEVERITY	EVIDENCE
AMITRIPTYLINE Concurrent use may result in hypertension, other cardiac effects, and CNS stimulation.	2	3	3

Onset: 0=Unspecified 1=Rapid 2=Delayed
Severity: 1=Contraindicated 2=Major 3=Moderate 4=Minor
Evidence: 1=Excellent 2=Good 3=Fair 4=Poor

INTERACTION	ONSET	SEVERITY	EVIDENCE
AMOXAPINE Concurrent use may result in hypertension, other cardiac effects, and CNS stimulation.	2	3	3
CLOMIPRAMINE Concurrent use may result in hypertension, other cardiac effects, and CNS stimulation.	2	3	3
CLORGYLINE Concurrent use may result in hypertensive crisis (headache, hyperpyrexia, hypertension).	0	1	3
DESIPRAMINE Concurrent use may result in hypertension, other cardiac effects, and CNS stimulation.	2	3	3
DOTHIEPIN Concurrent use may result in hypertension, other cardiac effects, and CNS stimulation.	2	3	3
DOXEPIN Concurrent use may result in hypertension, other cardiac effects, and CNS stimulation.	2	3	3
FURAZOLIDONE Concurrent use may result in hypertensive crisis (headache, hyperpyrexia, hypertension).	0	2	3
IMIPRAMINE Concurrent use may result in hypertension, other cardiac effects, and CNS stimulation.	2	3	3
IPRONIAZID Concurrent use may result in hypertensive crisis (headache, hyperpyrexia, hypertension).	0	1	3
ISOCARBOXAZID Concurrent use may result in hypertensive crisis (headache, hyperpyrexia, hypertension).	0	1	3
LOFEPRAMINE Concurrent use may result in hypertension, other cardiac effects, and CNS stimulation.	2	3	3
MOCLOBEMIDE Concurrent use may result in hypertensive crisis (headache, hyperpyrexia, hypertension).	0	1	3
NIALAMIDE Concurrent use may result in hypertensive crisis (headache, hyperpyrexia, hypertension).	0	1	3
NORTRIPTYLINE Concurrent use may result in hypertension, other cardiac effects, and CNS stimulation.	2	3	3
OPIPRAMOL Concurrent use may result in hypertension, other cardiac effects, and CNS stimulation.	2	3	3

INTERACTION	ONSET	SEVERITY	EVIDENCE
PARGYLINE Concurrent use may result in hypertensive crisis (headache, hyperpyrexia, hypertension).	0	1	3
PHENELZINE Concurrent use may result in hypertensive crisis (headache, hyperpyrexia, hypertension).	0	1	3
PROCARBAZINE Concurrent use may result in hypertensive crisis (headache, hyperpyrexia, hypertension).	0	1	3
PROTRIPTYLINE Concurrent use may result in hypertension, other cardiac effects, and CNS stimulation.	2	3	3
RASAGILINE Concurrent use may result in hypertensive crisis (headache, hyperpyrexia, hypertension).	0	1	3
SELEGILINE Concurrent use may result in hypertensive crisis (headache, hyperpyrexia, hypertension).	0	1	3
TOLOXATONE Concurrent use may result in hypertensive crisis (headache, hyperpyrexia, hypertension).	0	1	3
TRANYLCYPROMINE Concurrent use may result in hypertensive crisis (headache, hyperpyrexia, hypertension).	0	1	3
TRIMIPRAMINE Concurrent use may result in hypertension, other cardiac effects, and CNS stimulation.	2	3	3

Lithium (Eskalith, Lithobid)

INTERACTION	ONSET	SEVERITY	EVIDENCE
ACETAZOLAMIDE Concurrent use may result in decreased lithium effectiveness or increased lithium concentrations and lithium toxicity (weakness, tremor, excessive thirst, confusion).	2	3	3
ACETOPHENAZINE Concurrent use may result in weakness, dyskinesias, increased extrapyramidal symptoms, encephalopathy, and brain damage.	2	2	1
AZOSEMIDE Concurrent use may result in increased lithium concentrations and lithium toxicity (weakness, tremor, excessive thirst, confusion).	2	2	3
BEMETIZIDE Concurrent use may result in lithium toxicity (weakness, tremor, excessive thirst, confusion).	2	2	3

Onset: 0=Unspecified 1=Rapid 2=Delayed
Severity: 1=Contraindicated 2=Major 3=Moderate 4=Minor
Evidence: 1=Excellent 2=Good 3=Fair 4=Poor

INTERACTION	ONSET	SEVERITY	EVIDENCE
BENDROFLUMETHIAZIDE Concurrent use may result in increased lithium concentrations and lithium toxicity (weakness, tremor, excessive thirst, confusion).	2	2	3
BENZTHIAZIDE Concurrent use may result in increased lithium concentrations and lithium toxicity (weakness, tremor, excessive thirst, confusion).	2	2	3
BROMPERIDOL Concurrent use may result in weakness, dyskinesias, increased extrapyramidal symptoms, encephalopathy, and brain damage.	2	2	1
BUMETANIDE Concurrent use may result in increased lithium concentrations and lithium toxicity (weakness, tremor, excessive thirst, confusion).	2	2	3
BUTHIAZIDE Concurrent use may result in increased lithium concentrations and lithium toxicity (weakness, tremor, excessive thirst, confusion).	2	2	3
CANRENOATE Concurrent use may result in increased lithium concentrations and an increased risk of lithium toxicity (weakness, tremor, excessive thirst, confusion).	2	2	3
CHLOROTHIAZIDE Concurrent use may result in increased lithium concentrations and lithium toxicity (weakness, tremor, excessive thirst, confusion).	2	2	3
CHLORPROMAZINE Concurrent use may result in weakness, dyskinesias, increased extrapyramidal symptoms, encephalopathy, and brain damage.	2	2	1
CHLORPROTHIXENE Concurrent use may result in weakness, dyskinesias, increased extrapyramidal symptoms, encephalopathy, and brain damage.	2	2	1
CHLORTHALIDONE Concurrent use may result in increased lithium concentrations and lithium toxicity (weakness, tremor, excessive thirst, confusion).	2	2	3
CLOZAPINE Concurrent use may result in weakness, dyskinesias, increased extrapyramidal symptoms, encephalopathy, and brain damage.	2	2	1
CYCLOTHIAZIDE Concurrent use may result in increased lithium concentrations and lithium toxicity (weakness, tremor, excessive thirst, confusion).	2	2	3

INTERACTION	ONSET	SEVERITY	EVIDENCE
DICLOFENAC Concurrent use may result in lithium toxicity (weakness, tremor, excessive thirst, confusion).	2	3	3
DILTIAZEM Concurrent use may result in neurotoxicity, psychosis.	2	3	3
DOMPERIDONE Concurrent use may result in weakness, dyskinesias, increased extrapyramidal symptoms, encephalopathy, and brain damage.	2	2	1
DROPERIDOL Concurrent use may result in weakness, dyskinesias, increased extrapyramidal symptoms, encephalopathy, and brain damage.	2	2	1
ESCITALOPRAM Concurrent use may result in possible lithium toxicity (weakness, tremor, excessive thirst, confusion, dizziness).	2	3	3
ETHACRYNIC ACID Concurrent use may result in increased lithium concentrations and lithium toxicity (weakness, tremor, excessive thirst, confusion).	2	2	3
ETHOPROPAZINE Concurrent use may result in weakness, dyskinesias, increased extrapyramidal symptoms, encephalopathy, and brain damage.	2	2	1
FILGRASTIM Concurrent use may result in a greater than expected increase in white blood cell count.	2	3	3
FLUPENTHIXOL Concurrent use may result in weakness, dyskinesias, increased extrapyramidal symptoms, encephalopathy, and brain damage.	2	2	1
FLUPHENAZINE Concurrent use may result in weakness, dyskinesias, increased extrapyramidal symptoms, encephalopathy, and brain damage.	2	2	1
FLUVOXAMINE Concurrent use may result in possible lithium toxicity (weakness, tremor, excessive thirst, confusion, dizziness).	2	3	3
FOOD Concurrent use may result in increased lithium concentrations.	1	3	3
FOSINOPRIL Concurrent use may result in lithium toxicity (weakness, tremor, excessive thirst, confusion) and/or nephrotoxicity.	2	3	3

Onset: 0=Unspecified 1=Rapid 2=Delayed
Severity: 1=Contraindicated 2=Major 3=Moderate 4=Minor
Evidence: 1=Excellent 2=Good 3=Fair 4=Poor

INTERACTION	ONSET	SEVERITY	EVIDENCE
FUROSEMIDE Concurrent use may result in increased lithium concentrations and lithium toxicity (weakness, tremor, excessive thirst, confusion).	2	2	3
GUARANA Concomitant administration may cause alterations in serum lithium levels.	2	3	3
HALOPERIDOL Concurrent use may result in weakness, dyskinesias, increased extrapyramidal symptoms, encephalopathy, and brain damage.	2	2	1
HYDROCHLOROTHIAZIDE Concurrent use may result in increased lithium concentrations and lithium toxicity (weakness, tremor, excessive thirst, confusion).	2	2	2
HYDROFLUMETHIAZIDE Concurrent use may result in increased lithium concentrations and lithium toxicity (weakness, tremor, excessive thirst, confusion).	2	2	3
IBUPROFEN Concurrent use may result in an increased risk of lithium toxicity (weakness, tremor, excessive thirst, confusion).	2	3	3
INDAPAMIDE Concurrent use may result in increased lithium concentrations and lithium toxicity (weakness, tremor, excessive thirst, confusion).	2	2	3
INDOMETHACIN Concurrent use may result in an increased risk of lithium toxicity (weakness, tremor, excessive thirst, confusion).	2	3	3
KETOROLAC Concurrent use may result in lithium toxicity (weakness, tremor, excessive thirst, confusion).	2	3	2
LISINOPRIL Concurrent use may result in lithium toxicity (weakness, tremor, excessive thirst, confusion) and/or nephrotoxicity.	2	3	3
LOXAPINE Concurrent use may result in weakness, dyskinesias, increased extrapyramidal symptoms, encephalopathy, and brain damage.	2	2	1
MEFENAMIC ACID Concurrent use may result in lithium toxicity (weakness, tremor, excessive thirst, confusion).	2	3	3
MELOXICAM Concurrent use may result in elevation of plasma lithium levels and reduced renal lithium clearance.	1	3	3
MELPERONE Concurrent use may result in weakness, dyskinesias, increased extrapyramidal symptoms, encephalopathy, and brain damage.	2	2	1

INTERACTION	ONSET	SEVERITY	EVIDENCE
MESORIDAZINE Concurrent use may result in weakness, dyskinesias, increased extrapyramidal symptoms, encephalopathy, and brain damage.	2	2	1
METHOTRIMEPRAZINE Concurrent use may result in weakness, dyskinesias, increased extrapyramidal symptoms, encephalopathy, and brain damage.	2	2	1
METHYCLOTHIAZIDE Concurrent use may result in increased lithium concentrations and lithium toxicity (weakness, tremor, excessive thirst, confusion).	2	2	3
METHYLDOPA Concurrent use may result in an increased risk of lithium toxicity (tremor, weakness, excessive thirst, confusion).	2	3	3
METOLAZONE Concurrent use may result in increased lithium concentrations and lithium toxicity (weakness, tremor, excessive thirst, confusion).	2	2	3
METRONIDAZOLE Concurrent use may result in elevated lithium plasma levels and lithium toxicity (weakness, tremor, excessive thirst, confusion).	2	3	3
MOLINDONE Concurrent use may result in weakness, dyskinesias, increased extrapyramidal symptoms, encephalopathy, and brain damage.	2	2	1
NAPROXEN Concurrent use may result in elevated lithium plasma levels and lithium toxicity (weakness, tremor, excessive thirst, confusion).	2	3	3
OLANZAPINE Concurrent use may result in weakness, dyskinesias, increased extrapyramidal symptoms, encephalopathy, and brain damage.	2	2	1
PEGFILGRASTIM Concurrent use may result in a greater than expected increase in white blood cell count.	2	3	3
PENFLURIDOL Concurrent use may result in weakness, dyskinesias, increased extrapyramidal symptoms, encephalopathy, and brain damage.	2	2	1
PERICIAZINE Concurrent use may result in weakness, dyskinesias, increased extrapyramidal symptoms, encephalopathy, and brain damage.	2	2	1

Onset: 0=Unspecified 1=Rapid 2=Delayed
Severity: 1=Contraindicated 2=Major 3=Moderate 4=Minor
Evidence: 1=Excellent 2=Good 3=Fair 4=Poor

INTERACTION	ONSET	SEVERITY	EVIDENCE
PERPHENAZINE Concurrent use may result in weakness, dyskinesias, increased extrapyramidal symptoms, encephalopathy, and brain damage.	2	2	1
PHENYLBUTAZONE Concurrent use may result in lithium toxicity (weakness, tremor, excessive thirst, confusion).	2	3	3
PIMOZIDE Concurrent use may result in weakness, dyskinesias, increased extrapyramidal symptoms, encephalopathy, and brain damage.	2	2	1
PIPAMPERONE Concurrent use may result in weakness, dyskinesias, increased extrapyramidal symptoms, encephalopathy, and brain damage.	2	2	1
PIPOTIAZINE Concurrent use may result in weakness, dyskinesias, increased extrapyramidal symptoms, encephalopathy, and brain damage.	2	2	1
PIRETANIDE Concurrent use may result in increased lithium concentrations and lithium toxicity (weakness, tremor, excessive thirst, confusion).	2	2	3
PIROXICAM Concurrent use may result in lithium toxicity (weakness, tremor, excessive thirst, confusion).	2	3	3
POLYTHIAZIDE Concurrent use may result in increased lithium concentrations and lithium toxicity (weakness, tremor, excessive thirst, confusion).	2	2	3
PROCHLORPERAZINE Concurrent use may result in weakness, dyskinesias, increased extrapyramidal symptoms, encephalopathy, and brain damage.	2	2	1
PROMAZINE Concurrent use may result in weakness, dyskinesias, increased extrapyramidal symptoms, encephalopathy, and brain damage.	2	2	1
PROMETHAZINE Concurrent use may result in weakness, dyskinesias, increased extrapyramidal symptoms, encephalopathy, and brain damage.	2	2	1
QUINETHAZONE Concurrent use may result in increased lithium concentrations and lithium toxicity (weakness, tremor, excessive thirst, confusion).	2	2	3

INTERACTION	ONSET	SEVERITY	EVIDENCE
REMOXIPRIDE Concurrent use may result in weakness, dyskinesias, increased extrapyramidal symptoms, encephalopathy, and brain damage.	2	2	1
RISPERIDONE Concurrent use may result in weakness, dyskinesias, increased extrapyramidal symptoms, encephalopathy, and brain damage.	2	2	1
SERTINDOLE Concurrent use may result in weakness, dyskinesias, increased extrapyramidal symptoms, encephalopathy, and brain damage.	2	2	1
SIBUTRAMINE Concurrent use may result in an increased risk of serotonin syndrome (hypertension, hypothermia, myoclonus, mental status changes).	1	2	3
SODIUM BICARBONATE Concurrent use may result in decreased lithium effectiveness.	2	3	3
SPIRONOLACTONE Concurrent use may result in increased lithium concentrations and lithium toxicity (weakness, tremor, excessive thirst, confusion).	2	2	3
SULPIRIDE Concurrent use may result in weakness, dyskinesias, increased extrapyramidal symptoms, encephalopathy, and brain damage.	2	2	1
TENIDAP Concurrent use may result in increased lithium serum levels and possible lithium toxicity (weakness, tremor, excessive thirst, confusion).	2	3	3
THEOPHYLLINE Concurrent use may result in decreased lithium effectiveness.	2	3	2
THIOPROPAZATE Concurrent use may result in weakness, dyskinesias, increased extrapyramidal symptoms, encephalopathy, and brain damage.	2	2	1
THIOPROPERAZINE Concurrent use may result in weakness, dyskinesias, increased extrapyramidal symptoms, encephalopathy, and brain damage.	2	2	1
THIORIDAZINE Concurrent use may result in weakness, dyskinesias, increased extrapyramidal symptoms, encephalopathy, and brain damage.	2	2	1

Onset: 0=Unspecified 1=Rapid 2=Delayed
Severity: 1=Contraindicated 2=Major 3=Moderate 4=Minor
Evidence: 1=Excellent 2=Good 3=Fair 4=Poor

INTERACTION	ONSET	SEVERITY	EVIDENCE
THIOTHIXENE Concurrent use may result in weakness, dyskinesias, increased extrapyramidal symptoms, encephalopathy, and brain damage.	2	2	1
TIAPRIDE Concurrent use may result in weakness, dyskinesias, increased extrapyramidal symptoms, encephalopathy, and brain damage.	2	2	1
TRICHLORMETHIAZIDE Concurrent use may result in increased lithium concentrations and lithium toxicity (weakness, tremor, excessive thirst, confusion).	2	2	3
TRIFLUOPERAZINE Concurrent use may result in weakness, dyskinesias, increased extrapyramidal symptoms, encephalopathy, and brain damage.	2	2	1
TRIFLUPROMAZINE Concurrent use may result in weakness, dyskinesias, increased extrapyramidal symptoms, encephalopathy, and brain damage.	2	2	1
TRIMEPRAZINE Concurrent use may result in weakness, dyskinesias, increased extrapyramidal symptoms, encephalopathy, and brain damage.	2	2	1
VALDECOXIB Concurrent use may result in increased lithium plasma concentrations and an increased risk of lithium toxicity (weakness, tremor, excessive thirst, confusion).	2	3	3
XIPAMIDE Concurrent use may result in increased lithium concentrations and lithium toxicity (weakness, tremor, excessive thirst, confusion).	2	2	3
ZOTEPINE Concurrent use may result in weakness, dyskinesias, increased extrapyramidal symptoms, encephalopathy, and brain damage.	2	2	1
ZUCLOPENTHIXOL Concurrent use may result in weakness, dyskinesias, increased extrapyramidal symptoms, encephalopathy, and brain damage.	2	2	1

Lorazepam (Ativan, Ativan Injection)

INTERACTION	ONSET	SEVERITY	EVIDENCE
CLOZAPINE Concurrent use may result in central nervous system depression.	1	4	3
ETHANOL Concurrent use may result in increased sedation.	1	3	1

INTERACTION	ONSET	SEVERITY	EVIDENCE
ORAL CONTRACEPTIVE Concurrent use may result in decreased lorazepam effectiveness.	2	4	3
THEOPHYLLINE Concurrent use may result in decreased lorazepam effectiveness.	1	3	2

Maprotiline

INTERACTION	ONSET	SEVERITY	EVIDENCE
CISAPRIDE Concurrent use may result in cardiotoxicity (QT prolongation, torsade de pointes, cardiac arrest).	1	1	3
CLORGYLINE Concurrent use may result in neurotoxicity, seizures.	2	1	3
IPRONIAZID Concurrent use may result in neurotoxicity, seizures.	2	1	3
ISOCARBOXAZID Concurrent use may result in neurotoxicity, seizures.	2	1	3
MOCLOBEMIDE Concurrent use may result in neurotoxicity, seizures.	2	1	3
NIALAMIDE Concurrent use may result in neurotoxicity, seizures.	2	1	3
PARGYLINE Concurrent use may result in neurotoxicity, seizures.	2	1	3
PHENELZINE Concurrent use may result in neurotoxicity, seizures.	2	1	3
PROCARBAZINE Concurrent use may result in neurotoxicity, seizures.	2	1	3
SELEGILINE Concurrent use may result in neurotoxicity, seizures.	2	1	3
TOLOXATONE Concurrent use may result in neurotoxicity, seizures.	2	1	3
TRANYLCYPROMINE Concurrent use may result in neurotoxicity, seizures.	2	1	3

Memantine (Namenda)

INTERACTION	ONSET	SEVERITY	EVIDENCE
ACETAZOLAMIDE Concurrent use may result in reduced clearance of memantine.	0	3	3
CIMETIDINE Concurrent use may result in altered plasma levels of memantine and cimetidine.	0	3	3

Onset: 0=Unspecified 1=Rapid 2=Delayed
Severity: 1=Contraindicated 2=Major 3=Moderate 4=Minor
Evidence: 1=Excellent 2=Good 3=Fair 4=Poor

INTERACTION	ONSET	SEVERITY	EVIDENCE
DICHLORPHENAMIDE Concurrent use may result in reduced clearance of memantine.	0	3	3
HYDROCHLOROTHIAZIDE Concurrent use may result in altered plasma levels of memantine and hydrochlorothiazide.	0	3	3
METHAZOLAMIDE Concurrent use may result in reduced clearance of memantine.	0	3	3
NICOTINE Concurrent use may result in altered plasma levels of memantine and nicotine.	0	3	3
QUINIDINE Concurrent use may result in altered plasma levels of memantine and quinidine.	0	3	3
RANITIDINE Concurrent use may result in altered plasma levels of memantine and ranitidine.	0	3	3
SODIUM BICARBONATE Concurrent use may result in reduced renal clearance of memantine.	0	3	3

Mephobarbital (Mebaral)

INTERACTION	ONSET	SEVERITY	EVIDENCE
ADINAZOLAM Concurrent use may result in additive respiratory depression.	0	2	2
ALFENTANIL Concurrent use may result in additive respiratory depression.	0	2	2
ALPRAZOLAM Concurrent use may result in additive respiratory depression.	0	2	2
AMITRIPTYLINE Concurrent use may result in possible decreased tricyclic antidepressant serum concentrations and possible additive adverse effects.	2	4	2
AMOBARBITAL Concurrent use may result in additive respiratory depression.	0	2	3
AMOXAPINE Concurrent use may result in possible decreased tricyclic antidepressant serum concentrations and possible additive adverse effects.	2	4	2
ANILERIDINE Concurrent use may result in additive respiratory depression.	0	2	2
ANISINDIONE Concurrent use may result in decreased anticoagulant effectiveness.	2	2	3

INTERACTION	ONSET	SEVERITY	EVIDENCE
APROBARBITAL Concurrent use may result in additive respiratory depression.	0	2	3
BROMAZEPAM Concurrent use may result in additive respiratory depression.	0	2	2
BROTIZOLAM Concurrent use may result in additive respiratory depression.	0	2	2
BUTABARBITAL Concurrent use may result in additive respiratory depression.	0	2	3
BUTALBITAL Concurrent use may result in additive respiratory depression.	0	2	3
CALAMUS Concurrent use may result in increased central nervous system depression.	1	3	3
CANNABIS Concurrent use may result in increased central nervous system depression.	1	3	2
CAPSAICIN Concurrent use may result in increased or decreased effectiveness of barbiturates.	1	3	3
CARISOPRODOL Concurrent use may result in additive respiratory depression.	0	2	3
CATNIP Concurrent use may result in increased risk of central nervous system depression.	1	3	3
CHLORAL HYDRATE Concurrent use may result in additive respiratory depression.	0	2	3
CHLORDIAZEPOXIDE Concurrent use may result in additive respiratory depression.	0	2	2
CHLORZOXAZONE Concurrent use may result in additive respiratory depression.	0	2	3
CLOBAZAM Concurrent use may result in additive respiratory depression.	0	2	2
CLOMIPRAMINE Concurrent use may result in possible decreased tricyclic antidepressant serum concentrations and possible additive adverse effects.	2	4	2
CLONAZEPAM Concurrent use may result in additive respiratory depression.	0	2	2
CLORAZEPATE Concurrent use may result in additive respiratory depression.	0	2	2
CODEINE Concurrent use may result in additive respiratory depression.	0	2	2

Onset: 0=Unspecified 1=Rapid 2=Delayed
Severity: 1=Contraindicated 2=Major 3=Moderate 4=Minor
Evidence: 1=Excellent 2=Good 3=Fair 4=Poor

INTERACTION	ONSET	SEVERITY	EVIDENCE
DANTROLENE Concurrent use may result in additive respiratory depression.	0	2	3
DESIPRAMINE Concurrent use may result in possible decreased tricyclic antidepressant serum concentrations and possible additive adverse effects.	2	4	2
DIAZEPAM Concurrent use may result in additive respiratory depression.	0	2	2
DICUMAROL Concurrent use may result in decreased anticoagulant effectiveness.	2	2	2
DOTHIEPIN Concurrent use may result in possible decreased tricyclic antidepressant serum concentrations and possible additive adverse effects.	2	4	2
DOXEPIN Concurrent use may result in possible decreased tricyclic antidepressant serum concentrations and possible additive adverse effects.	2	4	2
ESTAZOLAM Concurrent use may result in additive respiratory depression.	0	2	2
ETHANOL Concurrent use may result in excessive CNS depression.	1	3	2
ETHCHLORVYNOL Concurrent use may result in additive respiratory depression.	0	2	3
EUCALYPTUS Concurrent use may result in decreased effectiveness of barbiturates.	1	3	3
EVENING PRIMROSE Concurrent use may result in reduced anticonvulsant effectiveness.	2	3	3
FENTANYL Concurrent use may result in additive respiratory depression.	0	2	2
FLUNITRAZEPAM Concurrent use may result in additive respiratory depression.	0	2	2
FLURAZEPAM Concurrent use may result in additive respiratory depression.	0	2	2
GINKGO Concurrent use may result in decreased anticonvulsant effectiveness.	2	3	2
HALAZEPAM Concurrent use may result in additive respiratory depression.	0	2	2
HOP Concurrent use may result in increased risk of central nervous system sedation.	1	3	3

INTERACTION	ONSET	SEVERITY	EVIDENCE
HYDROCODONE Concurrent use may result in additive respiratory depression.	0	2	2
HYDROMORPHONE Concurrent use may result in additive respiratory depression.	0	2	2
IMIPRAMINE Concurrent use may result in possible decreased tricyclic antidepressant serum concentrations and possible additive adverse effects.	2	4	2
KAVA Concurrent use may result in increased central nervous system depression.	1	3	3
KETAZOLAM Concurrent use may result in additive respiratory depression.	0	2	2
LEVORPHANOL Concurrent use may result in additive respiratory depression.	0	2	2
LOFEPRAMINE Concurrent use may result in possible decreased tricyclic antidepressant serum concentrations and possible additive adverse effects.	2	4	2
LORAZEPAM Concurrent use may result in additive respiratory depression.	0	2	2
LORMETAZEPAM Concurrent use may result in additive respiratory depression.	0	2	2
MEDAZEPAM Concurrent use may result in additive respiratory depression.	0	2	2
MEPERIDINE Concurrent use may result in additive respiratory depression.	0	2	2
MEPHENESIN Concurrent use may result in additive respiratory depression.	0	2	3
MEPHOBARBITAL Concurrent use may result in additive respiratory depression.	0	2	3
MEPROBAMATE Concurrent use may result in additive respiratory depression.	0	2	3
METAXALONE Concurrent use may result in additive respiratory depression.	0	2	3
METHOCARBAMOL Concurrent use may result in additive respiratory depression.	0	2	3
METHOHEXITAL Concurrent use may result in additive respiratory depression.	0	2	3
MIDAZOLAM Concurrent use may result in additive respiratory depression.	0	2	2
MORPHINE Concurrent use may result in additive respiratory depression.	0	2	2

Onset: 0=Unspecified 1=Rapid 2=Delayed
Severity: 1=Contraindicated 2=Major 3=Moderate 4=Minor
Evidence: 1=Excellent 2=Good 3=Fair 4=Poor

INTERACTION	ONSET	SEVERITY	EVIDENCE
MORPHINE SULFATE LIPOSOME Concurrent use may result in additive respiratory depression.	0	2	2
NITRAZEPAM Concurrent use may result in additive respiratory depression.	0	2	2
NORDAZEPAM Concurrent use may result in additive respiratory depression.	0	2	2
NORTRIPTYLINE Concurrent use may result in possible decreased tricyclic antidepressant serum concentrations and possible additive adverse effects.	2	4	2
OPIPRAMOL Concurrent use may result in possible decreased tricyclic antidepressant serum concentrations and possible additive adverse effects.	2	4	2
OXAZEPAM Concurrent use may result in additive respiratory depression.	0	2	2
OXYCODONE Concurrent use may result in additive respiratory depression.	0	2	2
OXYMORPHONE Concurrent use may result in additive respiratory depression.	0	2	2
PASSIONFLOWER Concurrent use may result in additive central nervous depression.	1	4	3
PENTOBARBITAL Concurrent use may result in additive respiratory depression.	0	2	3
PHENINDIONE Concurrent use may result in decreased anticoagulant effectiveness.	2	2	3
PHENOBARBITAL Concurrent use may result in additive respiratory depression.	0	2	3
PHENPROCOUMON Concurrent use may result in decreased anticoagulant effectiveness.	2	2	2
PIPERINE Concurrent use may result in increased central nervous system depression.	1	4	3
PRAZEPAM Concurrent use may result in additive respiratory depression.	0	2	2
PREDNISOLONE Concurrent use may result in decreased therapeutic effect of prednisolone.	2	3	3
PREDNISONE Concurrent use may result in decreased therapeutic effect of prednisone.	2	3	2
PRIMIDONE Concurrent use may result in additive respiratory depression.	0	2	3

INTERACTION	ONSET	SEVERITY	EVIDENCE
PROCARBAZINE Concurrent use may result in CNS depression.	0	3	3
PROPOXYPHENE Concurrent use may result in additive respiratory depression.	0	2	2
PROTRIPTYLINE Concurrent use may result in possible decreased tricyclic antidepressant serum concentrations and possible additive adverse effects.	2	4	2
QUAZEPAM Concurrent use may result in additive respiratory depression.	0	2	2
QUETIAPINE Concurrent use may result in decreased serum quetiapine concentrations.	0	2	2
REMIFENTANIL Concurrent use may result in additive respiratory depression.	0	2	2
SECOBARBITAL Concurrent use may result in additive respiratory depression.	0	2	3
SEVOFLURANE Concurrent use may result in increased concentrations of plasma inorganic fluoride.	1	3	3
SODIUM OXYBATE Concurrent use may result in additive respiratory depression.	0	2	3
ST JOHN'S WORT Concurrent use may result in decreased central nervous system depressive effect of barbiturates.	1	4	2
SUFENTANIL Concurrent use may result in additive respiratory depression.	0	2	2
TEMAZEPAM Concurrent use may result in additive respiratory depression.	0	2	2
THIOPENTAL Concurrent use may result in additive respiratory depression.	0	2	3
TRIAZOLAM Concurrent use may result in additive respiratory depression.	0	2	2
TRIMIPRAMINE Concurrent use may result in possible decreased tricyclic antidepressant serum concentrations and possible additive adverse effects.	2	4	2
TYLOPHORA Concurrent use may result in increased sedation.	1	3	3
VALERIAN Concurrent use may result in increased central nervous system depression.	1	3	3

Onset: 0=Unspecified 1=Rapid 2=Delayed
Severity: 1=Contraindicated 2=Major 3=Moderate 4=Minor
Evidence: 1=Excellent 2=Good 3=Fair 4=Poor

INTERACTION	ONSET	SEVERITY	EVIDENCE
VORICONAZOLE Concurrent use may result in reduced systemic exposure to voriconazole.	0	1	3
WARFARIN Concurrent use may result in decreased anticoagulant effectiveness.	2	3	2
ZOTEPINE Concurrent use may result in increased risk of barbiturate-induced respiratory depression; decreased zotepine plasma concentrations.	1	3	3

Meprobamate

INTERACTION	ONSET	SEVERITY	EVIDENCE
ETHANOL Concurrent use may result in increased sedation.	1	3	1

Methamphetamine (Desoxyn)

INTERACTION	ONSET	SEVERITY	EVIDENCE
CLORGYLINE Concurrent use may result in hypertensive crisis.	1	1	3
GUANETHIDINE Concurrent use may result in decreased guanethidine effectiveness.	1	3	2
IPRONIAZID Concurrent use may result in hypertensive crisis.	1	1	3
ISOCARBOXAZID Concurrent use may result in hypertensive crisis.	1	1	3
MOCLOBEMIDE Concurrent use may result in hypertensive crisis.	1	1	3
NIALAMIDE Concurrent use may result in hypertensive crisis.	1	1	3
PARGYLINE Concurrent use may result in hypertensive crisis.	1	1	3
PHENELZINE Concurrent use may result in hypertensive crisis.	1	1	3
PROCARBAZINE Concurrent use may result in hypertensive crisis.	1	1	3
SELEGILINE Concurrent use may result in hypertensive crisis.	1	1	3
TOLOXATONE Concurrent use may result in hypertensive crisis.	1	1	3
TRANYLCYPROMINE Concurrent use may result in hypertensive crisis.	1	1	3

Methylphenidate (Concerta, Daytrana, Metadate CD, Metadate ER, Methylin, Methylin ER, Ritalin, Ritalin-SR, Ritalin LA)

INTERACTION	ONSET	SEVERITY	EVIDENCE
CLORGYLINE Concurrent use may result in hypertensive crisis (headache, palpitation, neck stiffness).	1	1	3
GUANETHIDINE Concurrent use may result in decreased guanethidine effectiveness.	1	3	3
IPRONIAZID Concurrent use may result in hypertensive crisis (headache, palpitation, neck stiffness).	1	1	3
ISOCARBOXAZID Concurrent use may result in hypertensive crisis (headache, palpitation, neck stiffness).	1	1	3
LAZABEMIDE Concurrent use may result in hypertensive crisis (headache, palpitation, neck stiffness).	1	1	3
MOCLOBEMIDE Concurrent use may result in hypertensive crisis (headache, palpitation, neck stiffness).	1	1	3
NIALAMIDE Concurrent use may result in hypertensive crisis (headache, palpitation, neck stiffness).	1	1	3
PARGYLINE Concurrent use may result in hypertensive crisis (headache, palpitation, neck stiffness).	1	1	3
PHENELZINE Concurrent use may result in hypertensive crisis (headache, palpitation, neck stiffness).	1	1	3
PROCARBAZINE Concurrent use may result in hypertensive crisis (headache, palpitation, neck stiffness).	1	1	3
SELEGILINE Concurrent use may result in hypertensive crisis (headache, palpitation, neck stiffness).	1	1	3
TOLOXATONE Concurrent use may result in hypertensive crisis (headache, palpitation, neck stiffness).	1	1	3
TRANYLCYPROMINE Concurrent use may result in hypertensive crisis (headache, palpitation, neck stiffness).	1	1	3

Onset: 0=Unspecified 1=Rapid 2=Delayed
Severity: 1=Contraindicated 2=Major 3=Moderate 4=Minor
Evidence: 1=Excellent 2=Good 3=Fair 4=Poor

Mirtazapine (Remeron, Remeron SolTab)

INTERACTION	ONSET	SEVERITY	EVIDENCE
CLONIDINE Concurrent use may result in hypertension, decreased antihypertensive effectiveness.	2	2	3
CLORGYLINE Concurrent use may result in neurotoxicity, seizures.	2	1	3
IPRONIAZID Concurrent use may result in neurotoxicity, seizures.	2	1	3
ISOCARBOXAZID Concurrent use may result in neurotoxicity, seizures.	2	1	3
MOCLOBEMIDE Concurrent use may result in neurotoxicity, seizures.	2	1	3
NIALAMIDE Concurrent use may result in neurotoxicity, seizures.	2	1	3
PARGYLINE Concurrent use may result in neurotoxicity, seizures.	2	1	3
PHENELZINE Concurrent use may result in neurotoxicity, seizures.	2	1	3
PROCARBAZINE Concurrent use may result in neurotoxicity, seizures.	2	1	3
SELEGILINE Concurrent use may result in neurotoxicity, seizures.	2	1	3
TOLOXATONE Concurrent use may result in neurotoxicity, seizures.	2	1	3
TRANYLCYPROMINE Concurrent use may result in neurotoxicity, seizures.	2	1	3

Modafinil (Provigil)

INTERACTION	ONSET	SEVERITY	EVIDENCE
CARBAMAZEPINE Concurrent use may result in decreased modafinil efficacy.	0	4	3
CLOMIPRAMINE Concurrent use may result in increased plasma levels of clomipramine and desmethylclomipramine.	2	3	2
CYCLOSPORINE Concurrent use may result in decreased cyclosporine efficacy.	2	3	2
DESIPRAMINE Concurrent use may result in increased plasma levels of desipramine.	0	3	3
DESOGESTREL Concurrent use may result in decreased contraceptive bioavailability and reduced contraceptive effectiveness.	2	3	2

INTERACTION	ONSET	SEVERITY	EVIDENCE
DIAZEPAM Concurrent use may result in increased plasma concentrations of diazepam.	0	3	3
ETHINYL ESTRADIOL Concurrent use may result in decreased contraceptive bioavailability and reduced contraceptive effectiveness.	2	3	2
ETHYNODIOL Concurrent use may result in decreased contraceptive bioavailability and reduced contraceptive effectiveness.	2	3	2
ETONOGESTREL Concurrent use may result in decreased contraceptive bioavailability and reduced contraceptive effectiveness.	2	3	2
ITRACONAZOLE Concurrent use may result in an increase in modafinil exposure.	0	4	3
KETOCONAZOLE Concurrent use may result in an increase in modafinil exposure.	0	4	3
LEVONORGESTREL Concurrent use may result in decreased contraceptive bioavailability and reduced contraceptive effectiveness.	2	3	2
MESTRANOL Concurrent use may result in decreased contraceptive bioavailability and reduced contraceptive effectiveness.	2	3	2
NORELGESTROMIN Concurrent use may result in decreased contraceptive bioavailability and reduced contraceptive effectiveness.	2	3	2
NORETHINDRONE Concurrent use may result in decreased contraceptive bioavailability and reduced contraceptive effectiveness.	2	3	2
NORGESTIMATE Concurrent use may result in decreased contraceptive bioavailability and reduced contraceptive effectiveness.	2	3	2
NORGESTREL Concurrent use may result in decreased contraceptive bioavailability and reduced contraceptive effectiveness.	2	3	2
PHENOBARBITAL Concurrent use may result in decreased modafinil efficacy.	0	4	3
PHENYTOIN Concurrent use may result in increased plasma concentrations of phenytoin.	0	3	3
PROPRANOLOL Concurrent use may result in increased plasma concentrations of propranolol.	0	3	3

Onset: 0=Unspecified 1=Rapid 2=Delayed
Severity: 1=Contraindicated 2=Major 3=Moderate 4=Minor
Evidence: 1=Excellent 2=Good 3=Fair 4=Poor

INTERACTION	ONSET	SEVERITY	EVIDENCE
RIFAMPIN Concurrent use may result in decreased modafinil efficacy.	0	4	3
TRIAZOLAM Concurrent use may result in loss of triazolam efficacy.	0	3	2

Molindone (Moban)

INTERACTION	ONSET	SEVERITY	EVIDENCE
DROPERIDOL Concurrent use may result in an increased risk of cardiotoxicity (QT prolongation, torsade de pointes, cardiac arrest).	1	1	3
LITHIUM Concurrent use may result in weakness, dyskinesias, increased extrapyramidal symptoms, encephalopathy, and brain damage.	2	2	1
TRAMADOL Concurrent use may result in an increased risk of seizures.	1	2	3

Naloxone (Suboxone)

INTERACTION	ONSET	SEVERITY	EVIDENCE
CLONIDINE Concurrent use may result in hypertension.	1	3	2
YOHIMBINE Concurrent use may result in increased adverse effects.	1	3	1

Naltrexone (ReVia, Vivitrol)

INTERACTION	ONSET	SEVERITY	EVIDENCE
ALPHAPRODINE Concurrent use may result in precipitation of opioid withdrawal symptoms; decreased opioid effectiveness.	1	1	2
ALFENTANIL Concurrent use may result in precipitation of opioid withdrawal symptoms; decreased opioid effectiveness.	1	1	2
CODEINE Concurrent use may result in precipitation of opioid withdrawal symptoms; decreased opioid effectiveness.	1	1	2
DIHYDROCODEINE Concurrent use may result in precipitation of opioid withdrawal symptoms; decreased opioid effectiveness.	1	1	2
ETHYLMORPHINE Concurrent use may result in precipitation of opioid withdrawal symptoms; decreased opioid effectiveness.	1	1	2
FENTANYL Concurrent use may result in precipitation of opioid withdrawal symptoms; decreased opioid effectiveness.	1	1	2
HYDROCODONE Concurrent use may result in precipitation of opioid withdrawal symptoms; decreased opioid effectiveness.	1	1	2

INTERACTION	ONSET	SEVERITY	EVIDENCE
HYDROMORPHONE Concurrent use may result in precipitation of opioid withdrawal symptoms; decreased opioid effectiveness.	1	1	2
LEVORPHANOL Concurrent use may result in precipitation of opioid withdrawal symptoms; decreased opioid effectiveness.	1	1	2
MEPERIDINE Concurrent use may result in precipitation of opioid withdrawal symptoms; decreased opioid effectiveness.	1	1	2
METHADONE Concurrent use may result in precipitation of opioid withdrawal symptoms; decreased opioid effectiveness.	1	1	2
MORPHINE Concurrent use may result in precipitation of opioid withdrawal symptoms; decreased opioid effectiveness.	1	1	2
MORPHINE SULFATE LIPOSOME Concurrent use may result in precipitation of opioid withdrawal symptoms; decreased opioid effectiveness.	1	1	2
OXYCODONE Concurrent use may result in precipitation of opioid withdrawal symptoms; decreased opioid effectiveness.	1	1	2
OXYMORPHONE Concurrent use may result in precipitation of opioid withdrawal symptoms; decreased opioid effectiveness.	1	1	2
PROPOXYPHENE Concurrent use may result in precipitation of opioid withdrawal symptoms; decreased opioid effectiveness.	1	1	2
SUFENTANIL Concurrent use may result in precipitation of opioid withdrawal symptoms; decreased opioid effectiveness.	1	1	2

Nefazodone

INTERACTION	ONSET	SEVERITY	EVIDENCE
ALMOTRIPTAN Concurrent use may result in weakness, hyperreflexia, and/or incoordination.	0	3	3
ALPRAZOLAM Concurrent use may result in psychomotor impairment and sedation.	1	3	2
AMITRIPTYLINE Concurrent use may result in increased risk of serotonin syndrome (hypertension, hyperthermia, myoclonus, mental status changes).	1	2	3
ASTEMIZOLE Concurrent use may result in cardiotoxicity (QT interval prolongation, torsades de pointes, cardiac arrest).	1	1	2

Onset: 0=Unspecified **1**=Rapid **2**=Delayed
Severity: **1**=Contraindicated **2**=Major **3**=Moderate **4**=Minor
Evidence: **1**=Excellent **2**=Good **3**=Fair **4**=Poor

INTERACTION	ONSET	SEVERITY	EVIDENCE
CARBAMAZEPINE Concurrent use may result in an increased risk of carbamazepine toxicity (ataxia, nystagmus, diplopia, headache, vomiting, apnea, seizures, coma).	2	3	3
CISAPRIDE Concurrent use may result in an increased risk of cardiotoxicity (QT prolongation, torsades de pointes, cardiac arrest).	1	1	2
DIHYDROERGOTAMINE Concurrent use may result in an increased risk of ergotism (nausea, vomiting, vasospastic ischemia).	1	1	2
DROPERIDOL Concurrent use may result in an increased risk of cardiotoxicity (QT prolongation, torsade de pointes, cardiac arrest).	1	2	3
ERGOLOID MESYLATES Concurrent use may result in an increased risk of ergotism (nausea, vomiting, vasospastic ischemia).	1	1	2
ERGONOVINE Concurrent use may result in an increased risk of ergotism (nausea, vomiting, vasospastic ischemia).	1	1	2
ERGOTAMINE Concurrent use may result in an increased risk of ergotism (nausea, vomiting, vasospastic ischemia).	1	1	2
FURAZOLIDONE Concurrent use may result in weakness, hyperreflexia, and incoordination.	2	1	3
METHYLERGONOVINE Concurrent use may result in an increased risk of ergotism (nausea, vomiting, vasospastic ischemia).	1	1	2
PHENELZINE Concurrent use may result in hyperthermia, rigidity, myoclonus, seizures, fluctuations of vital signs, or mental status changes.	1	1	2
PIMOZIDE Concurrent use may result in an increased risk of cardiotoxicity (QT prolongation, torsades de pointes, cardiac arrest).	1	1	2
SELEGILINE Concurrent use may result in hyperthermia, rigidity, myoclonus, seizures, fluctuations of vital signs, or mental status changes.	1	2	2
SIBUTRAMINE Concurrent use may result in an increased risk of serotonin syndrome (hypertension, hypothermia, myoclonus, mental status changes).	1	2	3

INTERACTION	ONSET	SEVERITY	EVIDENCE
TERFENADINE Concurrent use may result in serious, even fatal, cardiovascular events (QT interval prolongation, torsades de pointes, or cardiac arrest).	1	1	2
TRANYLCYPROMINE Concurrent use may result in hyperthermia, rigidity, myoclonus, seizures, fluctuations of vital signs, or mental status changes.	1	2	2
TRIAZOLAM Concurrent use may result in psychomotor impairment and excessive sedation.	1	3	2

Nortriptyline (Aventyl, Pamelor)

INTERACTION	ONSET	SEVERITY	EVIDENCE
ACENOCOUMAROL Concurrent use may result in an increased risk of bleeding.	2	3	3
AMPRENAVIR Concurrent use may result in increased nortriptyline serum concentrations and potential toxicity (anticholinergic effects, sedation, confusion, cardiac arrhythmias).	2	2	3
ANISINDIONE Concurrent use may result in an increased risk of bleeding.	2	3	3
BEPRIDIL Concurrent use may result in an increased risk of cardiotoxicity (QT prolongation, torsade de pointes, cardiac arrest).	1	1	3
BETHANIDINE Concurrent use may result in decreased antihypertensive effectiveness.	1	3	3
CIMETIDINE Concurrent use may result in nortriptyline toxicity (dry mouth, blurred vision, urinary retention).	2	3	2
CISAPRIDE Concurrent use may result in cardiotoxicity (QT prolongation, torsade de pointes, cardiac arrest).	1	1	3
CLONIDINE Concurrent use may result in decreased antihypertensive effectiveness.	2	2	3
CLORGYLINE Concurrent use may result in neurotoxicity, seizures, or serotonin syndrome (hypertension, hyperthermia, myoclonus, mental status changes).	2	2	3
DICUMAROL Concurrent use may result in an increased risk of bleeding.	2	3	3

Onset: 0=Unspecified 1=Rapid 2=Delayed
Severity: 1=Contraindicated 2=Major 3=Moderate 4=Minor
Evidence: 1=Excellent 2=Good 3=Fair 4=Poor

INTERACTION	ONSET	SEVERITY	EVIDENCE
DROPERIDOL Concurrent use may result in an increased risk of cardiotoxicity (QT prolongation, torsade de pointes, cardiac arrest).	0	2	3
EPINEPHRINE Concurrent use may result in hypertension, cardiac arrhythmias, and tachycardia.	1	2	2
ETILEFRINE Concurrent use may result in hypertension, cardiac arrhythmias, and tachycardia.	1	2	2
FLUOXETINE Concurrent use may result in nortriptyline antidepressant toxicity (dry mouth, urinary retention, sedation) and an increased risk of cardiotoxicity (QT prolongation, torsade de pointes, cardiac arrest).	0	2	3
GREPAFLOXACIN Concurrent use may result in an increased risk of cardiotoxicity (QT prolongation, torsade de pointes, cardiac arrest).	2	1	3
GUANADREL Concurrent use may result in decreased antihypertensive effectiveness.	2	3	3
GUANETHIDINE Concurrent use may result in decreased antihypertensive effectiveness.	2	3	2
HALOFANTRINE Concurrent use may result in an increased risk of cardiotoxicity (QT prolongation, torsade de pointes, cardiac arrest).	2	2	3
ISOCARBOXAZID Concurrent use may result in neurotoxicity, seizures, or serotonin syndrome (hypertension, hyperthermia, myoclonus, mental status changes).	2	1	3
LEVOMETHADYL Concurrent use may result in an increased risk of cardiotoxicity (QT prolongation, torsade de pointes, cardiac arrest).	2	1	3
METHOXAMINE Concurrent use may result in hypertension, cardiac arrhythmias, and tachycardia.	1	2	2
MIDODRINE Concurrent use may result in hypertension, cardiac arrhythmias, and tachycardia.	1	2	2
MOCLOBEMIDE Concurrent use may result in neurotoxicity, seizures, or serotonin syndrome (hypertension, hyperthermia, myoclonus, mental status changes).	2	2	3

INTERACTION	ONSET	SEVERITY	EVIDENCE
NOREPINEPHRINE Concurrent use may result in hypertension, cardiac arrhythmias, and tachycardia.	1	2	2
OXILOFRINE Concurrent use may result in hypertension, cardiac arrhythmias, and tachycardia.	1	2	2
PHENELZINE Concurrent use may result in neurotoxicity, seizures, or serotonin syndrome (hypertension, hyperthermia, myoclonus, mental status changes).	2	2	3
PHENINDIONE Concurrent use may result in an increased risk of bleeding.	2	3	3
PHENPROCOUMON Concurrent use may result in an increased risk of bleeding.	2	3	3
PHENYLEPHRINE Concurrent use may result in hypertension, cardiac arrhythmias, and tachycardia.	1	2	2
PIMOZIDE Concurrent use may result in an increased risk of cardiotoxicity (QT prolongation, torsade de pointes, cardiac arrest).	0	1	3
PROCARBAZINE Concurrent use may result in neurotoxicity, seizures.	2	2	3
SELEGILINE Concurrent use may result in neurotoxicity, seizures, or serotonin syndrome (hypertension, hyperthermia, myoclonus, mental status changes).	2	2	3
SERTRALINE Concurrent use may result in elevated nortriptyline serum levels or possible serotonin syndrome (hypertension, hyperthermia, myoclonus, mental status changes).	2	2	3
SPARFLOXACIN Concurrent use may result in prolongation of the QTc interval and/or torsade de pointes.	2	1	3
TRAMADOL Concurrent use may result in an increased risk of seizures.	1	2	3
TRANYLCYPROMINE Concurrent use may result in neurotoxicity, seizures, or serotonin syndrome (hypertension, hyperthermia, myoclonus, mental status changes).	2	2	3
WARFARIN Concurrent use may result in an increased risk of bleeding.	2	3	3

Onset: 0=Unspecified 1=Rapid 2=Delayed
Severity: 1=Contraindicated 2=Major 3=Moderate 4=Minor
Evidence: 1=Excellent 2=Good 3=Fair 4=Poor

Olanzapine (Symbyax, Zyprexa, Zyprexa IntraMuscular, Zyprexa Zydis)

INTERACTION	ONSET	SEVERITY	EVIDENCE
CLOMIPRAMINE Concurrent use may result in an increased risk of seizures.	2	2	2
ETHANOL Concurrent use may result in excessive central nervous system depression.	1	3	3
FLUVOXAMINE Concurrent use may result in an increased risk of olanzapine adverse effects.	2	3	3
LEVOMETHADYL Concurrent use may result in an increased risk of cardiotoxicity (QT prolongation, torsade de pointes, cardiac arrest).	2	1	3
LITHIUM Concurrent use may result in weakness, dyskinesias, increased extrapyramidal symptoms, encephalopathy, and brain damage.	2	2	1

Oxazepam

INTERACTION	ONSET	SEVERITY	EVIDENCE
CABBAGE Concurrent use may result in reduced oxazepam effectiveness.	1	3	3
ECONAZOLE Concurrent use may result in increased oxazepam serum concentrations and potential oxazepam toxicity (sedation, slurred speech, central nervous system depression).	2	1	3
FOSPHENYTOIN Concurrent use may result in loss of oxazepam efficacy.	2	4	3
KAVA Concurrent use may result in increased central nervous system depression.	2	3	3
PHENYTOIN Concurrent use may result in loss of oxazepam efficacy.	2	4	3
ST. JOHN'S WORT Concurrent use may result in reduced oxazepam effectiveness.	2	3	2
THEOPHYLLINE Concurrent use may result in decreased oxazepam effectiveness.	1	3	2

Paliperidone (Invega)

INTERACTION	ONSET	SEVERITY	EVIDENCE
ACECAINIDE Concurrent use may result in an increased risk of cardiotoxicity (QT prolongation, torsades de pointes, cardiac arrest).	0	2	3

INTERACTION	ONSET	SEVERITY	EVIDENCE
AJMALINE Concurrent use may result in an increased risk of cardiotoxicity (QT prolongation, torsades de pointes, cardiac arrest).	0	2	2
AMIODARONE Concurrent use may result in an increased risk of cardiotoxicity (QT prolongation, torsades de pointes, cardiac arrest).	0	2	3
ARSENIC TRIOXIDE Concurrent use may result in prolongation of the QTc interval and/or torsades de pointes.	0	2	3
AZIMILIDE Concurrent use may result in an increased risk of cardiotoxicity (QT prolongation, torsades de pointes, cardiac arrest).	0	2	3
BRETYLIUM Concurrent use may result in an increased risk of cardiotoxicity (QT prolongation, torsades de pointes, cardiac arrest).	0	2	3
CHLORPROMAZINE Concurrent use may result in an increased risk of cardiotoxicity (QT prolongation, torsades de pointes, cardiac arrest).	0	2	3
DISOPYRAMIDE Concurrent use may result in an increased risk of cardiotoxicity (QT prolongation, torsades de pointes, cardiac arrest).	0	2	2
DOFETILIDE Concurrent use may result in an increased risk of cardiotoxicity (QT prolongation, torsades de pointes, cardiac arrest).	0	2	3
GATIFLOXACIN Concurrent use may result in an increased risk of cardiotoxicity (QT prolongation, torsades de pointes, cardiac arrest).	0	2	3
HYDROQUINIDINE Concurrent use may result in an increased risk of cardiotoxicity (QT prolongation, torsades de pointes, cardiac arrest).	0	2	2
IBUTILIDE Concurrent use may result in an increased risk of cardiotoxicity (QT prolongation, torsades de pointes, cardiac arrest).	0	2	3
LEVODOPA Concurrent use may result in loss of levodopa efficacy.	0	3	3

Onset: 0=Unspecified 1=Rapid 2=Delayed
Severity: 1=Contraindicated 2=Major 3=Moderate 4=Minor
Evidence: 1=Excellent 2=Good 3=Fair 4=Poor

INTERACTION	ONSET	SEVERITY	EVIDENCE
MESORIDAZINE Concurrent use may result in an increased risk of cardiotoxicity (QT prolongation, torsades de pointes, cardiac arrest).	0	1	3
METHADONE Concurrent use may result in an increased risk of QT interval prolongation.	0	2	3
MOXIFLOXACIN Concurrent use may result in an increased risk of cardiotoxicity (QT prolongation, torsades de pointes, cardiac arrest).	0	2	3
PIRMENOL Concurrent use may result in an increased risk of cardiotoxicity (QT prolongation, torsades de pointes, cardiac arrest).	0	2	2
PRAJMALINE Concurrent use may result in an increased risk of cardiotoxicity (QT prolongation, torsades de pointes, cardiac arrest).	0	2	2
PROCAINAMIDE Concurrent use may result in an increased risk of cardiotoxicity (QT prolongation, torsades de pointes, cardiac arrest).	0	2	2
PROCHLORPERAZINE Concurrent use may result in an increased risk of cardiotoxicity (QT prolongation, torsades de pointes, cardiac arrest).	0	2	3
QUINIDINE Concurrent use may result in an increased risk of cardiotoxicity (QT prolongation, torsades de pointes, cardiac arrest).	0	2	2
RANOLAZINE Concurrent use may result in an increased risk of QT interval prolongation.	0	1	3
SEMATILIDE Concurrent use may result in an increased risk of cardiotoxicity (QT prolongation, torsades de pointes, cardiac arrest).	0	2	3
SOTALOL Concurrent use may result in an increased risk of cardiotoxicity (QT prolongation, torsades de pointes, cardiac arrest).	0	2	3
TEDISAMIL Concurrent use may result in an increased risk of cardiotoxicity (QT prolongation, torsades de pointes, cardiac arrest).	0	2	3

INTERACTION	ONSET	SEVERITY	EVIDENCE
THIORIDAZINE Concurrent use may result in an increased risk of cardiotoxicity (QT prolongation, torsades de pointes, cardiac arrest).	0	1	3
TRIFLUOPERAZINE Concurrent use may result in an increased risk of cardiotoxicity (QT prolongation, torsades de pointes, cardiac arrest).	0	2	3

Paroxetine (Paxil, Paxil CR, Pexeva)

INTERACTION	ONSET	SEVERITY	EVIDENCE
ALMOTRIPTAN Concurrent use may result in weakness, hyperreflexia, and/or incoordination.	0	3	3
CIMETIDINE Concurrent use may result in increased paroxetine serum concentrations and possibly paroxetine toxicity (dizziness, somnolence, nausea, headache).	2	3	3
CLORGYLINE Concurrent use may result in central nervous system toxicity or serotonin syndrome (hypertension, hyperthermia, myoclonus, mental status changes).	1	1	2
DEXFENFLURAMINE Concurrent use may result in serotonin syndrome (hypertension, hyperthermia, myoclonus, mental status changes).	1	2	3
DEXTROMETHORPHAN Concurrent use may result in possible dextromethorphan toxicity (nausea, vomiting, blurred vision, hallucinations) or serotonin syndrome (hypertension, hyperthermia, myoclonus, mental status changes).	1	2	3
DROPERIDOL Concurrent use may result in an increased risk of cardiotoxicity (QT prolongation, torsade de pointes, cardiac arrest).	1	2	3
ENCAINIDE Concurrent use may result in an increased risk of encainide toxicity (cardiac arrhythmia).	1	3	3
ETHANOL Concurrent use may result in an increased risk of impairment of mental and motor skills.	1	4	3
FENFLURAMINE Concurrent use may result in serotonin syndrome (hypertension, hyperthermia, myoclonus, mental status changes).	1	2	3

Onset: 0=Unspecified 1=Rapid 2=Delayed
Severity: 1=Contraindicated 2=Major 3=Moderate 4=Minor
Evidence: 1=Excellent 2=Good 3=Fair 4=Poor

INTERACTION	ONSET	SEVERITY	EVIDENCE
FOSPHENYTOIN Concurrent use may result in reduced paroxetine efficacy.	2	3	3
FURAZOLIDONE Concurrent use may result in weakness, hyperreflexia, and incoordination.	2	1	3
HYDROXYTRYPTOPHAN Concurrent use may result in an increased risk of serotonin syndrome (hypertension, hyperthermia, myoclonus, mental status changes).	1	3	3
IPRONIAZID Concurrent use may result in central nervous system toxicity or serotonin syndrome (hypertension, hyperthermia, myoclonus, mental status changes).	1	1	2
ISOCARBOXAZID Concurrent use may result in central nervous system toxicity or serotonin syndrome (hypertension, hyperthermia, myoclonus, mental status changes).	1	1	2
MOCLOBEMIDE Concurrent use may result in central nervous system toxicity or serotonin syndrome (hypertension, hyperthermia, myoclonus, mental status changes).	1	1	2
NIALAMIDE Concurrent use may result in central nervous system toxicity or serotonin syndrome (hypertension, hyperthermia, myoclonus, mental status changes).	1	1	2
PARGYLINE Concurrent use may result in central nervous system toxicity or serotonin syndrome (hypertension, hyperthermia, myoclonus, mental status changes).	1	1	2
PERPHENAZINE Concurrent use may result in increased plasma concentrations and side effects of perphenazine.	1	3	3
PHENELZINE Concurrent use may result in central nervous system toxicity or serotonin syndrome (hypertension, hyperthermia, myoclonus, mental status changes).	1	1	2
PHENOBARBITAL Concurrent use may result in reduced paroxetine effectiveness.	1	4	3
PHENYTOIN Concurrent use may result in reduced phenytoin and paroxetine efficacy.	2	3	3
PIMOZIDE Concurrent use may result in an increased risk of pimozide toxicity including cardiotoxicity (QT prolongation, torsades de pointes, cardiac arrest).	1	1	2

INTERACTION	ONSET	SEVERITY	EVIDENCE
PROCARBAZINE Concurrent use may result in central nervous system toxicity or serotonin syndrome (hypertension, hyperthermia, myoclonus, mental status changes).	1	1	2
PROCYCLIDINE Concurrent use may result in an increased risk of anticholinergic effects (dry mouth, sedation, mydriasis).	1	3	3
PROPAFENONE Concurrent use may result in an increased risk of propafenone toxicity (cardiac arrhythmia).	1	3	3
RISPERIDONE Concurrent use may result in an increased risk for serotonin syndrome (hypertension, hyperthermia, myoclonus, mental status changes).	2	2	2
SELEGILINE Concurrent use may result in central nervous system toxicity or serotonin syndrome (hypertension, hyperthermia, myoclonus, mental status changes).	1	1	2
SIBUTRAMINE Concurrent use may result in an increased risk of serotonin syndrome (hypertension, hypothermia, myoclonus, mental status changes).	1	2	3
THEOPHYLLINE Concurrent use may result in an increased risk of theophylline toxicity.	2	3	3
THIORIDAZINE Concurrent use may result in an increased risk of thioridazine toxicity, cardiotoxicity (QT prolongation, torsade de pointes, cardiac arrest).	1	1	3
TOLOXATONE Concurrent use may result in central nervous system toxicity or serotonin syndrome (hypertension, hyperthermia, myoclonus, mental status changes).	1	1	2
TRAMADOL Concurrent use may result in an increased risk of seizures and serotonin syndrome (hypertension, hyperthermia, myoclonus, mental status changes).	1	2	2
TRANYLCYPROMINE Concurrent use may result in central nervous system toxicity or serotonin syndrome (hypertension, hyperthermia, myoclonus, mental status changes).	1	1	2
TRYPTOPHAN Concurrent use may result in serotonin syndrome (hypertension, hyperthermia, myoclonus, mental status changes).	2	2	3

Onset: 0=Unspecified 1=Rapid 2=Delayed
Severity: 1=Contraindicated 2=Major 3=Moderate 4=Minor
Evidence: 1=Excellent 2=Good 3=Fair 4=Poor

Pentobarbital (Nembutal)

INTERACTION	ONSET	SEVERITY	EVIDENCE
ALPRENOLOL Concurrent use may result in decreased alprenolol effectiveness.	2	3	2
DICUMAROL Concurrent use may result in decreased anticoagulant effectiveness.	2	2	2
ETHANOL Concurrent use may result in excessive central nervous system depression.	1	3	1
METOPROLOL Concurrent use may result in decreased metoprolol effectiveness.	2	3	3
PREDNISOLONE Concurrent use may result in decreased therapeutic effect of prednisolone.	2	3	2
PREDNISONE Concurrent use may result in decreased therapeutic effect of prednisone.	2	3	2
THEOPHYLLINE Concurrent use may result in decreased theophylline effectiveness.	2	3	3
VALERIAN Concurrent use may result in increased central nervous system depression.	1	3	3

Perphenazine

INTERACTION	ONSET	SEVERITY	EVIDENCE
BELLADONNA Concurrent use may result in increased manic, agitated reactions, or enhanced anticholinergic effects resulting in cardiorespiratory failure, especially in cases of belladonna overdose.	1	3	2
BENZTROPINE Concurrent use may result in decreased perphenazine serum concentrations, decreased perphenazine effectiveness, enhanced anticholinergic effects (ileus, hyperpyrexia, sedation, dry mouth).	2	3	3
CABERGOLINE Concurrent use may result in the decreased therapeutic effect of both drugs.	1	3	3
CISAPRIDE Concurrent use may result in cardiotoxicity (QT prolongation, torsade de pointes, cardiac arrest).	1	1	3
DROPERIDOL Concurrent use may result in an increased risk of cardiotoxicity (QT prolongation, torsade de pointes, cardiac arrest).	1	1	3

INTERACTION	ONSET	SEVERITY	EVIDENCE
ETHANOL Concurrent use may result in increased central nervous system depression and an increased risk of extrapyramidal reactions.	1	3	2
FOSPHENYTOIN Concurrent use may result in increased or decreased phenytoin levels and possibly reduced perphenazine levels.	2	4	3
GREPAFLOXACIN Concurrent use may result in an increased risk of cardiotoxicity (QT prolongation, torsade de pointes, cardiac arrest).	2	1	3
LEVODOPA Concurrent use may result in loss of levodopa efficacy.	1	3	2
LITHIUM Concurrent use may result in weakness, dyskinesias, increased extrapyramidal symptoms, encephalopathy, and brain damage.	2	2	1
MEPERIDINE Concurrent use may result in an increase in central nervous system and respiratory depression.	1	3	2
ORPHENADRINE Concurrent use may result in decreased perphenazine serum concentrations, decreased perphenazine effectiveness, enhanced anticholinergic effects (ileus, hyperpyrexia, sedation, dry mouth).	2	3	3
PAROXETINE Concurrent use may result in increased plasma concentrations and side effects of perphenazine.	1	3	3
PHENYTOIN Concurrent use may result in increased or decreased phenytoin levels and possibly reduced perphenazine levels.	2	4	3
PORFIMER Concurrent use may result in excessive intracellular damage in photosensitized tissues.	2	3	3
PROCYCLIDINE Concurrent use may result in decreased perphenazine serum concentrations, decreased perphenazine effectiveness, enhanced anticholinergic effects (ileus, hyperpyrexia, sedation, dry mouth).	2	3	3
TRAMADOL Concurrent use may result in an increased risk of seizures.	1	2	3
TRIHEXYPHENIDYL Concurrent use may result in decreased perphenazine serum concentrations, decreased perphenazine effectiveness, enhanced anticholinergic effects (ileus, hyperpyrexia, sedation, dry mouth).	2	3	3

Onset: 0=Unspecified 1=Rapid 2=Delayed
Severity: 1=Contraindicated 2=Major 3=Moderate 4=Minor
Evidence: 1=Excellent 2=Good 3=Fair 4=Poor

Phenelzine (Nardil)

INTERACTION	ONSET	SEVERITY	EVIDENCE
ACARBOSE Concurrent use may result in excessive hypoglycemia, central nervous system depression, and seizures.	1	3	2
ACETOHEXAMIDE Concurrent use may result in excessive hypoglycemia, central nervous system depression, and seizures.	1	3	2
ALBUTEROL Concurrent use may result in an increased risk of tachycardia, agitation, or hypomania.	2	2	2
AMITRIPTYLINE Concurrent use may result in neurotoxicity, seizures, or serotonin syndrome (hypertension, hyperthermia, myoclonus, mental status changes).	2	1	3
AMOXAPINE Concurrent use may result in neurotoxicity, seizures, or serotonin syndrome (hypertension, hyperthermia, myoclonus, mental status changes).	2	2	3
AMPHETAMINE Concurrent use may result in hypertensive crisis (headache, hyperpyrexia, hypertension).	1	1	2
APRACLONIDINE Concurrent use may result in potentiation of phenelzine effects.	1	1	3
BAMBUTEROL Concurrent use may result in an increased risk of tachycardia, agitation, or hypomania.	2	2	2
BENFLUOREX Concurrent use may result in excessive hypoglycemia, central nervous system depression, and seizures.	1	3	2
BENZPHETAMINE Concurrent use may result in hypertensive crisis (headache, hyperpyrexia, hypertension).	1	1	2
BITOLTEROL Concurrent use may result in an increased risk of tachycardia, agitation, or hypomania.	2	2	2
BROXATEROL Concurrent use may result in an increased risk of tachycardia, agitation, or hypomania.	2	2	2
BUPROPION Concurrent use may result in bupropion toxicity (seizures, agitation, psychotic changes).	1	1	3
BUSPIRONE Concurrent use may result in hypertensive crisis.	1	1	3
CARBAMAZEPINE Concurrent use may result in hypertensive urgency, hyperpyrexia, and seizures.	1	1	3

INTERACTION	ONSET	SEVERITY	EVIDENCE
CHLORPROPAMIDE Concurrent use may result in excessive hypoglycemia, central nervous system depression, and seizures.	1	3	2
CITALOPRAM Concurrent use may result in central nervous system toxicity or serotonin syndrome (hypertension, hyperthermia, myoclonus, mental status changes).	1	1	3
CLENBUTEROL Concurrent use may result in an increased risk of tachycardia, agitation, or hypomania.	2	2	2
CLOMIPRAMINE Concurrent use may result in neurotoxicity, seizures, or serotonin syndrome (hypertension, hyperthermia, myoclonus, mental status changes).	2	2	3
CLORGYLINE Concurrent use may result in hypertensive crisis (headache, palpitation, neck stiffness).	1	1	3
CLOVOXAMINE Concurrent use may result in central nervous system toxicity or serotonin syndrome (hypertension, hyperthermia, myoclonus, mental status changes).	1	1	3
COCAINE Concurrent use may result in hypertensive crisis (headache, hyperpyrexia, hypertension).	1	1	3
CYCLOBENZAPRINE Concurrent use may result in hypertensive crises (headache, hyperpyrexia, hypertension) or severe convulsive seizures.	1	1	3
CYPROHEPTADINE Concurrent use may result in prolonged and intensified anticholinergic effects.	2	1	3
DESIPRAMINE Concurrent use may result in neurotoxicity, seizures, or serotonin syndrome (hypertension, hyperthermia, myoclonus, mental status changes).	2	2	3
DEXFENFLURAMINE Concurrent use may result in central nervous system toxicity or serotonin syndrome (hypertension, hyperthermia, myoclonus, mental status changes).	1	1	3
DEXMETHYLPHENIDATE Concurrent use may result in hypertensive crisis (headache, palpitation, neck stiffness).	1	1	3
DEXTROAMPHETAMINE Concurrent use may result in a hypertensive crisis (headache, hyperpyrexia, hypertension).	1	1	3

Onset: 0=Unspecified 1=Rapid 2=Delayed
Severity: 1=Contraindicated 2=Major 3=Moderate 4=Minor
Evidence: 1=Excellent 2=Good 3=Fair 4=Poor

INTERACTION	ONSET	SEVERITY	EVIDENCE
DEXTROMETHORPHAN Concurrent use may result in an increased risk of serotonin syndrome (hypertension, hyperthermia, myoclonus, mental status changes).	1	1	3
DIETHYLPROPION Concurrent use may result in hypertensive crisis (headache, hyperpyrexia, hypertension).	1	1	2
DOPAMINE Concurrent use may result in hypertensive crisis (headache, hyperpyrexia, hypertension).	1	1	1
DOPAMINE FOODS Concurrent use may result in increased blood pressure.	1	1	1
DOTHIEPIN Concurrent use may result in neurotoxicity, seizures, or serotonin syndrome (hypertension, hyperthermia, myoclonus, mental status changes).	2	2	3
DOXEPIN Concurrent use may result in neurotoxicity, seizures, or serotonin syndrome (hypertension, hyperthermia, myoclonus, mental status changes).	2	2	3
DROPERIDOL Concurrent use may result in an increased risk of cardiotoxicity (QT prolongation, torsade de pointes, cardiac arrest).	1	2	3
DULOXETINE Concurrent use may result in central nervous system toxicity or serotonin syndrome (hypertension, hyperthermia, myoclonus, mental status changes).	1	1	2
EPHEDRINE Concurrent use may result in hypertensive crisis (headache, hyperpyrexia, hypertension).	1	2	3
EPINEPHRINE Concurrent use may result in increased hypertensive effects.	1	1	3
FEMOXETINE Concurrent use may result in central nervous system toxicity or serotonin syndrome (hypertension, hyperthermia, myoclonus, mental status changes).	1	1	3
FENFLURAMINE Concurrent use may result in serotonin syndrome (hypertension, hyperthermia, myoclonus, mental status changes).	1	1	3
FENOTEROL Concurrent use may result in an increased risk of tachycardia, agitation, or hypomania.	2	2	2
FLUOXETINE Concurrent use may result in central nervous system toxicity or serotonin syndrome (hypertension, hyperthermia, myoclonus, mental status changes).	1	1	2

INTERACTION	ONSET	SEVERITY	EVIDENCE
FLUVOXAMINE Concurrent use may result in central nervous system toxicity or serotonin syndrome (hypertension, hyperthermia, myoclonus, mental status changes).	1	1	2
FORMOTEROL Concurrent use may result in an increased risk of tachycardia, agitation, or hypomania.	2	2	2
FURAZOLIDONE Concurrent use may result in hypertensive crisis (headache, palpitation, neck stiffness).	1	1	3
GLICLAZIDE Concurrent use may result in excessive hypoglycemia, central nervous system depression, and seizures.	1	3	2
GLIMEPIRIDE Concurrent use may result in excessive hypoglycemia, central nervous system depression, and seizures.	1	3	2
GLIPIZIDE Concurrent use may result in excessive hypoglycemia, central nervous system depression, and seizures.	1	3	2
GLIQUIDONE Concurrent use may result in excessive hypoglycemia, central nervous system depression, and seizures.	1	3	2
GLYBURIDE Concurrent use may result in excessive hypoglycemia, central nervous system depression, and seizures.	1	3	2
GUANADREL Concurrent use may result in decreased antihypertensive response to guanadrel or hypertensive crisis when guanadrel is initiated in a patient already receiving phenelzine.	1	1	3
GUAR GUM Concurrent use may result in excessive hypoglycemia, central nervous system depression, and seizures.	1	3	2
HEXOPRENALINE Concurrent use may result in an increased risk of tachycardia, agitation, or hypomania.	2	2	2
IMIPRAMINE Concurrent use may result in neurotoxicity, seizures, or serotonin syndrome (hypertension, hyperthermia, myoclonus, mental status changes).	2	2	3
INSULIN Concurrent use may result in excessive hypoglycemia, central nervous system depression, and seizures.	1	3	2
IPRONIAZID Concurrent use may result in hypertensive crisis (headache, palpitation, neck stiffness).	1	1	3

Onset: 0=Unspecified 1=Rapid 2=Delayed
Severity: 1=Contraindicated 2=Major 3=Moderate 4=Minor
Evidence: 1=Excellent 2=Good 3=Fair 4=Poor

INTERACTION	ONSET	SEVERITY	EVIDENCE
ISOCARBOXAZID Concurrent use may result in hypertensive crisis (headache, palpitation, neck stiffness).	1	1	3
ISOETHARINE Concurrent use may result in an increased risk of tachycardia, agitation, or hypomania.	2	2	2
ISOMETHEPTENE Concurrent use may result in severe headache, hypertensive crisis, cardiac arrhythmias.	1	1	1
ISOPROTERENOL Concurrent use may result in increased hypertensive effects.	1	3	3
LAZABEMIDE Concurrent use may result in hypertensive crisis (headache, palpitation, neck stiffness).	1	1	3
LEVALBUTEROL Concurrent use may result in an increased risk of tachycardia, agitation, or hypomania.	2	2	2
LEVODOPA Concurrent use may result in hypertensive response.	1	1	3
LEVOMETHADYL Concurrent use may result in increased levels of levomethadyl or its active metabolites.	2	1	3
LOFEPRAMINE Concurrent use may result in neurotoxicity, seizures, or serotonin syndrome (hypertension, hyperthermia, myoclonus, mental status changes).	2	2	3
MA HUANG Concurrent use may result in increased risk for excessive phenelzine activity including headache, hyperpyrexia, arrhythmias, and hypertensive crisis.	1	2	3
MEPHENTERMINE Concurrent use may result in hypertensive crisis (headache, hyperpyrexia, hypertension).	1	1	2
MAPROTILINE Concurrent use may result in neurotoxicity, seizures.	2	1	3
MAZINDOL Concurrent use may result in hypertensive crisis.	1	1	3
MEPERIDINE Concurrent use may result in cardiovascular instability, hyperpyrexia, coma, or death.	1	1	2
METARAMINOL Concurrent use may result in hypertensive crisis (headache, hyperpyrexia, hypertension).	1	2	3
METFORMIN Concurrent use may result in excessive hypoglycemia, central nervous system depression, and seizures.	1	3	2

INTERACTION	ONSET	SEVERITY	EVIDENCE
METHAMPHETAMINE Concurrent use may result in hypertensive crisis.	1	1	3
METHOTRIMEPRAZINE Concurrent use may result in possibly prolonged effect of methotrimeprazine, with potentially increased side effects.	2	1	3
METHYLDOPA Concurrent use may result in hypertensive crisis (headache, palpitation, neck stiffness).	1	1	3
METHYLPHENIDATE Concurrent use may result in hypertensive crisis (headache, palpitation, neck stiffness).	1	1	3
MIGLITOL Concurrent use may result in excessive hypoglycemia, central nervous system depression, and seizures.	1	3	2
MIRTAZAPINE Concurrent use may result in neurotoxicity, seizures.	2	1	3
MOCLOBEMIDE Concurrent use may result in hypertensive crisis (headache, palpitation, neck stiffness).	1	1	3
MORPHINE Concurrent use may result in hypotension and exaggeration of central nervous system and respiratory depressant effects.	1	1	3
NEFAZODONE Concurrent use may result in hyperthermia, rigidity, myoclonus, seizures, fluctuations of vital signs, or mental status changes.	1	1	2
NEFOPAM Concurrent use may result in an increased risk of central nervous system excitation.	1	1	2
NIALAMIDE Concurrent use may result in hypertensive crisis (headache, palpitation, neck stiffness).	1	1	3
NOREPINEPHRINE Concurrent use may result in increased hypertensive effects.	1	1	3
NORTRIPTYLINE Concurrent use may result in neurotoxicity, seizures, or serotonin syndrome (hypertension, hyperthermia, myoclonus, mental status changes).	2	2	3
OPIPRAMOL Concurrent use may result in neurotoxicity, seizures, or serotonin syndrome (hypertension, hyperthermia, myoclonus, mental status changes).	2	1	3
OXYCODONE Concurrent use may result in anxiety, confusion and significant respiratory depressant effects or coma.	2	2	3

Onset: 0=Unspecified 1=Rapid 2=Delayed
Severity: 1=Contraindicated 2=Major 3=Moderate 4=Minor
Evidence: 1=Excellent 2=Good 3=Fair 4=Poor

INTERACTION	ONSET	SEVERITY	EVIDENCE
PARGYLINE Concurrent use may result in hypertensive crisis (headache, palpitation, neck stiffness).	1	1	3
PAROXETINE Concurrent use may result in central nervous system toxicity or serotonin syndrome (hypertension, hyperthermia, myoclonus, mental status changes).	1	1	2
PHENDIMETRAZINE Concurrent use may result in hypertensive crisis (headache, hyperpyrexia, hypertension).	1	1	2
PHENMETRAZINE Concurrent use may result in hypertensive crisis (headache, hyperpyrexia, hypertension).	1	1	2
PHENTERMINE Concurrent use may result in hypertensive crisis (headache, hyperpyrexia, hypertension).	1	1	1
PHENYLALANINE Concurrent use may result in hypertensive crisis (headache, palpitation, neck stiffness).	1	1	3
PHENYLEPHRINE Concurrent use may result in hypertensive crisis (headache, hyperpyrexia, hypertension).	1	1	2
PHENYLPROPANOLAMINE Concurrent use may result in hypertensive crisis (headache, hyperpyrexia, hypertension).	1	1	1
PIRBUTEROL Concurrent use may result in an increased risk of tachycardia, agitation, or hypomania.	2	2	2
PROCARBAZINE Concurrent use may result in hypertensive crisis (headache, palpitation, neck stiffness).	1	1	3
PROCATEROL Concurrent use may result in an increased risk of tachycardia, agitation, or hypomania.	2	2	2
PROTRIPTYLINE Concurrent use may result in neurotoxicity, seizures, or serotonin syndrome (hypertension, hyperthermia, myoclonus, mental status changes).	2	2	3
PSEUDOEPHEDRINE Concurrent use may result in hypertensive crisis (headache, hyperpyrexia, hypertension).	1	1	3
REBOXETINE Concurrent use may result in hyperthermia, rigidity, myoclonus, seizures, fluctuations of vital signs, or mental status changes.	1	2	3
RESERPINE Concurrent use may result in elevated catecholamine levels.	1	1	3

INTERACTION	ONSET	SEVERITY	EVIDENCE
RIMITEROL Concurrent use may result in an increased risk of tachycardia, agitation, or hypomania.	2	2	2
RITODRINE Concurrent use may result in an increased risk of tachycardia, agitation, or hypomania.	2	2	2
SALMETEROL Concurrent use may result in an increased risk of tachycardia, agitation, or hypomania.	2	2	2
SELEGILINE Concurrent use may result in hypertensive crisis (headache, palpitation, neck stiffness).	1	1	3
SERTRALINE Concurrent use may result in central nervous system toxicity or serotonin syndrome (hypertension, hyperthermia, myoclonus, mental status changes).	1	1	2
SIBUTRAMINE Concurrent use may result in central nervous system toxicity or serotonin syndrome (hypertension, hyperthermia, myoclonus, mental status changes).	1	1	3
SUMATRIPTAN Concurrent use may result in an increased risk of serotonin syndrome (hypertension, hyperthermia, myoclonus, mental status changes).	1	1	2
TERBUTALINE Concurrent use may result in an increased risk of tachycardia, agitation, or hypomania.	2	2	2
TOLAZAMIDE Concurrent use may result in excessive hypoglycemia, central nervous system depression, and seizures.	1	3	2
TOLBUTAMIDE Concurrent use may result in excessive hypoglycemia, central nervous system depression, and seizures.	1	3	2
TOLCAPONE Concurrent use may result in decreased catecholamine metabolism.	1	2	3
TOLOXATONE Concurrent use may result in hypertensive crisis (headache, palpitation, neck stiffness).	1	1	3
TRAMADOL Concurrent use may result in nausea, vomiting, cardiovascular collapse, respiratory depression, seizures.	1	2	3
TRANYLCYPROMINE Concurrent use may result in hypertensive crisis (headache, palpitation, neck stiffness).	1	1	3

Onset: 0=Unspecified 1=Rapid 2=Delayed
Severity: 1=Contraindicated 2=Major 3=Moderate 4=Minor
Evidence: 1=Excellent 2=Good 3=Fair 4=Poor

INTERACTION	ONSET	SEVERITY	EVIDENCE
TRIMIPRAMINE Concurrent use may result in neurotoxicity, seizures, or serotonin syndrome (hypertension, hyperthermia, myoclonus, mental status changes).	2	2	3
TROGLITAZONE Concurrent use may result in excessive hypoglycemia, central nervous system depression, and seizures.	1	3	2
TRYPTOPHAN Concurrent use may result in delirium and serotonin syndrome (hypertension, hyperthermia, myoclonus, mental status changes).	1	1	3
TULOBUTEROL Concurrent use may result in an increased risk of tachycardia, agitation, or hypomania.	2	2	2
TYRAMINE FOODS Concurrent use may result in increased blood pressure.	1	1	1
VENLAFAXINE Concurrent use may result in central nervous system toxicity or serotonin syndrome (hypertension, hyperthermia, myoclonus, mental status changes).	1	1	2

Phenobarbital

INTERACTION	ONSET	SEVERITY	EVIDENCE
ACENOCOUMAROL Concurrent use may result in decreased anticoagulant effectiveness.	2	2	2
ALPRENOLOL Concurrent use may result in decreased alprenolol effectiveness.	2	3	3
ANISINDIONE Concurrent use may result in decreased anticoagulant effectiveness.	2	2	2
BETAMETHASONE Concurrent use may result in decreased betamethasone effectiveness.	2	3	3
CHLORPROMAZINE Concurrent use may result in decreased chlorpromazine effectiveness.	1	3	3
CLOZAPINE Concurrent use may result in decreased clozapine plasma levels associated with marked worsening of psychosis.	2	3	3
CORTISONE Concurrent use may result in decreased cortisone effectiveness.	2	3	3
CYCLOSPORINE Concurrent use may result in decreased cyclosporine effectiveness.	2	3	3

INTERACTION	ONSET	SEVERITY	EVIDENCE
DEFLAZACORT Concurrent use may result in decreased corticosteroid effectiveness.	2	3	2
DEXAMETHASONE Concurrent use may result in decreased dexamethasone effectiveness.	2	3	2
DEXMETHYLPHENIDATE Concurrent use may result in an increase in phenobarbital plasma concentrations.	1	3	3
DICUMAROL Concurrent use may result in decreased anticoagulant effectiveness.	2	2	2
DIGITOXIN Concurrent use may result in decreased digitoxin levels.	2	3	3
DISOPYRAMIDE Concurrent use may result in decreased disopyramide effectiveness.	2	3	3
ETHANOL Concurrent use may result in excessive central nervous system depression.	1	3	1
ETHOSUXIMIDE Concurrent use may result in decreased ethosuximide serum concentrations.	2	3	3
FELODIPINE Concurrent use may result in decreased felodipine effectiveness.	2	3	3
FLUDROCORTISONE Concurrent use may result in decreased corticosteroid effectiveness.	2	3	2
FOSPHENYTOIN Concurrent use may result in increased or decreased phenytoin levels.	2	4	3
GRISEOFULVIN Concurrent use may result in decreased effectiveness of griseofulvin.	1	3	3
GUANFACINE Concurrent use may result in decreased guanfacine effectiveness.	2	3	3
HYDROCORTISONE Concurrent use may result in decreased corticosteroid effectiveness.	2	3	2
ITRACONAZOLE Concurrent use may result in loss of itraconazole efficacy.	2	3	3

Onset: 0=Unspecified 1=Rapid 2=Delayed
Severity: 1=Contraindicated 2=Major 3=Moderate 4=Minor
Evidence: 1=Excellent 2=Good 3=Fair 4=Poor

INTERACTION	ONSET	SEVERITY	EVIDENCE
LAMOTRIGINE Concurrent use may result in reduced lamotrigine efficacy, loss of seizure control.	2	3	2
METHOXYFLURANE Concurrent use may result in nephrotoxicity.	1	2	3
METHYLPREDNISOLONE Concurrent use may result in decreased methylprednisolone effectiveness.	2	3	2
METOPROLOL Concurrent use may result in decreased metoprolol effectiveness.	2	3	3
METRONIDAZOLE Concurrent use may result in decreased metronidazole effectiveness.	2	4	3
ORAL CONTRACEPTIVE Concurrent use may result in decreased contraceptive effectiveness.	2	2	2
PARAMETHASONE Concurrent use may result in decreased corticosteroid effectiveness.	2	3	2
PAROXETINE Concurrent use may result in reduced paroxetine effectiveness.	1	4	3
PHENINDIONE Concurrent use may result in decreased anticoagulant effectiveness.	2	2	2
PHENPROCOUMON Concurrent use may result in decreased anticoagulant effectiveness.	2	2	2
PHENYTOIN Concurrent use may result in increased or decreased phenytoin levels.	2	4	3
PREDNISOLONE Concurrent use may result in decreased prednisolone effectiveness.	2	3	2
PREDNISONE Concurrent use may result in decreased therapeutic effect of prednisone.	2	3	2
PROPRANOLOL Concurrent use may result in decreased propranolol effectiveness.	2	3	3
QUINIDINE Concurrent use may result in decreased quinidine effectiveness.	2	3	2
TACROLIMUS Concurrent use may result in decreased tacrolimus efficacy.	2	3	3

INTERACTION	ONSET	SEVERITY	EVIDENCE
TENIPOSIDE Concurrent use may result in increased teniposide clearance.	2	3	3
THEOPHYLLINE Concurrent use may result in decreased theophylline effectiveness.	2	3	2
TOPIRAMATE Concurrent use may result in a decrease in serum concentrations of topiramate.	2	3	3
TRIAMCINOLONE Concurrent use may result in decreased corticosteroid effectiveness.	2	3	2
VALERIAN Concurrent use may result in increased central nervous system depression.	1	3	3
VALPROIC ACID Concurrent use may result in phenobarbital toxicity or decreased valproic acid effectiveness.	2	3	1
VERAPAMIL Concurrent use may result in decreased verapamil effectiveness.	2	3	3
WARFARIN Concurrent use may result in decreased anticoagulant effectiveness.	2	3	1

Prochlorperazine

INTERACTION	ONSET	SEVERITY	EVIDENCE
BELLADONNA Concurrent use may result in increased manic, agitated reactions, or enhanced anticholinergic effects resulting in cardiorespiratory failure, especially in cases of belladonna overdose.	1	3	2
BENZTROPINE Concurrent use may result in decreased prochlorperazine serum concentrations, decreased prochlorperazine effectiveness, and enhanced anticholinergic effects (ileus, hyperpyrexia, sedation, dry mouth).	2	3	3
CABERGOLINE Concurrent use may result in the decreased therapeutic effect of both drugs.	1	3	3
CISAPRIDE Concurrent use may result in cardiotoxicity (QT prolongation, torsade de pointes, cardiac arrest).	1	1	3
ETHANOL Concurrent use may result in increased central nervous system depression and an increased risk of extrapyramidal reactions.	1	3	2

Onset: 0=Unspecified 1=Rapid 2=Delayed
Severity: 1=Contraindicated 2=Major 3=Moderate 4=Minor
Evidence: 1=Excellent 2=Good 3=Fair 4=Poor

INTERACTION	ONSET	SEVERITY	EVIDENCE
FOSPHENYTOIN Concurrent use may result in increased or decreased phenytoin levels and possibly reduced prochlorperazine levels.	2	4	3
GREPAFLOXACIN Concurrent use may result in an increased risk of cardiotoxicity (QT prolongation, torsade de pointes, cardiac arrest).	2	1	3
GUANETHIDINE Concurrent use may result in decreased guanethidine effectiveness.	1	3	2
HALOFANTRINE Concurrent use may result in an increased risk of cardiotoxicity (QT prolongation, torsade de pointes, cardiac arrest).	0	2	3
LEVODOPA Concurrent use may result in loss of levodopa efficacy.	1	3	2
LITHIUM Concurrent use may result in weakness, dyskinesias, increased extrapyramidal symptoms, encephalopathy, and brain damage.	2	2	1
MEPERIDINE Concurrent use may result in an increase in central nervous system and respiratory depression.	1	3	2
ORPHENADRINE Concurrent use may result in decreased prochlorperazine serum concentrations, decreased prochlorperazine effectiveness, and enhanced anticholinergic effects (ileus, hyperpyrexia, sedation, dry mouth).	2	3	3
PHENYTOIN Concurrent use may result in increased or decreased phenytoin levels and possibly reduced prochlorperazine levels.	2	4	3
PORFIMER Concurrent use may result in excessive intracellular damage in photosensitized tissues.	2	3	3
PROCYCLIDINE Concurrent use may result in decreased prochlorperazine serum concentrations, decreased prochlorperazine effectiveness, enhanced anticholinergic effects (ileus, hyperpyrexia, sedation, dry mouth).	2	3	3
TRIHEXYPHENIDYL Concurrent use may result in decreased prochlorperazine serum concentrations, decreased prochlorperazine effectiveness, and enhanced anticholinergic effects (ileus, hyperpyrexia, sedation, dry mouth).	2	3	3

Promethazine (Phenergan)

INTERACTION	ONSET	SEVERITY	EVIDENCE
BELLADONNA Concurrent use may result in increased manic, agitated reactions, or enhanced anticholinergic effects resulting in cardiorespiratory failure, especially in cases of belladonna overdose.	1	3	2
BENZTROPINE Concurrent use may result in decreased promethazine serum concentrations, decreased promethazine effectiveness, and enhanced anticholinergic effects (ileus, hyperpyrexia, sedation, dry mouth).	2	3	3
CABERGOLINE Concurrent use may result in the decreased therapeutic effect of both drugs.	1	3	3
CISAPRIDE Concurrent use may result in cardiotoxicity (QT prolongation, torsade de pointes, cardiac arrest).	1	1	3
FOSPHENYTOIN Concurrent use may result in increased or decreased phenytoin levels and possibly reduced phenothiazine levels.	2	4	3
GREPAFLOXACIN Concurrent use may result in an increased risk of cardiotoxicity (QT prolongation, torsade de pointes, cardiac arrest).	2	1	3
LITHIUM Concurrent use may result in weakness, dyskinesias, increased extrapyramidal symptoms, encephalopathy, and brain damage.	2	2	1
MEPERIDINE Concurrent use may result in an increase in central nervous system and respiratory depression.	1	3	2
ORPHENADRINE Concurrent use may result in decreased promethazine serum concentrations, decreased promethazine effectiveness, and enhanced anticholinergic effects (ileus, hyperpyrexia, sedation, dry mouth).	2	3	3
PHENYTOIN Concurrent use may result in increased or decreased phenytoin levels and possibly reduced promethazine levels.	2	4	3
PORFIMER Concurrent use may result in excessive intracellular damage in photosensitized tissues.	2	3	3

Onset: 0=Unspecified 1=Rapid 2=Delayed
Severity: 1=Contraindicated 2=Major 3=Moderate 4=Minor
Evidence: 1=Excellent 2=Good 3=Fair 4=Poor

INTERACTION	ONSET	SEVERITY	EVIDENCE
PROCYCLIDINE Concurrent use may result in decreased promethazine serum concentrations, decreased promethazine effectiveness, and enhanced anticholinergic effects (ileus, hyperpyrexia, sedation, dry mouth).	2	3	3
SPARFLOXACIN Concurrent use may result in prolongation of the QTc interval and/or torsades de pointes.	2	1	2
TRAMADOL Concurrent use may result in an increased risk of seizures.	1	2	3
TRIHEXYPHENIDYL Concurrent use may result in decreased promethazine serum concentrations, decreased promethazine effectiveness, and enhanced anticholinergic effects (ileus, hyperpyrexia, sedation, dry mouth).	2	3	3

Protriptyline (Vivactil)

INTERACTION	ONSET	SEVERITY	EVIDENCE
ACENOCOUMAROL Concurrent use may result in increased risk of bleeding.	2	3	3
AJMALINE Concurrent use may result in an increased risk of cardiotoxicity (QT prolongation, torsade de pointes, cardiac arrest).	0	2	3
AMISULPRIDE Concurrent use may result in an increased risk of cardiotoxicity (QT prolongation, torsade de pointes, cardiac arrest).	0	2	3
AMPRENAVIR Concurrent use may result in increased protriptyline serum concentrations and potential toxicity (anticholinergic effects, sedation, confusion, cardiac arrhythmias).	2	2	3
ANISINDIONE Concurrent use may result in increased risk of bleeding.	2	3	3
ASTEMIZOLE Concurrent use may result in an increased risk of cardiotoxicity (QT prolongation, torsade de pointes, cardiac arrest).	0	2	3
BEPRIDIL Concurrent use may result in an increased risk of cardiotoxicity (QT prolongation, torsade de pointes, cardiac arrest).	1	1	3
BETHANIDINE Concurrent use may result in decreased antihypertensive effectiveness.	1	3	2

INTERACTION	ONSET	SEVERITY	EVIDENCE
CARBAMAZEPINE Concurrent use may result in decreased protriptyline plasma concentrations and increased carbamazepine plasma concentrations and possible toxicity (ataxia, nystagmus, apnea, seizures, coma).	2	3	3
CIMETIDINE Concurrent use may result in protriptyline toxicity (dry mouth, blurred vision, urinary retention).	2	3	3
CISAPRIDE Concurrent use may result in cardiotoxicity (QT prolongation, torsade de pointes, cardiac arrest).	1	1	3
CLONIDINE Concurrent use may result in decreased antihypertensive effectiveness.	2	2	3
CLORGYLINE Concurrent use may result in neurotoxicity, seizures, or serotonin syndrome (hypertension, hyperthermia, myoclonus, mental status changes).	2	2	3
DICUMAROL Concurrent use may result in increased risk of bleeding.	2	3	3
DISOPYRAMIDE Concurrent use may result in an increased risk of cardiotoxicity (QT prolongation, torsade de pointes, cardiac arrest).	0	2	3
DROPERIDOL Concurrent use may result in an increased risk of cardiotoxicity (QT prolongation, torsade de pointes, cardiac arrest).	0	2	3
EPINEPHRINE Concurrent use may result in hypertension, cardiac arrhythmias, and tachycardia.	1	2	2
ETILEFRINE Concurrent use may result in hypertension, cardiac arrhythmias, and tachycardia.	1	2	2
FOSCARNET Concurrent use may result in an increased risk of cardiotoxicity (QT prolongation, torsade de pointes, cardiac arrest).	0	2	3
GREPAFLOXACIN Concurrent use may result in an increased risk of cardiotoxicity (QT prolongation, torsade de pointes, cardiac arrest).	2	1	3
GUANADREL Concurrent use may result in decreased antihypertensive effectiveness.	2	3	3

Onset: 0=Unspecified 1=Rapid 2=Delayed
Severity: 1=Contraindicated 2=Major 3=Moderate 4=Minor
Evidence: 1=Excellent 2=Good 3=Fair 4=Poor

INTERACTION	ONSET	SEVERITY	EVIDENCE
GUANETHIDINE Concurrent use may result in decreased antihypertensive effectiveness.	2	3	1
HALOFANTRINE Concurrent use may result in an increased risk of cardiotoxicity (QT prolongation, torsade de pointes, cardiac arrest).	2	2	3
HALOPERIDOL Concurrent use may result in an increased risk of cardiotoxicity (QT prolongation, torsade de pointes, cardiac arrest).	0	2	3
HYDROQUINIDINE Concurrent use may result in an increased risk of cardiotoxicity (QT prolongation, torsade de pointes, cardiac arrest).	0	2	3
IPRONIAZID Concurrent use may result in neurotoxicity, seizures, or serotonin syndrome (hypertension, hyperthermia, myoclonus, mental status changes).	2	2	3
ISOCARBOXAZID Concurrent use may result in neurotoxicity, seizures, or serotonin syndrome (hypertension, hyperthermia, myoclonus, mental status changes).	2	1	3
LEVOMETHADYL Concurrent use may result in an increased risk of cardiotoxicity (QT prolongation, torsade de pointes, cardiac arrest).	0	1	3
MESORIDAZINE Concurrent use may result in an increased risk of cardiotoxicity (QT prolongation, torsade de pointes, cardiac arrest).	0	1	3
METHOXAMINE Concurrent use may result in hypertension, cardiac arrhythmias, and tachycardia.	1	2	2
MIDODRINE Concurrent use may result in hypertension, cardiac arrhythmias, and tachycardia.	1	2	2
MOCLOBEMIDE Concurrent use may result in neurotoxicity, seizures, or serotonin syndrome (hypertension, hyperthermia, myoclonus, mental status changes).	2	2	3
NIALAMIDE Concurrent use may result in neurotoxicity, seizures, or serotonin syndrome (hypertension, hyperthermia, myoclonus, mental status changes).	2	2	3
NOREPINEPHRINE Concurrent use may result in hypertension, cardiac arrhythmias, and tachycardia.	1	2	2

INTERACTION	ONSET	SEVERITY	EVIDENCE
OXILOFRINE Concurrent use may result in hypertension, cardiac arrhythmias, and tachycardia.	1	2	2
PARGYLINE Concurrent use may result in neurotoxicity, seizures, or serotonin syndrome (hypertension, hyperthermia, myoclonus, mental status changes).	2	2	3
PAROXETINE Concurrent use may result in protriptyline toxicity (dry mouth, sedation, urinary retention).	2	3	3
PHENELZINE Concurrent use may result in neurotoxicity, seizures, or serotonin syndrome (hypertension, hyperthermia, myoclonus, mental status changes).	2	2	3
PHENINDIONE Concurrent use may result in increased risk of bleeding.	2	3	3
PHENPROCOUMON Concurrent use may result in increased risk of bleeding.	2	3	3
PHENYLEPHRINE Concurrent use may result in hypertension, cardiac arrhythmias, and tachycardia.	1	2	2
PIMOZIDE Concurrent use may result in an increased risk of cardiotoxicity (QT prolongation, torsade de pointes, cardiac arrest).	0	1	3
PIRMENOL Concurrent use may result in an increased risk of cardiotoxicity (QT prolongation, torsade de pointes, cardiac arrest).	0	2	3
PRAJMALINE Concurrent use may result in an increased risk of cardiotoxicity (QT prolongation, torsade de pointes, cardiac arrest).	0	2	3
PROCAINAMIDE Concurrent use may result in an increased risk of cardiotoxicity (QT prolongation, torsade de pointes, cardiac arrest).	0	2	3
PROCARBAZINE Concurrent use may result in neurotoxicity, seizures.	2	2	3
QUETIAPINE Concurrent use may result in an increased risk of cardiotoxicity (QT prolongation, torsade de pointes, cardiac arrest).	0	2	3

Onset: 0=Unspecified 1=Rapid 2=Delayed
Severity: 1=Contraindicated 2=Major 3=Moderate 4=Minor
Evidence: 1=Excellent 2=Good 3=Fair 4=Poor

INTERACTION	ONSET	SEVERITY	EVIDENCE
QUINIDINE Concurrent use may result in protriptyline toxicity (dry mouth, sedation) and an increased risk of cardiotoxicity (QT prolongation, torsade de pointes, cardiac arrest).	2	3	3
QUINIDINE Concurrent use may result in an increased risk of cardiotoxicity (QT prolongation, torsade de pointes, cardiac arrest).	0	2	3
RISPERIDONE Concurrent use may result in an increased risk of cardiotoxicity (QT prolongation, torsade de pointes, cardiac arrest).	0	2	3
S-ADENOSYLMETHIONINE Concurrent use may result in an increased risk of serotonin syndrome (hypertension, hyperthermia, myoclonus, mental status changes).	2	3	3
SELEGILINE Concurrent use may result in neurotoxicity, seizures, or serotonin syndrome (hypertension, hyperthermia, myoclonus, mental status changes).	2	2	3
SERTINDOLE Concurrent use may result in an increased risk of cardiotoxicity (QT prolongation, torsade de pointes, cardiac arrest).	0	2	3
SERTRALINE Concurrent use may result in modest elevations in protriptyline serum levels or possible serotonin syndrome (hypertension, hyperthermia, myoclonus, mental status changes).	2	2	3
SULTOPRIDE Concurrent use may result in an increased risk of cardiotoxicity (QT prolongation, torsade de pointes, cardiac arrest).	0	2	3
THIORIDAZINE Concurrent use may result in an increased risk of cardiotoxicity (QT prolongation, torsade de pointes, cardiac arrest).	0	1	3
TOLOXATONE Concurrent use may result in neurotoxicity, seizures, or serotonin syndrome (hypertension, hyperthermia, myoclonus, mental status changes).	2	2	3
TRAMADOL Concurrent use may result in an increased risk of seizures.	1	2	3
TRANYLCYPROMINE Concurrent use may result in neurotoxicity, seizures, or serotonin syndrome (hypertension, hyperthermia, myoclonus, mental status changes).	2	2	3

INTERACTION	ONSET	SEVERITY	EVIDENCE
WARFARIN Concurrent use may result in an increased risk of bleeding.	2	3	3
ZIPRASIDONE Concurrent use may result in an increased risk of cardiotoxicity (QT prolongation, torsade de pointes, cardiac arrest).	0	1	3
ZOTEPINE Concurrent use may result in an increased risk of cardiotoxicity (QT prolongation, torsade de pointes, cardiac arrest).	0	2	3

Quazepam (Doral)

INTERACTION	ONSET	SEVERITY	EVIDENCE
CIMETIDINE Concurrent use may result in quazepam toxicity (central nervous system depression).	1	4	3
THEOPHYLLINE Concurrent use may result in decreased quazepam effectiveness.	1	3	2

Quetiapine (Seroquel, Seroquel XR)

INTERACTION	ONSET	SEVERITY	EVIDENCE
ETHANOL Concurrent use may result in potentiation of the cognitive and motor effects of alcohol.	1	3	3

Ramelteon (Rozerem)

INTERACTION	ONSET	SEVERITY	EVIDENCE
FLUCONAZOLE Concurrent use may result in increased exposure to ramelteon with increased risk of side effects.	2	3	2
FLUVOXAMINE Concurrent use may result in profoundly increased exposure to ramelteon with increased risk of side effects.	2	2	2
KETOCONAZOLE Concurrent use may result in increased exposure to ramelteon with increased risk of side effects.	2	3	2
RIFAMPIN Concurrent use may result in decreased bioavailability of ramelteon.	0	4	2

Reserpine

INTERACTION	ONSET	SEVERITY	EVIDENCE
CLORGYLINE Concurrent use may result in elevated catecholamine levels.	1	1	3

Onset: 0=Unspecified 1=Rapid 2=Delayed
Severity: 1=Contraindicated 2=Major 3=Moderate 4=Minor
Evidence: 1=Excellent 2=Good 3=Fair 4=Poor

INTERACTION	ONSET	SEVERITY	EVIDENCE
IOBENGUANE Concurrent use may result in false-negative results of scintigraphy.	1	3	3
IPRONIAZID Concurrent use may result in elevated catecholamine levels.	1	1	3
ISOCARBOXAZID Concurrent use may result in elevated catecholamine levels.	1	1	3
MA HUANG Concurrent use may result in reduced hypotensive effect of reserpine.	1	3	3
MOCLOBEMIDE Concurrent use may result in elevated catecholamine levels.	1	1	3
NIALAMIDE Concurrent use may result in elevated catecholamine levels.	1	1	3
PARGYLINE Concurrent use may result in elevated catecholamine levels.	1	1	3
PHENELZINE Concurrent use may result in elevated catecholamine levels.	1	1	3
PROCARBAZINE Concurrent use may result in elevated catecholamine levels.	1	1	3
SELEGILINE Concurrent use may result in elevated catecholamine levels.	1	1	3
ST JOHN'S WORT Concurrent use may result in reduced reserpine effectiveness.	0	3	3
TOLOXATONE Concurrent use may result in elevated catecholamine levels.	1	1	3
TRANYLCYPROMINE Concurrent use may result in elevated catecholamine levels.	1	1	3
YOHIMBINE Concurrent use may result in reduced reserpine effectiveness.	1	3	2

Risperidone (Risperdal, Risperdal Consta, Risperdal M-Tab)

INTERACTION	ONSET	SEVERITY	EVIDENCE
DROPERIDOL Concurrent use may result in an increased risk of cardiotoxicity (QT prolongation, torsade de pointes, cardiac arrest).	0	2	3
LEVOMETHADYL Concurrent use may result in an increased risk of cardiotoxicity (QT prolongation, torsade de pointes, cardiac arrest).	2	1	3
LITHIUM Concurrent use may result in weakness, dyskinesias, increased extrapyramidal symptoms, encephalopathy, and brain damage.	2	2	1

INTERACTION	ONSET	SEVERITY	EVIDENCE
PAROXETINE Concurrent use may result in an increased risk for serotonin syndrome (hypertension, hyperthermia, myoclonus, mental status changes).	2	2	2
TRAMADOL Concurrent use may result in an increased risk of seizures.	1	2	3

Rivastigmine (Exelon)

No drug interactions have been reported by the manufacturer.

Secobarbital (Seconal)

INTERACTION	ONSET	SEVERITY	EVIDENCE
DICUMAROL Concurrent use may result in decreased anticoagulant effectiveness.	2	2	2
ETHANOL Concurrent use may result in excessive central nervous system depression.	1	3	1
FOSPHENYTOIN Concurrent use may result in increased or decreased phenytoin levels.	2	3	3
METHOXYFLURANE Concurrent use may result in nephrotoxicity.	1	3	3
ORAL CONTRACEPTIVE Concurrent use may result in decreased contraceptive effectiveness.	2	2	2
PHENYTOIN Concurrent use may result in increased or decreased phenytoin levels.	2	4	3
PREDNISOLONE Concurrent use may result in decreased therapeutic effect of prednisolone.	2	3	2
PREDNISONE Concurrent use may result in decreased therapeutic effect of prednisone.	2	3	2
THEOPHYLLINE Concurrent use may result in decreased theophylline effectiveness.	2	3	3
VALERIAN Concurrent use may result in increased central nervous system depression.	1	3	3
WARFARIN Concurrent use may result in decreased anticoagulant effectiveness.	2	3	1

Onset: 0=Unspecified 1=Rapid 2=Delayed
Severity: 1=Contraindicated 2=Major 3=Moderate 4=Minor
Evidence: 1=Excellent 2=Good 3=Fair 4=Poor

Selegiline (Emsam)

INTERACTION	ONSET	SEVERITY	EVIDENCE
DEXTROMETHORPHAN Concurrent use may result in serotonin syndrome (hypertension, hyperthermia, myoclonus, mental status changes).	1	1	2
DULOXETINE Concurrent use may result in central nervous system toxicity or serotonin syndrome (hypertension, hyperthermia, myoclonus, mental status changes).	1	1	2
ISOMETHEPTENE Concurrent use may result in severe headache, hypertensive crisis, cardiac arrhythmias.	1	1	2
LEVODOPA Concurrent use may result in hypertension or increased mortality.	2	1	2
MEPERIDINE Concurrent use may result in cardiovascular instability, hyperpyrexia, coma or serotonin syndrome (hypertension, hyperthermia, myoclonus, mental status changes).	1	1	2
METHOTRIMEPRAZINE Concurrent use may result in possibly prolonged effect of the phenothiazine, with potentially increased side effects.	2	1	2
NEFOPAM Concurrent use may result in an increased risk of central nervous system excitation.	1	1	2

Sertraline (Zoloft)

INTERACTION	ONSET	SEVERITY	EVIDENCE
ALMOTRIPTAN Concurrent use may result in weakness, hyperreflexia, and/or incoordination.	0	3	3
AMITRIPTYLINE Concurrent use may result in elevated amitriptyline serum levels or possible serotonin syndrome (hypertension, hyperthermia, myoclonus, mental status changes).	2	2	3
CARBAMAZEPINE Concurrent use may result in an increased risk of carbamazepine toxicity (ataxia, nystagmus, diplopia, headache, vomiting, apnea, seizures, coma) and decreased sertraline efficacy.	2	3	3
CIMETIDINE Concurrent use may result in elevated sertraline serum concentrations and increased risk of adverse side effects.	1	3	3
CLORGYLINE Concurrent use may result in central nervous system toxicity or serotonin syndrome (hypertension, hyperthermia, myoclonus, mental status changes).	1	1	2

INTERACTION	ONSET	SEVERITY	EVIDENCE
CLOZAPINE Concurrent use may result in an increased risk of clozapine toxicity (sedation, seizures, hypotension).	2	3	3
DEXFENFLURAMINE Concurrent use may result in serotonin syndrome (hypertension, hyperthermia, myoclonus, mental status changes).	1	2	3
DROPERIDOL Concurrent use may result in an increased risk of cardiotoxicity (QT prolongation, torsade de pointes, cardiac arrest).	1	2	3
FENFLURAMINE Concurrent use may result in serotonin syndrome (hypertension, hyperthermia, myoclonus, mental status changes).	1	2	3
FURAZOLIDONE Concurrent use may result in weakness, hyperreflexia, and incoordination.	2	1	3
HYDROXYTRYPTOPHAN Concurrent use may result in an increased risk of serotonin syndrome (hypertension, hyperthermia, myoclonus, mental status changes).	1	3	3
IPRONIAZID Concurrent use may result in central nervous system toxicity or serotonin syndrome (hypertension, hyperthermia, myoclonus, mental status changes).	1	1	2
ISOCARBOXAZID Concurrent use may result in central nervous system toxicity or serotonin syndrome (hypertension, hyperthermia, myoclonus, mental status changes).	1	1	2
LEVOMETHADYL Concurrent use may result in an increased risk of cardiotoxicity (QT prolongation, torsade de pointes, cardiac arrest).	2	1	3
MOCLOBEMIDE Concurrent use may result in central nervous system toxicity or serotonin syndrome (hypertension, hyperthermia, myoclonus, mental status changes).	1	1	2
NIALAMIDE Concurrent use may result in central nervous system toxicity or serotonin syndrome (hypertension, hyperthermia, myoclonus, mental status changes).	1	1	2
NORTRIPTYLINE Concurrent use may result in elevated nortriptyline serum levels or possible serotonin syndrome (hypertension, hyperthermia, myoclonus, mental status changes).	2	2	3

Onset: 0=Unspecified 1=Rapid 2=Delayed
Severity: 1=Contraindicated 2=Major 3=Moderate 4=Minor
Evidence: 1=Excellent 2=Good 3=Fair 4=Poor

INTERACTION	ONSET	SEVERITY	EVIDENCE
PARGYLINE Concurrent use may result in central nervous system toxicity or serotonin syndrome (hypertension, hyperthermia, myoclonus, mental status changes).	1	1	2
PHENELZINE Concurrent use may result in central nervous system toxicity or serotonin syndrome (hypertension, hyperthermia, myoclonus, mental status changes).	1	1	2
PIMOZIDE Concurrent use may result in an increase in plasma pimozide levels.	0	1	2
PROCARBAZINE Concurrent use may result in central nervous system toxicity or serotonin syndrome (hypertension, hyperthermia, myoclonus, mental status changes).	1	1	2
SELEGILINE Concurrent use may result in central nervous system toxicity or serotonin syndrome (hypertension, hyperthermia, myoclonus, mental status changes).	1	1	2
SIBUTRAMINE Concurrent use may result in an increased risk of serotonin syndrome (hypertension, hypothermia, myoclonus, mental status changes).	1	2	3
TERFENADINE Concurrent use may result in cardiotoxicity (QT prolongation, torsade de pointes, cardiac arrest).	1	2	3
TOLOXATONE Concurrent use may result in central nervous system toxicity or serotonin syndrome (hypertension, hyperthermia, myoclonus, mental status changes).	1	1	2
TRAMADOL Concurrent use may result in an increased risk of seizures and serotonin syndrome (hypertension, hyperthermia, myoclonus, mental status changes).	1	2	2
TRANYLCYPROMINE Concurrent use may result in central nervous system toxicity or serotonin syndrome (hypertension, hyperthermia, myoclonus, mental status changes).	1	1	2

Tacrine (Cognex)

INTERACTION	ONSET	SEVERITY	EVIDENCE
CIMETIDINE Concurrent use may result in tacrine toxicity (nausea, vomiting, loss of appetite).	1	4	2
FLUVOXAMINE Concurrent use may result in an increase in the plasma concentration of tacrine.	1	3	3

INTERACTION	ONSET	SEVERITY	EVIDENCE
THEOPHYLLINE Concurrent use may result in theophylline toxicity (nausea, vomiting, palpitations, seizures).	2	3	3

Temazepam (Restoril)

INTERACTION	ONSET	SEVERITY	EVIDENCE
ETHANOL Concurrent use may result in impaired psychomotor functions.	1	3	2
THEOPHYLLINE Concurrent use may result in decreased temazepam effectiveness.	1	3	2

Thioridazine

INTERACTION	ONSET	SEVERITY	EVIDENCE
ACETYLCHOLINE Concurrent use may result in an increased risk of cardiotoxicity (QT prolongation, torsade de pointes, cardiac arrest).	2	1	3
AJMALINE Concurrent use may result in an increased risk of cardiotoxicity (QT prolongation, torsade de pointes, cardiac arrest).	0	1	3
AMIODARONE Concurrent use may result in an increased risk of cardiotoxicity (QT prolongation, torsade de pointes, cardiac arrest).	0	1	3
APRINDINE Concurrent use may result in an increased risk of cardiotoxicity (QT prolongation, torsade de pointes, cardiac arrest).	0	1	3
ARSENIC TRIOXIDE Concurrent use may result in an increased risk of cardiotoxicity (QT prolongation, torsade de pointes, cardiac arrest).	0	1	3
ASTEMIZOLE Concurrent use may result in an increased risk of cardiotoxicity (QT prolongation, torsade de pointes, cardiac arrest).	0	1	3
BELLADONNA Concurrent use may result in increased manic, agitated reactions, or enhanced anticholinergic effects resulting in cardiorespiratory failure, especially in cases of belladonna overdose.	1	3	2

Onset: 0=Unspecified 1=Rapid 2=Delayed
Severity: 1=Contraindicated 2=Major 3=Moderate 4=Minor
Evidence: 1=Excellent 2=Good 3=Fair 4=Poor

INTERACTION	ONSET	SEVERITY	EVIDENCE
BENZTROPINE Concurrent use may result in decreased thioridazine serum concentrations, decreased thioridazine effectiveness, enhanced anticholinergic effects (ileus, hyperpyrexia, sedation, dry mouth).	2	3	3
CABERGOLINE Concurrent use may result in the decreased therapeutic effect of both drugs.	1	3	3
CISAPRIDE Concurrent use may result in cardiotoxicity (QT prolongation, torsade de pointes, cardiac arrest).	1	1	3
DIETHYLPROPION Concurrent use may result in an increased risk of cardiotoxicity (QT prolongation, torsade de pointes, cardiac arrest).	2	1	3
DROPERIDOL Concurrent use may result in an increased risk of cardiotoxicity (QT prolongation, torsade de pointes, cardiac arrest).	0	1	3
DULOXETINE Concurrent use may result in increased thioridazine serum concentrations and risk of cardiac arrhythmia.	0	1	2
ETHANOL Concurrent use may result in increased central nervous system depression and an increased risk of extrapyramidal reactions.	1	3	2
FLUOXETINE Concurrent use may result in an increased risk of cardiotoxicity (QT prolongation, torsade de pointes, cardiac arrest).	1	1	3
FLUVOXAMINE Concurrent use may result in an increased risk of thioridazine toxicity, cardiotoxicity (QT prolongation, torsade de pointes, cardiac arrest).	1	1	3
FOSPHENYTOIN Concurrent use may result in increased or decreased phenytoin levels and possibly reduced thioridazine levels.	2	4	3
GEMIFLOXACIN Concurrent use may result in an increased risk of cardiotoxicity (QT prolongation, torsades de pointes, cardiac arrest).	0	1	2
GREPAFLOXACIN Concurrent use may result in an increased risk of cardiotoxicity (QT prolongation, torsade de pointes, cardiac arrest).	2	1	3
HALOFANTRINE Concurrent use may result in an increased risk of cardiotoxicity (QT prolongation, torsade de pointes, cardiac arrest).	0	1	3

INTERACTION	ONSET	SEVERITY	EVIDENCE
IOPAMIDOL Concurrent use may result in an increased risk of cardiotoxicity (QT prolongation, torsade de pointes, cardiac arrest).	2	1	3
KETANSERIN Concurrent use may result in an increased risk of cardiotoxicity (QT prolongation, torsade de pointes, cardiac arrest).	2	1	3
LEVODOPA Concurrent use may result in loss of levodopa efficacy.	1	3	2
LEVOMETHADYL Concurrent use may result in an increased risk of cardiotoxicity (QT prolongation, torsade de pointes, cardiac arrest).	0	1	3
LITHIUM Concurrent use may result in weakness, dyskinesias, increased extrapyramidal symptoms, encephalopathy, and brain damage.	2	2	1
LUBELUZOLE Concurrent use may result in an increased risk of cardiotoxicity (QT prolongation, torsade de pointes, cardiac arrest).	2	1	3
MEPERIDINE Concurrent use may result in an increase in central nervous system and respiratory depression.	1	3	2
ORPHENADRINE Concurrent use may result in decreased thioridazine serum concentrations, decreased thioridazine effectiveness, enhanced anticholinergic effects (ileus, hyperpyrexia, sedation, dry mouth).	2	3	3
PAROXETINE Concurrent use may result in an increased risk of thioridazine toxicity, cardiotoxicity (QT prolongation, torsade de pointes, cardiac arrest).	1	1	3
PENTAMIDINE Concurrent use may result in an increased risk of cardiotoxicity (QT prolongation, torsade de pointes, cardiac arrest).	0	1	3
PHENYTOIN Concurrent use may result in increased or decreased phenytoin levels and possibly reduced thioridazine levels.	2	4	3
PINDOLOL Concurrent use may result in an increased risk of thioridazine toxicity, cardiotoxicity (QT prolongation, torsades de pointes, cardiac arrest).	2	1	2

Onset: 0=Unspecified 1=Rapid 2=Delayed
Severity: 1=Contraindicated 2=Major 3=Moderate 4=Minor
Evidence: 1=Excellent 2=Good 3=Fair 4=Poor

INTERACTION	ONSET	SEVERITY	EVIDENCE
PORFIMER Concurrent use may result in excessive intracellular damage in photosensitized tissues.	2	3	3
PROBUCOL Concurrent use may result in an increased risk of cardiotoxicity (QT prolongation, torsade de pointes, cardiac arrest).	2	1	3
PROCATEROL Concurrent use may result in an increased risk of cardiotoxicity (QT prolongation, torsade de pointes, cardiac arrest).	2	1	3
PROCYCLIDINE Concurrent use may result in decreased thioridazine serum concentrations, decreased thioridazine effectiveness, enhanced anticholinergic effects (ileus, hyperpyrexia, sedation, dry mouth).	2	3	3
PROPRANOLOL Concurrent use may result in an increased risk of thioridazine toxicity, cardiotoxicity (QT prolongation, torsade de pointes, cardiac arrest).	2	1	3
PROTIRELIN Concurrent use may result in decreased TSH response.	2	3	3
ROXITHROMYCIN Concurrent use may result in an increased risk of cardiotoxicity (QT prolongation, torsade de pointes, cardiac arrest).	2	1	3
SEMATILIDE Concurrent use may result in an increased risk of cardiotoxicity (QT prolongation, torsade de pointes, cardiac arrest).	0	1	3
SPARFLOXACIN Concurrent use may result in prolongation of the QTc interval and/or torsade de pointes.	2	1	3
SPIRAMYCIN Concurrent use may result in an increased risk of cardiotoxicity (QT prolongation, torsade de pointes, cardiac arrest).	0	1	3
TERFENADINE Concurrent use may result in an increased risk of cardiotoxicity (QT prolongation, torsade de pointes, cardiac arrest).	2	1	3
TRAMADOL Concurrent use may result in an increased risk of seizures.	1	2	3
TRIHEXYPHENIDYL Concurrent use may result in decreased thioridazine serum concentrations, decreased thioridazine effectiveness, enhanced anticholinergic effects (ileus, hyperpyrexia, sedation, dry mouth).	2	3	3

INTERACTION	ONSET	SEVERITY	EVIDENCE
ZIPRASIDONE Concurrent use may result in an increased risk of cardiotoxicity (QT prolongation, torsade de pointes, cardiac arrest).	0	1	3

Thiothixene (Navane)

INTERACTION	ONSET	SEVERITY	EVIDENCE
CABERGOLINE Concurrent use may result in the decreased therapeutic effect of both drugs.	1	3	3
LITHIUM Concurrent use may result in weakness, dyskinesias, increased extrapyramidal symptoms, encephalopathy, and brain damage.	2	2	1
TRAMADOL Concurrent use may result in an increased risk of seizures.	1	2	3

Tranylcypromine (Parnate)

INTERACTION	ONSET	SEVERITY	EVIDENCE
ACARBOSE Concurrent use may result in excessive hypoglycemia, central nervous system depression, and seizures.	1	3	2
ACETOHEXAMIDE Concurrent use may result in excessive hypoglycemia, central nervous system depression, and seizures.	1	3	2
ALBUTEROL Concurrent use may result in an increased risk of tachycardia, agitation, or hypomania.	2	2	2
ALTRETAMINE Concurrent use may result in an increased risk of severe orthostatic hypotension.	2	2	3
AMITRIPTYLINE Concurrent use may result in neurotoxicity, seizures, or serotonin syndrome (hypertension, hyperthermia, myoclonus, mental status changes).	2	1	3
AMOXAPINE Concurrent use may result in neurotoxicity, seizures, or serotonin syndrome (hypertension, hyperthermia, myoclonus, mental status changes).	2	2	3
AMPHETAMINE Concurrent use may result in hypertensive crisis (headache, hyperpyrexia, hypertension).	1	1	2
APRACLONIDINE Concurrent use may result in potentiation of tranylcypromine effects.	1	1	3

Onset: 0=Unspecified 1=Rapid 2=Delayed
Severity: 1=Contraindicated 2=Major 3=Moderate 4=Minor
Evidence: 1=Excellent 2=Good 3=Fair 4=Poor

INTERACTION	ONSET	SEVERITY	EVIDENCE
ATOMOXETINE Concurrent use may result in an increased risk of serotonin syndrome (hypertension, hyperthermia, myoclonus, mental status changes).	0	1	3
BAMBUTEROL Concurrent use may result in an increased risk of tachycardia, agitation, or hypomania.	2	2	2
BENFLUOREX Concurrent use may result in excessive hypoglycemia, central nervous system depression, and seizures.	1	3	2
BENZPHETAMINE Concurrent use may result in hypertensive crisis (headache, hyperpyrexia, hypertension).	1	1	2
BITOLTEROL Concurrent use may result in an increased risk of tachycardia, agitation, or hypomania.	2	2	2
BROXATEROL Concurrent use may result in an increased risk of tachycardia, agitation, or hypomania.	2	2	2
BUPROPION Concurrent use may result in bupropion toxicity (seizures, agitation, psychotic changes).	1	1	3
BUSPIRONE Concurrent use may result in hypertensive crisis.	1	1	3
CARBAMAZEPINE Concurrent use may result in hypertensive urgency, hyperpyrexia, and seizures.	1	1	3
CHLORPROPAMIDE Concurrent use may result in excessive hypoglycemia, central nervous system depression, and seizures.	1	3	2
CITALOPRAM Concurrent use may result in central nervous system toxicity or serotonin syndrome (hypertension, hyperthermia, myoclonus, mental status changes).	1	1	3
CLENBUTEROL Concurrent use may result in an increased risk of tachycardia, agitation, or hypomania.	2	2	2
CLOMIPRAMINE Concurrent use may result in neurotoxicity, seizures, or serotonin syndrome (hypertension, hyperthermia, myoclonus, mental status changes).	2	2	3
CLOVOXAMINE Concurrent use may result in central nervous system toxicity or serotonin syndrome (hypertension, hyperthermia, myoclonus, mental status changes).	1	1	3
CYCLOBENZAPRINE Concurrent use may result in hypertensive crises (headache, hyperpyrexia, hypertension) or severe convulsive seizures.	1	1	3

INTERACTION	ONSET	SEVERITY	EVIDENCE
CYPROHEPTADINE Concurrent use may result in prolonged and intensified anticholinergic effects.	2	1	3
DESIPRAMINE Concurrent use may result in neurotoxicity, seizures, or serotonin syndrome (hypertension, hyperthermia, myoclonus, mental status changes).	2	2	3
DEXFENFLURAMINE Concurrent use may result in central nervous system toxicity or serotonin syndrome (hypertension, hyperthermia, myoclonus, mental status changes).	1	1	3
DEXMETHYLPHENIDATE Concurrent use may result in hypertensive crisis (headache, palpitation, neck stiffness).	1	1	3
DEXTROAMPHETAMINE Concurrent use may result in hypertensive crisis (headache, hyperpyrexia, hypertension).	1	1	3
DEXTROMETHORPHAN Concurrent use may result in an increased risk of serotonin syndrome (hypertension, hyperthermia, myoclonus, mental status changes).	1	1	3
DIETHYLPROPION Concurrent use may result in hypertensive crisis (headache, hyperpyrexia, hypertension).	1	1	2
DOPAMINE Concurrent use may result in hypertensive crisis (headache, hyperpyrexia, hypertension).	1	1	1
DOTHIEPIN Concurrent use may result in neurotoxicity, seizures, or serotonin syndrome (hypertension, hyperthermia, myoclonus, mental status changes).	2	2	3
DOXEPIN Concurrent use may result in neurotoxicity, seizures, or serotonin syndrome (hypertension, hyperthermia, myoclonus, mental status changes).	2	2	3
DROPERIDOL Concurrent use may result in an increased risk of cardiotoxicity (QT prolongation, torsade de pointes, cardiac arrest).	1	2	3
DULOXETINE Concurrent use may result in central nervous system toxicity or serotonin syndrome (hypertension, hyperthermia, myoclonus, mental status changes).	1	1	2
ENTACAPONE Concurrent use may result in decreased catecholamine metabolism.	1	2	3

Onset: 0=Unspecified 1=Rapid 2=Delayed
Severity: 1=Contraindicated 2=Major 3=Moderate 4=Minor
Evidence: 1=Excellent 2=Good 3=Fair 4=Poor

INTERACTION	ONSET	SEVERITY	EVIDENCE
EPHEDRINE Concurrent use may result in hypertensive crisis (headache, hyperpyrexia, hypertension).	1	2	3
EPINEPHRINE Concurrent use may result in increased hypertensive effects.	1	3	3
ESCITALOPRAM Concurrent use may result in central nervous system toxicity or serotonin syndrome (hypertension, hyperthermia, myoclonus, mental status changes).	1	1	3
FEMOXETINE Concurrent use may result in central nervous system toxicity or serotonin syndrome (hypertension, hyperthermia, myoclonus, mental status changes).	1	1	3
FENFLURAMINE Concurrent use may result in serotonin syndrome (hypertension, hyperthermia, myoclonus, mental status changes).	1	1	3
FENOTEROL Concurrent use may result in an increased risk of tachycardia, agitation, or hypomania.	2	2	2
FLUOXETINE Concurrent use may result in central nervous system toxicity or serotonin syndrome (hypertension, hyperthermia, myoclonus, mental status changes).	1	1	2
FLUVOXAMINE Concurrent use may result in central nervous system toxicity or serotonin syndrome (hypertension, hyperthermia, myoclonus, mental status changes).	1	2	2
FORMOTEROL Concurrent use may result in an increased risk of tachycardia, agitation, or hypomania.	2	2	2
FURAZOLIDONE Concurrent use may result in an increased risk of a hypertensive crisis or convulsive seizures.	1	1	3
GLICLAZIDE Concurrent use may result in excessive hypoglycemia, central nervous system depression, and seizures.	1	3	2
GLIMEPIRIDE Concurrent use may result in excessive hypoglycemia, central nervous system depression, and seizures.	1	3	2
GLIPIZIDE Concurrent use may result in excessive hypoglycemia, central nervous system depression, and seizures.	1	3	2
GLIQUIDONE Concurrent use may result in excessive hypoglycemia, central nervous system depression, and seizures.	1	3	2

INTERACTION	ONSET	SEVERITY	EVIDENCE
GLYBURIDE Concurrent use may result in excessive hypoglycemia, central nervous system depression, and seizures.	1	3	2
GUANADREL Concurrent use may result in decreased antihypertensive response to guanadrel or hypertensive crisis when guanadrel is initiated in a patient already receiving tranylcypromine therapy.	1	1	3
GUANETHIDINE Concurrent use may result in decreased antihypertensive response to guanethidine or hypertensive crisis when guanethidine is initiated in a patient already receiving tranylcypromine therapy.	1	1	3
GUAR GUM Concurrent use may result in excessive hypoglycemia, central nervous system depression, and seizures.	1	3	2
HEXOPRENALINE Concurrent use may result in an increased risk of tachycardia, agitation, or hypomania.	2	2	2
IMIPRAMINE Concurrent use may result in neurotoxicity, seizures, or serotonin syndrome (hypertension, hyperthermia, myoclonus, mental status changes).	2	2	3
INSULIN Concurrent use may result in excessive hypoglycemia, central nervous system depression, and seizures.	1	3	2
INSULIN LISPRO, HUMAN Concurrent use may result in excessive hypoglycemia, central nervous system depression, and seizures.	1	3	2
ISOCARBOXAZID Concurrent use may result in an increased risk of a hypertensive crisis or convulsive seizures.	1	1	3
ISOETHARINE Concurrent use may result in an increased risk of tachycardia, agitation, or hypomania.	2	2	2
ISOMETHEPTENE Concurrent use may result in severe headache, hypertensive crisis, cardiac arrhythmias.	1	1	1
ISOPROTERENOL Concurrent use may result in increased hypertensive effects.	1	3	3
LEVALBUTEROL Concurrent use may result in an increased risk of tachycardia, agitation, or hypomania.	2	2	2
LEVODOPA Concurrent use may result in hypertensive crisis.	1	1	3

Onset: 0=Unspecified 1=Rapid 2=Delayed
Severity: 1=Contraindicated 2=Major 3=Moderate 4=Minor
Evidence: 1=Excellent 2=Good 3=Fair 4=Poor

INTERACTION	ONSET	SEVERITY	EVIDENCE
LEVOMETHADYL Concurrent use may result in increased levels of levomethadyl or its active metabolites.	2	1	3
LOFEPRAMINE Concurrent use may result in neurotoxicity, seizures, or serotonin syndrome (hypertension, hyperthermia, myoclonus, mental status changes).	2	2	3
MA HUANG Concurrent use may result in increased risk for excessive tranylcypromine activity including headache, hyperpyrexia, arrhythmias, and hypertensive crisis.	1	2	3
MAPROTILINE Concurrent use may result in neurotoxicity, seizures.	2	1	3
MAZINDOL Concurrent use may result in hypertensive crisis.	1	1	3
MEPERIDINE Concurrent use may result in cardiovascular instability, hyperpyrexia, coma.	1	1	2
MEPHENTERMINE Concurrent use may result in hypertensive crisis (headache, hyperpyrexia, hypertension).	1	1	2
METARAMINOL Concurrent use may result in hypertensive crisis (headache, hyperpyrexia, hypertension).	1	2	3
METFORMIN Concurrent use may result in excessive hypoglycemia, central nervous system depression, and seizures.	1	3	2
METHAMPHETAMINE Concurrent use may result in hypertensive crisis.	1	1	3
METHOTRIMEPRAZINE Concurrent use may result in possibly prolonged effect of the methotrimeprazine, with potentially increased side effects.	2	1	3
METHOXAMINE Concurrent use may result in hypertensive crisis (headache, hyperpyrexia, hypertension).	1	2	3
METHYLDOPA Concurrent use may result in hypertensive crisis (headache, palpitation, neck stiffness).	1	1	3
METHYLPHENIDATE Concurrent use may result in hypertensive crisis (headache, palpitation, neck stiffness).	1	1	3
MIGLITOL Concurrent use may result in excessive hypoglycemia, central nervous system depression, and seizures.	1	3	2
MIRTAZAPINE Concurrent use may result in neurotoxicity, seizures.	2	1	3

INTERACTION	ONSET	SEVERITY	EVIDENCE
MORPHINE Concurrent use may result in hypotension and exaggeration of central nervous system and respiratory depressant effects.	1	1	3
NEFAZODONE Concurrent use may result in hyperthermia, rigidity, myoclonus, seizures, fluctuations of vital signs, or mental status changes.	1	2	2
NEFOPAM Concurrent use may result in an increased risk of central nervous system excitation.	1	1	2
NOREPINEPHRINE Concurrent use may result in increased hypertensive effects.	1	3	3
NORTRIPTYLINE Concurrent use may result in neurotoxicity, seizures, or serotonin syndrome (hypertension, hyperthermia, myoclonus, mental status changes).	2	2	3
OPIPRAMOL Concurrent use may result in neurotoxicity, seizures, or serotonin syndrome (hypertension, hyperthermia, myoclonus, mental status changes).	2	1	3
OXYCODONE Concurrent use may result in anxiety, confusion and significant respiratory depressant effects or coma.	2	2	3
PARGYLINE Concurrent use may result in an increased risk of a hypertensive crisis or convulsive seizures.	1	1	3
PAROXETINE Concurrent use may result in central nervous system toxicity or serotonin syndrome (hypertension, hyperthermia, myoclonus, mental status changes).	1	1	2
PHENDIMETRAZINE Concurrent use may result in hypertensive crisis (headache, hyperpyrexia, hypertension).	1	1	2
PHENELZINE Concurrent use may result in hypertensive crisis (headache, palpitation, neck stiffness).	1	1	3
PHENMETRAZINE Concurrent use may result in hypertensive crisis (headache, hyperpyrexia, hypertension).	1	1	2
PHENTERMINE Concurrent use may result in hypertensive crisis (headache, hyperpyrexia, hypertension).	1	1	1
PHENYLEPHRINE Concurrent use may result in hypertensive crisis (headache, hyperpyrexia, hypertension).	1	1	3

Onset: 0=Unspecified 1=Rapid 2=Delayed
Severity: 1=Contraindicated 2=Major 3=Moderate 4=Minor
Evidence: 1=Excellent 2=Good 3=Fair 4=Poor

INTERACTION	ONSET	SEVERITY	EVIDENCE
PHENYLPROPANOLAMINE Concurrent use may result in hypertensive crisis (headache, hyperpyrexia, hypertension).	1	1	3
PIRBUTEROL Concurrent use may result in an increased risk of tachycardia, agitation, or hypomania.	2	2	2
PROCARBAZINE Concurrent use may result in an increased risk of hypertensive crisis or convulsive seizures.	1	1	3
PROCATEROL Concurrent use may result in an increased risk of tachycardia, agitation, or hypomania.	2	2	2
PROTRIPTYLINE Concurrent use may result in neurotoxicity, seizures, or serotonin syndrome (hypertension, hyperthermia, myoclonus, mental status changes).	2	2	3
PSEUDOEPHEDRINE Concurrent use may result in severe hypertension, hyperpyrexia, headache.	1	1	3
REBOXETINE Concurrent use may result in hyperthermia, rigidity, myoclonus, seizures, fluctuations of vital signs, or mental status changes.	1	2	3
RESERPINE Concurrent use may result in elevated catecholamine levels.	1	1	3
RIMITEROL Concurrent use may result in an increased risk of tachycardia, agitation, or hypomania.	2	2	2
RITODRINE Concurrent use may result in an increased risk of tachycardia, agitation, or hypomania.	2	2	2
RIZATRIPTAN Concurrent use may result in serotonin syndrome (hypertension, hyperthermia, myoclonus, mental status changes).	2	1	3
SALMETEROL Concurrent use may result in an increased risk of tachycardia, agitation, or hypomania.	2	2	2
SERTRALINE Concurrent use may result in central nervous system toxicity or serotonin syndrome (hypertension, hyperthermia, myoclonus, mental status changes).	1	1	2
SIBUTRAMINE Concurrent use may result in central nervous system toxicity or serotonin syndrome (hypertension, hyperthermia, myoclonus, mental status changes).	1	1	3

INTERACTION	ONSET	SEVERITY	EVIDENCE
SUMATRIPTAN Concurrent use may result in an increased risk of serotonin syndrome (hypertension, hyperthermia, myoclonus, mental status changes).	1	1	3
SUMATRIPTAN Concurrent use may result in serotonin syndrome (hypertension, hyperthermia, myoclonus, mental status changes).	1	1	2
TERBUTALINE Concurrent use may result in an increased risk of tachycardia, agitation, or hypomania.	2	2	2
TOLAZAMIDE Concurrent use may result in excessive hypoglycemia, central nervous system depression, and seizures.	1	3	2
TOLBUTAMIDE Concurrent use may result in excessive hypoglycemia, central nervous system depression, and seizures.	1	3	2
TOLCAPONE Concurrent use may result in decreased catecholamine metabolism.	1	2	3
TRAMADOL Concurrent use may result in nausea, vomiting, cardiovascular collapse, respiratory depression, seizures.	1	2	3
TRIMIPRAMINE Concurrent use may result in neurotoxicity, seizures, or serotonin syndrome (hypertension, hyperthermia, myoclonus, mental status changes).	2	2	3
TROGLITAZONE Concurrent use may result in excessive hypoglycemia, central nervous system depression, and seizures.	1	3	2
TRYPTOPHAN Concurrent use may result in an increased risk of hypertension, memory impairment, and disorientation.	1	1	3
TULOBUTEROL Concurrent use may result in an increased risk of tachycardia, agitation, or hypomania.	2	2	2
TYRAMINE FOODS Concurrent use may result in increased blood pressure.	1	1	1
VENLAFAXINE Concurrent use may result in central nervous system toxicity or serotonin syndrome (hypertension, hyperthermia, myoclonus, mental status changes).	1	1	2
ZOLMITRIPTAN Concurrent use may result in serotonin syndrome (hypertension, hyperthermia, myoclonus, mental status changes).	2	1	3

Onset: 0=Unspecified 1=Rapid 2=Delayed
Severity: 1=Contraindicated 2=Major 3=Moderate 4=Minor
Evidence: 1=Excellent 2=Good 3=Fair 4=Poor

Trazodone (Desyrel)

INTERACTION	ONSET	SEVERITY	EVIDENCE
DROPERIDOL Concurrent use may result in an increased risk of cardiotoxicity (QT prolongation, torsade de pointes, cardiac arrest).	1	2	3
FLUOXETINE Concurrent use may result in trazodone toxicity (sedation, dry mouth, urinary retention) or serotonin syndrome (hypertension, hyperthermia, myoclonus, mental status changes).	2	2	3
FOOD Concurrent use may result in increased time to peak levels.	1	4	2

Triazolam (Halcion)

INTERACTION	ONSET	SEVERITY	EVIDENCE
AMPRENAVIR Concurrent use may result in an increased risk of triazolam toxicity (excessive sedation, confusion).	1	1	3
AZITHROMYCIN Concurrent use may result in decreased clearance of triazolam and increased pharmacologic effect of triazolam.	0	4	3
CIMETIDINE Concurrent use may result in triazolam toxicity (excessive sedation, confusion).	1	4	3
CLARITHROMYCIN Concurrent use may result in increased triazolam toxicity (central nervous system depression, ataxia, lethargy).	2	3	3
DEHYDROEPIANDROSTERONE Concurrent use may result in increased central nervous system depression.	1	3	2
EFAVIRENZ Concurrent use may result in an increased risk of triazolam toxicity (excessive sedation, confusion).	2	1	3
ETHANOL Concurrent use may result in increased sedation.	1	3	1
FLUCONAZOLE Concurrent use may result in increased triazolam serum concentrations and potential triazolam toxicity (sedation, slurred speech, central nervous system depression).	2	1	3
FLUVOXAMINE Concurrent use may result in elevated serum triazolam concentrations.	2	3	3
FOSAMPRENAVIR Concurrent use may result in an increased risk of triazolam toxicity (excessive sedation, confusion, respiratory depression).	1	1	2

INTERACTION	ONSET	SEVERITY	EVIDENCE
GRAPEFRUIT JUICE Concurrent use may result in increased bioavailability of triazolam.	1	4	3
INDINAVIR Concurrent use may result in an increased risk of serious triazolam adverse effects (excessive or prolonged sedation).	1	1	3
ITRACONAZOLE Concurrent use may result in increased triazolam serum concentrations and potential triazolam toxicity (sedation, slurred speech, central nervous system depression).	2	1	3
JOSAMYCIN Concurrent use may result in increased triazolam toxicity (central nervous system depression, ataxia, lethargy).	2	3	3
KETOCONAZOLE Concurrent use may result in increased triazolam serum concentrations and potential triazolam toxicity (sedation, slurred speech, central nervous system depression).	2	1	3
MIBEFRADIL Concurrent use may result in an increased risk of triazolam toxicity (excessive sedation, confusion).	1	2	3
NELFINAVIR Concurrent use may result in prolonged and excessive sedation.	2	1	2
NEFAZODONE Concurrent use may result in psychomotor impairment and excessive sedation.	1	3	2
OMEPRAZOLE Concurrent use may result in triazolam toxicity (central nervous system depression, ataxia, lethargy).	2	3	3
RIFAMPIN Concurrent use may result in loss of triazolam efficacy.	1	3	3
RITONAVIR Concurrent use may result in an increased risk of extreme sedation and respiratory depression.	2	1	3
ROXITHROMYCIN Concurrent use may result in increased triazolam toxicity (central nervous system depression, ataxia, lethargy).	2	3	3
SAQUINAVIR Concurrent use may result in an increased risk of triazolam toxicity (excessive sedation, respiratory depression).	1	1	3
THEOPHYLLINE Concurrent use may result in decreased triazolam effectiveness.	1	3	2

Onset: 0=Unspecified 1=Rapid 2=Delayed
Severity: 1=Contraindicated 2=Major 3=Moderate 4=Minor
Evidence: 1=Excellent 2=Good 3=Fair 4=Poor

INTERACTION	ONSET	SEVERITY	EVIDENCE
TROLEANDOMYCIN Concurrent use may result in increased triazolam toxicity (central nervous system depression, ataxia, lethargy).	2	3	3

Trifluoperazine

INTERACTION	ONSET	SEVERITY	EVIDENCE
BELLADONNA Concurrent use may result in increased manic, agitated reactions, or enhanced anticholinergic effects resulting in cardiorespiratory failure, especially in cases of belladonna overdose.	1	3	2
BENZTROPINE Concurrent use may result in decreased trifluoperazine serum concentrations, decreased trifluoperazine effectiveness, enhanced anticholinergic effects (ileus, hyperpyrexia, sedation, dry mouth).	2	3	3
CABERGOLINE Concurrent use may result in the decreased therapeutic effect of both drugs.	1	3	3
CISAPRIDE Concurrent use may result in cardiotoxicity (QT prolongation, torsade de pointes, cardiac arrest).	1	1	3
DROPERIDOL Concurrent use may result in an increased risk of cardiotoxicity (QT prolongation, torsade de pointes, cardiac arrest).	0	2	3
ETHANOL Concurrent use may result in increased central nervous system depression and an increased risk of extrapyramidal reactions.	1	3	2
FOSPHENYTOIN Concurrent use may result in increased or decreased phenytoin levels and possibly reduced trifluoperazine levels.	2	4	3
GREPAFLOXACIN Concurrent use may result in an increased risk of cardiotoxicity (QT prolongation, torsade de pointes, cardiac arrest).	2	1	3
HALOFANTRINE Concurrent use may result in an increased risk of cardiotoxicity (QT prolongation, torsade de pointes, cardiac arrest).	0	2	3
LEVODOPA Concurrent use may result in loss of levodopa efficacy.	1	3	2
LEVOMETHADYL Concurrent use may result in an increased risk of cardiotoxicity (QT prolongation, torsade de pointes, cardiac arrest).	2	2	3

INTERACTION	ONSET	SEVERITY	EVIDENCE
LITHIUM Concurrent use may result in weakness, dyskinesias, increased extrapyramidal symptoms, encephalopathy, and brain damage.	2	2	1
MEPERIDINE Concurrent use may result in an increase in central nervous system and respiratory depression.	1	3	2
ORPHENADRINE Concurrent use may result in decreased trifluoperazine serum concentrations, decreased trifluoperazine effectiveness, enhanced anticholinergic effects (ileus, hyperpyrexia, sedation, dry mouth).	2	3	3
PHENYTOIN Concurrent use may result in increased or decreased phenytoin levels and possibly reduced trifluoperazine levels.	2	4	3
PORFIMER Concurrent use may result in excessive intracellular damage in photosensitized tissues.	2	3	3
PROCYCLIDINE Concurrent use may result in decreased trifluoperazine serum concentrations, decreased trifluoperazine effectiveness, enhanced anticholinergic effects (ileus, hyperpyrexia, sedation, dry mouth).	2	3	3
TRAMADOL Concurrent use may result in an increased risk of seizures.	1	2	3
TRIHEXYPHENIDYL Concurrent use may result in decreased trifluoperazine serum concentrations, decreased trifluoperazine effectiveness, enhanced anticholinergic effects (ileus, hyperpyrexia, sedation, dry mouth).	2	3	3
VENLAFAXINE Concurrent use may result in an increased risk of neuroleptic malignant syndrome and an increased risk of cardiotoxicity (QT prolongation, torsades de pointes, cardiac arrest)	1	1	2

Trihexyphenidyl

INTERACTION	ONSET	SEVERITY	EVIDENCE
ACETOPHENAZINE Concurrent use may result in decreased phenothiazine serum concentrations, decreased phenothiazine effectiveness, enhanced anticholinergic effects (ileus, hyperpyrexia, sedation, dry mouth).	2	3	3
BELLADONNA Concurrent use may result in excessive anticholinergic activity (severe dry mouth, constipation, decreased urination, excessive sedation, blurred vision).	1	4	3

Onset: 0=Unspecified 1=Rapid 2=Delayed
Severity: 1=Contraindicated 2=Major 3=Moderate 4=Minor
Evidence: 1=Excellent 2=Good 3=Fair 4=Poor

INTERACTION	ONSET	SEVERITY	EVIDENCE
BELLADONNA ALKALOIDS Concurrent use may result in excessive anticholinergic activity (severe dry mouth, constipation, decreased urination, excessive sedation, blurred vision).	1	4	3
BETEL NUT Concurrent use may result in reduced anticholinergic effect of trihexyphenidyl.	2	3	2
CHLORPROMAZINE Concurrent use may result in decreased phenothiazine s erum concentrations, decreased phenothiazine effectiveness, enhanced anticholinergic effects (ileus, hyperpyrexia, sedation, dry mouth).	2	3	2
CISAPRIDE Concurrent use may result in loss of cisapride efficacy.	2	4	3
ETHOPROPAZINE Concurrent use may result in decreased phenothiazine serum concentrations, decreased phenothiazine effectiveness, enhanced anticholinergic effects (ileus, hyperpyrexia, sedation, dry mouth).	2	3	3
FLUPHENAZINE Concurrent use may result in decreased phenothiazine serum concentrations, decreased phenothiazine effectiveness, enhanced anticholinergic effects (ileus, hyperpyrexia, sedation, dry mouth).	2	3	3
HALOPERIDOL Concurrent use may result in excessive anticholinergic effects (sedation, constipation, dry mouth).	2	3	2
MESORIDAZINE Concurrent use may result in decreased phenothiazine serum concentrations, decreased phenothiazine effectiveness, enhanced anticholinergic effects (ileus, hyperpyrexia, sedation, dry mouth).	2	3	3
METHOTRIMEPRAZINE Concurrent use may result in decreased phenothiazine serum concentrations, decreased phenothiazine effectiveness, enhanced anticholinergic effects (ileus, hyperpyrexia, sedation, dry mouth).	2	3	3
PERPHENAZINE Concurrent use may result in decreased phenothiazine serum concentrations, decreased phenothiazine effectiveness, enhanced anticholinergic effects (ileus, hyperpyrexia, sedation, dry mouth).	2	3	2
PIPOTIAZINE Concurrent use may result in decreased phenothiazine serum concentrations, decreased phenothiazine effectiveness, enhanced anticholinergic effects (ileus, hyperpyrexia, sedation, dry mouth).	2	3	3

INTERACTION	ONSET	SEVERITY	EVIDENCE
PROCHLORPERAZINE Concurrent use may result in decreased phenothiazine serum concentrations, decreased phenothiazine effectiveness, and enhanced anticholinergic effects (ileus, hyperpyrexia, sedation, dry mouth).	2	3	3
PROMAZINE Concurrent use may result in decreased phenothiazine serum concentrations, decreased phenothiazine effectiveness, enhanced anticholinergic effects (ileus, hyperpyrexia, sedation, dry mouth).	2	3	3
PROMETHAZINE Concurrent use may result in decreased phenothiazine serum concentrations, decreased phenothiazine effectiveness, and enhanced anticholinergic effects (ileus, hyperpyrexia, sedation, dry mouth).	2	3	3
PROPIOMAZINE Concurrent use may result in decreased phenothiazine serum concentrations, decreased phenothiazine effectiveness, enhanced anticholinergic effects (ileus, hyperpyrexia, sedation, dry mouth).	2	3	3
THIETHYLPERAZINE Concurrent use may result in decreased phenothiazine serum concentrations, decreased phenothiazine effectiveness, enhanced anticholinergic effects (ileus, hyperpyrexia, sedation, dry mouth).	2	3	3
THIORIDAZINE Concurrent use may result in decreased phenothiazine serum concentrations, decreased phenothiazine effectiveness, enhanced anticholinergic effects (ileus, hyperpyrexia, sedation, dry mouth).	2	3	3
TRIFLUOPERAZINE Concurrent use may result in decreased phenothiazine serum concentrations, decreased phenothiazine effectiveness, enhanced anticholinergic effects (ileus, hyperpyrexia, sedation, dry mouth).	2	3	3
TRIFLUPROMAZINE Concurrent use may result in decreased phenothiazine serum concentrations, decreased phenothiazine effectiveness, enhanced anticholinergic effects (ileus, hyperpyrexia, sedation, dry mouth).	2	3	3

Trimipramine (Surmontil)

INTERACTION	ONSET	SEVERITY	EVIDENCE
ACENOCOUMAROL Concurrent use may result in increased risk of bleeding.	2	3	3

Onset: 0=Unspecified 1=Rapid 2=Delayed
Severity: 1=Contraindicated 2=Major 3=Moderate 4=Minor
Evidence: 1=Excellent 2=Good 3=Fair 4=Poor

INTERACTION	ONSET	SEVERITY	EVIDENCE
AMPRENAVIR Concurrent use may result in increased trimipramine serum concentrations and potential toxicity (anticholinergic effects, sedation, confusion, cardiac arrhythmias).	2	2	3
ANISINDIONE Concurrent use may result in an increased risk of bleeding.	2	3	3
BEPRIDIL Concurrent use may result in an increased risk of cardiotoxicity (QT prolongation, torsade de pointes, cardiac arrest).	1	1	3
BETHANIDINE Concurrent use may result in decreased antihypertensive effectiveness.	1	3	3
CISAPRIDE Concurrent use may result in cardiotoxicity (QT prolongation, torsade de pointes, cardiac arrest).	1	1	3
CLONIDINE Concurrent use may result in decreased antihypertensive effectiveness.	2	2	3
CLORGYLINE Concurrent use may result in neurotoxicity, seizures, or serotonin syndrome (hypertension, hyperthermia, myoclonus, mental status changes).	2	2	3
DICUMAROL Concurrent use may result in an increased risk of bleeding.	2	3	3
DROPERIDOL Concurrent use may result in an increased risk of cardiotoxicity (QT prolongation, torsade de pointes, cardiac arrest).	0	2	3
EPINEPHRINE Concurrent use may result in hypertension, cardiac arrhythmias, and tachycardia.	1	2	2
ETILEFRINE Concurrent use may result in hypertension, cardiac arrhythmias, and tachycardia.	1	2	2
FLUOXETINE Concurrent use may result in trimipramine antidepressant toxicity (dry mouth, urinary retention, sedation) and an increased risk of cardiotoxicity (QT prolongation, torsade de pointes, cardiac arrest).	0	2	3
GREPAFLOXACIN Concurrent use may result in an increased risk of cardiotoxicity (QT prolongation, torsade de pointes, cardiac arrest).	2	1	3
GUANADREL Concurrent use may result in decreased antihypertensive effectiveness.	2	3	3

INTERACTION	ONSET	SEVERITY	EVIDENCE
HALOFANTRINE Concurrent use may result in an increased risk of cardiotoxicity (QT prolongation, torsade de pointes, cardiac arrest).	2	2	3
ISOCARBOXAZID Concurrent use may result in neurotoxicity, seizures, or serotonin syndrome (hypertension, hyperthermia, myoclonus, mental status changes).	2	1	3
LEVOMETHADYL Concurrent use may result in an increased risk of cardiotoxicity (QT prolongation, torsade de pointes, cardiac arrest).	2	1	3
METHOXAMINE Concurrent use may result in hypertension, cardiac arrhythmias, and tachycardia.	1	2	2
MIDODRINE Concurrent use may result in hypertension, cardiac arrhythmias, and tachycardia.	1	2	2
MOCLOBEMIDE Concurrent use may result in neurotoxicity, seizures, or serotonin syndrome (hypertension, hyperthermia, myoclonus, mental status changes).	2	2	3
NOREPINEPHRINE Concurrent use may result in hypertension, cardiac arrhythmias, and tachycardia.	1	2	2
OXILOFRINE Concurrent use may result in hypertension, cardiac arrhythmias, and tachycardia.	1	2	2
PHENELZINE Concurrent use may result in neurotoxicity, seizures, or serotonin syndrome (hypertension, hyperthermia, myoclonus, mental status changes).	2	2	3
PHENINDIONE Concurrent use may result in an increased risk of bleeding.	2	3	3
PHENPROCOUMON Concurrent use may result in an increased risk of bleeding.	2	3	3
PHENYLEPHRINE Concurrent use may result in hypertension, cardiac arrhythmias, and tachycardia.	1	2	2
PIMOZIDE Concurrent use may result in an increased risk of cardiotoxicity (QT prolongation, torsade de pointes, cardiac arrest).	0	1	3

Onset: 0=Unspecified **1**=Rapid **2**=Delayed
Severity: **1**=Contraindicated **2**=Major **3**=Moderate **4**=Minor
Evidence: **1**=Excellent **2**=Good **3**=Fair **4**=Poor

INTERACTION	ONSET	SEVERITY	EVIDENCE
PROCARBAZINE Concurrent use may result in neurotoxicity, seizures.	2	2	3
SELEGILINE Concurrent use may result in neurotoxicity, seizures, or serotonin syndrome (hypertension, hyperthermia, myoclonus, mental status changes).	2	2	3
TRANYLCYPROMINE Concurrent use may result in neurotoxicity, seizures, or serotonin syndrome (hypertension, hyperthermia, myoclonus, mental status changes).	2	2	3
WARFARIN Concurrent use may result in an increased risk of bleeding.	2	3	3

Valproic acid (Depakote, Depakote ER)

INTERACTION	ONSET	SEVERITY	EVIDENCE
CHOLESTYRAMINE Concurrent use may result in decreased serum valproic acid concentrations.	1	3	3
FELBAMATE Concurrent use may result in increased valproic acid concentrations.	2	3	3
FOSPHENYTOIN Concurrent use may result in altered valproate levels or altered phenytoin levels.	2	3	3
LAMOTRIGINE Concurrent use increased elimination half-life of lamotrigine leading to lamotrigine toxicity (fatigue, drowsiness, ataxia) and an increased risk of life-threatening rashes.	2	2	3
PHENOBARBITAL Concurrent use may result in phenobarbital toxicity or decreased valproic acid effectiveness.	2	3	1
PHENYTOIN Concurrent use may result in altered valproate levels or altered phenytoin levels.	2	3	3
PRIMIDONE Concurrent use may result in severe central nervous system depression.	1	2	3
TOPIRAMATE Concurrent use may result in decreased topiramate or valproic acid concentrations.	2	3	3
ZIDOVUDINE Concurrent use may result in increased zidovudine plasma concentrations and potential zidovudine toxicity (asthenia, fatigue, nausea, hematologic abnormalities).	2	3	3

Varenicline (Chantix)

No drug interactions have been reported by the manufacturer.

Venlafaxine (Effexor, Effexor XR)

INTERACTION	ONSET	SEVERITY	EVIDENCE
ALMOTRIPTAN Concurrent use may result in weakness, hyperreflexia, and/or incoordination.	0	3	3
CIMETIDINE Concurrent use may result in an increased risk of venlafaxine toxicity (nausea, drowsiness, dizziness, ejaculatory disturbances).	2	4	3
DEXFENFLURAMINE Concurrent use may result in serotonin syndrome (hypertension, hyperthermia, myoclonus, mental status changes).	1	2	3
ETHANOL Concurrent use may result in an increased risk of central nervous system effects.	1	4	3
FENFLURAMINE Concurrent use may result in serotonin syndrome (hypertension, hyperthermia, myoclonus, mental status changes).	1	2	3
FURAZOLIDONE Concurrent use may result in weakness, hyperreflexia, and incoordination.	2	1	3
IPRONIAZID Concurrent use may result in central nervous system toxicity or serotonin syndrome (hypertension, hyperthermia, myoclonus, mental status changes).	1	1	2
ISOCARBOXAZID Concurrent use may result in central nervous system toxicity or serotonin syndrome (hypertension, hyperthermia, myoclonus, mental status changes).	1	1	2
MOCLOBEMIDE Concurrent use may result in central nervous system toxicity or serotonin syndrome (hypertension, hyperthermia, myoclonus, mental status changes).	1	1	2
NIALAMIDE Concurrent use may result in central nervous system toxicity or serotonin syndrome (hypertension, hyperthermia, myoclonus, mental status changes).	1	1	2
PARGYLINE Concurrent use may result in central nervous system toxicity or serotonin syndrome (hypertension, hyperthermia, myoclonus, mental status changes).	1	1	2

Onset: 0=Unspecified 1=Rapid 2=Delayed
Severity: 1=Contraindicated 2=Major 3=Moderate 4=Minor
Evidence: 1=Excellent 2=Good 3=Fair 4=Poor

INTERACTION	ONSET	SEVERITY	EVIDENCE
PHENELZINE Concurrent use may result in central nervous system toxicity or serotonin syndrome (hypertension, hyperthermia, myoclonus, mental status changes).	1	1	2
PROCARBAZINE Concurrent use may result in central nervous system toxicity or serotonin syndrome (hypertension, hyperthermia, myoclonus, mental status changes).	1	1	2
SELEGILINE Concurrent use may result in central nervous system toxicity or serotonin syndrome (hypertension, hyperthermia, myoclonus, mental status changes).	1	1	2
SIBUTRAMINE Concurrent use may result in an increased risk of serotonin syndrome (hypertension, hypothermia, myoclonus, mental status changes).	1	2	3
TOLOXATONE Concurrent use may result in central nervous system toxicity or serotonin syndrome (hypertension, hyperthermia, myoclonus, mental status changes).	1	1	2
TRAMADOL Concurrent use may result in an increased risk of seizures and serotonin syndrome (hypertension, hyperthermia, myoclonus, mental status changes).	1	2	2
TRANYLCYPROMINE Concurrent use may result in central nervous system toxicity or serotonin syndrome (hypertension, hyperthermia, myoclonus, mental status changes).	1	1	2
TRIFLUOPERAZINE Concurrent use may result in an increased risk of neuroleptic malignant syndrome and an increased risk of cardiotoxicity (QT prolongation, torsades de pointes, cardiac arrest).	1	1	2

Zaleplon (Sonata)

INTERACTION	ONSET	SEVERITY	EVIDENCE
ETHANOL Concurrent use may result in impaired psychomotor functions.	1	3	3

Ziprasidone (Geodon)

INTERACTION	ONSET	SEVERITY	EVIDENCE
ACECAINIDE Concurrent use may result in an increased risk of cardiotoxicity (QT prolongation, torsade de pointes, cardiac arrest).	0	1	3
AJMALINE Concurrent use may result in an increased risk of cardiotoxicity (QT prolongation, torsade de pointes, cardiac arrest).	0	1	3

INTERACTION	ONSET	SEVERITY	EVIDENCE
AMIODARONE			
Concurrent use may result in an increased risk of cardiotoxicity (QT prolongation, torsade de pointes, cardiac arrest).	0	1	3
ARSENIC TRIOXIDE			
Concurrent use may result in an increased risk of cardiotoxicity (QT prolongation, torsade de pointes, cardiac arrest).	0	1	3
AZIMILIDE			
Concurrent use may result in an increased risk of cardiotoxicity (QT prolongation, torsade de pointes, cardiac arrest).	0	1	3
BRETYLIUM			
Concurrent use may result in an increased risk of cardiotoxicity (QT prolongation, torsade de pointes, cardiac arrest).	0	1	3
CHLORPROMAZINE			
Concurrent use may result in an increased risk of cardiotoxicity (QT prolongation, torsade de pointes, cardiac arrest).	0	1	3
DISOPYRAMIDE			
Concurrent use may result in an increased risk of cardiotoxicity (QT prolongation, torsade de pointes, cardiac arrest).	0	1	3
DOFETILIDE			
Concurrent use may result in an increased risk of cardiotoxicity (QT prolongation, torsade de pointes, cardiac arrest).	0	1	3
DOLASETRON			
Concurrent use may result in an increased risk of cardiotoxicity (QT prolongation, torsade de pointes, cardiac arrest).	2	1	3
DROPERIDOL			
Concurrent use may result in an increased risk of cardiotoxicity (QT prolongation, torsade de pointes, cardiac arrest).	0	1	3
GATIFLOXACIN			
Concurrent use may result in an increased risk of cardiotoxicity (QT prolongation, torsade de pointes, cardiac arrest).	2	1	3
GEMIFLOXACIN			
Concurrent use may result in an increased risk of cardiotoxicity (QT prolongation, torsades de pointes, cardiac arrest).	0	1	2

Onset: 0=Unspecified 1=Rapid 2=Delayed
Severity: 1=Contraindicated 2=Major 3=Moderate 4=Minor
Evidence: 1=Excellent 2=Good 3=Fair 4=Poor

INTERACTION	ONSET	SEVERITY	EVIDENCE
HALOFANTRINE Concurrent use may result in an increased risk of cardiotoxicity (QT prolongation, torsade de pointes, cardiac arrest).	0	1	3
IBUTILIDE Concurrent use may result in an increased risk of cardiotoxicity (QT prolongation, torsade de pointes, cardiac arrest).	0	1	3
LEVOMETHADYL Concurrent use may result in an increased risk of cardiotoxicity (QT prolongation, torsade de pointes, cardiac arrest).	2	1	3
MEFLOQUINE Concurrent use may result in an increased risk of cardiotoxicity (QT prolongation, torsade de pointes, cardiac arrest).	2	1	3
MESORIDAZINE Concurrent use may result in an increased risk of cardiotoxicity (QT prolongation, torsade de pointes, cardiac arrest).	0	1	3
MOXIFLOXACIN Concurrent use may result in an increased risk of cardiotoxicity (QT prolongation, torsade de pointes, cardiac arrest).	2	1	3
PENTAMIDINE Concurrent use may result in an increased risk of cardiotoxicity (QT prolongation, torsade de pointes, cardiac arrest).	0	1	3
PIMOZIDE Concurrent use may result in an increased risk of cardiotoxicity (QT prolongation, torsade de pointes, cardiac arrest).	2	1	3
PIRMENOL Concurrent use may result in an increased risk of cardiotoxicity (QT prolongation, torsade de pointes, cardiac arrest).	0	1	3
PRAJMALINE Concurrent use may result in an increased risk of cardiotoxicity (QT prolongation, torsade de pointes, cardiac arrest).	0	1	3
PROBUCOL Concurrent use may result in an increased risk of cardiotoxicity (QT prolongation, torsade de pointes, cardiac arrest).	2	1	3
PROCAINAMIDE Concurrent use may result in an increased risk of cardiotoxicity (QT prolongation, torsade de pointes, cardiac arrest).	0	1	3

INTERACTION	ONSET	SEVERITY	EVIDENCE
QUINIDINE Concurrent use may result in an increased risk of cardiotoxicity (QT prolongation, torsade de pointes, cardiac arrest).	0	1	3
SEMATILIDE Concurrent use may result in an increased risk of cardiotoxicity (QT prolongation, torsade de pointes, cardiac arrest).	0	1	3
SOTALOL Concurrent use may result in an increased risk of cardiotoxicity (QT prolongation, torsade de pointes, cardiac arrest).	0	1	3
SPARFLOXACIN Concurrent use may result in an increased risk of cardiotoxicity (QT prolongation, torsade de pointes, cardiac arrest).	2	1	3
TACROLIMUS Concurrent use may result in an increased risk of cardiotoxicity (QT prolongation, torsade de pointes, cardiac arrest).	2	1	3
TEDISAMIL Concurrent use may result in an increased risk of cardiotoxicity (QT prolongation, torsade de pointes, cardiac arrest).	0	1	3
THIORIDAZINE Concurrent use may result in an increased risk of cardiotoxicity (QT prolongation, torsade de pointes, cardiac arrest).	0	1	3

Zolpidem (Ambien, Ambien CR)

INTERACTION	ONSET	SEVERITY	EVIDENCE
ETHANOL Concurrent use may result in increased sedation.	1	3	3
KETOCONAZOLE Concurrent use may result in increased plasma concentrations and pharmacodynamic effects of zolpidem.	1	3	3
RIFAMPIN Concurrent use may result in decreased plasma concentration and pharmacodynamic effect of zolpidem.	1	3	3

Onset: 0=Unspecified 1=Rapid 2=Delayed
Severity: 1=Contraindicated 2=Major 3=Moderate 4=Minor
Evidence: 1=Excellent 2=Good 3=Fair 4=Poor

Section 3

Street Drug Profiles

Individuals who are prescribed psychotropic medications can also have problems with substance abuse. To aid clinicians in this area, the *PDR® Drug Guide for Mental Health Professionals* has included this section on street drugs. More than 100 substances of abuse are discussed, divided into four categories:

- *Part 1:* Commercial products, including alcohol, nitrites, and inhaled substances such as aerosol propellants and gases.
- *Part 2:* Over-the-counter drugs, including commonly used antihistamines and cough medicines.
- *Part 3:* Commonly abused prescription drugs, including benzodiazepines and other central nervous system depressants, barbiturates, stimulants, narcotic analgesics, and anabolic steroids. Some of the drugs discussed in this category may no longer be commercially available in the U.S. However, they are included because it may still be possible to obtain them from foreign countries or illegal sources.
- *Part 4*: Illegal drugs, including cannabis, cocaine, heroin, and hallucinogens such as LSD.

Each profile is listed alphabetically by generic name and includes brand names (if available), common street names, a detailed description, common side effects of abuse, symptoms of overdose and withdrawal, and other pertinent facts. Please note that while every attempt has been made to provide the most current information, the data on street drugs are constantly changing in all of the related aspects discussed.

The profiles also include the Drug Enforcement Administration (DEA) classification, which is based on the Controlled Substances Act of 1970. **Class I** drugs are illegal, have a high potential for abuse, and have no accepted medical use in the United States. Drugs in the remaining classes are legal and have a currently accepted medical or research use, along with the following designations: **Class II** drugs have a high potential for abuse; **Class III** drugs have some potential for abuse; **Class IV** drugs have a relatively low potential for abuse; and **Class V** have the lowest potential for abuse.

This section does not include information on drug screening, due to numerous variations in laboratory testing methods and collection procedures. The window of opportunity to detect a drug is dependent on many factors, including the user's metabolic rate, dose size, how the drug was taken, and the cutoff concentration used by the laboratory to detect the drug. Generally, the drugs chosen for workplace screenings are detectable for several days after use. For specific information, contact the Substance Abuse and Mental Health Services Administration at 800-967-5752 or the website at www.workplace.samhsa.gov; and the DEA at 202-307-1000 or www.dea.gov.

Part 1.
Commercial Products

AEROSOLS AND GASES
COMMON STREET NAMES: Air blast, discorama, huff, laughing gas, moon gas, Oz, toncho, whippets
DEA CLASS: Not classified
PHARMACOLOGIC CLASS: Inhalants

Description: Except for medical anesthetics, aerosols and gases are not classified as drugs because they are not manufactured for pharmacologic use. Abused substances include household and commercial products such as butane lighters, propane tanks, and refrigerant gases; household aerosol propellants such as spray paints, hair or deodorant sprays, cooking oil, whipping cream, and fabric protectors; and medical anesthetic gases such as ether, chloroform, halothane, and nitrous oxide or "laughing gas." Most of these products produce short-term psychoactive effects similar to alcohol.

Method of use: Inhaled through the mouth or nose. In addition to inhaling directly from aerosol cans, users sniff the fumes from a plastic bag or through a cloth saturated with the substance (known as huffing). Users also inhale directly from balloons filled with nitrous oxide.

Duration of action: Onset is rapid but effects last only a short time. Inhaled nitrous oxide is rapidly eliminated by the lungs as unchanged gas.

Psychological effects: Aggressive behavior, apathy, delusions, distorted perception of reality, euphoria, hallucinations, impaired thinking and spatial judgment, loss of coordination, and loss of inhibition.

Physical effects: Depressed reflexes, dizziness, drowsiness, gait disturbance, head rush, headache, inattentiveness, limb spasm, loss of equilibrium and coordination, loss of sensation, nausea, rapid heartbeat followed by lethargy, slurred speech, vomiting, and wheezing. Long-term use may cause irreversible brain or nervous system damage, hearing loss, certain types of anemia, and bone marrow damage. Frequent use can cause tolerance and physical dependence. Serious burn injuries were reported because of the highly flammable nature of these products.

Overdose symptoms: Because these products are short-acting, users tend to inhale the fumes repeatedly for several hours, which increases the risk of overdosing. Symptoms may include impaired muscle tone, numbness and tingling in the extremities, respiratory depression, and heart and lung damage. Chronic exposure may induce heart failure and death within minutes of use, known as sudden sniffing death (SSD). High concentrations of inhalants can cause death from suffocation by displacing oxygen in the lungs. Nitrous oxide may cause sudden death by restricting oxygen to the brain. Death is usually related to asphyxia rather than a specific nitrous oxide level.

Withdrawal symptoms: Withdrawal symptoms may develop within several hours to a few days after the last use. Symptoms may include profuse sweating, rapid pulse, weight loss, disorientation, irritability, depression, sleeplessness, nausea, vomiting, physical agitation, anxiety, tremors, hallucinations, and seizures.

ALCOHOL
COMMON STREET NAMES: Booze, hooch
DEA CLASS: Not classified
PHARMACOLOGIC CLASS: CNS depressant

Description: Alcohol is a liquid made by yeast fermentation of carbohydrates such as grain or fruit. There are many varieties of alcohol, but ethanol (ethyl alcohol) is the type used to make alcoholic beverages and the one that is most commonly abused.

Method of use: Ingested

Duration of action: Onset and duration depend on various factors: the amount ingested, the type(s) of alcohol used, whether it was taken with or without food, and whether the individual is a chronic or occasional user.

Detection in blood screening: Alcohol use is best confirmed by breath or blood analysis. Blood alcohol content (BAC) helps determine the individual's intoxication level. BAC is influenced by the individual's weight, gender, height, tolerance, how quickly the alcohol was consumed, and whether it was taken with or without food. Most of the alcohol consumed is processed by the liver. A healthy liver metabolizes about 0.015 grams per deciliter per hour, which means that three-fourths of an ounce of pure alcohol is metabolized in 2 hours (this is equivalent to one 5-ounce glass of wine, one 12-ounce can of beer, or one 1.5-ounce shot of hard liquor). If the BAC is more than 100 milligrams per deciliter, the individual is considered intoxicated. Heavy drinkers have more active livers and may be able to metabolize up to three drinks an hour.

Psychological effects: Initial effects may include confusion, euphoria, and a false sense of well-being, which is replaced by anxiety, restlessness, mood changes, and depression as the BAC increases. Chronic use can cause psychological dependence.

Physical effects: Chronic alcohol abuse may cause anemia and other blood disorders, color-blindness, constipation, diarrhea, elevated blood pressure, inflammation of the pancreas, inflammation of the stomach lining, irregular heart rhythm, liver damage, low blood sugar, muscle weakness, and seizures. Chronic use can cause tolerance and physical dependence.

Overdose symptoms: The effects of alcohol intoxication vary among users. Some individuals may become intoxicated at a much lower BAC than others. The following data are based on clinical studies:

1. BAC of 0.02-0.03: Slight euphoria and loss of shyness.
2. BAC of 0.04-0.06: Sense of well-being, relaxation, lowered inhibitions, euphoria, and minor impairment of memory.
3. BAC of 0.07-0.09: Slight impairment of balance, speech, vision, reaction time, memory, and hearing. Loss of judgment and self-control are also noticeable at this stage.
4. BAC of 0.10-0.125: Significant impairment of balance, motor coordination, vision, speech, reaction time, and hearing. Euphoria is still apparent.
5. BAC of 0.13-0.15: Lack of physical control, blurred vision, and major loss of balance. Euphoria is reduced and replaced by anxiety and restlessness.
6. BAC of 0.16-0.20: Significant anxiety and restlessness, glossy eyes, and nausea. Pupils are slow to respond to stimuli.
7. BAC of 0.25: Significant anxiety and restlessness, nausea and vomiting, irregular "drunken" gait, loss of fine motor coordination, and mental confusion.
8. BAC of 0.30: Loss of consciousness.
9. BAC of 0.40 and up: Onset of stupor, coma, and possibly death due to respiratory depression.

Other symptoms of intoxication include constricted pupils, decreased heart rate, low blood pressure and respiration rate, diminished reflexes, and profuse sweating. Binge drinking is the most dangerous way to get severely intoxicated and is alarmingly prevalent among high school and college students. A binge is usually defined as having four or more drinks (for women) or five or more drinks (for men) in about 2 hours.

Withdrawal symptoms: Abruptly stopping use may cause strong alcohol cravings, nausea, excessive sweating, shakiness, depression, mood changes, headache, insomnia, unstable heart rate or blood pressure, tremors, anxiety or panic attacks, confusion and/or hallucinations (delirium tremens), and in extreme cases, seizures.

NITRITES (nonprescription products)

COMMON STREET NAMES: Ames, Amys, aroma of men, bolt, boppers, climax, hardware, pearls, poppers, quicksilver, rush, snappers, thrust, whiteout
DEA CLASS: Not classified
PHARMACOLOGIC CLASS: Inhalants

Description: Nitrites are volatile liquids that are readily absorbed from the lungs. Unlike other inhalants, they work primarily by dilating blood vessels and relaxing the muscles. Amyl nitrite and glyceryl trinitrate are used medically to treat acute chest pain (angina) and severe heart murmurs (see the prescription nitrites entry listed on page 484. Industrial nitrites that are reportedly abused are cyclohexyl nitrite, an ingredient found in room deodorizers, and butyl nitrite, which was used previously in the manufacturing of perfumes and antifreeze but is now considered illegal. Most of these products are used as sexual enhancers.

Method of use: Inhaled through the mouth or nose. In addition to inhaling directly from aerosol cans, users sniff the fumes from a plastic bag or through a cloth saturated with the substance (known as huffing).

Duration of action: Onset is rapid but effects last only a short time, usually 30 to 60 minutes.

Psychological effects: Loss of inhibition, distorted perception of reality, aggressive behavior, apathy, impaired judgment, euphoria, hallucinations, loss of coordination, and delusions.

Physical effects: Rapid heartbeat followed by lethargy, head rush, headaches, nausea, vomiting, slurred speech, loss of coordination, and wheezing. Frequent use can cause tolerance and physical dependence. Serious but reversible physical effects may include liver or kidney damage and blood oxygen depletion. Chronic use can cause serious damage to the heart and lungs and suppress the immune system, increasing the risk of infection. Prolonged use can also lead to poor muscle tone, muscle wasting, and numbness and tingling in the extremities.

Overdose symptoms: Because these products are short-acting, users tend to inhale the fumes repeatedly for several hours, which increases the risk of overdosing. Prolonged inhalation of nitrites may cause irregular and rapid heart rhythm, heart failure, and death within minutes of use.

Withdrawal symptoms: Abrupt discontinuation of use may cause sweating, rapid pulse, hand tremors, insomnia, nausea, vomiting, physical agitation, anxiety, hallucinations, and seizures.

Part 2.
Over-the-Counter Drugs

DEXTROMETHORPHAN
BRAND NAMES: Delsym, Robitussin DM, Benylin DM, Triaminic DM,
Vicks 44 Cough Relief, and others
COMMON STREET NAMES: Robotripping, Robo, Triple C
DEA CLASS: Not classified
PHARMACOLOGIC CLASS: Antitussive

Description: This medication is indicated for the temporary symptomatic
relief of nonproductive cough occurring with colds and inhaled irritants.
There are many cough and cold combination products that contain dextromethorphan as an active ingredient.

Method of use: Ingested

Duration of action: The antitussive effects last up to 6 hours.

Psychological effects of abuse: Subjective effects reported with abuse of
dextromethorphan include euphoria, floating/flying sensation, hallucinations (auditory and visual), increased self-awareness, increased perception, increased sense of self, increased sociability, modification of
sounds, and synesthesia (association of sounds with color). Other mental
and emotional effects associated with dextromethorphan abuse include
anxiety, panic, dysphoria, depression, fear of sleep, loss of memory, for-
getfulness, stupor, confusion, restlessness, agitation, irritability, paranoia,
and psychosis. May result in drug abuse or dependency, although this is
very infrequent.

Physical effects of abuse: Euphoria and restlessness, persisting for 15
minutes to 2 hours, followed by depression, tiredness, and dizziness.
Some other effects include nausea, vomiting, drowsiness, and fatigue
(with chronic use).

Overdose symptoms: CNS effects are more prevalent and include shakiness and unsteady walk, blurred vision, coma, confusion, drowsiness or
dizziness, respiratory depression, severe nausea and vomiting, unusual
excitement, restlessness, irritability, and difficulty in urination.

Withdrawal symptoms: Abrupt discontinuation is not associated with
physical withdrawal symptoms; however, intense cravings for the drug
have been reported.

DIMENHYDRINATE
BRAND NAME: Dramamine, Driminate
DEA CLASS: Not classified
PHARMACOLOGIC CLASS: Antihistamine

Description: Dimenhydrinate is primarily used in the prevention and treatment of vertigo, motion sickness, and nausea and vomiting during pregnancy.

Method of use: Ingested

Duration of action: The antiemetic effects last 3 to 6 hours.

Psychological effects of abuse: Abuse of dimenhydrinate has resulted in psychotic-like reactions, including delirium and hallucinations.

Physical effects of abuse: Hypertension, increased heart rate, and drying of mucous membranes. Dimenhydrinate may frequently be used by women with anorexia or bulimia, because of the drug's sedative, anorexic, and emetic properties.

Overdose symptoms: Overdose may result in CNS depression and/or stimulation and may resemble anticholinergic overdose. Effects may include fixed and dilated pupils, flushed face, dry mouth, excitation, hallucinations, and tonic-clonic seizures. In young children, CNS stimulation is the predominant overdose symptom.

Withdrawal symptoms: Withdrawal of the drug resulted in enhanced excitability, increased heart rate, hypertension, and mydriasis.

DIPHENHYDRAMINE
BRAND NAMES: Benadryl, Benylin Decongestant Cough, Diphenist, Diphenyl, Nytol, and others
DEA CLASS: Not classified
PHARMACOLOGIC CLASS: Antihistamine

Description: Diphenhydramine is an antihistamine with many therapeutic applications. Some oral dosage forms are available without a prescription for use as an antitussive, a nighttime sleep aid, or to relieve allergy symptoms. There are many combination products that contain diphenhydramine as an active ingredient.

Method of use: Ingested

Duration of action: Effects have been noted to last 4 to 6 hours.

Psychological effects of abuse: Anticholinergic side effects such as insomnia, tremors, nervousness, psychomotor agitation, and dyskinesias. A combination of butorphanol and diphenhydramine is being increasingly used as a drug of abuse. Tolerance develops and progressively higher doses are needed to reach the desired state, which is described as "being on the nod."

Physical effects of abuse: Sedation and mild euphoria, irritability, palpitations, blurred vision, constipation, urinary retention, tachycardia, and dryness of the mouth, nose and throat.

Overdose symptoms: The following symptoms have been observed: **Mild/Moderate:** tachycardia, dry flushed skin, hallucinations, mydriasis, decreased bowel sounds, urinary retention. **Severe:** seizures, coma, electrocardiogram QRS-wave widening, dysrhythmias, torsades de pointes. **Rare:** rhabdomyolysis, renal failure.

Withdrawal symptoms: Chronic abuse has resulted in withdrawal symptoms, including recurrence of insomnia, increased daytime restlessness, irritability and excessive blinking

Part 3.
Prescription Drugs

ACETAMINOPHEN WITH CODEINE PHOSPHATE
BRAND NAME: Tylenol with Codeine
COMMON STREET NAMES: Dreamer, God's drug, mister blue
DEA CLASS: Class III (tablets) and Class V (suspensions and elixirs)
PHARMACOLOGIC CLASS: Antipyretic analgesic, narcotic analgesic

Description: This medication is a fixed-dose combination of acetaminophen, an antipyretic (fever-reducing) analgesic; and codeine, a narcotic analgesic. It is prescribed for the relief of mild to moderately severe pain.

Method of use: Ingested

Duration of action: The analgesic effects usually last 4 to 6 hours after ingestion.

Psychological effects of abuse: Euphoria alternating with depression, confusion, nervousness, and hallucinations. The psychological dependence associated with narcotic addiction is complex. Long after physical dependence has ended, the addict may continue to think and talk about the drug and feel unable to manage daily activities without it.

Physical effects of abuse: Light-headedness, dizziness, nausea, vomiting, constipation, stomach discomfort, shortness of breath, and elevated blood pressure. Physical dependence can occur after prolonged use. Chronic use of acetaminophen is associated with liver damage. Abusing codeine may lead to breathing difficulties followed by respiratory arrest.

Overdose symptoms: Tolerance develops rapidly, and the progressively higher doses needed are often in the toxic range. Acute acetaminophen overdose can potentially result in fatal liver toxicity. Early symptoms include nausea, vomiting, sweating, and weakness. Clinical and laboratory evidence of liver toxicity may not be apparent until 48 to 72 hours after ingestion.

Overdose symptoms related to codeine include cold and clammy skin, severe drowsiness, constricted pupils, severe weakness, low blood pressure, respiratory depression, and coma.

Withdrawal symptoms: Although withdrawal is painful physically and emotionally, it is rarely life-threatening if adequate hydration and nutritional support are maintained. Withdrawal symptoms are similar to those of morphine but are considerably less intense. Abruptly stopping use can cause excessive tearing, yawning, and sweating in about 12 to 14 hours after the last dose. Additional symptoms may include diminished appetite, irritability, tremor, seizures, and loss of consciousness.

Adderall *see Dextroamphetamine, page 450*

Adipex-P *see Phentermine, page 498*

ALPRAZOLAM
BRAND NAME: Xanax
COMMON STREET NAMES: Candy, downers, sleeping pills, tranks, xanies
DEA CLASS: Class IV
PHARMACOLOGIC CLASS: Benzodiazepine, antianxiety

Description: Alprazolam is used to treat anxiety disorders with or without depression, acute stress reactions such as anxiety prior to surgery, and panic attacks with or without irrational fear. Abuse of benzodiazepines is particularly high among heroin and cocaine users.

Method of use: Ingested

Duration of action: 6 to 12 hours, but may persist longer in obese individuals.

Psychological effects of abuse: Amnesia, depression, difficulty concentrating, diminished sexual desire, impaired judgment, reduced inhibition, pressured speech, and suicidal ideation. Paradoxical reactions may include aggressive and agitated behavior. Prolonged use leads to psychological dependence and may cause behavior problems such as extreme aggression and hostility.

Physical effects of abuse: Change in appetite, constipation, difficulty urinating, dizziness, impaired muscle coordination, irregular gait, lightheadedness, low blood pressure, menstrual irregularities, and slurred speech. Long-term use may cause physical dependence.

Overdose symptoms: The most severe signs of overdose are respiratory depression and loss of consciousness. Other symptoms may include confusion, rapid and slurred speech, extreme sleepiness, diminished reflexes, and loss of muscle coordination. Death from overdose of a single benzodiazepine is extremely rare. However, there is an increased risk of toxicity when benzodiazepines are combined with alcohol and/or other CNS depressants. Fatalities have been reported in individuals who have overdosed with a combination of a single benzodiazepine and alcohol.

Withdrawal symptoms: Abrupt termination following long-term use may precipitate withdrawal symptoms and require hospitalization. Symptoms may include abdominal and muscle cramps, depression, insomnia, sweating, vomiting, tremors, and seizures.

Alurate *see Aprobarbital, page 439*

Ambien *see Zolpidem, page 511*

AMOBARBITAL SODIUM
BRAND NAME: Amytal sodium
COMMON STREET NAMES: Blue heavens, dolls, downers, goofballs, M&Ms, rainbows, red and blues, red devils, yellows
DEA CLASS: Class II
PHARMACOLOGIC CLASS: Barbiturate, hypnotic, sedative, anticonvulsant

Description: Barbiturates depress the sensory cortex, decrease motor activity, alter brain function, and produce drowsiness, sedation, and hypnosis. Amobarbital is used for the short-term treatment of insomnia. It is also used as a sedating agent for reducing anxiety prior to surgery.

Method of use: Injected IV or IM

Duration of action: 6 to 8 hours following a standard therapeutic dose.

Psychological effects of abuse: Barbiturates can cause psychological dependence, especially following prolonged use of high doses. Principal psychological effects include confusion, alternating euphoria and depression, and memory loss.

Physical effects of abuse: The most frequent physical effects are due to CNS depression, including dizziness, headache, excessive sleepiness, drowsiness, and irregular gait. Other physical symptoms may include headache, stomach pain, and skin rash. Paradoxical excitement and irritability may also occur. In chronic users, blood disorders such as megaloblastic anemia may develop. Physical dependence is a significant risk, since it can develop after short-term use.

Overdose symptoms: Overdosing with amobarbital may result in severe CNS depression. Initial symptoms include eye gazing, contracted pupils, slurred speech, irregular gait, and interrupted breathing. More serious overdose may result in respiratory and cardiovascular depression, severely low blood pressure and body temperature, coma, and shock that can lead to death. Reddish, bleeding blisters ("barb-burns") may occur on the hands, buttocks, and back of knees in about 6 percent of users; however, barbiturate overdose is not the sole cause of such blisters. All harmful effects are enhanced when barbiturates are taken with alcohol and/or other CNS depressants.

Withdrawal symptoms: Amobarbital is one of the most commonly abused barbiturates. Symptoms are similar to those of alcohol withdrawal and characterized by severe apprehension, weakness, elevated anxiety, irritability, dizziness, headache, sleeplessness, muscle twitching, nausea and vomiting, distortion of visual perception, and rapid pulse. Severely low blood pressure and convulsions may develop after a day or two, which eventually leads to hallucinations, delirium, and continuous seizures, followed by coma and death.

AMOBARBITAL AND SECOBARBITAL

COMMON STREET NAMES: Dolls, downers, goofballs, M&Ms, rainbows, red and blues, red birds, red devils, yellows
DEA CLASS: Class II
PHARMACOLOGIC CLASS: Barbiturate

Not commercially available in the U.S.

Description: Barbiturates depress the sensory cortex, decrease motor activity, alter brain function, and produce drowsiness, sedation, and hypnosis. This drug combination is used as a sedative to relieve anxiety before surgery and as a supplemental agent for the short-term treatment of insomnia.

Method of use: Ingested

Duration of action: 6 to 8 hours following a standard therapeutic dose.

Psychological effects of abuse: Barbiturates may cause psychological dependence, especially following prolonged use of high doses. Psychological effects may include confusion, alternating euphoria and depression, and memory loss.

Physical effects of abuse: The most frequent physical effects are due to CNS depression, including dizziness, headache, excessive sleepiness, drowsiness, and irregular gait. Other symptoms may include headache, stomach pain, and skin rash. Paradoxical excitement and irritability may also occur. In chronic users, blood disorders such as megaloblastic anemia may develop. Physical dependence is a significant risk, since it can develop after short-term use.

Overdose symptoms: Overdosing with this drug may result in severe CNS depression. Initial symptoms include eye gazing, constricted pupils, slurred speech, irregular gait, and interrupted breathing. More serious overdose may result in respiratory and cardiovascular depression, severely low blood pressure and body temperature, coma, and shock that can lead to death. Reddish, bleeding blisters ("barb-burns") may occur on the hands, buttocks, and back of the knees in about 6 percent of users; however, barbiturate overdose is not the sole cause of such blisters. All harmful effects are enhanced when barbiturates are taken with alcohol and/or other CNS depressants.

Withdrawal symptoms: Amobarbital, one of the ingredients in Tuinal, is a commonly abused barbiturate. Symptoms are similar to those of alcohol withdrawal and characterized by severe apprehension, weakness, elevated anxiety, irritability, dizziness, headache, sleeplessness, muscle twitching, nausea and vomiting, distortion of visual perception, and rapid pulse. Severely low blood pressure and convulsions may develop after a day or two, which eventually leads to hallucinations, delirium, and continuous seizures, followed by coma and death.

Amytal *see Amobarbital, page 437*

Anadrol *see Oxymetholone, page 490*

Android *see Methyltestosterone, page 477*

Anolor *see Butalbital, page 442*

APROBARBITAL
COMMON STREET NAMES: Dolls, downers, goofballs, M&Ms, rainbows, red and blues, red devils, yellows
DEA CLASS: Class III
PHARMACOLOGIC CLASS: Barbiturate, hypnotic, sedative

Description: Aprobarbital is used for the short-term treatment of insomnia. It is also used as a sedating agent for reducing anxiety prior to surgery.

Method of use: Ingested

Duration of action: About 6 to 8 hours following a standard therapeutic dose.

Psychological effects of abuse: Barbiturates may cause psychological dependence, especially following prolonged use of high doses. Principal psychological effects may include confusion, alternating euphoria and depression, and memory loss.

Physical effects of abuse: The most frequent physical effects are due to CNS depression, including dizziness, headache, excessive sleepiness, drowsiness, and irregular gait. Other symptoms may include headache, stomach pain, and skin rash. Paradoxical excitement and irritability may also occur. In chronic users, blood disorders such as megaloblastic anemia may develop. Physical dependence is a significant risk, since it can develop after short-term use.

Overdose symptoms: Overdosing with aprobarbital can cause severe CNS depression. Initial symptoms may include eye gazing, contracted pupils, slurred speech, irregular gait, and interrupted breathing. More serious overdose may result in respiratory and cardiovascular depression, severely low blood pressure and body temperature, coma, and shock that can lead to death. Reddish, bleeding blisters ("barb-burns") may occur on the hands, buttocks, and back of knees in about 6 percent of users; however, barbiturate overdose is not the sole cause of such blisters. All harmful effects are enhanced when barbiturates are taken with alcohol and/or other CNS depressants.

Withdrawal symptoms: Aprobarbital is one of the most commonly abused barbiturates. Symptoms are similar to those of alcohol withdrawal and characterized by severe apprehension, weakness, elevated anxiety, irritability, dizziness, headache, sleeplessness, muscle twitching, nausea and vomiting, distortion of visual perception, and rapid pulse. Severely low blood pressure and convulsions may develop after a day or two, which eventually leads to hallucinations, delirium, and continuous seizures, followed by coma and death.

Aquachloral *see Chloral hydrate, page 444*

Astramorph PF *see Morphine, page 481*

Ativan *see Lorazepam, page 469*

Avinza *see Morphine, page 481*

BENZPHETAMINE HYDROCHLORIDE
BRAND NAME: Didrex
COMMON STREET NAMES: Chalk, crystal, crank, glass, meth, ice, speed
DEA CLASS: Class III
PHARMACOLOGIC CLASS: Amphetamine, CNS stimulant

Description: Benzphetamine is prescribed as a supplemental agent for weight loss. It is meant to be used along with caloric restriction, exercise, and behavior modification.

Method of use: Ingested and snorted

Duration of action: 8 to 24 hours

Psychological effects of abuse: Depression, hyperactivity, irritability, personality changes, and restlessness. Psychological dependence develops with chronic use.

Physical effects of abuse: Abdominal cramps, diarrhea, fatigue, insomnia, nausea, and vomiting. Long-term use may lead to physical dependence.

Overdose symptoms: Tolerance develops rapidly in chronic users, and progressively higher doses are needed to obtain the same effects as before. Overdose symptoms may include confusion, aggressiveness, hallucinations, panic state, severely elevated body temperature, tremors, rapid breathing, and muscle rigidity. Cardiovascular effects may include irregular heartbeat, severely low or high blood pressure, and circulatory collapse. The most severe symptom is psychosis that is clinically indistinguishable from schizophrenia. A fatal overdose is usually preceded by convulsions and coma.

Withdrawal symptoms: Benzphetamine is highly addictive, and physical dependence develops rapidly. Abrupt cessation of use may cause anxiety, extreme fatigue, paranoia, aggressive behavior, and strong drug cravings. Severe depression and suicidal ideation have also been reported.

Bontril *see Phendimetrazine, page 495*

BUTABARBITAL SODIUM
BRAND NAME: Butisol sodium
COMMON STREET NAMES: Barbs, downers, goofballs
DEA CLASS: Class III
PHARMACOLOGIC CLASS: Barbiturate, sedative, hypnotic

Description: Barbiturates depress the sensory cortex, decrease motor activity, alter brain function, and produce drowsiness, sedation, and hypnosis. Butabarbital is used primarily for daytime sedation.

Method of use: Ingested

Duration of action: Effects start within an hour and last for about 6 to 8 hours.

Psychological effects of abuse: Alternating euphoria and depression, confusion, and memory loss. Barbiturates may cause psychological dependence, especially following prolonged use of high doses.

Physical effects of abuse: Decreased blood pressure, unusual tiredness, nausea and vomiting, dizziness, drowsiness, heartburn, excessive sleepiness, shortness of breath, and dose-dependent respiratory depression. Prolonged use may cause tolerance and physical dependence.

Overdose symptoms: Unsteady gait, slurred speech, eye gazing, confusion, low blood pressure and body temperature, rapid heartbeat, and dose-dependent respiratory depression. All toxic effects are enhanced when butabarbital is taken with alcohol and/or other CNS depressant drugs.

Withdrawal symptoms: Symptoms are similar to those of alcohol withdrawal and characterized by severe apprehension, weakness, heightened anxiety, irritability, dizziness, headache, sleeplessness, muscle twitching, nausea and vomiting, distortion of visual perception, and rapid pulse. Severely low blood pressure and convulsions may develop after a day or two, which eventually leads to hallucinations, delirium, and continuous seizures, followed by coma and death.

BUTALBITAL COMBINATION PRODUCTS

GENERIC NAMES: Butalbital, aspirin, and caffeine (Fiorinal); butalbital, codeine phosphate, aspirin, and caffeine (Fiorinal with Codeine); Butalbital, codeine phosphate, acetominophen, and caffeine (Fioricet with Codeine) and butalbital, acetaminophen, and caffeine (Anolor, Esgic, Fioricet, Repan, Zebutal)

COMMON STREET NAMES: Barbs, downers, goofballs

DEA CLASS: Class III (Fiorinal, Fiornal with Codeine, Fioricet with codeine)

PHARMACOLOGIC CLASS: Barbiturate, sedative, hypnotic

Description: These products are used primarily to relieve muscle and tension headache.

Method of use: Ingested

Duration of action: Effects start within an hour and last for about 12 hours.

Psychological effects of abuse: Confusion, hallucinations, depression, and feelings of intoxication. Barbiturates may cause psychological dependence, especially following prolonged use of high doses.

Physical effects of abuse: Decreased blood pressure, unusual tiredness, nausea and vomiting, dizziness, drowsiness, heartburn, excessive sleepiness, shortness of breath, and dose-dependent respiratory depression. Prolonged use may cause tolerance and physical dependence.

Overdose symptoms: Symptoms may include unsteady gait, slurred speech, eye gazing, confusion, low blood pressure and body temperature, rapid heart rate, and dose-dependent respiratory depression. All toxic effects are enhanced when these products are taken with alcohol and/or other CNS depressants. In cases of serious overdose, respiratory depression may lead to Cheyne-Stokes respiration (abnormal breathing patterns characterized by alternating periods of shallow and deep breathing) as well as respiratory arrest and coma, followed by death. In extreme cases, electrical activities in the brain may cease and electroencephalogram (EEG) readings may be "flat," although this does not necessarily indicate clinical death and may be fully reversible.

Withdrawal symptoms: Symptoms are similar to those of alcohol withdrawal and characterized by severe apprehension, strong drug cravings, weakness, heightened anxiety, irritability, dizziness, headache, sleeplessness, muscle twitching, nausea and vomiting, distortion of visual perception, and rapid pulse. Severely low blood pressure and convulsions may develop after a day or two, which eventually leads to hallucinations, delirium, and continuous seizures, followed by coma and death.

Butisol sodium *see Butabarbital, page 441*

BUTORPHANOL TARTRATE
BRAND NAME: Stadol
COMMON STREET NAMES: Not known
DEA CLASS: Class IV
PHARMACOLOGIC CLASS: Narcotic analgesic

Description: Butorphanol is a mixed narcotic agonist/antagonist and produces generalized CNS depression. It is used to help manage moderate to severe pain, as a sedative prior to surgery, and as a supplemental agent during anesthesia.

Method of use: Injected IV or IM and sniffed via nasal spray

Duration of action: Depends on dose and method of use. The effects persist for about 3 to 4 hours after injection, and about 4 to 5 hours after nasal application.

Psychological effects of abuse: Anxiety, apathy, confusion, depression, euphoria, general sense of well-being, hallucinations, inability to concentrate, nightmares, paradoxical excitement, and psychological dependence (after prolonged use). The psychological dependence associated with narcotic addiction is complex. Long after physical dependence has ended, the addict may continue to think and talk about the drug and feel unable to manage daily activities without it.

Physical effects of abuse: Blurred vision, constipation, dizziness, drowsiness, constricted pupils, excessive sleepiness, excessive sweating, flu-like symptoms, headache, light-headedness, low blood pressure, nausea, respiratory depression, respiratory tract infection, shortness of breath, slow pulse, tremors, unpleasant taste, vomiting, and weakness. Prolonged use may cause tolerance and physical dependence. Signs of tolerance include euphoria, sedation, shorter duration of action, and weaker painkilling effect.

Overdose symptoms: Chronic use can lead to tolerance, with the user needing progressively higher doses to obtain the same effects as before. Signs of overdose include constricted pupils, cold and clammy skin, confusion, severe drowsiness, slow or labored breathing, CNS and cardiac depression, and convulsions.

Withdrawal symptoms: Abruptly stopping the drug after long-term use may precipitate withdrawal symptoms. Intensity of symptoms is directly related to total daily dose, frequency and duration of use, and health of the user. Withdrawal from narcotics is rarely life-threatening. Without medical intervention, most of the physical symptoms of butorphanol withdrawal disappear within 7 to 10 days. Early symptoms may include watery eyes, runny nose, repeated yawning, and excessive sweating. Later-stage symptoms may include nervousness, muscle twitching, drug cravings, restlessness, irritability, loss of appetite, chills alternating with flushing, nausea, vomiting, bone and muscle pain in the back and extremities, tremors, elevated heart rate and blood pressure, and severe depression.

CHLORAL HYDRATE

BRAND NAMES: Aquachloral, Somnote
COMMON STREET NAMES: Jellies, jellybeans, joy juice, knockout drops, Mickey, Mickey Finn, Peter, torpedo
DEA CLASS: Class IV
PHARMACOLOGIC CLASS: Sedative, hypnotic

Description: Chloral hydrate has properties similar to those of barbiturates. It is used for short-term sedation before diagnostic procedures, as a supplemental agent to manage pain following surgery, and for the short-term treatment of insomnia.

Method of use: Ingested or administered rectally

Duration of action: Chloral hydrate usually takes effect within 30 minutes and will induce sleep in about an hour following administration. The effects may last 4 to 8 hours.

Psychological effects of abuse: Confusion, disorientation, hallucinations, "hangover" effects, impaired judgment and concentration, nightmares, and paradoxical excitement.

Physical effects of abuse: Diarrhea, dizziness, headache, light-headedness, nausea, slow reflexes, stomach pain, unsteadiness, and vomiting.

Chronic use can lead to addiction, severe withdrawal symptoms, and possibly liver damage.

Overdose symptoms: Tolerance develops rapidly after prolonged use, and the progressively higher doses needed are often in the toxic range. Signs of overdose may include severe drowsiness, nausea, vomiting, severe stomach pain, slurred speech, irregular gait, difficulty swallowing, severe weakness, dilated pupils, shortness of breath or other breathing problems, low blood pressure, irregular heart rate, low body temperature, respiratory depression, convulsions, and coma.

Withdrawal symptoms: Abruptly stopping use may precipitate withdrawal symptoms such as anorexia, nausea, vomiting, muscle weakness, low blood pressure, tremors, and seizures.

CLORAZEPATE DIPOTASSIUM
BRAND NAME: Tranxene
COMMON STREET NAMES: Candy, downers, sleeping pills, tranks
DEA CLASS: Class IV
PHARMACOLOGIC CLASS: Benzodiazepine, sedative, anticonvulsant

Description: Clorazepate is used to treat anxiety disorders, alcohol withdrawal, and as a supplemental agent in certain types of seizure disorders. Abuse of benzodiazepines is particularly high among heroin and cocaine users.

Method of use: Ingested

Duration of action: 8 to 24 hours

Psychological effects of abuse: Confusion, depression, impaired judgment and thinking abilities, mild euphoria, pressured speech, reduced inhibition, and suicidal ideation. Prolonged use may cause psychological dependence.

Physical effects of abuse: Change in appetite, constipation, difficulty urinating, dizziness, drowsiness, dry mouth, impaired muscle coordination, insomnia, irregular gait, light-headedness, low blood pressure, menstrual irregularities, nausea, slurred speech, tremor, and vomiting. Long-term use may cause physical dependence.

Overdose symptoms: The most severe signs of overdose are respiratory depression and coma. Other symptoms may include confusion, diminished reflexes, paradoxical euphoria, extreme sleepiness, and impaired coordination. Death from overdose of a single benzodiazepine is extremely rare. However, there is an increased risk of toxicity when benzodiazepines are combined with alcohol and/or other CNS depressants.

Fatalities have been reported in individuals who have overdosed with a combination of a single benzodiazepine and alcohol.

Withdrawal symptoms: Abrupt termination following long-term use may precipitate withdrawal symptoms and require hospitalization. Symptoms may include abdominal and muscle cramps, depression, insomnia, sweating, vomiting, tremors, and seizures.

CHLORDIAZEPOXIDE
BRAND NAME: Librium
COMMON STREET NAMES: Candy, downers, sleeping pills, tranks
DEA CLASS: Class IV
PHARMACOLOGIC CLASS: Benzodiazepine, sedative, hypnotic

Description: Chlordiazepoxide is used to treat anxiety disorders with or without depression, alcohol withdrawal, and acute stress reactions such as anxiety prior to surgery. Abuse of benzodiazepines is particularly high among heroin and cocaine users.

Method of use: Ingested and injected IM or IV

Duration of action: 5 to 30 hours

Psycological effects of abuse: Confusion, depression, impaired judgment, mild euphoria, pressured speech, reduced inhibition, and suicidal ideation. Long-term use may cause psychological dependence.

Physical effects of abuse: Changes in appetite and body weight, dizziness, drowsiness, dry mouth, impaired muscle coordination, insomnia, irregular gait, light-headedness, low blood pressure, menstrual irregularities, nausea, slurred speech, and vomiting. Long-term use may cause physical dependence.

Overdose symptoms: The most severe signs of overdose are respiratory depression and coma. Other symptoms may include confusion, diminished reflexes, extreme sleepiness, unrealistic euphoria, and impaired muscle coordination. Death from overdose of a single benzodiazepine is extremely rare. However, there is an increased risk of toxicity when benzodiazepines are combined with alcohol and/or other CNS depressants. Fatalities have been reported in individuals who have overdosed with a combination of a single benzodiazepine and alcohol.

Withdrawal symptoms: Abrupt termination following long-term use may precipitate withdrawal symptoms and require hospitalization. Symptoms may include abdominal and muscle cramps, depression, insomnia, sweating, vomiting, tremors, and seizures.

CLONAZEPAM

BRAND NAME: Klonopin
COMMON STREET NAMES: Candy, downers, sleeping pills, tranks
DEA CLASS: Class IV
PHARMACOLOGIC CLASS: Benzodiazepine, anticonvulsant

Description: Clonazepam is used to treat panic disorder with or without irrational fears. It is also prescribed for certain types of seizures, either as monotherapy or an adjunct. Abuse of benzodiazepines is particularly high among heroin and cocaine users.

Method of use: Ingested

Duration of action: 18 to 50 hours

Psychological effects of abuse: Amnesia, confusion, depression, impaired judgment and thinking abilities, reduced inhibition, and suicidal ideation. Paradoxical effects include euphoria, hyperactivity, and extreme aggression. Prolonged use may cause psychological dependence.

Physical effects of abuse: Changes in sexual desire, constipation, decreased blood pressure, dizziness, drowsiness, fatigue, impaired physical capabilities, irregular gait, loss of muscle tone, sleepiness, slowed psychomotor performance, urinary retention, and visual disturbances. Prolonged use may cause physical dependence.

Overdose symptoms: The most severe signs of overdose are respiratory depression, loss of consciousness, and coma. Other symptoms may include confusion, diminished reflexes, slurred speech, impaired coordination, apnea, extreme sleepiness, loss of muscle tone, and severely low blood pressure. Death from overdose of a single benzodiazepine is extremely rare. However, there is an increased risk of toxicity when benzodiazepines are combined with alcohol and/or other CNS depressants. Fatalities have been reported in patients who have overdosed with a combination of a single benzodiazepine and alcohol.

Withdrawal symptoms: Abrupt termination following long-term use may precipitate withdrawal symptoms and require hospitalization. Symptoms may include abdominal and muscle cramps, depression, insomnia, sweating, vomiting, tremors, and seizures.

CODEINE PHOSPHATE AND CODEINE SULFATE

BRAND NAMES: Capital with Codeine, Tylenol with Codeine
COMMON STREET NAMES: Hillbilly heroin, killers, percs, poor man's heroin, schoolboy
DEA CLASS: Class II (single agent), Class III (combined with Tylenol), and Class V (cough suppressant products)
PHARMACOLOGIC CLASS: Narcotic analgesic, cough suppressant

Description: Codeine is produced by the chemical manipulation of morphine. However, codeine produces less analgesia and sedation than morphine, and is less likely to cause respiratory depression. Codeine is indicated for mild to moderate pain. In lower doses, it is used as a cough suppressant. Codeine is also indicated for the symptomatic relief of acute diarrhea.

Method of use: Ingested and injected IM or SC

Duration of action: Depends on the dose and method of use. In general, codeine's analgesic effects last 4 to 6 hours following administration.

Psychological effects of abuse: Confusion, false sense of well-being, inability to concentrate, and psychological dependence (after prolonged use). The psychological dependence associated with narcotic addiction is complex. Long after physical dependence has ended, the addict may continue to think and talk about the drug and feel unable to manage daily activities without it.

Physical effects of abuse: Blurred vision, change in heart rhythm, constipation, constriction of pupils, drowsiness, dry mouth, flushing of the face, low blood pressure, headache, nausea, respiratory depression, urinary urgency or retention, and vomiting. *High doses:* Lethargy, seizures, and coma may occur. Prolonged use can cause physical dependence, but codeine produces less euphoria and sedation than morphine.

Overdose symptoms: Tolerance can develop rapidly, and progressively higher doses are needed to obtain the same effects as before. Signs of overdose may include constipation, stomach cramps, nausea, vomiting, drowsiness, dizziness, slurred speech, extreme sleepiness, low body temperature, low blood pressure, swelling, cold and clammy skin, nonreactive pupils, pulmonary edema, CNS and respiratory depression, convulsions, and coma. Death may result from respiratory failure 2 to 4 hours postingestion. Risk of overdose increases significantly when the drug is taken with alcohol.

Withdrawal symptoms: Although withdrawal is painful physically and emotionally, it's rarely life-threatening if adequate hydration and nutritional support are maintained. The symptoms are similar to those of morphine withdrawal but are considerably less intense. Abruptly stopping use can cause excessive tearing, yawning, and sweating about 12 to 14 hours after the last dose. Additional symptoms may include diminished appetite, gooseflesh, irritability, tremors, seizures, and loss of consciousness.

Concerta *see Methylphenidate, page 476*

Dalmane *see Flurazepam, page 462*

Darvon *see Propoxyphene, page 500*

Delatestryl *see Testosterone, page 506*

Demerol *see Meperidine, page 470*

Desoxyn *see Methamphetamine, page 474*

Dexedrine *see Dextroamphetamine, page 450*

DEXMETHYLPHENIDATE HYDROCHLORIDE
BRAND NAME: Focalin, Focalin XR
COMMON STREET NAME: Working man's cocaine
DEA CLASS: Class II
PHARMACOLOGIC CLASS: CNS stimulant, nonamphetamine

Description: This drug has pharmacologic actions similar to those of dextroamphetamine. It is used to treat attention deficit hyperactivity disorder (ADHD) and excessive daytime sleepiness (narcolepsy). Severe complications can occur when dexmethylphenidate tablets are crushed and diluted in water for injection. The tablets contain insoluble fillers that can block small blood vessels, causing serious damage to the lungs and eye retina. In addition, there have been reports of fatalities among drug users who combined dexmethylphenidate with pentazocine, a narcotic analgesic.

Method of use: Ingested; tablets are also crushed and snorted or diluted in water and injected.

Duration of action: 4 to 5 hours following a standard therapeutic dose.

Psychological effects of abuse: Depression, nervousness, and psychotic behavior.

Physical effects of abuse: Abdominal cramps, chronic insomnia, diarrhea, loss of appetite, nausea, rapid heart rate, tiredness, vomiting, and weight loss. Severe blockage in the blood vessels of the lungs and eye retina can occur when the drug is injected.

Overdose symptoms: Signs of overdose may include excessive sweating and hyperactivity, vomiting, agitation, tremors, severely elevated body temperature and blood pressure, rapid heart rate, and hallucinations.

Withdrawal symptoms: Withdrawal reactions are less common than with other CNS stimulants. Symptoms may include severe fatigue, depression, nausea, vomiting, stomach cramps, insomnia, and nightmares.

DEXTROAMPHETAMINE
BRAND NAMES: Adderall, Dexedrine, DextroStat, Adderal XR
COMMON STREET NAMES: Bennies, black beauties, crosses, hearts, LA turn-around, speed, truck drivers, uppers
DEA CLASS: Class II
PHARMACOLOGIC CLASS: Amphetamine, CNS stimulant, anorexiant

Description: Dextroamphetamine has a marked CNS stimulant effect, particularly on the cerebral cortex. It is used to treat excessive daytime sleepiness (narcolepsy) and attention deficit hyperactivity disorder (ADHD).

Method of use: Ingested, snorted, smoked, and injected

Duration of action: About 4 hours for short-acting forms and 6 to 12 hours for long-acting forms.

Psychological effects of abuse: Aggression, confusion, depression, anxiety, delusions, agitation, paranoia, hallucinations, drug craving, and impulsive behavior. Tolerance and psychological dependence may develop after chronic use.

Physical effects of abuse: Blood-vessel inflammation in the brain, elevated blood pressure, fever, muscle pain, poor blood circulation, rapid heart rate, and weight loss.

Overdose symptoms: Overdose syndromes are characterized by circulatory collapse, seizures, irregular heart rate, significantly elevated body temperature, severe muscle weakness and pain, kidney and liver injuries, and coma. In some cases, severe psychosis was reported within 24 hours following IV administration.

Withdrawal symptoms: Abruptly stopping the drug after long-term use may cause extreme fatigue, overeating, depression, and stupor.

DIAZEPAM
BRAND NAME: Valium
COMMON STREET NAMES: Candy, downers, sleeping pills, tranks
DEA CLASS: Class IV
PHARMACOLOGIC CLASS: Benzodiazepine, sedative, antianxiety, anticonvulsant

Description: Diazepam is used to treat anxiety disorders with or without depression, acute stress reactions such as anxiety prior to surgery, panic attacks with or without irrational fear, alcohol withdrawal, and certain types of seizure disorders. Abuse of benzodiazepines is particularly high among heroin and cocaine users.

Method of use: Ingested and injected IM or IV

Duration of action: Effects can linger up to 4 days, but may persist longer in chronic users.

Psychological effects of abuse: Confusion, impaired judgment and thinking abilities, irritability, mild euphoria, pressured speech, reduced inhibition, and suicidal ideation. Long-term use may cause psychological dependence.

Physical effects of abuse: Changes in appetite and body weight, constipation, dizziness, impaired muscle coordination, low blood pressure, and vertigo. Long-term use may cause physical dependence.

Overdose symptoms: The most severe signs of overdose are respiratory depression and coma. Other symptoms may include confusion, diminished reflexes, unrealistic euphoria, extreme sleepiness, and impaired muscle coordination. Death from overdose of a single benzodiazepine is extremely rare. However, there is an increased risk of toxicity when benzodiazepines are combined with alcohol and/or other CNS depressants. Fatalities have been reported in individuals who have overdosed with a combination of a single benzodiazepine and alcohol.

Withdrawal symptoms: Abrupt termination following long-term use may precipitate withdrawal symptoms and require hospitalization. Symptoms may include abdominal and muscle cramps, depression, insomnia, sweating, vomiting, tremors, and seizures.

Didrex *see Benzphetamine, page 440*

DIETHYLPROPION HYDROCHLORIDE
BRAND NAMES: Tenuate
COMMON STREET NAMES: Bam, bambita, beans, black beauties, Christmas trees, dolls, jellybeans, little bomb
DEA CLASS: Class IV
PHARMACOLOGIC CLASS: CNS stimulant and indirect-acting sympathomimetic, anorexiant

Description: Diethylpropion is related to amphetamines both chemically and pharmacologically. It is used as a supplemental agent to help promote weight loss in conjunction with caloric restriction, exercise, and behavior modification.

Method of use: Ingestion

Duration of action: 6 to 8 hours

Psychological effects of abuse: Mental depression, restlessness, talkativeness, uncontrollable excitement, personality changes, and psychosis.

Physical effects of abuse: Constipation, dry mouth, nausea, vomiting, stomach cramps, dizziness, light-headedness, sleeplessness, headache, elevated blood pressure, rapid heartbeat, blurred vision, dilated pupils, and intermittent or painful urination.

Overdose symptoms: Signs of overdose include confusion, restlessness, rapid breathing, stomach cramps, exaggerated reflexes, extremely high fever, irregular heartbeat, elevated blood pressure, hallucinations, panic state, convulsions, and coma.

Withdrawal symptoms: Physical dependence is not common. However, abruptly stopping use can occasionally cause insomnia, tiredness, depression, stomach cramps, convulsions, and nightmares.

Dilaudid *see Hydromorphone, page 466*

Dolophine *see Methadone, page 473*

Dopram *see Doxapram, page 452*

Doral *see Quazepam, page 501*

DOXAPRAM HYDROCHLORIDE
BRAND NAME: Dopram
COMMON STREET NAMES: Not known
DEA CLASS: Not classified
PHARMACOLOGIC CLASS: CNS and respiratory stimulant, nonamphetamine

Description: This drug is used to manage respiratory depression due to anesthesia. It is also used to manage abnormally high levels of carbon monoxide in the blood secondary to chronic obstructive pulmonary disease (COPD). Doxapram may raise blood pressure and stimulate the nervous system.

Method of use: Ingested and injected IV

Duration of action: About 6 to 8 hours

Psychological effects of abuse: Confusion, delirium, and hallucinations.

Physical effects of abuse: Shortness of breath, coughing, respiratory problems such as hyperventilation, convulsions, headache, dizziness, hiccup, hyperactivity, sweating, flushing, fever, nausea, vomiting, diarrhea, excessive sweating, flushing, difficulty urinating, and sudden high or low blood pressure.

Overdose symptoms: Signs of overdose include anorexia, high fever, excessive sweating, flushing, muscle rigidity, delirium, hallucinations, seizures, coma, and respiratory failure.

Withdrawal symptoms: To date, there are no reports of withdrawal effects following a standard therapeutic dose.

DRONABINOL AND NABILONE

BRAND NAME: Marinol (dronabinol); also known as delta-9-tetrahydro-cannabinol (THC)
COMMON STREET NAMES: Bud, endo, grass, herb, kind bud, Mary Jane, pot, shake, sinsemilla, weed
DEA CLASS: Class III
PHARMACOLOGIC CLASS: Antiemetic

Description: Dronabinol and nabilone are chemically related to THC, the active ingredient in marijuana. They are used to treat the nausea and vomiting associated with cancer chemotherapy and are prescribed only when other antiemetic drugs have failed to work. Dronabinol is also used to treat anorexia associated with weight loss in AIDS patients.

Method of use: Ingested

Duration of action: Onset of action occurs within 1 hour after ingestion and effects persist for 20 to 24 hours.

Psychological effects of abuse: Anxiety, confusion, depression, detachment from reality, hallucinations, memory loss, and mood changes.

Physical effects of abuse: Blurred vision, diarrhea, dizziness, drowsiness, dry eyes, dry mouth, feeling faint, headache, high blood pressure, increased appetite, irregular gait, rapid heartbeat, ringing in the ears, and vertigo. Chronic users may develop tolerance and physical dependence.

Overdose symptoms: Heavy users may develop tolerance rapidly and need progressively larger doses to obtain the same effects as before. Signs of overdose may include dizziness, drowsiness, slurred speech, irregular gait, decreased motor coordination and muscle strength, extreme tiredness or weakness, rapid heartbeat, high or low blood pressure, and rarely, psychosis.

Withdrawal symptoms: Abruptly stopping use may cause drug cravings, irritability, agitation, apprehension, insomnia, excessive sweating, aggressiveness, and extreme anxiety.

Duramorph PF *see Morphine, page 481*

Esgic *See Butalbital, page 442*

ESTAZOLAM

BRAND NAME: ProSom
COMMON STREET NAMES: Candy, downers, sleeping pills, tranks
DEA CLASS: Class IV
PHARMACOLOGIC CLASS: Benzodiazepine, sedative, hypnotic

Description: Estazolam is used for the short-term treatment of sleep disorders such as difficulty falling asleep or staying asleep. Abuse of benzodiazepines is particularly high among heroin and cocaine users.

Method of use: Ingested

Duration of action: Up to 30 hours

Psychological effects of abuse: Confusion, impaired judgment and thinking abilities, irritability, mild euphoria, pressured speech, reduced inhibition, and suicidal ideation. Long-term use may cause psychological dependence.

Physical effects of abuse: Changes in appetite and body weight, constipation, dizziness, impaired muscle coordination, and low blood pressure. Long-term use may cause physical dependence.

Overdose symptoms: The most severe signs of overdose are respiratory depression and coma. Other symptoms may include confusion, diminished reflexes, extreme sleepiness, unrealistic euphoria, and impaired muscle coordination. Death from overdose of a single benzodiazepine is extremely rare. However, there is an increased risk of toxicity when benzodiazepines are combined with alcohol and/or other CNS depressants. Fatalities have been reported in patients who have overdosed with a combination of a single benzodiazepine and alcohol.

Withdrawal symptoms: Abrupt termination following long-term use may precipitate withdrawal symptoms and require hospitalization. Symptoms may include abdominal and muscle cramps, depression, insomnia, sweating, vomiting, tremors, and seizures.

ETHCHLORVYNOL

COMMON STREET NAMES: Not known
DEA CLASS: Class IV
PHARMACOLOGIC CLASS: Sedative, hypnotic

Not commercially available in the U.S.

Description: Ethchlorvynol is used for the short-term treatment of sleep disorders, but it is not superior to the benzodiazepines. For the most part, benzodiazepines have replaced the use of ethchlorvynol because of its high potential for causing addiction and toxic overdose.

Methodic of use: Ingested

Duration of action: Hypnotic effects last about 5 hours following ingestion of a single therapeutic dose. If given in high doses, the effects may persist for up to 35 hours.

Psychological effects of abuse: Confusion, feelings of intoxication, hallucinations, and depression. Prolonged use of high doses may cause psychological dependence.

Physical effects of abuse: Dizziness, irregular gait, facial numbness, low blood pressure, vomiting, nausea, visual changes, cough, shortness of breath, respiratory distress, and accumulation of fluid in the lungs (with IV injections only). Prolonged use may cause intense physical addiction and withdrawal symptoms.

Overdose symptoms: Tolerance develops rapidly, and the progressively higher doses needed are often in the toxic range. Symptoms include severely low blood pressure, accumulation of fluid in the lungs, and liver damage.

Withdrawal symptoms: Abrupt cessation of use may cause weakness, heightened anxiety, irritability, dizziness, headache, sleeplessness, nausea and vomiting, distortion of visual perception, rapid pulse, and convulsions.

ETHINAMATE
COMMON STREET NAMES: Not known
DEA CLASS: Class IV
PHARMACOLOGIC CLASS: Sedative, hypnotic

Not commercially available in the U.S.

Description: Ethinamate is marketed in other countries for the short-term treatment of insomnia. The drug was withdrawn from the U.S. market in 1990 after safer and more effective agents became available.

Method of use: Ingested

Duration of action: The hypnotic effects start within 20 minutes and last 3 to 5 hours.

Psychological effects of abuse: Behavioral changes, excessive irritability, and paradoxical excitement. Prolonged use may cause psychological dependence.

Physical effects of abuse: Dizziness, drowsiness, confusion, irregular gait, nausea, vomiting, and "hangover" effects. Prolonged use may cause tolerance and physical dependence.

Overdose symptoms: Tolerance develops rapidly, and the progressively higher doses needed are often in the toxic range. Toxicity reactions are similar to barbiturates. Major symptoms of overdose are CNS and respiratory depression, severely low blood pressure, and coma (after high doses). Additional symptoms include severe weakness, confusion, slurred speech, irregular gait, shortness of breath, breathing difficulties, and slowed heartbeat.

Withdrawal symptoms: Abrupt cessation of use may cause confusion, restlessness, nervousness, irritability, trembling, sleeplessness, agitation, dizziness, hyperactive reflexes, hallucinations, and seizures.

ETHYLESTRENOL
COMMON STREET NAMES: Arnolds, gym candy, juice, pumpers, roids, stackers, weight trainers
DEA CLASS: Class III
PHARMACOLOGIC CLASS: Anabolic-androgenic steroid

Not commercially available in the U.S.

Description: Androgens are steroid hormones that develop and maintain male sex characteristics. They are used primarily to replace insufficient levels of testosterone due to poor functioning of the testes. When used in combination with exercise and a high-protein diet, androgens can promote increased muscle size and strength, improve stamina, and decrease recovery time between workouts. Androgens are also used to promote the development of puberty in males with clearly delayed onset. Additionally, androgens are sometimes prescribed for women with advancing, inoperable metastatic breast cancer who are 1 to 5 years postmenopausal.

Method of use: Ingested. Chronic users tend to rotate steroids using various methods known as cycling, stacking, and pyramiding. Sporadic discontinuation of use is believed to allow testosterone levels and sperm counts to return to normal. Taking steroids regularly with periodic "drug-free times" is called cycling. Stacking refers to the concomitant use of two or more steroids at high doses. Pyramiding is when the dose, frequency, or number of steroids taken is gradually increased, followed by progressive tapering of the drug(s).

Duration of action: Depends on the formulation, frequency, and method of use. In general, effects may last up to 6 days.

Psychological effects of abuse: Mood changes, depression, uncontrollable aggressive behavior, euphoria, anxiety, irritability, increased sex drive, and rarely, psychosis. Psychological dependence may also occur.

Physical effects of abuse: Angry or hostile feelings, elevated blood pressure and cholesterol, headache, insomnia, premature balding, psychotic reactions, severe acne, sexual dysfunction, and violent behavior. *In men:* Breast development, impotence, intermittent or painful urination, painful or persistent erections, reduced sperm production, and shrinking of the testicles. *In women:* Decreased body fat and breast size, deepening of the voice, enlarged clitoris, excessive growth of body hair, and menstrual changes. *In adolescents:* Premature termination of growth.

Prolonged use can lead to tolerance. While the long-term effects are not completely known, chronic steroid abuse has been associated with damage to the heart, liver, and brain.

Overdose symptoms: There have been no reports of serious overdose with this drug. Chronic use of high doses may cause excessive sexual stimulation, reduced sperm production, enlarged breasts in males, uncontrolled painful erection, jaundice, and deteriorating liver function. Excessive fluid retention may occur in users who have heart, liver, or kidney disease.

Withdrawal symptoms: Abrupt discontinuation may cause mood changes, tiredness, restlessness, loss of appetite, dissatisfaction with body image, sleeplessness, reduced sex drive, paranoia, and severe depression that can lead to suicide attempts.

FENFLURAMINE
COMMON STREET NAMES: Pep pills, speed, uppers
DEA CLASS: Class IV
PHARMACOLOGIC CLASS: CNS stimulant

Not commercially available in the U.S.

Description: Fenfluramine was previously used as a supplemental agent to help promote weight loss. It was withdrawn from the market worldwide due to its serious adverse effect on heart valves, but can still be found among drug users. Fenfluramine is an indirect-acting sympathomimetic agent related to amphetamines, but at standard doses it usually depresses rather than stimulates the central nervous system.

Method of use: Ingested

Duration of action: Following a single dose, effects may last 4 to 6 hours.

Psychological effects of abuse: Confusion, agitation, depression, restlessness, combative behavior, and hallucinations. Acute paranoia and other psychotic behavior were also reported with the use of this product.

Physical effects of abuse: Constipation, dry mouth, nausea, vomiting, stomach cramps, dizziness, light-headedness, sleeplessness, headache, elevated blood pressure, rapid heartbeat, blurred vision, dilated pupils, and intermittent or painful urination. Valvular heart disease was reported with prolonged use, particularly when ingested with phentermine.

Overdose symptoms: Tolerance may develop after 12 weeks of chronic use, and progressively larger doses are needed to obtain the same effects as before. Toxicity can persist for up to 3 days following a single large dose. Overdose symptoms may include dilated and nonreactive pupils, double vision, rapid and irregular pulse, irregular heart rhythm, respiratory failure, seizures, and coma.

Withdrawal symptoms: Withdrawal symptoms following cessation of fenfluramine are rare, but agitation, irritability, hyperactivity, and interrupted sleep patterns have been reported.

FENTANYL and FENTANYL CITRATE
BRAND NAMES: Actiq, Duragesic, Sublimaze
COMMON STREET NAMES: China girl, China white, dance fever, friend, goodfellas, king ivory
DEA CLASS: Class II
PHARMACOLOGIC CLASS: Narcotic analgesic

Description: Fentanyl is used as a sedative prior to surgery, as a supplemental agent to induce general or local anesthesia, and to help manage moderate to severe pain. Transdermal fentanyl is used for chronic pain. Actiq, a raspberry-flavored lozenge, is indicated only for treating breakthrough cancer pain in opiate-tolerant individuals. Actiq is about 80 times more potent than morphine. Although the pharmacologic effects of fentanyl are the same as those of heroin, fentanyl is 50 to 100 times more potent. U.S. authorities have identified at least 12 analogues of fentanyl being produced clandestinely.

Method of use: The most common method is IV injection; other methods include transdermal (absorbed through the skin), transmucosal (buccal, or absorbed through the gums), smoked, and snorted.

Duration of action: Depends on dose and method of use. In general, the effects last for only 1 to 2 hours following administration. However, repeated administration of large doses may result in accumulation and a longer duration of action.

Psychological effects of abuse: Confusion, depression, and hallucinations. Psychological dependence can result after prolonged use, especially with high doses. The psychological dependence associated with narcotic addiction is complex. Long after physical dependence has ended, the addict may continue to think and talk about the drug and feel unable to manage daily activities without it.

Physical effects of abuse: Low blood pressure, drowsiness, dizziness, headache, restlessness, fatigue, muscle rigidity, seizures, paradoxical CNS stimulation, nausea, constipation, vomiting, diminished appetite, dry mouth, stomach cramps, decreased urination, and shortness of breath. Chronic use may cause physical dependence.

Overdose symptoms: The main symptoms are constricted pupils, CNS depression, and slow or labored breathing. Severe overdose may result in interrupted breathing, circulatory depression, severely low blood pressure, muscle rigidity, slow heart rate, seizures, delirium, and shock. Physical activity, such as strenuous exercise or dancing, may cause increased absorption of transdermal fentanyl. Toxicity has been reported with transdermal patches due to heat-induced changes in the delivery system. Risk of overdose increases significantly when the drug is taken with alcohol.

Withdrawal symptoms: Abruptly stopping the drug after chronic use may precipitate withdrawal. The intensity of symptoms is directly related to the total daily dose, frequency and duration of use, and the health of the user. Although withdrawal from narcotics is painful physically and emotionally, it is rarely life-threatening if adequate hydration and nutritional support are maintained. Early symptoms include watery eyes, runny nose, repeated yawning, and excessive sweating. Later-stage symptoms may include restlessness, irritability, loss of appetite, nausea, vomiting, diarrhea, shivering, drug cravings, tremors, and severe depression. Advanced withdrawal symptoms may include chills alternating with flushing, muscle and bone pain in the back and extremities, and elevated heart rate and blood pressure.

Fioricet *see Butalbital, page 442*

Fiorinal *see Butalbital, page 442*

FLUNITRAZEPAM
COMMON STREET NAMES: Forget-me pill, Mexican valium, R2, Roche, roofies, roofinol, rope, rophies
DEA CLASS: Class IV
PHARMACOLOGIC CLASS: Benzodiazepine, sedative, hypnotic

Not commercially available in the U.S.

Description: Flunitrazepam is neither approved nor manufactured in the U.S. It is used in other countries for the short-term treatment of insomnia, as a muscle relaxant prior to surgery, and as an aid in the induction of anesthesia. There is widespread abuse of flunitrazepam among drug users, especially those who use opioids or cocaine. Flunitrazepam has also gained a reputation as a "date rape" drug. Victims who are unknowingly given the drug become incapacitated and unable to resist sexual assault.

Method of use: Ingested, snorted, and injected IM or IV

Duration of action: 9 to 30 hours, depending on method of use and dose size.

Psychological effects of abuse: Amnesia, confusion, impaired mental capabilities, mania or hypomania, and suicidal ideation. Long-term use may cause psychological dependence.

Physical effects of abuse: Constipation, decreased blood pressure, dizziness, drowsiness, impaired physical capabilities, loss of muscle tone, sleepiness, slowed psychomotor performance, urinary retention, and visual disturbances. Long-term use may cause physical dependence. Neurological effects can persist for years, particularly in older people.

Overdose symptoms: Overdose with flunitrazepam is particularly dangerous since respiratory arrest can develop rapidly. Other symptoms may include confusion, diminished reflexes, disorientation, impaired coordination, extreme sleepiness, slurred speech, visual disturbances, loss of muscle tone, lowered blood pressure and pulse, and loss of consciousness. Death from overdose of a single benzodiazepine is extremely rare. However, there is an increased risk of toxicity when benzodiazepines are combined with alcohol and/or other CNS depressants. Fatalities have been reported in patients who have overdosed with a combination of a single benzodiazepine and alcohol.

Withdrawal symptoms: Abrupt termination following long-term use may precipitate withdrawal symptoms and require hospitalization. Symptoms may include abdominal and muscle cramps, agitation, delirium, depression, insomnia, rapid pulse, sweating, vomiting, hallucinations, tremors, and seizures.

FLUOXYMESTERONE
BRAND NAME: Halotestin
COMMON STREET NAMES: Arnolds, gym candy, juice, pumpers, roids, stackers, weight trainers
DEA CLASS: Class III
PHARMACOLOGIC CLASS: Anabolic-androgenic steroid

Description: Androgens are steroid hormones that develop and maintain male sex characteristics. They are used primarily to replace insufficient levels of testosterone due to poor functioning of the testes. When used in combination with exercise and a high-protein diet, androgens can promote increased muscle size and strength, improve stamina, and decrease recovery time between workouts. Androgens are also used to promote the development of puberty in males with clearly delayed onset. Additionally, androgens are sometimes prescribed for women with advancing, inoperable metastatic breast cancer who are 1 to 5 years postmenopausal. Fluoxymesterone has also been used in the management of anemias caused by certain cancers or chemotherapy.

Method of use: Ingested. Chronic users tend to rotate steroids using various methods known as cycling, stacking, and pyramiding. Sporadic discontinuation of use is believed to allow testosterone levels and sperm counts to return to normal. Taking steroids regularly with periodic "drug-free times" is called cycling. Stacking refers to the concomitant use of two or more steroids at high doses. Pyramiding is when the dose, frequency, or number of steroids taken is gradually increased, followed by progressive tapering of the drug(s).

Duration of action: Depends on the formulation, frequency, and method of use. In general, effects may last up to 6 days.

Psychological effects of abuse: Anxiety, changes in sex drive, and depression. Psychological dependence may also occur.

Physical effects of abuse: Angry or hostile feelings, elevated blood pressure and cholesterol, headache, insomnia, premature balding, psychotic reactions, severe acne, sexual dysfunction, and violent behavior. *In men:* Breast development, impotence, intermittent or painful urination, painful or persistent erections, reduced sperm production, and shrinking of the testicles. *In women:* Decreased body fat and breast size, deepening of the voice, enlarged clitoris, excessive growth of body hair, and menstrual changes. *In adolescents:* Premature termination of growth.

Prolonged use can lead to tolerance. While the long-term effects are not completely known, chronic steroid abuse has been associated with damage to the heart, liver, and brain.

Overdose symptoms: There have been no reports of serious overdose with this drug. Chronic use of high doses may cause excessive sexual stimulation, reduced sperm production, enlarged breasts in males, uncontrolled painful erection, jaundice, and deteriorating liver function. Excessive fluid retention may occur in users who have heart, liver, or kidney disease.

Withdrawal symptoms: Abrupt discontinuation may cause mood changes, tiredness, restlessness, loss of appetite, dissatisfaction with body image, sleeplessness, reduced sex drive, paranoia, and severe depression that can lead to suicide attempts.

FLURAZEPAM
BRAND NAME: Dalmane
COMMON STREET NAMES: Candy, downers, sleeping pills, tranks
DEA CLASS: Class IV
PHARMACOLOGIC CLASS: Benzodiazepine, sedative, hypnotic

Description: Flurazepam is used for the short-term treatment of sleep disorders such as insomnia. Abuse of benzodiazepines is particularly high among heroin and cocaine users.

Method of use: Ingested

Duration of action: 6 to 8 hours

Psychological effects of abuse: Confusion, impaired judgment and thinking abilities, irritability, mild euphoria, pressured speech, reduced inhibition, and suicidal ideation. Long-term use may cause psychological dependence.

Physical effects of abuse: Changes in appetite and body weight, constipation, dizziness, impaired muscle coordination, and low blood pressure. Long-term use may cause physical dependence.

Overdose symptoms: The most severe signs of overdose are respiratory depression and coma. Other symptoms may include confusion, diminished reflexes, unsteady gait, unrealistic euphoria, extreme sleepiness, and impaired muscle coordination. Death from overdose of a single benzodiazepine is extremely rare. However, there is an increased risk of toxicity when benzodiazepines are combined with alcohol and/or other CNS depressants. Fatalities have been reported in patients who have overdosed with a combination of a single benzodiazepine and alcohol.

Withdrawal symptoms: Abrupt termination following long-term use may precipitate withdrawal symptoms and require hospitalization. Symptoms may include abdominal and muscle cramps, depression, insomnia, sweating, vomiting, tremors, and seizures.

Focalin *see Dexmethylphenidate, page 449*

GHB (GAMMA HYDROXYBUTYRATE or SODIUM OXYBATE)
BRAND NAME: Xyrem
COMMON STREET NAMES: Bodily harm, cherry meth, fantasy, Georgia home boy, grievous bodily harm, liquid ecstasy, liquid E, liquid X, organic quaalude, salty water, scoop, sleep-500, somatomaz, vita-G
DEA CLASS: GHB is Class I; Xyrem is Class III for medical use.
PHARMACOLOGIC CLASS: CNS depressant

Description: GHB is produced naturally in small amounts by the body, but its function is unclear. The drug is used in Europe as a supplemental agent during anesthesia. It is also marketed as a drug that promotes muscle growth. In 2002, the FDA approved GHB to help reduce the number of cataplexy attacks (a condition marked by weak or paralyzed muscles) in patients with narcolepsy, but only under strict distribution control. When produced in clandestine laboratories, its effects are unpredictable. Drug abusers use GHB to reduce the stimulant effects of cocaine, methamphetamine, ephedrine, LSD, and mescaline, as well as to prevent the withdrawal symptoms of these agents. According to government reports, GHB has surpassed Rohypnol as the most common substance used in drug-facilitated sexual assaults. GBL (gamma butyrolactone), an analog of GHB, is also abused.

Method of use: Ingested

Duration of action: GHB is extremely short-acting and quickly leaves the user's system.

Psychological effects of abuse: Agitation, amnesia, confusion, delusion, depression, hallucinations, paranoia, and psychosis.

Physical effects of abuse: GHB is highly addictive, particularly with prolonged use. Early physical effects may include breathing problems, dizziness, excessive sweating, headache, loss of muscle tone, lowered blood pressure, nausea, reduced inhibition, sleepiness, sleepwalking, slowed heart rate and respiration, vertigo, and vomiting. Higher doses may cause complete loss of muscle coordination, decreased level of consciousness, slurred speech, seizures, coma, and death. Mixing GHB with alcohol greatly increases the CNS depressant effects, including respiratory arrest, unconsciousness, and coma.

Overdose symptoms: GHB is frequently combined with alcohol, which increases the risk of severe overdose. Symptoms depend on the amount ingested, whether any other CNS depressants were taken concurrently, and whether the drug was taken with or without food. Signs of overdose may include confusion, agitation, increased combativeness, excessive sweating, headache, impaired coordination, irregular gait, vomiting, blurred vision, memory loss, shortness of breath, respiratory depression, hallucinations, lowered body temperature, slow heart rate, seizures, and death.

Withdrawal symptoms: Abruptly stopping use may cause anxiety, agitation, insomnia, tremors, abnormally fast heart rate, and delirium within 1 to 6 hours after the last dose was taken, and the symptoms can last for months afterward.

GLUTETHIMIDE

COMMON STREET NAMES: Doors; when combined with codeine: doors & fours, loads, pancakes and syrup
DEA CLASS: Class II
PHARMACOLOGIC CLASS: Sedative, hypnotic

Not commercially available in the U.S.

Description: Glutethimide has properties similar to those of barbiturates. It was used previously for the short-term treatment of insomnia, but safer and more effective products have now replaced it. Currently, there is little medical use of the drug in the U.S.

Method of use: Ingested

Duration of action: Sedation occurs 15 to 30 minutes following ingestion, with peak serum levels occurring 1 to 6 hours later.

Psychological effects of abuse: Confusion, false sense of well-being, and impaired perception. Psychological dependence may occur with prolonged use of high doses.

Physical effects of abuse: Anxiety, difficulty swallowing, excessive sleepiness, low blood pressure, loss of coordination, sexual dysfunction, and slowed heart rate and breathing. Excessive use leads to tolerance, physical dependence, and withdrawal symptoms similar to those of the barbiturates.

Overdose symptoms: Tolerance develops rapidly, and progressively higher doses are needed to obtain the same effects as before. Signs of overdose may include extreme tiredness, irregular gait, muscle rigidity, muscular hyperactivity, rapid heart rate, low blood pressure, respiratory failure, heart failure, seizures, and possibly coma.

Withdrawal symptoms: Severity of withdrawal symptoms are similar to those of barbiturates, including weakness, abdominal cramps, nausea, vomiting, disorientation, anxiety, restlessness, elevated body temperature, rapid heart rate, stupor, delirium, visual hallucinations, tremors, seizures, and possibly death.

Halcion *see Triazolam, page 509*

Halotestin *see Fluoxymesterone, page 460*

HYDROCODONE COMBINATION PRODUCTS

GENERIC NAMES: Hydrocodone with acetaminophen (Anexsia, Lorcet, Lortab, Maxidone, Norco, Vicodin, Zydone); hydrocodone with chlorpheniramine (Tussionex); hydrocodone with guaifenesin (Vicodin Tuss); hydrocodone with ibuprofen (Vicoprofen)

COMMON STREET NAMES: Hillbilly heroin, killers, percs, poor man's heroin, schoolboy

DEA CLASS: Class III for combination products; Class II for hydrocodone

PHARMACOLOGIC CLASS: Narcotic analgesic (hydrocodone as a single agent); combination products are classified as cough suppressant, decongestant, expectorant, or antihistamine.

Description: Hydrocodone is used to manage mild to moderate pain and as a cough suppressant.

Method of use: Ingested

Duration of action: Depends on the dose and drug(s) used. In general, when hydrocodone is combined with other analgesics, the painkilling effects may last for up to 8 hours following ingestion.

Psychological effects of abuse: Anxiety, confusion, false sense of well-being, inability to concentrate, mood changes, psychological dependence (after prolonged use). The psychological dependence associated with narcotic addiction is complex. Long after physical dependence has ended, the addict may continue to think and talk about the drug and feel unable to manage daily activities without it.

Physical effects of abuse: Constipation, dizziness, irregular breathing, light-headedness, nausea, respiratory depression, urinary retention, and vomiting. Physical tolerance develops rapidly and is marked by euphoria, sedation, shorter duration of action, and weaker painkilling effects.

Overdose symptoms: Chronic use leads to tolerance, and progressively higher doses are needed to obtain the same effects as before. Signs of overdose may include bluish skin, cold and clammy skin, excessive perspiration, limp muscles, low blood pressure, slow heartbeat, breathing problems, and extreme sleepiness that could progress to a state of nonresponsiveness or coma. Risk of overdose increases significantly when the drug is taken with alcohol.

Withdrawal symptoms: Although the symptoms are similar to those of morphine withdrawal, they are considerably less intense. Abruptly stopping use may cause excessive tearing, yawning, and sweating about 12 to 14 hours after the last dose. Additional symptoms may include diminished appetite, gooseflesh, irritability, confusion, irregular breathing, tremors, seizures and loss of consciousness.

HYDROMORPHONE
BRAND NAMES: Dilaudid, Dilaudid-HP
COMMON STREET NAMES: D, dillies, dust, juice, smack
DEA CLASS: Class II
PHARMACOLOGIC CLASS: Narcotic analgesic, cough suppressant

Description: Hydromorphone is used to help manage moderate to severe pain. In lower doses, it's used as a cough suppressant. Compared with morphine, hydromorphone is two to eight times more potent, has a shorter duration of action, and produces more sedation.

Method of use: Ingested, used rectally, and injected IM, IV, or SC. Narcotic addicts often dissolve the tablets and inject the solution as a substitute for heroin.

Duration of action: About 4 to 5 hours

Psychological effects of abuse: Confusion, depression, hallucination, moodiness, nervousness, psychological dependence (after prolonged use), restlessness, and paradoxical CNS stimulation. The psychological dependence associated with narcotic addiction is complex. Long after physical dependence has ended, the addict may continue to think and talk about the drug and feel unable to manage daily activities without it.

Physical effects of abuse: Constricted pupils, decreased urination, diminished appetite, dry mouth, dizziness, headache, irregular breathing, low blood pressure, light-headedness, nausea, paradoxical CNS stimulation, rash, respiratory depression, seizures, severe constipation, stomach cramps, tiredness, and vomiting. Physical dependence may develop after prolonged use.

Overdose symptoms: Although tolerance develops slowly, the risk of overdose eventually increases as progressively larger doses are needed to obtain the same effects as before. Symptoms of overdose may include severe drowsiness, clammy skin, confusion, constricted pupils, low blood pressure, interrupted breathing, slow pulse, tremors, respiratory depression, convulsions, and coma. Risk of overdose increases significantly when the drug is taken with alcohol.

Withdrawal symptoms: Withdrawal begins slowly, with peak effects occurring 5 days after the last dose; however, sleep disturbances can persist for 13 days afterward. Although withdrawal is painful physically and emotionally, it's rarely life-threatening if adequate hydration and nutritional support are maintained. Early symptoms may include irritability, insomnia, diminished appetite, severe yawning, severe sneezing, tearing, and cold-like symptoms. Later-stage symptoms include nausea, vomiting, diarrhea, abdominal cramps, paradoxical excitability, bone and muscle pain in the back and extremities, fever, chills, excessive sweating, depression, and elevated heart rate and blood pressure.

Infumorph *see Morphine, page 481*

Intensol *see Oxycodone, page 488*

Ionamin *see Phentermine, page 498*

Kadian *see Morphine, page 481*

KETAMINE
BRAND NAME: Ketalar
COMMON STREET NAMES: Cat Valiums, jet, K, K-hole, keets, Lady K, new ecstasy, Special K, super C, vitamin K
DEA CLASS: Class III
PHARMACOLOGIC CLASS: General anesthetic; also identified as a dissociative anesthetic

Description: Ketamine's chemical structure and pharmacologic action are similar to those of phencyclidine (PCP), but it is significantly less potent. The drug's delusional effects are similar to LSD and mescaline. Ketamine produces "dissociative anesthesia," characterized by pain relief and amnesia without causing loss of consciousness. Legally, it is used to induce and maintain general anesthesia, especially when a cardiovascular depression needs to be prevented. Due to its disassociative effects and the fact that it is tasteless and odorless, ketamine is reportedly used as a date-rape drug.

Method of use: Ingested, snorted, used rectally, smoked, and rarely, injected IM or IV

Duration of action: About 2 to 4 hours following the standard dose. Effects of chronic use may take anywhere from several months to 2 years to wear off completely.

Psychological effects of abuse: Visual hallucinations, out-of-body experience, confusion, anxiety, depression, delirium, long-term memory loss, amnesia, aggressive or violent behavior, and vivid dreams. Long-term use may cause tolerance and psychological dependence.

Physical effects of abuse: Ketamine's physical effects are similar to PCP, and it has the same visual effects as LSD. The drug causes impaired motor function, exaggerated sense of strength, elevated blood pressure, rapid heart rate, tremors, slurred speech, nausea, vomiting, loss of appetite, rapid eye movement, and respiratory depression. Rarely, seizures and respiratory arrest may occur.

Overdose symptoms: Disorientation, irrational behavior, hallucinations, rapid heart rate, elevated blood pressure, convulsions, muscle rigidity, respiratory depression, and coma. Death is rare following ketamine abuse or overdose, but 1 gram may cause death.

Withdrawal symptoms: None are reported, since no evidence of physical dependence can be detected when the drug is abruptly withdrawn.

Klonopin *see Clonazepam, page 447*

Levo-Dromoran *see Levorphanol, page 468*

LEVORPHANOL TARTRATE
BRAND NAME: Levo-Dromoran
COMMON STREET NAMES: Dreamer, M, Miss Emma, morph
DEA CLASS: Class II
PHARMACOLOGIC CLASS: Narcotic analgesic

Description: Levorphanol is a potent synthetic opioid that is classified as a morphine derivative. It is used to help manage moderate to severe pain, as a sedative prior to surgery, and as a supplemental agent to nitrous oxide/oxygen anesthesia.

Method of use: Ingested, snorted, and injected IV, IM, or SC

Duration of action: Depends on the dose. Effects generally last 4 to 8 hours but can persist significantly longer in chronic users.

Psychological effects of abuse: Confusion, depression, hallucinations, mood changes, psychological dependence (after prolonged use), and restlessness. The psychological dependence associated with narcotic addiction is complex. Long after physical dependence has ended, the addict may continue to think and talk about the drug and feel unable to manage daily activities without it.

Physical effects of abuse: Blurred vision, constipation, dizziness, excessive sleepiness, low blood pressure, nausea, respiratory depression, slow pulse, and vomiting.

Overdose symptoms: Signs of overdose may include anxiety, cold and clammy skin, confusion, weakness, severe drowsiness and dizziness, constricted pupils, low blood pressure, slow heart rate, CNS and cardiac depression, convulsions, respiratory depression, and unconsciousness.

Withdrawal symptoms: Abruptly stopping the drug after long-term use may precipitate withdrawal symptoms. The intensity and duration of symptoms are directly related to the total daily dose, frequency of use, and health of the user. Although withdrawal from narcotics is painful physically and emotionally, it is rarely life-threatening if adequate hydration and nutritional support are maintained. Early withdrawal symptoms may include watery eyes, runny nose, repeated yawning, and excessive sweating. Later-stage symptoms may include nervousness, muscle twitching, drug cravings, restlessness, irritability, loss of appetite, chills alternating with flushing, nausea, vomiting, bone and muscle pain in the back and extremities, tremors, elevated heart rate and blood pressure, and severe depression.

Librium *see Chlordiazepoxide, page 446*

LORAZEPAM
BRAND NAME: Ativan
COMMON STREET NAMES: Candy, downers, sleeping pills, tranks
DEA CLASS: Class IV
PHARMACOLOGIC CLASS: Benzodiazepine, sedative, antianxiety, antiemetic, anticonvulsant

Description: Lorazepam is used to treat anxiety disorders, including anxiety associated with depression. In addition, it is used intravenously to treat severe epileptic seizures, as a sedative to induce relaxation before anesthesia, and as a supplemental therapy to prevent vomiting. Abuse of benzodiazepines is particularly high among heroin and cocaine users.

Method of use: Ingested and injected IM or IV

Duration of action: 8 to 25 hours

Psychological effects of abuse: Confusion, impaired judgment and thinking abilities, irritability, mild euphoria, pressured speech, reduced inhibition, and suicidal ideation. Long-term use may cause psychological dependence.

Physical effects of abuse: Changes in appetite and body weight, constipation, dizziness, impaired muscle coordination, labored breathing, and low blood pressure. Long-term use may cause physical dependence.

Overdose symptoms: The most severe signs of overdose are respiratory depression and coma. Other symptoms may include confusion, diminished reflexes, unrealistic euphoria, extreme sleepiness, and impaired muscle coordination. Death from overdose of a single benzodiazepine is extremely rare. However, there is an increased risk of toxicity when benzodiazepines are combined with alcohol and/or other CNS depressants. Fatalities have been reported in patients who have overdosed with a combination of a single benzodiazepine and alcohol.

Withdrawal symptoms: Abrupt termination following long-term use may precipitate withdrawal symptoms and require hospitalization. Symptoms may include abdominal and muscle cramps, depression, insomnia, sweating, vomiting, tremors, and seizures.

Lorcet *see Hydrocodone, page 465*

Lortab *see Hydrocodone, page 465*

Luminal *see Phenobarbital, page 497*

Marinol *see Dronabinol, page 453*

Maxidone *see Hydrocodone, page 465*

Mebaral *see Mephobarbital, page 471*

MEPERIDINE HYDROCHLORIDE
BRAND NAMES: Demerol, Meperitab
COMMON STREET NAMES: D, dillies, dust, juice, smack
DEA CLASS: Class II
PHARMACOLOGIC CLASS: Narcotic analgesic

Description: Meperidine is used as a sedative before surgery, as a supplemental agent to induce anesthesia, and to help manage moderate to severe pain. Although it has effects similar to morphine, meperidine has a shorter duration of action and weaker cough suppressing and antidiarrheal activities.

Method of use: Ingested and injected IM, IV, or SC

Duration of action: Depends on the dose and method of use. In general, effects persist 2 to 4 hours following administration.

Psychological effects of abuse: Confusion, depression, and hallucinations. The psychological dependence associated with narcotic addiction is complex. Long after physical dependence has ended, the addict may continue to think and talk about the drug and feel unable to manage daily activities without it. Psychological addiction is a major problem with meperidine, particularly when used in higher doses for prolonged periods.

Physical effects of abuse: Low blood pressure, drowsiness, dizziness, headache, light-headedness, feeling faint, restlessness, fatigue, seizures, nausea, constipation, vomiting, diminished appetite, dry mouth, abdominal cramps, stomach cramps, urine retention, and shortness of breath. Higher doses and long-term use is associated with paradoxical CNS excitement, tremors, and seizures due to the accumulation of the active metabolite normeperidine. Meperidine use has also been associated with symptoms that resemble Parkinson's disease, including jerky movements and tremors. Physical tolerance and addiction can develop, particularly when used in higher doses for prolonged periods.

Overdose symptoms: Chronic use leads to tolerance, and progressively larger doses are needed to obtain the same effects as before. Symptoms of overdose may include severe drowsiness, constricted pupils, clammy skin, confusion, slow pulse, slow or labored breathing, CNS depression, tremors, and seizures. Risk of overdose increases significantly when the drug is taken with alcohol.

Withdrawal symptoms: The intensity of symptoms is directly related to the total daily dose, frequency and duration of use, and the health of the user. Withdrawal symptoms may persist for up to 5 days after the last dose. Although withdrawal from narcotics is painful physically and emotionally, it is rarely life-threatening. Early symptoms appear within 3 hours after the last dose and may include watery eyes, runny nose, yawning, and sweating. Later-stage symptoms may include nervousness, muscle twitching, drug cravings, restlessness, irritability, loss of appetite, chills alternating with flushing, excessive sweating, nausea, vomiting, bone and muscle pain in the back and extremities, tremors, rapid heart rate, elevated blood pressure, and severe depression.

Meperitab *see Meperidine, page 470*

MEPHOBARBITAL
BRAND NAME: Mebaral
COMMON STREET NAME: Downers
DEA CLASS: Class IV
PHARMACOLOGIC CLASS: Barbiturate, sedative, anticonvulsant

Description: Barbiturates depress the sensory cortex, decrease motor activity, alter brain function, and produce drowsiness, sedation, and hypnosis. Mephobarbital is used primarily for daytime sedation and the management of seizure disorders.

Method of use: Ingested

Duration of action: Effects start within an hour and last for about 12 hours.

Psychological effects of abuse: Barbiturates may cause psychological dependence, especially following prolonged use of high doses. Effects may include confusion, alternating euphoria and depression, memory loss, impaired judgment, nervousness, nightmares, and hallucinations.

Physical effects of abuse: The most frequent physical effects are due to CNS depression, including dizziness, headache, excessive sleepiness, drowsiness, and irregular gait. Other symptoms may include headache, stomach pain, and skin rash. Paradoxical excitement and irritability may also occur. In chronic users, blood disorders such as megaloblastic anemia may develop. Short-term therapy has been associated with the development of Stevens-Johnson syndrome and toxic skin eruptions. Rarely, necrotic ulcer of the mouth may occur within 10 days of ingestion. Physical dependence is a significant risk, since it can develop after short-term use.

Overdose symptoms: Unsteady gait, slurred speech, confusion, low body temperature and blood pressure, and dose-dependent respiratory depression. Toxic effects are enhanced when the drug is taken with alcohol and/or other CNS depressants.

Withdrawal symptoms: Symptoms are similar to those of alcohol withdrawal and characterized by severe apprehension, weakness, heightened anxiety, irritability, dizziness, headache, sleeplessness, muscle twitching, nausea and vomiting, distortion of visual perception, and rapid pulse. Severely low blood pressure and convulsions may develop after a day or two, which eventually leads to hallucinations and delirium followed by coma and death.

MEPROBAMATE and CARISOPRODOL

BRAND NAMES: Soma (carisoprodol)
COMMON STREET NAMES: Not known
DEA CLASS: Class IV (meprobamate only)
PHARMACOLOGIC CLASS: Antianxiety agent (meprobamate); muscle relaxant (carisoprodol)

Description: Meprobamate is used to treat anxiety, tension, and muscle spasms associated with tension. Carisoprodol is a muscle relaxant that the body metabolically converts to meprobamate, which probably accounts for some of the drug's pharmacologic properties as well as its tendency to be abused.

Method of use: Ingested

Duration of action: Onset and duration of action of meprobamate are similar to those of the intermediate-acting barbiturates. Its effects peak 2 hours following ingestion and persist for about 10 hours.

Psychological effects of abuse: Confusion, euphoria, and impaired mental abilities. Psychological dependence may develop after prolonged use.

Physical effects of abuse: Chills, diarrhea, drowsiness, elevated heart rate, feeling faint, headache, impaired physical abilities, loss of appetite, nausea, numbness in the extremities, slurred speech, stomach pain, vertigo, and vomiting. Tolerance and physical dependence may develop after excessive use.

Overdose symptoms: Overdose can cause death due to respiratory failure and/or severely low blood pressure. Other signs of overdose may include drowsiness, irregular gait, tiredness, weakness, nausea, vomiting, blurred vision, low blood pressure, shock, and coma.

Withdrawal symptoms: Abruptly stopping use may cause confusion, memory loss, excessive sweating, nervousness, elevated blood pressure, hallucinations, and psychosis.

Metadate *see Methylphenidate, page 476.*

METHADONE

BRAND NAMES: Dolophine, Methadone Intensol, Methadose
COMMON STREET NAMES: D, dillies, dolls, done, dust, frizzies, juice, smack
DEA CLASS: Class II
PHARMACOLOGIC CLASS: Narcotic analgesic

Description: Although methadone's chemical structure is different from morphine and heroin, its pharmacologic effects are the same. It's used for detoxification and maintenance treatment of narcotic addiction and to help manage severe pain. High-dose methadone is useful for treating heroin addicts because it can block the drug's effects.

Method of use: Ingested and injected IM, IV, or SC

Duration of action: About 6 to 8 hours, although effects can last 24 to 48 hours in chronic users.

Psychological effects of abuse: Agitation, change in sexual desires, confusion, depression, disorientation, euphoria, and psychological depedence (after prolonged use). The psychological dependence associated with narcotic addiction is complex. Long after physical dependence has ended, the addict may continue to think and talk about the drug and feel unable to manage daily activities without it.

Physical effects of abuse: Blurred vision, CNS and respiratory depression, constricted pupils, constipation, diminished appetite, dizziness, drowsiness, faintness, headache, insomnia, light-headedness, loss of appetite, low blood pressure, nausea, seizures, slow heartbeat, slow or troubled breathing, stomach cramps, tremors, and vomiting. Chronic use results in tolerance and physical dependence.

Overdose symptoms: Chronic use leads to tolerance, and progressively higher doses are needed to obtain the same effects as before. Signs of overdose include low body temperature, constricted pupils, cold and clammy skin, confusion, severe drowsiness, slow or troubled breathing, CNS and respiratory depression, slow heartbeat, tremors, and seizures.

Withdrawal symptoms: Abruptly stopping the drug after chronic use may precipitate withdrawal symptoms. Although withdrawal from narcotics is painful physically and emotionally, it is rarely life-threatening if adequate hydration and nutritional support are maintained. Methadone withdrawal starts 24 hours after the last dose and can persist for several weeks. The intensity of symptoms is directly related to the total daily dose, frequency and duration of use, and the health of the user.

Early withdrawal symptoms may include watery eyes, runny nose, repeated yawning, and excessive sweating. Later-stage symptoms include restlessness, irritability, loss of appetite, nausea, vomiting, diarrhea, tremors, severe depression, shivering, and drug cravings. Advanced withdrawal symptoms may include elevated heart rate and blood pressure, chills alternating with flushing, and bone and muscle pain in the back and extremities.

Methadone Intensol *see Methadone, page 473*

Methadose *see Methadone, page 473*

METHAMPHETAMINE HYDROCHLORIDE
BRAND NAME: Desoxyn
COMMON STREET NAMES: Chalk, crank, crystal, fire, glass, go fast, ice, meth, speed
DEA CLASS: Class II
PHARMACOLOGIC CLASS: Amphetamine, CNS stimulant

Description: Amphetamine, methamphetamine, and dextroamphetamine are collectively referred to as amphetamines; they have similar chemical properties and pharmacologic actions. Methamphetamine is used as a supplemental agent for treating attention deficit hyperactivity disorder (ADHD). It is also used as a short-term aid for weight loss when combined with caloric restriction, exercise, and behavior modification.

Method of use: Ingested, snorted, smoked (most common use), and injected IV

Duration of action: 8 to 24 hours

Psychological effects of abuse: Anxiety, heightened energy, increased alertness, irritability, restlessness, and talkativeness. Large doses can cause confusion, delusion, rage, violence, visual and auditory hallucinations, delirium, self-destructive behavior, aggressiveness, and panic. Chronic use leads to psychotic behavior, including paranoia, hallucinations, and psychotic rages that may result in violence. Psychological dependence develops rapidly in chronic users.

Physical effects of abuse: Amphetamines are known to increase energy and decrease appetite. Other physical symptoms may include diarrhea, dilated pupils, elevated body temperature, excessive sweating, headache, insomnia, muscle rigidity, rapid heartbeat, rapid breathing, stomach cramps, tremors, and vomiting. Chronic abuse may lead to permanent brain damage. There are characteristic sores on the bodies of chronic users from scratching at "bugs" (the delusional belief that bugs are crawling under the skin). Acute lead poisoning may also develop due to the method of production of methamphetamines that uses lead acetate as a reagent.

Overdose symptoms: Tolerance to the anorectic effect of methamphetamine usually develops within a few weeks. Individuals may need progressively larger doses to obtain the same effects as before. Symptoms of overdose may include nausea, vomiting, diarrhea, restlessness, severe high blood pressure, dangerously high body temperature, tremors, hyperactivity, rapid and irregular heartbeat, rapid breathing, muscle rigidity, severe psychosis, serotonin syndrome, seizures, and coma. High doses may cause stroke. Fatality rates increase significantly if high blood pressure and seizures occur.

Withdrawal symptoms: Methamphetamine is a powerfully addictive drug, and physical and psychological dependence develop rapidly. Abrupt cessation of use may cause anxiety, fatigue, paranoia, aggressive behavior, and strong drug cravings. Severe depression and suicidal ideation have also been reported. Psychotic behavior may persist for months or years after discontinuation of use.

METHENOLONE
COMMON STREET NAMES: Arnolds, gym candy, juice, pumpers, roids, stackers, weight trainers
DEA CLASS: Class III
PHARMACOLOGIC CLASS: Anabolic-androgenic steroid

Not commercially available in the U.S.

Description: Androgens are steroid hormones that develop and maintain male sex characteristics. They are used primarily to replace insufficient levels of testosterone due to poor functioning of the testes. When used in combination with exercise and a high-protein diet, androgens can promote increased muscle size and strength, improve stamina, and decrease recovery time between workouts. Androgens are also used to promote the development of puberty in males with clearly delayed onset. Additionally, androgens are sometimes prescribed for women with advancing, inoperable metastatic breast cancer who are 1 to 5 years postmenopausal. Methenolone has also been effective in the management of aplastic anemia.

Method of use: Ingested and injected IM

Duration of action: Not entirely known but is believed to remain in the body for at least a week.

Psychological effects of abuse: Mood changes, depression, uncontrollable aggressive behavior, euphoria, anxiety, irritability, increased sex drive, and rarely, psychosis. Psychological dependence may also occur.

Physical effects of abuse: Angry or hostile feelings, elevated blood pressure and cholesterol, headache, insomnia, premature balding, psychotic reactions, severe acne, sexual dysfunction, and violent behavior. *In men:* Breast development, impotence, intermittent or painful urination, painful or persistent erections, reduced sperm production, and shrinking of the testicles. *In women:* Decreased body fat and breast size, deepening of the voice, enlarged clitoris, excessive growth of body hair, and menstrual changes. *In adolescents:* Premature termination of growth.

Prolonged use can lead to tolerance. While the long-term effects are not completely known, chronic steroid abuse has been associated with damage to the heart, liver, and brain.

Overdose symptoms: There have been no reports of serious overdose with androgenic steroids. Chronic use of high doses may cause excessive sexual stimulation, reduced sperm production, enlarged breasts in males, uncontrollable painful erection, jaundice, and deteriorating liver function. Excessive fluid retention may occur in users who have heart, liver, or kidney disease.

Withdrawal symptoms: Abrupt discontinuation may cause mood changes, tiredness, restlessness, loss of appetite, dissatisfaction with body image, sleeplessness, reduced sex drive, paranoia, and severe depression that can lead to suicide attempts.

Methitest *see Methyltestosterone, page 477*

Methylin *see Methylphenidate, page 476*

METHYLPHENIDATE HYDROCHLORIDE
BRAND NAMES: Concerta, Metadate, Methylin, Ritalin, Ritalin LA
COMMON STREET NAMES: R-ball, Rit, vitamin R, working man's cocaine
DEA CLASS: Class II
PHARMACOLOGIC CLASS: CNS stimulant, nonamphetamine

Description: Methylphenidate is used to treat attention deficit hyperactivity disorder (ADHD). In addition, it is the preferred drug for treating excessive daytime sleepiness (narcolepsy) due to its rapid action and fewer side effects than other CNS stimulants. Severe complications can occur when methylphenidate tablets are crushed and diluted in water for injection. The tablets contain soluble fibers that can block small blood vessels, causing serious damage to the lungs and eye retina.

Method of use: Ingested; tablets are also crushed and snorted or diluted in water and injected.

Duration of action: 4 to 5 hours following a standard therapeutic dose.

Psychological effects of abuse: Depression, nervousness, and psychotic behavior.

Physical effects of abuse: Anorexia, blurred vision, dizziness, elevated blood pressure, elevated or lowered pulse, headache, high body temperature, insomnia, irregular heart rhythm, nausea, stomach pain, Tourette's syndrome, toxic psychosis, vomiting, and weight loss. Severe blockage in the blood vessels of the lungs and eye retina can occur when the drug is injected.

Overdose symptoms: Signs of overdose include excessive sweating and hyperactivity, vomiting, agitation, tremors, severely elevated body temperature and blood pressure, rapid heart rate, and hallucinations.

Withdrawal symptoms: Withdrawal reactions are less common than with other CNS stimulants. Symptoms may include severe fatigue, depression, nausea, vomiting, stomach cramps, insomnia, and nightmares.

METHYLTESTOSTERONE
BRAND NAMES: Android, Methitest, Testred, Virilon
COMMON STREET NAMES: Arnolds, gym candy, juice, pumpers, roids, stackers, weight trainers
DEA CLASS: Class III
PHARMACOLOGIC CLASS: Anabolic-androgenic steroid

Description: Androgens are steroid hormones that develop and maintain male sex characteristics. They are used primarily to replace insufficient levels of testosterone due to poor functioning of the testes. When used in combination with exercise and a high-protein diet, androgens can promote increased muscle size and strength, improve stamina, and decrease recovery time between workouts. Androgens are also used to promote the development of puberty in males with clearly delayed onset. Additionally, androgens are sometimes prescribed for women with advancing, inoperable metastatic breast cancer who are 1 to 5 years postmenopausal.

Method of use: Ingested and absorbed through the cheek and gum (buccal administration). Chronic users tend to rotate steroids using various methods known as cycling, stacking, and pyramiding. Sporadic discontinuation of use is believed to allow testosterone levels and sperm counts to return to normal. Taking steroids regularly with periodic "drug-free times" is called cycling. Stacking refers to the concomitant use of two or more steroids at high doses. Pyramiding is when the dose, frequency, or number of steroids taken is gradually increased, followed by progressive tapering of the drug(s).

Duration of action: Depends on the dose and method of use. Methyltestosterone remains active for up to 22 hours following use.

Psychological effects of abuse: Mood changes, depression, uncontrollable aggressive behavior, euphoria, anxiety, irritability, increased sex drive, and rarely, psychosis. Psychological dependence may occur.

Physical effects of abuse: Angry or hostile feelings, elevated blood pressure and cholesterol, headache, insomnia, premature balding, psychotic reactions, severe acne, sexual dysfunction, and violent behavior. *In men:* Breast development, impotence, intermittent or painful urination, painful or persistent erections, reduced sperm production, and shrinking of the testicles. *In women:* Decreased body fat and breast size, deepening of the voice, enlarged clitoris, excessive growth of body hair, and menstrual changes. *In adolescents:* Premature termination of growth.

Prolonged use can lead to tolerance. While the long-term effects are not completely known, chronic steroid abuse has been associated with damage to the heart, liver, and brain.

Overdose symptoms: There are no documented reports of overdose with androgens. Chronic use of high doses may cause excessive sexual stimulation, reduced sperm production, enlarged breasts in males, uncontrollable painful erection, jaundice, and deteriorating liver function. Excessive fluid retention may occur in users who have heart, liver, or kidney disease.

Withdrawal symptoms: Abrupt discontinuation may cause mood changes, tiredness, restlessness, loss of appetite, dissatisfaction with body image, sleeplessness, reduced sex drive, paranoia, and severe depression that can lead to suicide attempts.

METHYPRYLON

COMMON STREET NAMES: Not known
DEA CLASS: Class III
PHARMACOLOGIC CLASS: Sedative, hypnotic (nonbarbiturate)

Description: Methyprylon is chemically related to glutethimide and causes CNS depression similar to barbiturates. The drug is marketed in other countries for the short-term treatment of insomnia. Methyprylon was withdrawn from the U.S. market after safer and more effective agents became available.

Method of use: Ingested, used rectally

Duration of action: Usually 5 to 8 hours following a standard therapeutic dose.

Psychological effects of abuse: Confusion, depression, paradoxical excitement, hallucinations, nightmares, and restlessness. Prolonged use may lead to psychological dependence.

Physical effects of abuse: Blurred or double vision, dizziness, drowsiness, fever, headache, insomnia, irregular gait, nausea, vomiting, diarrhea, constipation, stomach cramps, trembling, and weakness. Prolonged use may cause liver damage and/or soft bones or rickets. Respiratory depression, seizures, and coma have also been reported. Prolonged use may lead to tolerance and physical dependence.

Overdose symptoms: Complications with sedative overdose—such as pneumonia, fluid accumulation in the lungs, heart arrhythmias, and heart or kidney failure—may occur in rare cases. Life-threatening signs of overdose include severe confusion, dilated pupils, rapid heartbeat, excessive CNS and respiratory depression, severe drowsiness, loss of reflexes, coma, respiratory arrest, and death. Additional symptoms may include constricted pupils, slurred speech, irregular gait, weakness, and low body temperature.

Withdrawal symptoms: Abrupt cessation of use may cause severe confusion, nightmares, restlessness, paradoxical excitement, sleeplessness, excessive sweating, hallucinations, and seizures. Death has also been reported in individuals not receiving medical treatment during withdrawal.

MIDAZOLAM HYDROCHLORIDE

COMMON STREET NAMES: Candy, downers, sleeping pills, tranks
DEA CLASS: Class IV
PHARMACOLOGIC CLASS: Benzodiazepine, sedative, hypnotic

Description: Midazolam is used to produce drowsiness and relieve anxiety before surgery or diagnostic procedures. It is also used to induce loss of consciousness and amnesia in patients having surgery or those in critical-care settings. It is three to four times more potent than Valium. Abuse of benzodiazepines is particularly high among heroin and cocaine users.

Method of use: Ingested, snorted, and injected IM or IV

Duration of action: Up to 6 hours

Psychological effects of abuse: Amnesia, confusion, depression, impaired judgment and thinking abilities, reduced inhibition, and suicidal ideation. Paradoxical effects include euphoria, hyperactivity, and extreme aggression. Prolonged use may cause psychological dependence.

Physical effects of abuse: Constipation, decreased blood pressure, dizziness, drowsiness, impaired physical capabilities, irregular gait, loss of muscle tone, sleepiness, slowed psychomotor performance, urinary retention, and visual disturbances. Prolonged use may cause physical dependence.

Overdose symptoms: The most severe signs of overdose are respiratory depression, loss of consciousness, and coma. Other symptoms may include confusion, depression, diminished reflexes, slurred speech, impaired coordination, apnea, extreme sleepiness, loss of muscle tone, and severely low blood pressure. Death from overdose of a single benzodiazepine is extremely rare. However, there is an increased risk of toxicity when benzodiazepines are combined with alcohol and/or other CNS depressants. Fatalities have been reported in patients who have overdosed with a combination of a single benzodiazepine and alcohol.

Withdrawal symptoms: Abrupt termination following long-term use may precipitate withdrawal symptoms and require hospitalization. Symptoms may include abdominal and muscle cramps, depression, insomnia, sweating, vomiting, tremors, and seizures.

MODAFINIL
BRAND NAME: Provigil
COMMON STREET NAMES: Not known
DEA CLASS: Class IV
PHARMACOLOGIC CLASS: CNS stimulant, nonamphetamine

Description: Modafinil is used to improve wakefulness in those with excessive daytime sleepiness (narcolepsy). It is also used to treat obstructive sleep apnea/hypopnea syndrome and shift work sleep disorder. The drug is chemically and pharmacologically unrelated to other CNS stimulants such as methylphenidate or amphetamines.

Method of use: Ingested

Duration of action: About 10 to 12 hours

Psychological effects of abuse: Psychoactive and euphoric effects, as well as alterations of mood and perception, are the most common psychological effects of modafinil. Other effects may include anxiety, depression, confusion, paranoid delusions, auditory hallucinations, and amnesia. Eye problems such as floaters and dryness have also been reported.

Physical effects of abuse: High or low blood pressure, irregular heartbeats, headache, nervousness, dizziness, sleeplessness, irregular gait, nausea, diarrhea, vomiting, dry mouth, reduced appetite, ejaculatory difficulties, urinary difficulties, neck pain, tremor, abnormal involuntary movements, tingling sensation, abnormal vision, increased liver enzymes, shortness of breath, and nasal congestion.

Overdose symptoms: Overdose information is limited. The following have been reported with high doses: agitation, irritability, confusion, nervousness, tremor, sleeplessness, and heart palpitations.

Withdrawal symptoms: To date, physical dependence on this drug has not been reported. However, experience with modafinil is limited, and the potential for dependence still exists.

MORPHINE SULFATE

BRAND NAMES: Astramorph PF, Avinza, Duramorph PF, Infumorph, Kadian, MS Contin, MSIR, Oramorph SR, RMS, Roxanol
COMMON STREET NAMES: Dreamer, M, Miss Emma, morph
DEA CLASS: Class II
PHARMACOLOGIC CLASS: Narcotic analgesic

Description: Morphine is the principal constituent of opium. It is used as a sedative prior to surgery, as a supplemental agent to induce anesthesia, and to manage moderate to severe pain. Morphine can also be used to relieve pain associated with heart attack and to relieve anxiety in patients who have shortness of breath due to pulmonary edema or acute heart failure.

Method of use: Ingested, used rectally, and injected IM, IV, or SC

Duration of action: Depends on the dose and method of use. In general, the effects last 3 to 6 hours following administration. However, in chronic users the effects may last significantly longer.

Psychological effects of abuse: Confusion, disorientation, false sense of well-being, hallucinations, and thought disturbances. The psychological dependence associated with narcotic addiction is complex. Long after physical dependence has ended, the addict may continue to think and talk about the drug and feel unable to manage daily activities without it. Psychological dependence on morphine is known to develop slowly.

Physical effects of abuse: Blurred vision, CNS and respiratory depression, constipation, diminished appetite, dizziness, drowsiness, dry mouth, flushing, headache, low blood pressure and pulse, muscle rigidity, nausea, paradoxical CNS stimulation, restlessness, seizures, shortness of breath, stomach cramps, tiredness, urine retention, and vomiting. Physical dependence on morphine develops progressively.

Overdose symptoms: Although tolerance develops slowly, the risk of overdose eventually increases as progressively larger doses are needed to obtain the same effects as before. Signs of overdose may include severe drowsiness, constricted pupils, clammy skin, confusion, low blood pressure, interrupted breathing, slow pulse, tremors, respiratory depression, convulsions, and coma. Risk of overdose increases significantly when the drug is taken with alcohol.

Withdrawal symptoms: Although withdrawal from morphine is painful physically and emotionally, it's rarely life-threatening if adequate hydration and nutritional support are maintained. Symptoms begin slowly, with peak effects observed 5 days after cessation of use; however, sleep disturbances can persist up to 13 days following the last dose. Early withdrawal symptoms may include irritability, sleeplessness, diminished appetite, excessive yawning, severe sneezing, tearing, and head cold. Later-stage symptoms may include nausea, vomiting, severe diarrhea, paradoxical excitability, abdominal cramps, bone and muscle pain in the back and extremities, fever and chills, excessive sweating, and depression. Muscle spasms and kicking movements can also occur, which may explain the expression "kicking the habit."

MS Contin *see Morphine, page 481*

MSIR *see Morphine, page 481*

Mysoline *see Primidone, page 499*

NANDROLONE DECANOATE

COMMON STREET NAMES: Arnolds, gym candy, juice, pumpers, roids, stackers, weight trainers
DEA CLASS: Class III
PHARMACOLOGIC CLASS: Anabolic-androgenic steroid

Description: Androgens are steroid hormones that develop and maintain male sex characteristics. They are used primarily to replace insufficient levels of testosterone due to poor functioning of the testes. When used in combination with exercise and a high-protein diet, androgens can promote increased muscle size and strength, improve stamina, and decrease recovery time between workouts. Androgens are also used to promote the development of puberty in males with clearly delayed onset. Additionally, androgens are sometimes prescribed for women with advancing, inoperable metastatic breast cancer who are 1 to 5 years postmenopausal. Nandrolone has also been shown to positively influence calcium metabolism and increase bone mass in people with osteoporosis.

Method of use: Injected IM. Chronic users tend to rotate steroids using various methods known as cycling, stacking, and pyramiding. Sporadic discontinuation of use is believed to allow testosterone levels and sperm counts to return to normal. Taking steroids regularly with periodic "drug-free times" is called cycling. Stacking refers to the concomitant use of two or more steroids at high doses. Pyramiding is when the dose, frequency, or number of steroids taken is gradually increased, followed by progressive tapering of the drug(s).

Duration of action: Approximately 3 to 4 weeks.

Psychological effects of abuse: Mood changes, depression, and increased sex drive. Psychological dependence may also develop.

Physical effects of abuse: Angry or hostile feelings, elevated blood pressure and cholesterol, headache, insomnia, premature balding, psychotic reactions, severe acne, sexual dysfunction, and violent behavior. *In men:* Breast development, impotence, intermittent or painful urination, painful or persistent erections, reduced sperm production, and shrinking of the testicles. *In women:* Decreased body fat and breast size, deepening of the voice, enlarged clitoris, excessive growth of body hair, and menstrual changes. *In adolescents:* Premature termination of growth.

Prolonged use can lead to tolerance. While the long-term effects are not completely known, chronic steroid abuse has been associated with damage to the heart, liver, and brain.

Overdose symptoms: There have been no reports of serious overdose with this product. Chronic exposure to high doses may cause serious acne, excessive growth of body hair, hoarseness, changes in sex drive, poor sperm production, and menstrual problems in women.

Withdrawal symptoms: Abrupt discontinuation can cause mood changes, tiredness, restlessness, loss of appetite, dissatisfaction with body image, sleeplessness, reduced sex drive, paranoia, and severe depression that can lead to suicide attempts.

Nembutal *see Pentobarbital, page 494*

NITRAZEPAM
COMMON STREET NAMES: Candy, downers, sleeping pills, tranks
DEA CLASS: Class IV
PHARMACOLOGIC CLASS: Benzodiazepine, sedative, hypnotic

Not commercially available in the U.S.

Description: Nitrazepam is neither approved nor manufactured in the U.S. It has similar pharmacologic properties as diazepam (Valium). Nitrazepam is used in other countries for the short-term treatment of insomnia. It has also been used in epilepsy, particularly in infants. Abuse of benzodiazepines is particularly high among heroin and cocaine users.

Method of use: Ingested and injected IM or IV

Duration of action: Up to 30 hours

Psychological effects of abuse: Amnesia, confusion, depression, euphoria, impaired judgment and thinking abilities, mild euphoria, pressured speech, reduced inhibition, and suicidal ideation. Long-term use may cause psychological dependence.

Physical effects of abuse: Constipation, decreased blood pressure, dizziness, drowsiness, impaired physical capabilities, loss of muscle tone, sleepiness, slowed psychomotor performance, urinary retention, and visual disturbances.

Overdose symptoms: The most severe signs of overdose are respiratory depression, loss of consciousness, and coma. Other symptoms may include sensitivity to light, diminished reflexes, slurred speech, impaired coordination, apnea, extreme sleepiness, loss of muscle tone, severely low blood pressure, and tremors. Death from overdose of a single benzodiazepine is extremely rare. However, there is an increased risk of toxicity when benzodiazepines are combined with alcohol and/or other CNS depressants. Fatalities have been reported in patients who have overdosed with a combination of a single benzodiazepine and alcohol.

Withdrawal symptoms: Abrupt termination following long-term use may precipitate withdrawal symptoms and require hospitalization. Symptoms may include abdominal and muscle cramps, depression, insomnia, severe drowsiness, sweating, vomiting, tremors, respiratory depression, seizures, and coma.

NITRITES (amyl nitrite and glyceryl trinitrate)
COMMON STREET NAME: Poppers
DEA CLASS: Not classified
PHARMACOLOGIC CLASS: Coronary vasodilator

Description: Nitrites are volatile liquids that are readily absorbed from the lungs. Amyl nitrite has an action similar to glyceryl trinitrate (also known as nitroglycerin). Nitrites relax and open the blood vessels to the heart and are used therapeutically to relieve acute chest pain (angina) and to help manage heart murmurs. In addition, nitrites are used as supplemental agents to counteract cyanide poisoning, although their effectiveness for this use is still in question. These drugs are often abused because users believe they expand creativity, stimulate music appreciation, promote a sense of abandon in dancing, and intensify sexual experiences.

Method of use: Inhalation

Duration of action: Therapeutic effects of short-acting products usually occur within 30 seconds and last for 3 to 5 minutes.

Psychological effects of abuse: Aggressive behavior, anxiety, restlessness, and rarely, psychosis.

Physical effects of abuse: Anemia and other blood disorders, blurred vision, coma, cough, dizziness, elevated pressure in the eye, face rash, flushing, loss of coordination, low blood pressure or pulse, nausea, paralysis of the face, throbbing headache, rapid heartbeat, shortness of breath, throat irritation, vomiting, weakness, and rarely, death. Cerebrovascular disease can occur due to severely low blood pressure. Tolerance may develop with prolonged use.

Overdose symptoms: Seizures have been reported following severe overdose. Fatalities from nitrite toxicity have occurred due to uncontrolled artery spasm (vasodilation) and/or methemoglobinemia, which causes dangerously low oxygenation of the tissues. Other signs of overdose include bluish skin color, fainting, shortness of breath, increased pressure in the eye, stomach irritation accompanied by nausea and vomiting, severe abdominal pain, muscular weakness, weakness that effects only one side of the body, psychosis, coma, and rarely, death.

Withdrawal symptoms: Sudden withdrawal may cause sharp or persistent contractions of the heart arteries (coronary vasospasm), possibly leading to reduced blood flow and heart damage.

Norco *see Hydrocodone, page 465*

Numorphan *see Oxymorphone, page 491*

OPIUM

BRAND NAMES: Opium Tincture (also known as deodorized tincture of opium), Paregoric
COMMON STREET NAMES: Gee, God's medicine, gondola, great tobacco, gum, gumma
DEA CLASS: Class II for extracts, tinctures, and poppy; Class III for opium combination products such as Paregoric (opium with camphor).
PHARMACOLOGIC CLASS: Narcotic analgesic, antidiarrheal

Description: In the U.S., opium is used in the paregoric form to treat severe diarrhea. Rarely, it's used to relieve pain. Drug traffickers harvest opium from the poppy plant and refine the drug to make morphine or heroin.

Method of use: Ingested

Duration of action: Generally 4 to 5 hours

Psychological effects of abuse: Anxiety, confusion, depression, false sense of well-being, mood changes, psychological dependence (after prolonged use), and restlessness. The psychological dependence associated with narcotic addiction is complex. Long after physical dependence has ended, the addict may continue to think and talk about the drug and feel unable to manage daily activities without it.

Physical effects of abuse: Constipation, dizziness, headache, irregular breathing, light-headedness, loss of appetite, muscle weakness, low blood pressure, nausea, respiratory depression, sleeplessness, slowed heart rate, stomach cramps, urinary retention, and vomiting. Prolonged use may cause physical dependence.

Overdose symptoms: Chronic use leads to tolerance, and progressively higher doses are needed to obtain the same effects as before. Signs of overdose may include constipation, stomach cramps, nausea, vomiting, extreme sleepiness, nonreactive pupils, drowsiness, dizziness, slurred speech, cold and clammy skin, lowered body temperature and blood pressure, CNS and respiratory depression, convulsions, and coma. Death rarely occurs.

Withdrawal symptoms: Opiate withdrawal is considered to be fairly mild. The symptoms begin slowly, with peak effects observed after about 5 days, although sleep disturbances can persist for 13 days following abrupt cessation of use. Symptoms may include excessive yawning, nasal congestion, nausea, vomiting, diarrhea, excessive perspiration, muscle and joint pain, anxiety, fear, mildly elevated blood pressure, and rapid heartbeat. Other signs of withdrawal may include excessive tearing, restlessness, dilated pupils, involuntary twitching, abdominal pain, dehydration, and elevated blood sugar levels.

Oramorph SR *see Morphine, page 481*

Oxandrin *see Oxandrolone, page 486*

OXANDROLONE
BRAND NAMES: Oxandrin
COMMON STREET NAMES: Arnolds, gym candy, juice, pumpers, roids, stackers, weight trainers
DEA CLASS: Class III
PHARMACOLOGIC CLASS: Anabolic-androgenic steroids

Description: Androgens are steroid hormones that develop and maintain male sex characteristics. Oxandrolone is used as a supplemental treatment to promote weight gain following extensive weight loss due to surgery, chronic infections, or severe trauma. It is also used to treat patients who fail to gain or maintain normal weight for unknown medical reasons.

Method of use: Ingested. Chronic users tend to rotate steroids using various methods known as cycling, stacking, and pyramiding. Sporadic discontinuation of use is believed to allow testosterone levels and sperm counts to return to normal. Taking steroids regularly with periodic "drug-free times" is called cycling. Stacking refers to the concomitant use of two or more steroids at high doses. Pyramiding is when the dose, frequency, or number of steroids taken is gradually increased, followed by progressive tapering of the drug(s).

Duration of action: Depends on the formulation, frequency, and method of use. In general, effects last up to 6 days.

Psychological effects of abuse: Altered sex drive, depression, and mood changes. Psychological dependence may also develop.

Physical effects of abuse: Angry or hostile feelings, elevated blood pressure and cholesterol, headache, insomnia, premature balding, psychotic reactions, severe acne, sexual dysfunction, and violent behavior. *In men:* Breast development, impotence, intermittent or painful urination, painful or persistent erections, reduced sperm production, and shrinking of the testicles. *In women:* Decreased body fat and breast size, deepening of the voice, enlarged clitoris, excessive growth of body hair, and menstrual changes. *In adolescents:* Premature termination of growth.

Prolonged use can lead to tolerance. While the long-term effects are not completely known, chronic steroid abuse has been associated with damage to the heart, liver, and brain.

Overdose symptoms: There have been no reports of serious overdose with this drug, but excessive sodium and water retention may occur.

Withdrawal symptoms: Abrupt discontinuation may cause mood changes, tiredness, restlessness, loss of appetite, dissatisfaction with body image, sleeplessness, reduced sex drive, paranoia, and severe depression that can lead to suicide attempts.

OXAZEPAM

COMMON STREET NAMES: Candy, downers, sleeping pills, tranks
DEA CLASS: Class IV
PHARMACOLOGIC CLASS: Benzodiazepine, antianxiety, anticonvulsant

Description: Oxazepam is used to treat anxiety disorders and alcohol withdrawal. Abuse of benzodiazepines is particularly high among heroin and cocaine users.

Method of use: Ingested

Duration of action: 5 to 15 hours

Psychological effects of abuse: Amnesia, confusion, impaired judgment and thinking capabilities, mania or hypomania, pressured speech, reduced inhibition, and suicidal ideation. Long-term use may cause psychological dependence.

Physical effects of abuse: Constipation, dizziness, drowsiness, impaired physical capabilities, low blood pressure, muscle relaxation, sleepiness, slowed psychomotor performance, urinary retention, and visual disturbances. Long-term use may cause physical dependence.

Overdose symptoms: The most severe signs of overdose are respiratory depression and loss of consciousness. Other symptoms may include confusion, diminished reflexes, impaired coordination, slurred speech, extreme sleepiness, and loss of muscle tone. Death from overdose of a single benzodiazepine is extremely rare. However, there is an increased risk of toxicity when benzodiazepines are combined with alcohol and/or other CNS depressants. Fatalities have been reported in patients who have overdosed with a combination of a single benzodiazepine and alcohol.

Withdrawal symptoms: Abrupt termination following long-term use may precipitate withdrawal symptoms and require hospitalization. Symptoms may include abdominal and muscle cramps, depression, insomnia, sweating, vomiting, tremors, and seizures.

OXYCODONE HYDROCHLORIDE
BRAND NAMES: Intensol, OxyContin, OxyDose, OxyFast, OxyIR, Percocet, Percodan, Roxicodone, Tylox
COMMON STREET NAMES: Hillbilly heroin, killers, OC's, Oxycotton, Oxy's, Percs, Poor man's heroin
DEA CLASS: Class II
PHARMACOLOGIC CLASS: Narcotic analgesic

Description: Oxycodone is a semisynthetic opioid derived from the opium alkaloid thebaine. It is used for the management of moderate to severe pain. Oxycodone has pharmacologic actions similar to codeine, heroin, and morphine. It elevates levels of the neurotransmitter dopamine, which is linked to pleasurable experiences. Opiate addicts use oxycodone to control withdrawal symptoms when heroin or morphine is unavailable. The brand OxyContin is especially prone to abuse because it contains higher doses of the medication in a timed-release tablet.

Method of use: Tablets are chewed or crushed into a powder that is snorted or diluted in water for injection. Chewing, crushing, or diluting long-acting tablets disables the timed-release action and allows high doses of the drug to enter the bloodstream quickly. Using oxycodone like this dramatically increases the risk of overdose.

Duration of action: Depends on the dose and method of use. In general, the effects last 4 to 6 hours following administration. The effects of timed-release tablets can persist for 12 hours or more.

Psychological effects of abuse: Abnormal dreams, anxiety, confusion, psychological dependence (after prolonged use), and thought disturbances. The psychological dependence associated with narcotic addiction is complex. Long after physical dependence has ended, the addict may continue to think and talk about the drug and feel unable to manage daily activities without it.

Physical effects of abuse: Abdominal cramps, constipation, decreased urination, diminished appetite, dizziness, dry mouth, euphoria, excessive sweating, gastrointestinal inflammation, headache, hiccups, light-headedness, low blood pressure, nausea, respiratory depression, restlessness, sedation, sleepiness, and vomiting. Chronic use may cause tolerance and physical dependence.

Overdose symptoms: Fatalities have been reported, mostly when the timed-release tablets were crushed and snorted. Signs of overdose include dizziness, constricted pupils, weakness, cold and clammy skin, CNS depression, slowed or interrupted breathing, seizures, loss of consciousness, and coma. Risk of overdose increases significantly when the drug is taken with alcohol.

Withdrawal symptoms: Although withdrawal from oxycodone is painful physically and emotionally, it's rarely life-threatening if adequate hydration and nutritional support are maintained. Although the symptoms are similar to those of morphine withdrawal, they are considerably less intense. Abruptly stopping use may cause excessive tearing, yawning, and sweating about 12 to 14 hours after the last dose. Additional symptoms may include diminished appetite, irritability, restless sleep (sometimes called the "yen"), confusion, irregular breathing, tremors, seizures, and loss of consciousness.

OxyContin *see Oxycodone, page 488*

OxyDose *see Oxycodone, page 488*

OxyFast *see Oxycodone, page 488*

OxyIR *see Oxycodone, page 488*

OXYMETHOLONE

BRAND NAME: Anadrol
COMMON STREET NAMES: Arnolds, gym candy, juice, pumpers, roids, stackers, weight trainers
DEA CLASS: Class III
PHARMACOLOGIC CLASS: Anabolic-androgenic steroid

Description: Oxymetholone is a synthetic derivative of testosterone. It is used for the treatment of anemias caused by weak red blood cell production or bone marrow failure.

Method of use: Ingested. Chronic users tend to rotate steroids using various methods known as cycling, stacking, and pyramiding. Sporadic discontinuation of use is believed to allow testosterone levels and sperm counts to return to normal. Taking steroids regularly with periodic "drug-free times" is called cycling. Stacking refers to the concomitant use of two or more steroids at high doses. Pyramiding is when the dose, frequency, or number of steroids taken is gradually increased, followed by progressive tapering of the drug(s).

Duration of action: Depends on the formulation, frequency, and method used. In general, effects may last up to 6 days following use.

Psychological effects of abuse: Mood changes, depression, and reduced sex drive. Psychological dependence may occur.

Physical effects of abuse: Angry or hostile feelings, elevated blood pressure and cholesterol, headache, insomnia, premature balding, psychotic reactions, severe acne, sexual dysfunction, and violent behavior. *In men:* Breast development, impotence, intermittent or painful urination, painful or persistent erections, reduced sperm production, and shrinking of the testicles. *In women:* Decreased body fat and breast size, deepening of the voice, enlarged clitoris, excessive growth of body hair, and menstrual changes. *In adolescents:* Premature termination of growth.

Prolonged use can lead to tolerance. While the long-term effects are not completely known, chronic steroid abuse has been associated with damage to the heart, liver, and brain.

Overdose symptoms: There have been no reports of severe overdose with this drug, and toxicity is unlikely following acute overdose. Chronic exposure to high doses may result in severe acne, excessive growth of body hair, hoarseness, change in sex drive, poor sperm production, and menstrual problems in women.

Withdrawal symptoms: Abrupt discontinuation may cause mood changes, tiredness, restlessness, loss of appetite, dissatisfaction with body image, sleeplessness, reduced sex drive, paranoia, and severe depression that can lead to suicide attempts.

OXYMORPHONE HYDROCHLORIDE

BRAND NAME: Numorphan
COMMON STREET NAMES: Dreamer, M, Miss Emma
DEA CLASS: Class II
PHARMACOLOGIC CLASS: Narcotic analgesic

Description: Oxymorphone is used to help manage moderate to severe pain, as a sedative prior to surgery, and as a supplemental agent during anesthesia. It's also used to relieve anxiety in patients who have difficulty breathing due to pulmonary edema caused by heart dysfunction.

Method of use: Rectal and injected IV, IM, or SC

Duration of action: Generally 3 to 6 hours (rectal and IV administration)

Psychological effects of abuse: Confusion, depression, hallucinations, and paradoxical CNS stimulation. The psychological dependence associated with narcotic addiction is complex. Long after physical dependence has ended, the addict may continue to think and talk about the drug and feel unable to manage daily activities without it.

Physical effects of abuse: Blurred vision, CNS and respiratory depression, constipation, diminished appetite, dizziness, drowsiness, dry mouth, flushing, headache, low blood pressure, lowered pulse, muscle rigidity, nausea, paradoxical CNS stimulation, restlessness, seizures, shortness of breath, stomach cramps, tiredness, urinary retention, and vomiting. Physical dependence develops progressively.

Overdose symptoms: Although tolerance develops slowly, the user eventually needs progressively larger doses to obtain the same effects as before. Symptoms of overdose may include severe drowsiness, clammy skin, confusion, constricted pupils, low blood pressure, interrupted breathing, slow pulse, tremors, respiratory depression, convulsions, and coma. Risk of overdose increases significantly when the drug is taken with alcohol.

Withdrawal symptoms: Although withdrawal from narcotics is painful physically and emotionally, it's rarely life-threatening if adequate hydration and nutritional support are maintained. Symptoms begin slowly, with peak effects observed 5 days after cessation of use; however, sleep disturbances can persist up to 13 days following the last dose. Early withdrawal symptoms may include irritability, sleeplessness, diminished appetite, excessive yawning, severe sneezing, tearing, and head cold. Later-stage symptoms may include nausea, vomiting, severe diarrhea, paradoxical excitability, abdominal cramps, bone and muscle pain in the back and extremities, fever and chills, excessive sweating, and depression. Elevated heart rate and blood pressure may also develop.

PARALDEHYDE

COMMON STREET NAMES: Blue angels, blue devils, downers, goofers, nebbies, Peter, pink ladies, rainbows, softballs, yellow bullets
DEA CLASS: Class IV
PHARMACOLOGIC CLASS: Sedative, hypnotic

Description: Paraldehyde is marketed in other countries for the short-term treatment of insomnia. It is also used for treating symptoms of alcohol, barbiturate, and opiate withdrawal. High doses have sometimes been used to treat delirium and seizures. Paraldehyde was withdrawn from the U.S. market after safer and more effective agents became available.

Method of use: Ingested, used rectally, and injected IM or IV. Intravenous administration is extremely hazardous and could cause internal bleeding, accumulation of fluid in the lungs, heart damage, and circulatory collapse. Intramuscular injections are painful and could cause severe tissue damage, skin infection, and nerve damage at the injection site. Oral use can cause mouth and stomach irritation; rectal use can also cause irritation.

Duration of action: Depends on method of use. Hypnotic effects generally last 8 to 12 hours following a standard therapeutic dose.

Psychological effects of abuse: Nervousness, restlessness, irritability, and severe anxiety. Prolonged use may cause psychological dependence.

Physical effects of abuse: Coughing, low blood pressure, rapid heartbeat, fluid in the lungs, increased blood clotting, infection at the injection site, drowsiness, dizziness, "hangover" effects, stomach pain, nausea, and seizures. Paraldehyde decomposes during long-term storage, and deaths from corrosive poisoning have occurred after use of the decomposed drug. Prolonged use can lead to tolerance and physical dependence, especially in alcoholics.

Overdose symptoms: Death due to heart failure has been reported. Signs of overdose include weakness, depression, nausea, vomiting, rapid or labored breathing, slowed heartbeat, severely low blood pressure, and kidney or liver damage. Severe overdose could lead to respiratory depression and stupor followed by coma.

Withdrawal symptoms: Abrupt discontinuation can cause muscle and stomach cramps, excessive sweating, nausea, vomiting, tremors, hallucinations, and convulsions.

PEMOLINE
COMMON STREET NAMES: Not known
DEA CLASS: Class IV
PHARMACOLOGIC CLASS: CNS stimulant, nonamphetamine

Not commercially available in the U.S.

Description: Pemoline works much like dextroamphetamine and is used to treat attention deficit hyperactivity disorder (ADHD). However, pemoline is not recommended as first-line therapy due to its possible connection with liver failure.

Method of use: Ingested

Duration of action: For children, 7 hours; in other patients effects may last up to 13 hours.

Psychological effects of abuse: Depression, irritability, mild euphoria, and paranoid psychosis.

Physical effects of abuse: Dizziness, drowsiness, seizures, sleeplessness, headache, hallucinations, liver problems, loss of appetite, movement disorders, nausea, stuttering, stomach discomfort, severe muscle weakness, Tourette's syndrome, and weight loss. Prolonged use can lead to physical dependence.

Overdose symptoms: Prolonged use can lead to tolerance, and the progressively higher doses needed are often in the toxic range. Signs of overdose include agitation, confusion, restlessness, excessive sweating, severe muscle weakness, vomiting, rapid heartbeat, high blood pressure or body temperature, and hallucinations.

Withdrawal symptoms: Abrupt cessation of use may cause severe fatigue, sleepiness, headache, nausea, vomiting, abdominal pain, depression, paranoid psychosis, and seizures.

PENTAZOCINE HYDROCHLORIDE
BRAND NAME: Talwin
COMMON STREET NAMES: Poor man's heroin, Ts and Bs, Ts and Blues
DEA CLASS: Class IV
PHARMACOLOGIC CLASS: Narcotic analgesic, sedative

Description: Pentazocine is an opioid-type pain medication. It is used to treat moderate to severe pain, as a sedative prior to surgery, and as a supplemental agent during anesthesia. Combined preparations with aspirin may also be used in the treatment of moderate pain.

Method of use: Ingested and injected IM, IV, or SC

Duration of action: After ingestion: 4 to 5 hours; after injection: 2 to 3 hours.

Psychological effects of abuse: Confusion, disorientation, hallucinations, nightmares, and thought disturbances. The psychological dependence associated with narcotic addiction is complex. Long after physical dependence has ended, the addict may continue to think and talk about the drug and feel unable to manage daily activities without it.

Physical effects of abuse: Abdominal pain, blurred vision, chills, constipation, diminished appetite, dry mouth, feeling faint, flushing, headache, light-headedness, low blood pressure, nausea, sleeplessness, and vomiting. High doses can lead to rapid heart rate and respiratory depression. Chronic use may cause physical dependence.

Overdose symptoms: Although tolerance develops slowly, the user eventually needs progressively larger doses to obtain the same effects as before. Signs of overdose may include severe drowsiness, constricted pupils, severe high blood pressure, interrupted breathing, slow pulse, tremors, respiratory depression, convulsions, and coma. Risk of overdose increases significantly when the drug is taken with alcohol.

Withdrawal symptoms: Although pentazocine may cause physical dependence, withdrawal symptoms are much less severe than those of morphine. Early withdrawal symptoms may include irritability, sleeplessness, diminished appetite, excessive yawning, severe sneezing, tearing, and head cold. Later-stage symptoms may include nausea, vomiting, severe diarrhea, abdominal cramps, bone and muscle pain in the back and extremities, fever and chills, excessive sweating, depression, and elevated heart rate and blood pressure.

Pentothal *see Thiopental, page 507*

PENTOBARBITAL SODIUM
BRAND NAME: Nembutal
COMMON STREET NAMES: Downers, jackets, yellows
DEA CLASS: Class II
PHARMACOLOGIC CLASS: Barbiturate, sedative, anticonvulsant

Description: Barbiturates depress the sensory cortex, decrease motor activity, alter cerebral function, and produce drowsiness, sedation, and hypnosis. Pentobarbital is used as a sedative prior to surgery and to help induce anesthesia and alleviate anxiety. In addition, it is used for the emergency treatment of acute convulsive episodes such as status epilepticus.

Method of use: Used rectally and injected IM or IV

Duration of action: 3 to 4 hours following administration of a standard therapeutic dose.

Psychological effects of abuse: Barbiturates may cause psychological dependence, especially following prolonged use of high doses. Principal side effects include confusion, alternating euphoria and depression, and memory loss.

Physical effects of abuse: The most frequent physical side effects are due to CNS depression, including dizziness, headache, excessive sleepiness, drowsiness, and irregular gait. Other symptoms may include headache, stomach pain, and skin rash. Paradoxical excitement and irritability may also occur. In chronic users, blood disorders such as megaloblastic anemia may develop. Physical dependence is a significant risk, since it can develop after short-term use.

Overdose symptoms: Pentobarbital overdose may be complicated by the development of kidney necrosis, muscle necrosis, skin lesions, pneumonia, and low blood sugar. Seizures are not expected, except upon abrupt withdrawal from the drug.

Withdrawal symptoms: Pentobarbital is one of the most commonly abused barbiturates. Severe and life-threatening symptoms may occur within 48 hours of abrupt withdrawal, including continuous seizures, acute delirium syndromes with toxic psychosis, and coma, eventually resulting in death.

Percocet *see Oxycodone, page 488*

Percodan *see Oxycodone, page 488*

PHENDIMETRAZINE TARTRATE
BRAND NAMES: Bontril
COMMON STREET NAMES: Not known
DEA CLASS: Class III
PHARMACOLOGIC CLASS: CNS stimulant, anorexiant

Description: Phendimetrazine is related to amphetamines both chemically and pharmacologically. It is a CNS stimulant and an indirect-acting sympathomimetic with actions similar to those of dextroamphetamine. Phendimetrazine is used as a short-term aid to help promote weight loss in conjunction with caloric restriction, exercise, and behavior modification.

Method of use: Ingested

Duration of action: 9 to 12 hours

Psychological effects of abuse: Agitation, paranoia, delusions, and hyperactivity. Rarely, psychotic episodes may occur following a single dose.

Physical effects of abuse: Elevated blood pressure, rapid heart rate, sleep disturbances, headache, dizziness, dry mouth, thirst, constipation, nausea, diarrhea, and increased urinary frequency. Effects of chronic abuse include hyperactivity, severe sleeplessness, severe irritability, personality changes, and psychosis. Pulmonary hypertension and valvular heart defects have been reported in patients receiving phendimetrazine in combination with other weight-loss-promoting drugs.

Overdose symptoms: Although overdose with phendimetrazine is rare, the following symptoms have been reported: agitation, hyperactivity, significantly elevated blood pressure and body temperature, and seizures.

Withdrawal symptoms: Although there are no reports of withdrawal reactions, the potential still exists for long-term users.

PHENMETRAZINE
BRAND NAME: Preludin
COMMON STREET NAMES: Black Cadillacs, beans, blue devils, bolt, cartwheels, fives, hearts, jellybeans, pep pills, snap
DEA CLASS: Class II
PHARMACOLOGIC CLASS: CNS stimulant, appetite suppressant

Not commercially available in the U.S.

Description: Phenmetrazine is related to amphetamines both chemically and pharmacologically. It is a CNS stimulant and indirect-acting sympathomimetic with actions similar to those of dextroamphetamine. It is used as a short-term aid to help promote weight loss in conjunction with caloric restriction, exercise, and behavior modification. Phenmetrazine is not recommended as first-line therapy due to the potential for serious CNS side effects.

Method of use: Ingested, used rectally, and injected IV

Duration of action: Depends on the formulation. The effects of shorter-acting agents can last 4 to 6 hours, while the sustained-release version can last for 24 hours or more.

Psychological effects of abuse: Mild euphoria, nervousness, irritability, altered sexual desire, depression, mania, and rarely, psychotic behavior. Prolonged use may cause psychological dependence.

Physical effects of abuse: Rapid heartbeat, high blood pressure, heart palpitations, sleeplessness, headache, tremor, dizziness, dry mouth, excessive thirst, constipation, stomach discomfort, diarrhea, frequent urination, impotence, and blurred vision. Severe physical effects may include pulmonary hypertension, heart murmurs, and valvular heart disease. Prolonged use may cause physical dependence.

Overdose symptoms: Tolerance develops rapidly, and the progressively higher doses needed are often in the toxic range. Overdose symptoms include sleeplessness, hyperactivity, personality changes, psychosis, hallucinations, irregular heart rhythm, aggressive behavior, panic state, elevated body temperature, hyperactive reflexes, convulsions, and coma. Fatalities due to heart failure have been reported with high doses.

Withdrawal symptoms: Abrupt cessation of high doses may cause extreme fatigue, depression, and sleeping problems. Additional symptoms include hyperactivity, irritability, nausea, vomiting, nightmares, and tremors.

PHENOBARBITAL SODIUM
BRAND NAME: Luminal sodium
COMMON STREET NAMES: Barbs, downers, goofballs
DEA CLASS: Class IV
PHARMACOLOGIC CLASS: Barbiturate, sedative, hypnotic, anticonvulsant

Description: Barbiturates depress the sensory cortex, decrease motor activity, alter brain function, and produce drowsiness, sedation, and hypnosis. Phenobarbital is used to treat grand-mal and partial seizures. In addition, the injected form is effective for inducing sedation prior to surgery and facilitating the induction of anesthesia.

Method of use: Ingested and injected IM, IV, or SC

Duration of action: Effects begin in 20 to 60 minutes and can last for days, depending on the dose.

Psychological effects of abuse: Barbiturates may cause psychological dependence, especially following prolonged use of high doses. Psychological side effects may include confusion, alternating euphoria and depression, memory loss, impaired judgment, nervousness, nightmares, and hallucinations.

Physical effects of abuse: The most frequent physical effects are due to CNS depression, including dizziness, headache, excessive sleepiness, drowsiness, and irregular gait. Other symptoms may include headache, stomach pain, and skin rash. Paradoxical excitement and irritability may also occur. Short-term therapy with phenobarbital has been associated with the development of Stevens-Johnson syndrome and toxic skin eruptions. Physical dependence is a significant risk, since it can develop after short-term use.

Overdose symptoms: Phenobarbital overdose is associated with unusual reactions, including red, blistering skin lesions and neurological problems, that can appear 1 to 2 hours after ingestion. Other symptoms of overdose may include unsteady gait, slurred speech, confusion, low body temperature and blood pressure, and dose-dependent respiratory depression. Toxic effects may be enhanced when the drug is taken with alcohol and/or other CNS depressant drugs.

Withdrawal symptoms: Phenobarbital is abused less frequently because it is a long-acting barbiturate. Nevertheless, abrupt withdrawal may cause continuous seizures. Withdrawal symptoms can occur following discontinuation of chronic phenobarbital use, but are rare following an acute overdose. Symptoms are similar to those of alcohol withdrawal and may include generalized weakness, heightened anxiety, irritability, dizziness, headache, sleeplessness, muscle twitching, nausea and vomiting, and rapid pulse. Severely low blood pressure and convulsions may develop after a day or two, which eventually leads to hallucinations and delirium followed by coma and death.

PHENTERMINE HYDROCHLORIDE
BRAND NAMES: Adipex-P, Ionamin
COMMON STREET NAMES: Pep pills, speed, uppers
DEA CLASS: Class IV
PHARMACOLOGIC CLASS: CNS stimulant, anorexiant

Description: Phentermine is related to amphetamines both chemically and pharmacologically. It is used as a short-term aid to help promote weight loss in conjunction with caloric restriction, exercise, and behavior modification.

Method of use: Ingested

Duration of action: Up to 20 hours

Psychological effects of abuse: Confusion, agitation, reduced sexual desire, and restlessness. Acute paranoia and other psychotic behavior have also been reported. Psychological dependence can occur after chronic abuse.

Physical effects of abuse: Elevated blood pressure, rapid heart rate, constipation, diarrhea, nausea, dry mouth, sleeplessness, headache, and dizziness. Pulmonary hypertension and valvular heart defects have been reported, particularly when given concomitantly with fenfluramine or dexfenfluramine. Ischemic cerebrovascular disease, severe headache, and numbness have been associated with the use of phentermine.

Overdose symptoms: Overdose with phentermine is rare, but symptoms may include agitation, hyperactivity, significantly elevated blood pressure and body temperature, and seizures.

Withdrawal symptoms: Abrupt withdrawal may cause extreme fatigue and depression.

PRIMIDONE
BRAND NAME: Mysoline
COMMON STREET NAMES: Barb, downers, goofers
DEA CLASS: Not classified
PHARMACOLOGIC CLASS: Barbiturate, anticonvulsant

Description: Primidone is used in the management of grand-mal, psychomotor, and focal seizures. One of its active metabolites is phenobarbital.

Method of use: Ingested

Duration of action: Effects are age- and dose-dependent, but usually persist for up to 5 days due to the drug's active metabolites.

Psychological effects of abuse: Barbiturates may cause psychological dependence, especially following prolonged use of high doses. Psychological side effects may include behavioral changes and excessive irritability.

Physical effects of abuse: Drowsiness, vertigo, tiredness, irregular gait, loss of appetite, nausea, vomiting, sexual dysfunction, double vision, and rapid eye movements.

Overdose symptoms: Unsteady gait, confusion, slurred speech, low blood pressure, lowered or elevated body temperature, dose-dependent respiratory depression, and coma. The drug's toxic effects are enhanced when taken with alcohol and/or other CNS depressants.

Withdrawal symptoms: Symptoms are similar to those of alcohol withdrawal and characterized by severe apprehension, weakness, heightened anxiety, irritability, dizziness, headache, sleeplessness, muscle twitching, nausea and vomiting, distortion of visual perception, and rapid pulse. Severely low blood pressure and convulsions may develop after a day or two, which eventually leads to hallucinations, delirium, and continuous seizures, followed by coma and death.

PROPOXYPHENE HYDROCHLORIDE and PROPOXYPHENE NAPSYLATE

BRAND NAME: Darvon
COMMON STREET NAMES: D, dillies, dust, juice, smack
DEA CLASS: Class IV
PHARMACOLOGIC CLASS: Narcotic analgesic

Description: Propoxyphene is an opioid analgesic that is structurally related to methadone. It is used to alleviate mild to moderate pain.

Method of use: Ingested

Duration of action: Generally, effects persist 6 to 12 hours following use, but can last 30 to 36 hours in chronic users.

Psychological effects of abuse: Confusion, depression, hallucinations, nervousness, and paradoxical excitement. The psychological dependence associated with narcotic addiction is complex. Long after physical dependence has ended, the addict may continue to think and talk about the drug and feel unable to manage daily activities without it.

Physical effects of abuse: Blurred vision, CNS and respiratory depression, constricted pupils, constipation, diminished appetite, dizziness, drowsiness, faintness, headache, insomnia, light-headedness, loss of appetite, low blood pressure, nausea, seizures, slow heartbeat, slow or troubled breathing, stomach cramps, tremors, and vomiting. Chronic use results in tolerance and physical dependence.

Overdose symptoms: Chronic use can lead to tolerance, and progressively higher doses are needed to obtain the same effects as before. Toxic accumulations of propoxyphene and its metabolites can occur quickly with repeated doses, and the effects are often complicated by the addition of alcohol or other drugs. A disturbing number of fatalities have occurred from accidental or intentional overdose with propoxyphene; death within an hour of overdosing is not uncommon. Psychotic reactions and possibly fatal CNS depression—including decreased or labored breathing, temporary stoppage of breathing, and decreased heart function—can develop rapidly. Other symptoms of propoxyphene overdose may include bluish skin, extreme sleepiness, pupil constriction later followed by dilation, irregular heartbeat, low blood pressure, stupor, seizures, and coma.

Withdrawal symptoms: Severe withdrawal syndromes have been reported, particularly in older individuals. Symptoms may include restlessness, muscle and bone pain, severe diarrhea, sleeplessness, involuntary leg movements, chills alternating with hot flashes, depression, nausea, vomiting, elevated heart rate and blood pressure, convulsions, and coma.

ProSom *see Estazolam, page 454*

Provigil *see Modafinil, page 480*

QUAZEPAM

BRAND NAME: Doral
COMMON STREET NAMES: Candy, downers, sleeping pills, tranks
DEA CLASS: Class IV
PHARMACOLOGIC CLASS: Benzodiazepine, sedative, hypnotic

Description: Quazepam is used for the short-term treatment of sleep disorders such as insomnia. Abuse of benzodiazepines is particularly high among heroin and cocaine users.

Method of use: Ingested

Duration of action: 25 to 41 hours

Psychological effects of abuse: Confusion, impaired judgment and thinking abilities, irritability, mild euphoria, pressured speech, reduced inhibition, and suicidal ideation. Long-term use may cause psychological dependence.

Physical effects of abuse: Changes in appetite and body weight, constipation, dizziness, impaired muscle coordination, and low blood pressure. Long-term use may cause physical dependence.

Overdose symptoms: The most severe signs of overdose are respiratory depression and coma. Other symptoms may include confusion, diminished reflexes, manic behavior, unrealistic euphoria, extreme sleepiness, and impaired muscle coordination. Death from overdose of a single benzodiazepine is extremely rare. However, there is an increased risk of toxicity when benzodiazepines are combined with alcohol and/or other CNS depressants. Fatalities have been reported in patients who have overdosed with a combination of a single benzodiazepine and alcohol.

Withdrawal symptoms: Abrupt termination may lead to withdrawal symptoms and require hospitalization. Symptoms may include abdominal and muscle cramps, depression, insomnia, sweating, vomiting, tremors, and seizures.

Repan *see Butalbital, page 442*

Restoril *see Temazepam, page 505*

Ritalin *see Methylphenidate, page 476*

RMS *see Morphine, page 481*

Roxanol *see Morphine, page 481*

Roxicodone *see Oxycodone, page 488*

SECOBARBITAL
BRAND NAME: Seconal
COMMON STREET NAMES: Downers, reds, red devils
DEA CLASS: Class II
PHARMACOLOGIC CLASS: Barbiturate (short-acting), sedative, hypnotic, anticonvulsant

Description: Barbiturates depress the sensory cortex, decrease motor activity, alter brain function, and produce drowsiness, sedation, and hypnosis. Secobarbital is used as an emergency aid in the management of acute convulsive episodes. In addition, it is used for the short-term treatment of insomnia and as a sedative before surgery to help induce anesthesia and alleviate anxiety.

Method of use: Ingested and injected IV or IM

Duration of action: 3 to 4 hours

Psychological effects of abuse: Barbiturates may cause psychological dependence, especially following prolonged use of high doses. Psychological effects may include confusion, alternating euphoria and depression, and memory loss.

Physical effects of abuse: The most frequent physical effects are due to CNS depression, including dizziness, headache, excessive sleepiness, drowsiness, and irregular gait. Other symptoms may include headache, stomach pain, and skin rash. Paradoxical excitement and irritability may also occur. In chronic users, blood disorders such as megaloblastic anemia may develop. Physical dependence is a significant risk, since it can develop after short-term use.

Overdose symptoms: Symptoms may include unsteady gait, slurred speech, confusion, low body temperature and blood pressure, and dose-dependent respiratory depression. Toxic effects are enhanced when secobarbital is taken with alcohol and/or other CNS depressant drugs.

Withdrawal symptoms: Addiction may result following chronic use. Withdrawal symptoms may include anorexia, nausea, vomiting, muscle weakness, tremors, and low blood pressure, followed by seizures within 16 to 24 hours after the last dose. Acute delirium with toxic psychosis may occur within 48 hours following termination of use.

Seconal *see Secobarbital, page 502*

Soma *see Meprobamate and Carisoprodol, page 472*

Somnote *see Chloral hydrate, page 444*

Sonata *see Zaleplon, page 510*

Stadol *see Butorphanol, page 443*

Sufenta *see Sufentanil, page 503*

SUFENTANIL CITRATE
BRAND NAME: Sufenta
COMMON STREET NAMES: China white, China girl, dance fever, friend, good-fellas, king ivory
DEA CLASS: Class II
PHARMACOLOGIC CLASS: Narcotic analgesic/agonist, general anesthetic

Description: Sufentanil has three main uses: 1) as a primary agent for induction and maintenance of anesthesia administered with oxygen; 2) as a supplemental agent during maintenance of general anesthesia; and 3) as a combined agent used with low-dose bupivacaine during labor.

Method of use: Injected IV

Duration of action: Depends on dose size and the user's weight (duration is longer in obese individuals). Effects generally last 2 to 3 hours, but repeated use of large doses may result in accumulation and a longer duration of action.

Psychological effects of abuse: Confusion, depression, hallucinations, and restlessness. Prolonged use causes psychological dependence, particularly when high doses are used.

Physical effects of abuse: Blurred vision, CNS depression, constipation, decreased urination, diminished appetite, dizziness, drowsiness, dry mouth, excessive sleepiness, headache, high blood pressure (depending on dose), muscle rigidity, nausea, respiratory depression (depending on dose), slow heart rate or pulse, stomach cramps, and vomiting. Chronic use may cause physical dependence.

Overdose symptoms: The primary signs of overdose include CNS and respiratory depression and constricted pupils. Serious overdose may result in interrupted breathing, circulatory depression, severely low blood pressure, muscle rigidity, slow heart rate, delirium, seizures, and shock.

Withdrawal symptoms: Abruptly stopping the drug after long-term use may precipitate withdrawal symptoms. The intensity of symptoms is directly related to the total daily dose, frequency and duration of use, and the health of the user. Although painful physically and emotionally, withdrawal from narcotics is rarely life-threatening. Early symptoms may include watery eyes, runny nose, yawning, and sweating. Later-stage symptoms may include nervousness, muscle twitching, drug cravings, restlessness, irritability, loss of appetite, chills alternating with flushing, nausea, vomiting, bone and muscle pain in the back and extremities, tremors, elevated heart rate and blood pressure, and severe depression.

STANOZOLOL
COMMON STREET NAMES: Arnolds, gym candy, juice, pumpers, roids, stackers, weight trainers
DEA CLASS: Class III
PHARMACOLOGIC CLASS: Anabolic-androgenic steroid

Description: Androgens are steroid hormones that develop and maintain male sex characteristics. They are used primarily to replace insufficient levels of testosterone due to poor functioning of the testes. When used in combination with exercise and a high-protein diet, androgens can promote increased muscle size and strength, improve stamina, and decrease recovery time between workouts. Androgens are also used to promote the development of puberty in males with clearly delayed onset. Additionally, androgens are sometimes prescribed for women with advancing, inoperable metastatic breast cancer who are 1 to 5 years postmenopausal. This product is also effective for treating excessive swelling and welts below the skin (angioedema).

Method of use: Ingested. Chronic users tend to rotate steroids using various methods known as cycling, stacking, and pyramiding. Sporadic discontinuation of use is believed to allow testosterone levels and sperm counts to return to normal. Taking steroids regularly with periodic "drug-free times" is called cycling. Stacking refers to the concomitant use of two or more steroids at high doses. Pyramiding is when the dose, frequency, or number of steroids taken is gradually increased, followed by progressive tapering of the drug(s).

Duration of action: Depends on the formulation, frequency, and method used. In general, effects can last up to 6 days following use.

Psychological effects of abuse: Mood changes, decreased or increased sexual drive, anxiety, and depression. Psychological dependence may occur.

Physical effects of abuse: Angry or hostile feelings, elevated blood pressure and cholesterol, headache, insomnia, premature balding, psychotic reactions, severe acne, sexual dysfunction, and violent behavior. *In men:* Breast development, impotence, intermittent or painful urination, painful or persistent erections, reduced sperm production, and shrinking of the testicles. *In women:* Decreased body fat and breast size, deepening of the voice, enlarged clitoris, excessive growth of body hair, and menstrual changes. *In adolescents:* Premature termination of growth.

Prolonged use can lead to tolerance. While the long-term effects are not completely known, chronic steroid abuse has been associated with damage to the heart, liver, and brain.

Overdose symptoms: There have been no reports of severe overdose with this product. Chronic abuse of high doses may result in acne, excessive body hair, changes in hormonal and lipid metabolism, nausea, vomiting, jaundice, behavioral changes, stroke, heart function deterioration, psychosis, and sudden death.

Withdrawal symptoms: Abrupt discontinuation may cause mood changes, tiredness, restlessness, loss of appetite, dissatisfaction with body image, sleeplessness, reduced sex drive, paranoia, and severe depression that can lead to suicide attempts.

Talwin *see Pentazocine, page 493*

TEMAZEPAM
BRAND NAME: Restoril
COMMON STREET NAMES: Candy, downers, sleeping pills, tranks
DEA CLASS: Class IV
PHARMACOLOGIC CLASS: Benzodiazepine, sedative, hypnotic

Description: Temazepam is used for the short-term treatment of sleep disorders such as insomnia. Abuse of benzodiazepines is particularly high among heroin and cocaine users.

Method of use: Ingested

Duration of action: 5 to 17 hours

Psychological effects of abuse: Confusion, impaired judgment and thinking abilities, irritability, mild euphoria, pressured speech, reduced inhibition, and suicidal ideation. Long-term use may cause psychological dependence.

Physical effects of abuse: Changes in appetite and body weight, constipation, dizziness, impaired muscle coordination, impaired physical capabilities, and low blood pressure. Long-term use may cause physical dependence.

Overdose symptoms: The most severe signs of overdose are respiratory depression and coma. Other symptoms may include confusion, diminished reflexes, manic behavior, unrealistic euphoria, extreme sleepiness, and impaired coordination. Death from overdose of a single benzodi-azepine is extremely rare. However, there is an increased risk of toxicity when benzodiazepines are combined with alcohol and/or other CNS depressants. Fatalities have been reported in patients who have overdosed with a combination of a single benzodiazepine and alcohol.

Withdrawal symptoms: Abrupt termination following long-term use may precipitate withdrawal symptoms and require hospitalization. Symptoms may include abdominal and muscle cramps, agitation, delirium, depression, insomnia, rapid pulse, sweating, vomiting, hallucinations, tremors, and seizures.

Tenuate *see Diethylpropion, page 451*

TESTOSTERONE ENANTHATE
BRAND NAME: Delatestryl
COMMON STREET NAMES: Arnolds, gym candy, juice, pumpers, roids, stackers, weight trainers
DEA CLASS: Class III
PHARMACOLOGIC CLASS: Anabolic-androgenic steroid

Description: Androgens are steroid hormones that develop and maintain male sex characteristics. Testosterone enanthate is a derivative of the male hormone testosterone. Androgens are used primarily to replace insufficient levels of testosterone due to poor functioning of the testes. When used in combination with exercise and a high-protein diet, androgens can promote increased muscle size and strength, improve stamina, and decrease recovery time between workouts. Androgens are also used to promote the development of puberty in males with clearly delayed onset. Additionally, androgens are sometimes prescribed for women with advancing, inoperable metastatic breast cancer who are 1 to 5 years post-menopausal. This product has also been used in premenopausal women with breast cancer who have benefited from removal of one or both ovaries and are considered to have a hormone-responsive tumor.

Method of use: Injected IM. Chronic users tend to rotate steroids using various methods known as cycling, stacking, and pyramiding. Sporadic discontinuation of use is believed to allow testosterone levels and sperm counts to return to normal. Taking steroids regularly with periodic "drug-free times" is called cycling. Stacking refers to the concomitant use of two or more steroids at high doses. Pyramiding is when the dose, frequency, or number of steroids taken is gradually increased, followed by progressive tapering of the drug(s).

Duration of action: Up to 24 hours following IM administration.

Psychological effects of abuse: Mood changes, depression, and reduced sex drive. Psychological dependence may occur.

Physical effects of abuse: Angry or hostile feelings, elevated blood pressure and cholesterol, headache, insomnia, premature balding, psychotic reactions, severe acne, sexual dysfunction, and violent behavior. *In men:* Breast development, impotence, intermittent or painful urination, painful or persistent erections, reduced sperm production, and shrinking of the testicles. *In women:* Decreased body fat and breast size, deepening of the voice, enlarged clitoris, excessive growth of body hair, and menstrual changes. *In adolescents:* Premature termination of growth.

Prolonged use can lead to tolerance. While the long-term effects are not completely known, chronic steroid abuse has been associated with damage to the heart, liver, and brain.

Overdose symptoms: There have been no reports of severe overdose with this product. Chronic abuse of high doses may result in blurred vision, headache, sudden and severe inability to speak, seizures, slurred speech, temporary blindness, and sudden, severe weakness in the arm and/or leg on one side of the body.

Withdrawal symptoms: Abrupt discontinuation may cause mood changes, tiredness, restlessness, loss of appetite, dissatisfaction with body image, sleeplessness, reduced sex drive, paranoia, and severe depression that can lead to suicide attempts.

Testred *see Methyltestosterone, page 477*

THIOPENTAL SODIUM
BRAND NAME: Pentothal
COMMON STREET NAMES:
DEA CLASS: Class III
PHARMACOLOGIC CLASS: Barbiturate, anticonvulsant, general anesthetic, sedative

Description: Barbiturates depress the sensory cortex, decrease motor activity, alter brain function, and produce drowsiness, sedation, and hypnosis. Thiopental is used to control convulsions by inducing anesthesia. It is also used to treat grand-mal, psychomotor, and focal seizures. One of the drug's active metabolites is phenobarbital.

Method of use: Ingested

Duration of action: Effects are age- and dose-dependent but are usually brief.

Psychological effects of abuse: Barbiturates may cause psychological dependence, especially following prolonged use of high doses. Effects may include behavioral changes, excessive irritability, nightmares, hallucinations, nervousness, anxiety, and impaired judgment.

Physical effects of abuse: Low heart rate and blood pressure, feeling faint, drowsiness, tiredness, dizziness, headache, chills, coughing, irregular gait, loss of appetite, excessive sleeplessness, nausea, vomiting, sexual dysfunction, double vision, rapid eye movements, respiratory depression, and interrupted breathing.

Overdose symptoms: Unsteady gait, confusion, slurred speech, low blood pressure, high or low body temperature, sleepiness, dose-dependent respiratory depression, shock, and coma. The drug's toxic effects are enhanced when taken with alcohol and/or other CNS depressants.

Withdrawal symptoms: Symptoms are similar to those of alcohol withdrawal and characterized by severe apprehension, weakness, heightened anxiety, irritability, dizziness, headache, sleeplessness, muscle twitching, nausea and vomiting, distortion of visual perception, and rapid pulse. Severely low blood pressure and convulsions may develop after a day or two, which eventually lead to hallucinations, delirium, and continuous seizures, followed by coma and death.

Tranxene *see Clorazepate, page 445*

TRENBOLONE ACETATE
COMMON STREET NAMES: Arnolds, gym candy, juice, pumpers, roids, stackers, weight trainers
DEA CLASS: Class III
PHARMACOLOGIC CLASS: Anabolic-androgenic steroid

Not commercially available in the U.S.

Description: Androgens are steroid hormones that develop and maintain male sex characteristics. They are used primarily to replace insufficient levels of testosterone due to poor functioning of the testes. When used in combination with exercise and a high-protein diet, androgens can promote increased muscle size and strength, improve stamina, and decrease recovery time between workouts. Androgens are also used to promote the development of puberty in males with clearly delayed onset. Additionally, androgens are sometimes precribed for women with advancing, inoperable metastatic breast cancer who are 1 to 5 years postmenopausal.

Method of use: Ingested. Chronic users tend to rotate steroids using various methods known as cycling, stacking, and pyramiding. Sporadic discontinuation of use is believed to allow testosterone levels and sperm counts to return to normal. Taking steroids regularly with periodic "drug-free times" is called cycling. Stacking refers to the concomitant use of two or more steroids at high doses. Pyramiding is when the dose, frequency, or number of steroids taken is gradually increased, followed by progressive tapering of the drug(s).

Duration of action: Depends on the formulation, frequency, and method of use. In general, effects may last up to 6 days.

Psychological effects of abuse: Mood changes, depression, uncontrollable aggressive behavior, euphoria, anxiety, irritability, increased sex drive, and rarely, psychosis. Psychological dependence may also occur.

Physical effects of abuse: Angry or hostile feelings, elevated blood pressure and cholesterol, headache, insomnia, premature balding, psychotic reactions, severe acne, sexual dysfunction, and violent behavior. ***In men:*** Breast development, impotence, intermittent or painful urination, painful or persistent erections, reduced sperm production, and shrinking of the testicles. ***In women:*** Decreased body fat and breast size, deepening of the voice, enlarged clitoris, excessive growth of body hair, and menstrual changes. ***In adolescents:*** Premature termination of growth.

Prolonged use can lead to tolerance. While the long-term effects are not completely known, chronic steroid abuse has been associated with damage to the heart, liver, and brain.

Overdose symptoms: There have been no reports of serious overdose with this drug. Chronic use of high doses may cause excessive sexual stimulation, reduced sperm production, enlarged breasts in males, uncontrolled painful erection, jaundice, and deteriorating liver function. Excessive fluid retention may occur in users who have heart, liver, or kidney disease.

Withdrawal symptoms: Abrupt discontinuation may cause mood changes, tiredness, restlessness, loss of appetite, dissatisfaction with body image, sleeplessness, reduced sex drive, paranoia, and severe depression that can lead to suicide attempts.

TRIAZOLAM
BRAND NAME: Halcion
COMMON STREET NAMES: Candy, downers, sleeping pills, tranks
DEA CLASS: Class IV
PHARMACOLOGIC CLASS: Benzodiazepine, sedative, hypnotic

Description: Triazolam is used for the short-term treatment of sleep disorders such as insomnia. Abuse of benzodiazepines is particularly high among heroin and cocaine users.

Method of use: Ingested

Duration of action: 6 to 7 hours

Psychological effects of abuse: Confusion, impaired judgment and thinking abilities, irritability, mild euphoria, pressured speech, reduced inhibition, and suicidal ideation. Long-term use may cause psychological dependence.

Physical effects of abuse: Changes in appetite and body weight, constipation, dizziness, impaired muscle coordination, and low blood pressure. Long-term use may cause physical dependence.

Overdose symptoms: The most severe signs of overdose are respiratory depression and coma. Other symptoms may include confusion, diminished reflexes, manic behavior, unrealistic euphoria, extreme sleepiness, and impaired coordination. Death from overdose of a single benzodiazepine is extremely rare. However, there is an increased risk of toxicity when benzodiazepines are combined with alcohol and/or other CNS depressants. Fatalities have been reported in patients who have overdosed with a combination of a single benzodiazepine and alcohol.

Withdrawal symptoms: Abrupt termination following long-term use may precipitate withdrawal symptoms and require hospitalization. Symptoms may include abdominal and muscle cramps, depression, insomnia, sweating, vomiting, tremors, and seizures.

Tylox *see Oxycodone, page 488*

Valium *see Diazepam, page 450*

Vicodin *see Hydrocodone, page 465*

Virilon *see Methyltestosterone, page 477*

Xanax *see Alprazolam, page 436*

Xyrem *see GHB, page 462*

ZALEPLON
BRAND NAME: Sonata
COMMON STREET NAMES: Candy, downers, sleeping pills, tranks
DEA CLASS: Class IV
PHARMACOLOGIC CLASS: Hypnotic (not a benzodiazepine, but interacts with the same receptors in the brain)

Description: Zaleplon is used for the short-term treatment of insomnia. Abuse of benzodiazepine-type hypnotics is particularly high among heroin and cocaine users.

Method of use: Ingested

Duration of action: 6 to 8 hours

Psychological effects of abuse: Abnormal dreams, amnesia, changes in sexual desire, confusion, depersonalization, depression, hallucinations, impaired judgment and thinking abilities, reduced inhibition, and suicidal ideation. Paradoxical effects include euphoria, hyperactivity, and extreme aggression. Prolonged use may cause psychological dependence.

Physical effects of abuse: Abdominal pain, constipation, decreased blood pressure, dizziness, drowsiness, fatigue, impaired physical capabilities, irregular gait, light-headedness, loss of appetite, menstrual irregularities, migraine, nausea, sleepiness, slowed psychomotor performance, urinary retention, vertigo, and visual disturbances. Prolonged use may cause physical dependence.

Overdose symptoms: The most severe signs of overdose with benzodi-azepine-type hypnotics are respiratory depression, loss of consciousness, and coma. Other symptoms may include sensitivity to light, confusion, diminished reflexes, slurred speech, impaired coordination, apnea, extreme sleepiness, loss of muscle tone, and severely low blood pressure. Death from overdose of a single benzodiazepine-type hypnotic is extremely rare. However, there is an increased risk of toxicity when ben-zodiazepine-type drugs are combined with alcohol and/or other CNS depressants. Fatalities have been reported in patients who have overdosed with a combination of a single benzodiazepine-type hypnotic and alcohol.

Withdrawal symptoms: Abrupt termination following long-term use may precipitate withdrawal symptoms and require hospitalization. Symptoms may include abdominal and muscle cramps, depression, insomnia, severe drowsiness, sweating, vomiting, tremors, respiratory depression, seizures, and coma.

Zebutal *see Butalbital, page 442*

ZOLPIDEM
BRAND NAME: Ambien, Ambien CR
COMMON STREET NAMES: Candy, downers, sleeping pills, tranks
DEA CLASS: Class IV
PHARMACOLOGIC CLASS: Hypnotic, sedative (not a benzodiazepine, but interacts with the same receptors in the brain)

Description: Zolpidem is used for the short-term treatment of insomnia. Abuse of benzodiazepine-type hypnotics is particularly high among heroin and cocaine users.

Method of use: Ingested

Duration of action: 6 to 8 hours

Psychological effects of abuse: Abnormal dreams, amnesia, confusion, depression, impaired judgment and thinking abilities, reduced inhibition, and suicidal ideation. Paradoxical effects include euphoria, hyperactivity, and extreme aggression. Prolonged use may cause psychological dependence.

Physical effects of abuse: Changes in sexual desire, constipation, decreased blood pressure, dizziness, drowsiness, fatigue, impaired physical capabilities, irregular gait, light-headedness, sleepiness, slowed psychomotor performance, urinary retention, and visual disturbances. Prolonged use may cause physical dependence.

Overdose symptoms: The most severe signs of overdose with benzodiazepine-type hypnotics are respiratory depression, loss of consciousness, and coma. Other symptoms may include confusion, diminished reflexes, slurred speech, impaired coordination, apnea, extreme sleepiness, loss of muscle tone, and severely low blood pressure. Death from overdose of a single benzodiazepine-type hypnotic is extremely rare. However, there is an increased risk of toxicity when benzodiazepine-type drugs are combined with alcohol and/or other CNS depressants. Fatalities have been reported in patients who have overdosed with a combination of a single benzodiazepine-type hypnotic and alcohol.

Withdrawal symptoms: Abrupt termination following long-term use may precipitate withdrawal symptoms and require hospitalization. Symptoms may include abdominal and muscle cramps, depression, insomnia, sweating, vomiting, tremors, and seizures.

Part 4.
Illegal Drugs

AMT (ALPHA-METHYLTRYPTAMINE)
COMMON STREET NAMES: Amthrax, Amtrak, spirals
DEA CLASS: Class I
PHARMACOLOGIC CLASS: Hallucinogen

Description: AMT is a chemical found in a variety of South American plants. The drug has a similar structure and pharmacologic characteristics as other tryptamine-based Class I hallucinogens.

Method of use: Ingested (often as a tea), smoked or used as snuff, and rarely, injected.

Duration of action: 1 to 6 hours, but in chronic users the effects can last 18 to 24 hours.

Psychological effects: AMT can produce similar psychological effects as other hallucinogens, including changes in perception, visual distortions, agitation, hyperactivity, confusion, euphoria, anxiety, mood alterations, slowed thinking, delirium, and unpredictable behavior. Long-term use may cause tolerance and psychological dependence.

Physical effects: AMT can produce similar physical effects as other hallucinogens, including CNS depression or stimulation, nausea, vomiting, diarrhea, elevated blood pressure and body temperature, abnormally fast heart rate, blurred vision, excessive salivation, irregular gait, loss of appetite, irregular breathing, numbness in the extremities, dizziness, drowsiness, decreased REM sleep, enhanced color awareness, and time distortion.

Overdose symptoms: AMT is not considered addictive; it does not produce compulsive drug-seeking behavior as do cocaine, amphetamines, heroin, and alcohol. However, it does produce tolerance, and chronic users must take progressively higher doses to achieve the same effects as before. This is particularly dangerous due to the unpredictability of the drug's effects. Symptoms of overdose may include irregular gait, rapid heart rate, tremors, and elevated blood pressure and body temperature.

Withdrawal symptoms: None are reported, since no evidence of physical dependence can be detected when the drug is abruptly withdrawn.

4-BROMO-2,5-DIMETHOXYPHENETHYLAMINE

COMMON STREET NAMES: 2C-B, B-DMPEA, bromo, MFT, Nexus, two's
DEA CLASS: Class I
PHARMACOLOGIC CLASS: CNS stimulant

Description: This drug is an illegally manufactured variation of mescaline and amphetamine and has the same pharmacologic actions as amphetamine. Because the drug is manufactured in clandestine laboratories, it's rarely pure, and the amount of active drug in an oral dose can vary considerably.

Method of use: Ingested and snorted

Duration of action: Up to 8 hours; effects begin 20 to 30 minutes after use and reach their peak within 1 to 2 hours.

Psychological effects: Aggressive and impulsive behavior, agitation, anxiety, confusion, delusions, depression, drug cravings, hallucinations, and paranoia. Psychological dependence can develop rapidly.

Physical effects: Dilated pupils, elevated heart rate, and increased blood pressure. Long-term effects may include psychiatric disturbances, impaired cognitive functions, and memory loss.

Overdose symptoms: In general, toxicity results in mild symptoms that may include agitation, dilated pupils, fatigue, poor concentration, excessive sweating, elevated blood pressure, and rapid heart rate. Occasionally, severe depression, anxiety, and delirium can occur. Severe overdose may cause dangerously high body temperature, blood-clotting problems, severe muscle weakness and pain, seizures, and acute kidney failure.

Withdrawal symptoms: Abruptly stopping the drug after long-term use may cause extreme fatigue, overeating, depression, and stupor.

COCAINE and CRACK COCAINE

COMMON STREET NAMES: Big C, blow, coke, crack, crank, flake, lady, nose candy, rocks, snow, snowbirds, white, zip
DEA CLASS: Class II
PHARMACOLOGIC CLASS: CNS stimulant

Description: Cocaine is prepared from an extract of the coca plant. It is one of the most potent CNS stimulants and is widely abused. Crack cocaine is processed with baking soda or ammonia to produce a form that can be smoked. Currently, controlled doses of cocaine can be administered by a doctor for legitimate medical use, primarily as a local anesthetic for certain eye, ear, and throat surgeries.

Method of use: Ingested, snorted, smoked (also called "freebasing"), and injected IV. Each method has significant health risks for the user.

Duration of action: Depends on the method of use. Snorting produces a slow onset that lasts 15 to 30 minutes. The effects of smoking or IV injection last 5 to 10 minutes and produce a more intense high.

Psychological effects: Cocaine use causes psychological dependence. *Moderate doses:* Agitation, argumentative behavior, irritability, nervousness, and talkativeness. *High doses:* Anxiety, delusions, extreme irritability, paranoia, and restlessness.

Physical effects: Cocaine is highly addictive due to its rapid onset of action. Compulsive use appears to develop more quickly in smokers than in users who snort. *Moderate doses:* Abdominal pain, constricted blood vessels, decreased appetite, dilated pupils, disturbances in heart rhythm, elevated blood pressure, headaches, increased body temperature, nausea, and rapid heart and respiratory rates. *High doses:* Abdominal pain, blurred vision, chest pain, coma, convulsions, dizziness, excessive sweating, headaches, heart attacks, muscle spasms, nausea, respiratory failure, shortness of breath, and stroke. *Warning:* Cocaine use can cause sudden death, even after the first time the drug is taken.

Overdose symptoms: An overdose can be fatal. Tolerance develops rapidly, and chronic users must take progressively higher doses to obtain the same effects as before. Cocaine-related deaths are usually caused by cardiac arrest or seizures followed by respiratory arrest. Other symptoms of overdose include high body temperature, hallucinations, and convulsions. Smoking or injecting cocaine is more dangerous than snorting it. Risk of harmful effects also increases when the drug is combined with alcohol.

Withdrawal symptoms: Abruptly stopping chronic use of high doses may produce relatively mild withdrawal symptoms, including depression, anxiety, sleep disturbances, and increased appetite. These usually occur within 24 to 48 hours following the last dose and can last 7 to 10 days. Long-term users may develop acute tolerance and can suffer from depression, headache, fatigue, and irritability after they stop using the drug. Crack cocaine users appear to develop a greater dependence on the drug and therefore have more severe withdrawal symptoms, including major psychiatric complications and severe depression.

DOM (4-METHYL-2,5-DIMETHOXYAMPHETAMINE) and DOB (4-BROMO-2,5-DIMETHOXYAMPHETAMINE)

COMMON STREET NAME: STP, an acronym for Serenity, Tranquility, and Peace
DEA CLASS: Class I
PHARMACOLOGIC CLASS: CNS stimulant

Description: These drugs are an illegally manufactured variation of mescaline and amphetamine. They are sold as drug-laced pieces of paper. Because these drugs are manufactured in clandestine laboratories, they are rarely pure, and the amount of active drug in an oral dose can vary considerably.

Method of use: Ingested, snorted, and rarely, injected IV

Duration of action: Depends on method of use. Effects can last 12 to 36 hours. Symptoms start about an hour after use and reach their peak after 4 to 10 hours.

Psychological effects: The main effects are perceptual distortions that can vary with dose, setting, and the user's mood. Tolerance and psychological dependence can develop rapidly following chronic use.

Physical effects: The most common effects are elevated heart rate, increased blood pressure, and dilated pupils. Because DOB and DOM are hallucinogens, their effects are unpredictable and could be substantially different each time they are used.

Overdose symptoms: In general, toxicity with these drugs results in mild symptoms that may include agitation, elevated blood pressure, rapid heart rate, dilated pupils, and excessive sweating. Fatigue and poor concentration are also common. Occasionally, severe depression, anxiety, and delirium can occur. Severe overdose may cause dangerously high body temperature, blood-clotting problems, muscle weakness, seizures, and acute kidney failure.

Withdrawal symptoms: These drugs are highly addictive, and physical and psychological dependence develops rapidly. Abrupt cessation of use may cause anxiety, paranoia, aggressive behavior, and strong drug cravings. Suicidal ideation has been reported. Psychotic behavior may persist for months or years after discontinuation of use.

HASHISH

COMMON STREET NAMES: Boom, chronic, gangster, hash, hash oil, hemp
DEA CLASS: Class I
PHARMACOLOGIC CLASS: Cannabinoid

Description: Hashish contains the psychoactive chemical delta-9-tetrahydrocannabinol (THC). It is made from the THC-rich resinous material of the cannabis plant, which is collected, dried, and then compressed into a variety of forms, such as balls, cakes, or cookie-like sheets. Pieces are then broken off, placed in pipes, and smoked. The Middle East, North Africa, Pakistan, and Afghanistan are the main sources of hashish.

Hashish (and hash oil) are stronger forms of marijuana. The drug's effects depend on the potency of the THC content. Hashish averages 2 to 8 percent THC, but it can contain as much as 20 percent. The drug has no legitimate medical use, but THC and a synthetic cannabinol (nabilone) are used to prevent vomiting in patients receiving cancer chemotherapy. In some studies, cannabis was found to have effects similar to analgesics, muscle relaxants, and appetite stimulants.

Hash oil is a tar-like solution distilled from hashish; it can contain anywhere from 15 to 70 percent THC. Cannabis growers usually try to maximize the plant's THC content.

Method of use: Hashish is usually smoked as a cigarette (called a joint or nail) or in a pipe (bong).

Duration of action: Hashish produces an effect almost immediately and reaches its peak in about 30 minutes. The effects usually wear off after 3 to 4 hours. Chronic users may not experience anything until 30 to 90 minutes after the first inhalation, but the effects can last for up to 8 hours.

Psychological effects: Distortion of time and space, loss of memory, impaired judgment, panic and anxiety attacks, and a false sense of well-being. Users taking cannabis in large doses have had psychotic episodes with paranoid or schizophrenic characteristics. Prolonged use of cannabis may lead to tolerance and psychological dependence.

Physical effects: Early physical effects may include nausea and vomiting. Later-stage effects may include memory loss, poor coordination, impaired learning skills, elevated heart rate and blood pressure, dry mouth, dry eyes, and blurred vision. Experts continue to debate whether physical dependence can occur.

Overdose symptoms: Heavy users rapidly develop tolerance and need progressively higher doses to obtain the same effects as before. Symptoms of overdose may include increased appetite, red and swollen eyes, dry mouth, poor motor coordination, and elevated heart rate and blood pressure.

Withdrawal symptoms: Withdrawal symptoms may include loss of appetite, anxiety, sleeplessness, irritability, restlessness, visual abnormalities, excessive sweating, headache, and stomach upset.

HEROIN
COMMON STREET NAMES: Brown sugar, cheese (black tar heroin), dope, H, horse, junk, skag, skunk, smack, white horse
DEA CLASS: Class I
PHARMACOLOGIC CLASS: Narcotic analgesic

Description: Heroin is derived from the resin of the poppy plant. Pure heroin is a white powder with a bitter taste but is rarely sold on the street. Most heroin is distributed as powder that varies in color due to additives and manufacturing impurities. Another form of heroin, "black tar," has become increasingly available in the United States. The color and consistency of black tar heroin results from the crude processing methods used to manufacture the substance in Mexico. When mixed with Tylenol PM and crushed into powder form, black tar heroin is sold very inexpensively to minors, who then snort it. Heroin, which is illegal in the United States, is used in very limited treatment applications in other countries.

Method of use: Ingested, snorted, smoked, and injected IV (also called mainlining), IM, or SC (also called skin popping). Injection is the most efficient way to administer low-purity heroin, and until recently was the preferred method of use. The availability of higher-purity heroin now allows users to snort or smoke the narcotic.

Duration of action: The euphoric effects usually occur 7 to 8 seconds after injection. IM injection produces a relatively slow onset, typically 5 to 8 minutes. When heroin is sniffed or smoked, the peak effects usually occur within 10 to 15 minutes.

Psychological effects: Enhanced sexual pleasure, euphoria, psychological dependence, and significantly impaired mental function. The psychological dependence associated with narcotic addiction is complex. Long after physical dependence has ended, the addict may continue to think and talk about the drug and feel unable to manage daily activities without it.

Physical effects: Short-term physical effects include drowsiness, dry mouth, flushing, and a heavy feeling in the extremities. Long-term effects may include alternating wakefulness and drowsiness, slowed breathing, and reduced mental functioning. The development of infectious diseases—such as HIV/AIDS, infection of the heart lining, various abscesses, pneumonia, and hepatitis—is a major problem in heroin users. In addition, the impurities in the drug—especially talc—may clog blood vessels and damage the lungs, liver, kidneys, and brain.

Overdose symptoms: Tolerance and physical dependence may develop after only 2 to 3 days of continued heroin use. This greatly increases the risk of overdose as progressively higher doses are needed to obtain the same effects as before. Overdose may cause shallow breathing, convulsions, coma, and possibly death. In addition, heroin suppresses breathing and can cause the lungs to fill with fluid, which may also lead to death. Since heroin is manufactured in clandestine laboratories and drug impurities are unknown, abusers are at great risk of overdose or death.

Withdrawal symptoms: Withdrawal from heroin is extremely painful and dangerous. Symptoms are worse in people who have used large doses for prolonged periods. Abrupt withdrawal of heroin in a chronic user may be fatal. Symptoms may begin to appear within 6 hours after the last dose and continue to manifest within 24 hours. Withdrawal symptoms reach their peak at 48 to 72 hours following the last dose but may continue for weeks. Early symptoms include irritability, insomnia, diminished appetite, goose-flesh, hot and cold flashes, dilated pupils, runny nose, severe yawning, severe sneezing, excessive tearing, and cold-like symptoms. Later-stage symptoms include abdominal cramps, bone and muscle pain in the back and extremities, pronounced depression, nausea, vomiting, diarrhea, alternating fever and chills, excessive sweating, and elevated heart rate and blood pressure. Muscle spasms and kicking movements can also occur, which may explain the expression "kicking the habit."

KHAT

COMMON STREET NAMES: Khat has more than 40 street names, including Cadillac express, cat, chat, ephedrine, gat, go fast, kat, qat, slick, sniff, superspeed, tohai, tschat, wonderstar
DEA CLASS: Class I (cathine, one of the ingredients in khat, is Class IV)
PHARMACOLOGIC CLASS: CNS stimulant

Description: Khat is a naturally occurring stimulant derived from the *Catha edulis* shrub. This shrub is cultivated mainly in East Africa and the Arabian Peninsula, where the use of khat is an established cultural tradition for many social occasions. Khat is illegal in the U.S. but is used in some countries to aid weight loss.

The stimulating effects of khat are due to cathinone (a phenylpropylamine agent) and, to a much lesser extent, cathine (a norpseudoephedrine agent). Cathinone is about 10 times more potent than cathine and is only present in fresh leaves. As the leaves mature or dry, cathinone is converted to cathine. The effects of these alkaloids resemble those of amphetamines, particularly cathinone.

Methcathinone is an illegal synthetic drug that is sold as an alternative to methamphetamine. It has a chemical structure similar to cathinone but has stronger addictive properties and side effects.

Method of use: Usually ingested but can be snorted. The leaves are often chewed like tobacco and the juice swallowed; occasionally the chewed leaves are also swallowed. In addition, khat can be brewed as a tea or crushed and mixed with honey to make a paste.

Duration of action: Several hours

Psychological effects: Aggressive verbal outbursts, behavioral changes, euphoria, pressured speech, and psychotic reactions. Rarely, schizophrenic behavior or manic-like psychosis may occur. Psychological dependence develops rapidly.

Physical effects: Anorexia, constipation, dilated pupils, dry mouth, elevated blood pressure and body temperature, headache, increased heart rate with palpitations, insomnia, mouth inflammation or infection, severe nausea, swollen cornea, and tremors. Rarely, abnormal heart rhythm and severe chest pain may occur. Cathinone is very addictive, and physical dependence develops rapidly with chronic use.

Overdose symptoms: The main symptoms are hyperactivity, severely elevated blood pressure and body temperature, and seizures. Serious overdose symptoms from chewing khat are due to the phenylpropylamine content of the leaves.

Withdrawal symptoms: Cathinone is highly addictive, and physical and psychological dependence develop rapidly. Abruptly stopping the drug may precipitate withdrawal symptoms such as anxiety, paranoia, aggressive behavior, and strong drug cravings. Suicidal ideation has also been reported. Psychotic behavior may persist for months or years after discontinuation of use.

LSD (LYSERGIC ACID DIETHYLAMIDE)

COMMON STREET NAMES: Acid, blotter, boomers, cubes, dots, L, mellow yello, microdots, tabs, trips, window pane, yellow sunshines
DEA CLASS: Class I
PHARMACOLOGIC CLASS: Hallucinogen

Description: LSD is a potent hallucinogenic substance. It has no legitimate medical use. LSD, commonly referred to as acid, is usually sold as "dots" on blotter paper, but it can also be found as tablets, square gel caps, and rarely, in liquid form. Rogue chemists manufacturer the drug as a crystalline powder that can be reduced to a clear liquid for dosing purposes.

Method of use: Ingested

Duration of action: Up to 12 hours

Psychological effects: Psychological effects depend on the individual. The user may feel various emotions at once or swing rapidly from one mood to another. Depending on the dose, the drug may produce delusions, visual hallucinations, flashbacks, severe depression, and panic attacks. The user often refers to this experience as a "bad trip." Some LSD users experience severe, terrifying thoughts, and become fearful of losing control, going insane, or dying. Long-term use may cause tolerance and psychological dependence.

Physical effects: The effects of LSD are unpredictable, but the drug is not physically addictive. Physical reactions to LSD depend on the dose; the user's personality, mood, and expectations; and the surroundings in which the drug is used. Initial effects may include dilated pupils, elevated body temperature, increased heart rate and blood pressure, excessive sweating, loss of appetite, sleeplessness, dry mouth, and tremors.

Overdose symptoms: LSD is not considered addictive; it does not produce compulsive drug-seeking behavior as do cocaine, amphetamines, heroin, and alcohol. However, it does produce tolerance, and chronic users must take progressively higher doses to achieve the same effects as before. This is particularly dangerous due to the unpredictability of LSD. Symptoms of overdose may include excessive tearing, irregular gait, dilated pupils, rapid heart rate, tremors, and elevated blood pressure and body temperature. Overdose with LSD can be frightening and cause panic. Injuries and fatal accidents have been reported during states of LSD intoxication.

Withdrawal symptoms: None are reported, since no evidence of physical dependence can be detected when the drug is abruptly withdrawn.

MARIJUANA
COMMON STREET NAMES: Blunt, budah, chronic, dope, ganja, grass, herb, homegrown, indo, joints, Mary Jane, pot, reefer, schwag, sinsemilla, skunk, weed
DEA CLASS: Class I
PHARMACOLOGIC CLASS: Cannabinoid

Description: Marijuana is a green, brown, or gray mixture of dried, shredded leaves, stems, seeds, and flowers of the hemp plant (*Cannabis sativa*). Cannabis is a term that refers to marijuana and other drugs made from the same plant. The active ingredient in marijuana is delta-9-tetrahydrocannabinol (THC), which is responsible for its psychoactive effects.

Method of use: Smoked as a cigarette (joint) or in a pipe (bong). Users also smoke blunts, the street name for cigars that have had their tobacco contents replaced with marijuana and other illicit drugs such as crack. Marijuana can also be mixed into foods or used to brew a tea.

Duration of action: Effects begin as soon as the drug enters the brain and can last from 1 to 3 hours.

Psychological effects: All cannabis products are mind-altering drugs. Users initially feel euphoric but then become extremely sleepy and depressed. Other effects include distorted perception, mood changes, anxiety or panic attacks, and difficulty with thinking and problem solving.

Physical effects: Short-term effects may include memory loss, poor coordination, impaired learning skills, elevated heart rate and blood pressure, dry mouth, dry eyes, and blurred vision. The potential for heart attack increases within the first hour of use due to the drug's effects on heart rate and blood pressure. Marijuana may also impair the immune system, which greatly increases the risk of bacterial infections. Tolerance and physical dependence may develop with long-term use.

In addition, smoking marijuana causes similar effects on the lungs as smoking tobacco, including daily cough and phlegm production, frequent chest illnesses, heightened risk of lung infections, and greater tendency toward obstructed airways. Marijuana contains 50 to 70 percent more carcinogenic hydrocarbons than tobacco, and cancer of the respiratory tract and lungs can result from marijuana smoking.

Overdose symptoms: Heavy users rapidly develop tolerance and need progressively higher doses to obtain the same effects as before. Serious health effects are more likely to be secondary to impaired judgment and behavioral problems rather than direct overdose effects. Early symptoms of overdose may include excessive sleepiness, mild euphoria, short-term memory loss, difficulty in accomplishing tasks, and lapses of attention. Serious overdose effects may include extreme tiredness, severe weakness and drowsiness, dizziness, slurred speech, irregular gait, decreased motor coordination and muscle strength, and rarely, psychosis.

Withdrawal symptoms: Abrupt discontinuation of use may cause drug cravings, irritability, agitation, apprehension, aggressiveness, tremulousness, sleeplessness, excessive sweating, and elevated anxiety. Additional symptoms may include increased aggression that reaches its peak effects about a week after the last smoked dose.

MDMA (3,4-METHYLENEDIOXYMETHAMPHETAMINE)

COMMON STREET NAMES: Adam, clarity, ecstasy, Eve, lover's speed, peace, STP, X, XTC

DEA CLASS: Class I

PHARMACOLOGIC CLASS: Amphetamine, CNS stimulant

Description: MDMA is an illegally manufactured variation of mescaline and amphetamine. It has both psychedelic and stimulant effects. It is a so-called "club drug" used at all-night dance parties known as "raves." Because MDMA is manufactured in clandestine laboratories, it is rarely pure, and the amount of active drug in an oral dose can vary considerably.

Method of use: Ingested and snorted

Duration of action: Psychedelic effects last 4 to 6 hours.

Psychological effects: Anxiety, confusion, depression, paranoia, drug craving, and aggressive and impulsive behavior. Tolerance and psychological dependence may develop with chronic use.

Physical effects: High blood pressure, increased heart rate, elevated body temperature, jaw and teeth clenching, muscle tension, chills and/or sweating, nausea, blurred vision, faintness, dizziness, and drug craving. MDMA can increase heart rate significantly during strenuous physical activity, but the heart does not respond normally. Since MDMA use is associated with such strenuous activities as dancing for hours, the drug's effects on the heart could increase the risk of heart damage and cardiovascular collapse.

Overdose symptoms: Large doses may cause extremely high fever, severely high blood pressure, rapid heart rate, and kidney and heart failure. *Warning:* Drinking too much water after taking MDMA can be lethal. MDMA significantly increases the blood levels of vasopressin (an antidiuretic hormone). Vasopressin causes the body to retain more water, which dilutes the amount of sodium and other salts in the blood. This can swell the brain, causing damage to the brain and nerve tissue.

Withdrawal symptoms: MDMA is a powerfully addictive drug, and physical and psychological dependence develops rapidly. Abrupt cessation may precipitate withdrawal symptoms such as anxiety, paranoia, aggressive behavior, and strong drug cravings. Suicidal ideation has been reported. Psychotic behavior may persist for months or years after discontinuation of use.

MESCALINE (PEYOTE CACTUS)
COMMON STREET NAMES: Buttons, cactus, mesc
DEA CLASS: Class I
PHARMACOLOGIC CLASS: Hallucinogen

Description: Peyote is a small cactus whose principal active ingredient is mescaline (3, 4, 5-trimethoxyphenethylamine), a compound that is structurally similar to amphetamines. It can be either extracted from the plant or produced synthetically.

Method of use: Ingested (sometimes brewed as a tea) and smoked

Duration of action: 6 to 12 hours

Psychological effects: Common effects include visual and auditory hallucinations, abnormal sensory perception, amnesia, and anxiety. The following may also occur: suicidal thoughts, emotional instability, fear, anxiety, paranoia, and flashbacks.

Physical effects: Dizziness, drowsiness, headache, light-headedness, excessive salivation, tremors, weakness, increased muscle tone, blurred vision, dilated pupils, irregular gait, elevated blood pressure, stomach cramps, nausea, vomiting, abnormal reflexes, shivering, feelings of hot or cold, and respiratory depression. The drug can also cause numbness of the tongue and mouth. Tolerance has been documented but decreases rapidly within a few days following cessation of use. Although physiological drug addiction generally does not occur, cross-tolerance with other hallucinogens can develop.

Overdose symptoms: Overdose can cause death due to homicidal, psychotic, or suicidal behavior. Signs of mescaline overdose resemble those of LSD. A wide range of symptoms can be present, since users often take other drugs simultaneously with mescaline. Concomitant administration of alcohol with mescaline may produce prolonged seizures and coma.

Withdrawal symptoms: None are reported, since no evidence of physical dependence can be detected when the drug is abruptly withdrawn.

METHAQUALONE
COMMON STREET NAMES: Ludes, mandrex, Quaalude, quad, quay
DEA CLASS: Class I
PHARMACOLOGIC CLASS: Sedative, hypnotic

Description: Methaqualone has properties similar to those of barbiturates. It was used previously for the short-term treatment of insomnia but was withdrawn from the market in the U.S. and other countries due to a high risk of abuse.

Method of use: Ingested

Duration of action: Methaqualone absorbs rapidly following ingestion. The drug reaches peak serum levels within 2 hours, with the effects lasting 5 to 8 hours.

Psychological effects: Anxiety, confusion, false sense of well-being, and impaired perception. Psychological dependence may occur with prolonged use of high doses.

Physical effects: Excessive sleepiness, loss of coordination, low blood pressure, sexual dysfunction, and slowed heart rate and breathing. Excessive use leads to tolerance, physical dependence, and withdrawal symptoms similar to those of barbiturates.

Overdose symptoms: Tolerance develops rapidly, and progressively higher doses are needed to obtain the same effects as before. Signs of overdose may include extreme tiredness, irregular gait, muscle rigidity, muscular hyperactivity, rapid heart rate, low blood pressure, respiratory failure, heart failure, seizures, and coma.

Withdrawal symptoms: Methaqualone withdrawal may lead to death if left untreated. Symptoms include weakness, abdominal cramps, nausea, vomiting, disorientation, anxiety, restlessness, rapid heart rate, visual hallucinations, stupor, delirium, tremors, and seizures.

5-MeO-DIPT (5-METHOXY-N, N-DIISOPROPYLTRYPTAMINE)
COMMON STREET NAMES: Foxy, foxy methoxy
DEA CLASS: Class I
PHARMACOLOGIC CLASS: Hallucinogen

Description: This drug has the same chemical properties and effects as other tryptamine-based Class I hallucinogens.

Method of use: Ingested, snorted, and smoked

Duration of action: 3 to 6 hours

Psychological effects: This drug can cause the same psychological effects as other hallucinogens, including changes in perception, visual distortions, agitation, hyperactivity, confusion, euphoria, anxiety, mood alterations, slowed thinking, delirium, and unpredictable behavior. Long-term use may cause tolerance and psychological dependence.

Physical effects: This drug can produce the same physical effects as other hallucinogens, including CNS depression or stimulation, nausea, vomiting, diarrhea, elevated blood pressure and body temperature, abnormally fast heart rate, blurred vision, excessive salivation, irregular gait, loss of appetite, irregular breathing, numbness in the extremities, dizziness, drowsiness, decreased REM sleep, enhanced color awareness, and time distortion.

Overdose symptoms: This drug is not considered addictive; it does not produce compulsive drug-seeking behavior as do cocaine, amphetamine, heroin, and alcohol. However, it does produce tolerance, and chronic users must take progressively higher doses to achieve the same effects as before. This is particularly dangerous due to the unpredictability of the drug's effects. Symptoms of overdose may include irregular gait, rapid heart rate, tremors, and elevated blood pressure and body temperature.

Withdrawal symptoms: None are reported, since no evidence of physical dependence can be detected when the drug is abruptly withdrawn.

PCP (PHENCYCLIDINE)

COMMON STREET NAMES: Angel dust, boat, hog, love boat, peace pill
DEA CLASS: Class I and II
PHARMACOLOGIC CLASS: Hallucinogen

Description: PCP is a dissociative anesthetic with sympathomimetic and hallucinogenic properties. It is a bitter-tasting, white crystalline powder that can dissolve in water and be mixed with dyes. PCP is manufactured illegally by rogue chemists in places known as "bucket labs." It is related chemically to ketamine and is a potent analgesic and anesthetic. The drug was originally developed as a tranquilizer for animals. PCP was former-ly used in humans as an intravenous anesthetic, but severe adverse effects—especially postoperative psychosis—precluded its use. However, the drug still has some veterinary applications.

Method of use: Ingested, smoked, snorted, and injected IV. The most pop-ular method is to apply the drug to a marijuana joint or menthol cigarette and smoke it, known as a "kool-dip."

Duration of action: If smoked, the effects start in 2 to 5 minutes and last about 15 to 30 minutes. In chronic users the effects can last 4 to 6 hours but may also linger for 1 to 2 days.

Psychological effects: PCP is a highly addictive drug that can cause psy-chological dependence. Frequent use can result in tolerance and drug craving. Effects may include mood and perception alteration, paranoia, panic attacks, anxiety, decreased awareness, compulsive drug-seeking behavior, and suicidal ideation. It can induce psychosis that is indistin-guishable from schizophrenia. The following have also been reported: hallucinations, euphoria, agitation, hyperactivity, disorientation, and vio-lent delusional behavior.

Physical effects: The physical effects of PCP are unpredictable, but the following have been reported: elevated pulse and heart rate, increased blood pressure and body temperature, muscle relaxation, dilated pupils, rapid eye movement, nausea, vomiting, blurred vision, dizziness, tremors, shallow breathing, loss of coordination, excessive salivation, excessive perspiration, convulsions, numbness and tingling in the extremities, and occasionally, excessively high fever. Constricted pupils and seizures are more common in children. Substantially increased blood pressure is the hallmark sign that usually resolves within 4 hours but can persist for more than 24 hours. Respiratory effects are uncommon without concur-rent use of sedatives, narcotics, or alcohol.

Overdose symptoms: An overdose can cause death due to respiratory depression and coma. Other symptoms include unpredictable behavior, depression, convulsions, flashbacks, psychosis, delusions, and dangerously high fever.

Withdrawal symptoms: None are reported, since no evidence of physical dependence can be detected when the drug is abruptly withdrawn.

PMA (PARAMETHOXYAMPHETAMINE)
COMMON STREET NAMES: Death, Mitsubishi, double-stack
DEA CLASS: Class I
PHARMACOLOGIC CLASS: Amphetamine, hallucinogen, CNS stimulant

Description: PMA is a synthetic hallucinogen that is structurally related to MDMA but is significantly more lethal, even in smaller doses. It is produced legally in the U.S. for limited commercial applications and scientific research.

Method of use: Ingested, but the powder form may be injected or snorted.

Duration of action: Up to 8 hours; effects begin 30 to 60 minutes after use and reach their peak after approximately 90 minutes.

Psychological effects: Initial feelings include a rush of euphoria followed by a general sense of happiness and well-being. These effects are followed by a "coming down" phase 3 to 6 hours later, resulting in depression, anxiety, and general negativity that can persist for several days. Prolonged use may cause tolerance and psychological dependence.

Physical effects: Depends on the dose. A single small dose can cause labored breathing, erratic eye movement, elevated pulse rate and body temperature, high blood pressure, muscle spasms, nausea, and heightened visual stimulation. Larger doses may cause irregular heart rhythm, serious breathing difficulties, severely elevated body temperature, vomiting, kidney failure, and cardiac arrest.

Overdose symptoms: Illicit drug makers sometimes stamp MDMA logos on their PMA "products" in order to pass them off as MDMA. This could increase the risk of fatal overdose because users may unknownly mix PMA with MDMA. Signs of overdose can include vomiting, severely elevated body temperature, convulsions, coma, and death.

Withdrawal symptoms: None are reported, since no evidence of physical dependence can be detected when the drug is abruptly withdrawn.

PSILOCYBIN
COMMON STREET NAMES: Magic mushroom, musk, purple passion, shrooms
DEA CLASS: Class I
PHARMACOLOGIC CLASS: Hallucinogen

Description: Psilocybin, or psilocyn, is obtained from certain mushrooms indigenous to tropical and subtropical regions of South America, Mexico, and the United States. These mushrooms are available fresh or dried. The effects produced by dried or brewed mushrooms are far less predictable and largely depend on the particular mushrooms used and the age and preservation of the extract. Psilocybin has properties similar to LSD but is less potent. It has no legitimate medical use.

Method of use: Ingested; the mushrooms are sometimes brewed as a tea or added to food to mask the bitter flavor.

Duration of action: 4 to 6 hours

Psychological effects: Vivid visual and auditory hallucinations, panic attacks, and emotional disturbances. Long-term use may cause tolerance and psychological dependence.

Physical effects: There are many species of mushrooms that contain varying amounts of psilocybin as well as uncertain amounts of other chemicals. It is nearly impossible to predict the physical effects of this compound. The most commonly reported effects include drowsiness, vomiting, muscle weakness, and panic attacks. The exact mechanism of action and extent of toxicity are unknown.

Overdose symptoms: Symptoms of overdose may occur 30 to 60 minutes (and sometimes as late as 3 hours) following ingestion. Signs include a pleasant yet apprehensive mood, impaired judgment, compulsive movements, vertigo, dilated pupils, irregular gait, tingling sensations, muscle weakness, loss of muscle tone, and drowsiness that almost progresses to sleep. Children may develop high temperatures with seizures.

Withdrawal symptoms: None are reported, since no evidence of physical dependence can be detected when the drug is abruptly withdrawn.

SALVIA DIVINORUM
COMMON STREET NAMES: Diviner's sage, herbal ecstasy, Mexican mint, ska Maria Pastora
DEA CLASS: Not classified
PHARMACOLOGIC CLASS: Hallucinogen

Description: S. divinorum is a perennial herb in the mint family. It's one of several vision-inducing plants used by the Mazatec Indians of Mexico.

The herb's active ingredient is Salvinorin A, a psychoactive chemical that can cause intense hallucinations.

Method of use: Ingested (usually as a tea), smoked, and chewed. The herb is most effective when it's vaporized and inhaled.

Duration of action: Hallucinogenic effects can last up to 1 hour.

Psychological effects: *S. divinorum* may cause similar psychological effects as ketamine, mescaline, and psilocybin, including changes in perception, hallucinations, and delirium. Long-term use may cause tolerance and psychological dependence.

Physical effects: *S. divinorum* may induce similar physical effects as ketamine, mescaline, and psilocybin, including CNS depression or stimulation, nausea, vomiting, diarrhea, elevated blood pressure, and abnormally fast heart rate.

Overdose symptoms: This drug is not considered addictive; it does not produce compulsive drug-seeking behavior as do cocaine, amphetamines, heroin, and alcohol. However, it does produce tolerance, and chronic users must take progressively higher doses to achieve the same effects as before. This is particularly dangerous due to the unpredictability of the drug's effects. Signs of overdose may include irregular gait, rapid heart rate, tremors, and elevated blood pressure and body temperature.

Withdrawal symptoms: None are reported, since no evidence of physical dependence can be detected when the drug is abruptly withdrawn.

Common Prescription Drugs

Because patients with psychological disorders are often under simultaneous treatment for other medical problems, this section presents you with brief descriptions of the most commonly prescribed drugs and their customary uses. Based on government-approved product labeling, the information is organized alphabetically by each medication's leading brand name and cross-referenced by the generic name. To see whether a drug is likely to interact with a patient's psychotropic regimen, check the appropriate listings in Section 2 of this book.

Abacavir *See Ziagen*

Abacavir, Lamivudine, and Zidovudine *See Trizivir*

Acarbose *See Precose*

ACCOLATE
Zafirlukast

Accolate is prescribed to prevent asthma attacks. Unlike some of the inhaled medications used to relieve attacks in progress, it is not a steroid. Instead, it works by blocking the action of certain types of leukotrienes—natural compounds that cause swelling and constriction in the lungs. Taken in tablet form, it is used for long-term treatment.

AccuNeb *See Proventil*

ACCUPRIL
Quinapril

Accupril is used in the treatment of high blood pressure. It can be taken alone or in combination with a thiazide type of water pill such as HydroDIURIL. Accupril is in a family of drugs known as "ACE inhibitors." It works by preventing a chemical in the blood called angiotensin I from converting into a more potent form that increases salt and water retention in the body. Accupril also enhances blood flow throughout the blood vessels. Along with other drugs, Accupril is also prescribed in the treatment of congestive heart failure.

ACCURETIC
Quinapril with Hydrochlorothiazide

Accuretic combines two types of blood pressure medication. The first, quinapril hydrochloride, is an ACE (angiotensin-converting enzyme) inhibitor. It works by preventing a chemical in the blood called angiotensin I from converting into a more potent form (angiotensin II) that increases salt and water retention in the body and causes the blood vessels to constrict—two actions that tend to increase blood pressure.

To aid in clearing excess water from the body, Accuretic also contains hydrochlorothiazide, a diuretic that promotes production of urine. Diuretics often wash too much potassium out of the body along with the water. However, the ACE inhibitor part of Accuretic tends to keep potassium in the body, thereby canceling this unwanted effect.

Accuretic is not used for the initial treatment of high blood pressure. It is saved for later use, when a single blood pressure medication is not sufficient for the job. In addition, some doctors are using Accuretic along with other drugs to treat congestive heart failure.

ACCUTANE
Isotretinoin
Other brand name: Amnesteem

Accutane, a chemical cousin of vitamin A, is prescribed for the treatment of severe, disfiguring cystic acne that has not cleared up in response to milder medications such as antibiotics. It works on the oil glands within the skin, shrinking them and diminishing their output. The patient takes Accutane orally every day for several months, then stops. The antiacne effect can last even after the course of medication is finished.

Acebutolol *See Sectral*

ACEON
Perindopril

Aceon is used in the treatment of high blood pressure. It can be taken alone or in combination with thiazide diuretics that help rid the body of excess water. Aceon belongs to a family of drugs called angiotensin converting enzyme (ACE) inhibitors. It works by preventing a chemical in the blood called angiotensin I from converting into a more potent form that increases salt and water retention in the body. Aceon also improves the flow of blood through the circulatory system.

Acetaminophen with Codeine *See Tylenol with Codeine*

Acetaminophen with Oxycodone *See Percocet*

Acetazolamide *See Diamox*

ACIPHEX
Rabeprazole

AcipHex blocks acid production in the stomach. It is prescribed for the short-term (4 to 8 weeks) treatment of sores and inflammation in the upper digestive canal (esophagus). This condition, known as gastro-esophageal reflux disease (GERD), is caused by the backflow of stomach acid into the esophagus over a prolonged period of time. Because GERD can be chronic, doctors sometimes continue to prescribe AcipHex to prevent a relapse after the initial course of treatment.

AcipHex can also be prescribed for the short-term (up to 4 weeks) treatment of duodenal ulcers (ulcers that form just outside the stomach at the top of the small intestine), and for Zollinger-Ellison syndrome, a disease which causes the stomach to produce too much acid. The drug is classified as a "proton pump inhibitor." It works by blocking a specific enzyme essential to the production of stomach acid. It begins reducing acid within an hour of administration.

AcipHex is sometimes combined with the antibiotics amoxicillin and clarithromycin to treat infections caused by *H. pylori*, a type of bacteria that lives in the digestive tract and is often associated with recurrent ulcers.

ACLOVATE
Alclometasone

Aclovate, a synthetic steroid medication of the cortisone family, is spread on the skin to relieve certain types of itchy rashes, including psoriasis.

ACTIVELLA AND FEMHRT
Estrogen with Progestin
Other brand name: Prefest

These medications are designed for use in hormone replacement therapy. Both combine a form of estrogen with a substance that acts like progesterone. Both relieve the symptoms of menopause, and both are prescribed to prevent osteoporosis in postmenopausal women. (Activella is also used for vaginal atrophy.)

Estrogen, when taken by itself, poses an increased risk of uterine cancer. The progestin in these products largely counteracts this effect.

ACTONEL
Risedronate
Other brand name: Actonel with Calcium

Although our bones seem solid and stable, they actually undergo constant renewal. Specialized cells called osteoclasts draw used calcium out of the bones while other cells called osteoblasts replace it. Especially after menopause, this process can get out of balance. Calcium starts to leach out of the bones faster than it can be replaced, leading to the brittle-bone disease called osteoporosis.

Actonel combats this problem by reducing the activity of the osteoclasts and slowing the loss of calcium from the bones. It is prescribed for postmenopausal women, both to prevent osteoporosis and to strengthen the bones once the disease has begun. It is also used to prevent or treat osteoporosis resulting from therapy with steroid medications, and it is used in the treatment of Paget's disease, a condition in which patches of bone become softened and enlarged.

Both Actonel and a similar drug called Fosamax are members of the family of drugs called bisphosphonates.

Actonel with Calcium is indicated for the treatment and prevention of postmenopausal osteoporosis. Actonel with Calcium is a co-packaged product containing Actonel for once weekly dosing and calcium carbonate tablets for daily dosing for the remaining 6 days of the week.

ACTOPLUS MET
Pioglitazone and Metformin

ACTO*plus* met is used to treat type 2 diabetes. It contains two medications, pioglitazone and metformin, which work together to help keep blood sugar levels under control. Type 2 diabetes usually stems from the body's inability to make good use of insulin, the natural hormone that helps to transfer sugar out of the blood and into the cells, where it's converted to energy. ACTO*plus* met works by improving the body's response to its own natural insulin supply. It also helps decrease sugar production and absorption.

ACTOS
Pioglitazone

Actos is used to control high blood sugar in type 2 diabetes. This form of the illness usually stems from the body's inability to make good use of insulin, the natural hormone that helps to transfer sugar out of the blood and into the cells, where it's converted to energy. Actos works by improving the body's response to its natural supply of insulin, rather than increasing its insulin output. Actos also reduces the production of unneeded sugar in the liver.

Actos (and the similar drug Avandia) can be used alone or in combination with insulin injections or other oral diabetes medications such as DiaBeta, Micronase, Glucotrol, or Glucophage.

ACULAR
Ketorolac, ocular

Acular relieves the itchy eyes brought on by seasonal allergies. Doctors also prescribe it to reduce inflammation after cataracts have been removed from the eyes. A preservative-free formulation (Acular PF) is used to reduce pain and light-sensitivity following operations to correct vision. Acular belongs to the class of medications called nonsteroidal anti-inflammatory drugs.

Acyclovir *See Zovirax*

ADALAT CC
Nifedipine

Adalat CC is used to treat angina (chest pain caused by lack of oxygen to the heart due to clogged arteries or spasm of the arteries). Adalat CC is a calcium channel blocker. It eases the workload of the heart by relaxing the muscles in the walls of the arteries, allowing them to dilate. This improves blood flow through the heart and throughout the body, reduces blood pressure, and helps prevent angina.

Adapalene *See Differin*

Adefovir *See Hepsera*

ADIPEX-P
Phentermine

Adipex-P, an appetite suppressant, is prescribed for short-term use (a few weeks) as part of an overall weight reduction program that also includes dieting, exercise, and counseling. The drug is for use only by excessively overweight individuals who have a condition—such as diabetes, high blood pressure, or high cholesterol—that could lead to serious medical problems.

ADVAIR DISKUS
Fluticasone and Salmeterol
Other brand name: Advair HFA

Advair Diskus is an oral inhaler that contains two types of asthma medication. One is fluticasone propionate, a steroid that reduces inflammation in the lungs. The other, salmeterol, is a long-acting bronchodilator that opens up the airways. Together, the two ingredients provide better control of asthma than either does individually.

ADVICOR
Lovastatin and Extended-Release niacin

Advicor is a cholesterol-lowering drug. Excess cholesterol in the bloodstream can lead to hardening of the arteries and heart disease. Advicor lowers total cholesterol and LDL ("bad") cholesterol, while raising the amount of HDL ("good") cholesterol.

Advicor is a combination of two cholesterol-fighting ingredients: extended-release niacin and lovastatin (Mevacor). It is prescribed only when other drugs and a program of diet, exercise, and weight reduction have been unsuccessful in lowering cholesterol levels.

Advil *See Motrin*

AEROBID
Flunisolide

AeroBid is prescribed for people who need long-term treatment to control and prevent the symptoms of asthma. It contains an anti-inflammatory steroid type of medication and may reduce or eliminate the need for other corticosteroids.

AGENERASE
Amprenavir

Agenerase is one of the many drugs now used to combat human immuno-deficiency virus (HIV) infection. HIV undermines the immune system, reducing the body's ability to fight off other infections and eventually leading to the deadly condition known as acquired immune deficiency syndrome (AIDS).

Agenerase slows the progress of HIV by interfering with an important step in the virus's reproductive cycle. The drug is a member of the group of "protease inhibitors" famous for having successfully halted the advance of the virus in many HIV-positive individuals. Agenerase is prescribed only as part of a "drug cocktail" that attacks the virus on several fronts. It is not used alone.

AGGRENOX
Aspirin with Extended-release dipyridamole

Aggrenox is prescribed to stave off a stroke in people who have had a "mini-stroke" (transient ischemic attack) or a full-scale stroke due to a blood clot blocking an artery in the brain.

Both the ingredients in Aggrenox prevent the formation of clots by interfering with the tendency of blood platelets to clump together. However, the two ingredients together are more effective at preventing strokes than either ingredient taken alone. Aggrenox doesn't eliminate the possibility of a stroke; but it does reduce the odds by almost six percentage points during the first two years of treatment.

Aktob *See Tobrex*

Albuterol *See Proair HFA or Proventil*

Alclometasone *See Aclovate*

ALDACTAZIDE
Spironolactone with Hydrochlorothiazide

Aldactazide is used in the treatment of high blood pressure and other conditions that require the elimination of excess fluid from the body. These conditions include congestive heart failure, cirrhosis of the liver, and kidney disease. Aldactazide combines two diuretic drugs that help the body produce and eliminate more urine. Spironolactone, one of the ingredients, helps to minimize the potassium loss that can be caused by the hydrochlorothiazide component.

ALDACT ONE
Spironolactone

Aldactone flushes excess salt and water from the body and controls high blood pressure. It is used in the diagnosis and treatment of hyperaldosteronism, a condition in which the adrenal gland secretes too much aldosterone (a hormone that regulates the body's salt and potassium levels). It is also used in treating other conditions that require the elimination of excess fluid from the body. These conditions include congestive heart failure, high blood pressure, cirrhosis of the liver, kidney disease, and unusually low potassium levels in the blood. When used for high blood pressure, Aldactone can be taken alone or with other high blood pressure medications.

ALDARA
Imiquimod

Aldara is used to treat external warts around the genital and rectal areas called condyloma acuminatum. It is not used on warts inside the vagina, penis, or rectum. Aldara is also used to treat a skin condition of the face and scalp called actinic keratoses. Aldara can also be used to treat certain types of skin cancer called superficial basal cell carcinoma (sBCC).

It works by aiding the immune system to help protect the body from viruses that cause warts. The medicine does not fight the viruses that cause warts directly. It does help to relieve and control wart production. It is not known how Aldara helps actinic keratoses or skin cancer.

ALDOMET
Methyldopa

Aldomet is used to treat high blood pressure. It is effective when used alone or with other high blood pressure medications.

Alendronate *See Fosamax*

Alesse *See Oral Contraceptives*

Aleve *See Anaprox*

Alfuzosin *See Uroxatral*

Aliskiren *See Tekturna*

ALLEGRA
Fexofenadine
Other brand name: Allegra-D

Allegra relieves the itchy, runny nose, sneezing, and itchy, red, watery eyes that come with hay fever. Its effect begins in 1 hour and lasts 12 hours, peaking around the second or third hour. Allegra is one of the new type of antihistamines that rarely cause drowsiness. It is also used to relieve the itching and welts of hives.

In addition to the antihistamine in Allegra, Allegra-D also contains the nasal decongestant pseudoephedrine.

Allopurinol *See Zyloprim*

Almotriptan *See Axert*

ALPHAGAN P
Brimonidine

Alphagan P lowers high pressure in the eye, a problem typically caused by the condition known as open-angle glaucoma. Alphagan P works in two ways: it reduces production of the liquid that fills the eyeball, and it promotes drainage of this liquid.

Alprostadil *See Caverject*

ALREX
Loteprednol

Alrex belongs to the group of medicines known as corticosteroids (cortisone-like medicines). It is used to treat inflammation (redness) of the eye, which may occur with certain eye problems or following eye surgery. This medicine is also used to temporarily treat the symptoms of the eye caused by a condition known as seasonal allergic conjunctivitis (seasonal eye allergy).

ALTACE
Ramipril

Altace is used in the treatment of high blood pressure. It is effective when used alone or in combination with other high blood pressure medications, especially thiazide-type water pills (diuretics). Altace works by preventing the conversion of a chemical in the blood called angiotensin I into a more potent substance that increases salt and water retention in the body. It also enhances blood flow in the circulatory system. It is a member of the group of drugs called ACE inhibitors.

Altace is also prescribed to reduce the chances of heart attack, stroke, and heart-related death in people 55 years or older who are in danger of such an event. Typical candidates include those who suffer from coronary artery disease, poor circulation, stroke, or diabetes and have at least one other risk factor, such as high blood pressure, high cholesterol levels, low HDL ("good") cholesterol, or cigarette smoking.

For those who do suffer a heart attack and develop heart failure, Altace can be prescribed to prevent the condition from getting worse.

ALTOPREV
Lovastatin

Altoprev is combined with a proper diet to treat high cholesterol levels in the blood. Using this medicine may help prevent medical problems caused by such substances clogging the blood vessels. This medicine may also be used to prevent certain types of heart problems in patients with risk factors for heart problems.

Altoprev belongs to the group of medicines called 3-hydroxy-3-methylglutaryl coenzyme A (HMG-CoA) reductase inhibitors. It works by blocking an enzyme that is needed by the body to make cholesterol, thereby reducing the amount of cholesterol in the blood.

Amantadine *See Symmetrel*

AMARYL
Glimepiride

Amaryl is an oral medication used to treat type 2 (non-insulin-dependent) diabetes when diet and exercise alone fail to control abnormally high levels of blood sugar. Like other diabetes drugs classified as sulfonylureas, Amaryl lowers blood sugar by stimulating the pancreas to produce more insulin. Amaryl is often prescribed along with the insulin-boosting drug Glucophage. It may also be used in conjunction with insulin and other diabetes drugs.

AMERGE
Naratriptan

Amerge is used for relief of classic migraine headaches. It's helpful whether or not the headache is preceded by an aura (visual disturbances, usually sensations of halos or flickering lights). The drug works only during an actual attack. It will not reduce the number of headaches that develop.

Amiloride with Hydrochlorothiazide *See Moduretic*

AMITIZA
Lubiprostone

Amitiza is used to treat chronic constipation in adults. This medicine works by increasing intestinal fluid secretion, which helps ease the passage of stool and helps relieve the symptoms associated with constipation.

Amlodipine *See Norvasc*

Amlodipine with Atorvastatin *See Caduet*

Amlodipine with Benazepril *See Lotrel*

Amnesteem *See Accutane*

Amoxicillin *See Amoxil*

Amoxicillin, Clarithromycin, and Lansoprazole *See Prevpac*

Amoxicillin with Clavulanate *See Augmentin*

AMOXIL
Amoxicillin

Amoxil, an antibiotic, is used to treat a wide variety of infections, including: gonorrhea, middle ear infections, skin infections, upper and lower respiratory tract infections, and infections of the genital and urinary tract. In combination with other drugs such as Prilosec, Prevacid, and/or Biaxin, it is also used to treat duodenal ulcers caused by *H. pylori* bacteria (sores in the wall of the small intestine near the exit from the stomach).

AMPICILLIN
Brand name: Principen

Ampicillin is a penicillin-like antibiotic prescribed for a wide variety of infections, including gonorrhea and other genital and urinary infections, respiratory infections, and gastrointestinal infections, as well as meningitis (inflamed membranes of the spinal cord or brain).

Amprenavir *See Agenerase*

Anakinra *See Kineret*

ANAPROX
Naproxen sodium
Other brand names: Aleve, Naprelan

Anaprox and Naprelan are nonsteroidal anti-inflammatory drugs used to relieve mild to moderate pain and menstrual cramps. They are also prescribed for relief of the inflammation, swelling, stiffness, and joint pain associated with rheumatoid arthritis and osteoarthritis (the most common form of arthritis), and for ankylosing spondylitis (spinal arthritis), tendinitis, bursitis, acute gout, and other conditions. Anaprox also may be prescribed for juvenile arthritis.

The over-the-counter form of naproxen sodium, Aleve, is used for temporary relief of minor aches and pains, and to reduce fever.

Anaspaz *See Levsin*

Anastrozole *See Arimidex*

ANDROGEL
Testosterone gel

AndroGel is a hormone replacement product for men suffering from hypo-gonadism, a low level of the male hormone testosterone. This condition is marked by symptoms such as impotence and decreased interest in sex, lowered mood, fatigue, and decreases in bone density and lean body mass. Testosterone replacement therapy helps correct these problems. AndroGel, applied daily to the skin, provides an especially convenient way of taking the hormone, which was previously administered only by injection or skin patch.

Anexsia *See Vicodin*

ANTARA
Fenofibrate

Antara is used to lower triglyceride (fat-like substances) levels and cholesterol levels in the blood. This may help prevent the development of pancreatitis (inflammation of the pancreas) caused by high levels of triglycerides in the blood.

ANTIVERT
Meclizine
Other brand name: Bonine

Antivert, an antihistamine, is prescribed for the management of nausea, vomiting, and dizziness associated with motion sickness.

Antivert may also be prescribed for the management of vertigo (a spinning sensation or a feeling that the ground is tilted) due to diseases affecting the vestibular system (the bony labyrinth of the ear, which contains the sensors that control balance).

Aprepitant *See Emend*

Apri *See Oral Contraceptives*

ARAVA
Leflunomide

Arava is used in the treatment of rheumatoid arthritis. It reduces the pain, stiffness, inflammation, and swelling associated with this disease, and staves off the joint damage that ultimately results.

Arformoterol *See Brovana*

ARIMIDEX
Anastrozole

Arimidex is a first-line treatment of breast cancer in postmenopausal women. It slows the growth of advanced cancer within the breast and cancer that has spread to other parts of the body. Arimidex is also used to treat advanced breast cancer in postmenopausal women whose disease has spread to other parts of the body following treatment with tamoxifen (Nolvadex), another anticancer drug. Arimidex can also be prescribed along with other drugs to treat the early stages of breast cancer in post-menopausal women.

Arimidex combats the kind of breast cancer that thrives on estrogen. One of the hormones produced by the adrenal gland is converted to a form of estrogen by an enzyme called aromatase. Arimidex suppresses this enzyme and thereby reduces the level of estrogen circulating in the body.

ARMOUR THYROID
Thyroid hormones

Armour Thyroid is prescribed when the thyroid gland is unable to produce enough hormone. It is also used to treat or prevent goiter (enlargement of the thyroid gland), and is given in a "suppression test" to diagnose an over-active thyroid.

AROMASIN
Exemestane

Aromasin is a medicine that is used to treat breast cancer in women whose disease has progressed while they were taking tamoxifen.

Many breast cancer tumors grow in response to estrogen. Aromasin interferes with the production of estrogen in the body. As a result, the amount of estrogen that the tumor is exposed to is reduced, limiting the growth of the tumor. This medicine is meant to be used only by women who have already stopped menstruating.

ARTHROTEC
Diclofenac with Misoprostol

Arthrotec is designed to relieve the symptoms of arthritis in people who are also prone to ulcers. It contains diclofenac, a nonsteroidal anti-inflammatory drug (NSAID) for control of the inflammation, swelling, stiffness, and joint pain associated with rheumatoid arthritis and osteoarthritis. However, since NSAIDs can cause stomach ulcers in susceptible people,

Arthrotec also contains misoprostol, a synthetic prostaglandin that serves to reduce the production of stomach acid, thereby protecting the stomach lining and thus preventing ulcers.

ASACOL
Mesalamine

Asacol is used to treat inflammatory bowel disease, such as ulcerative colitis. It works inside the bowel by helping to reduce the inflammation and other symptoms of the disease.

ASMANEX
Mometasone

Asmanex belongs to the family of medicines known as corticosteroids (cortisone-like medicines). It is used to help prevent the symptoms of asthma. When used regularly every day, inhaled Asmanex decreases the number and severity of asthma attacks. However, it will not relieve an asthma attack that has already started.

Inhaled Asmanex works by preventing certain cells in the lungs and breathing passages from releasing substances that cause asthma symptoms.

Aspirin with Extended-release dipyridamole *See Aggrenox*

ASTELIN
Azelastine nasal spray

Astelin is an antihistamine nasal spray. It is prescribed for the relief of hay fever symptoms such as itchy, runny nose and sneezing, and can also be used to relieve cases of congested, runny nose and postnasal drip unrelated to allergies.

ATACAND
Candesartan

Atacand controls high blood pressure. It works by blocking the effect of a hormone called angiotensin II. Unopposed, this substance prompts the blood vessels to contract, an action that tends to raise blood pressure. Atacand relaxes and expands the blood vessels, allowing pressure to drop. The drug may be prescribed alone or with other blood pressure medications.

ATACAND HCT
Candesartan with Hydrochlorothiazide

Atacand HCT is a combination medication used in the treatment of high blood pressure. One component, candesartan, belongs to a class of blood pressure medications that work by preventing the hormone angiotensin II from constricting the blood vessels. This allows the blood to flow more freely and helps keep blood pressure down. The other component, hydrochlorothiazide, is a diuretic that increases the output of urine. This removes excess fluid from the body and helps lower blood pressure. Doctors usually prescribe Atacand HCT in place of its individual components. It can also be prescribed along with other blood pressure medications.

Atazanavir *See Reyataz*

Atenolol *See Tenormin*

Atenolol with Chlorthalidone *See Tenoretic*

Atorvastatin *See Lipitor*

ATROVENT
Ipratropium
Other brand name: Atrovent HFA

Atrovent HFA is prescribed for long-term treatment of bronchial spasms (wheezing) associated with chronic obstructive pulmonary disease, including chronic bronchitis and emphysema. When inhaled, Atrovent opens the air passages, allowing more oxygen to reach the lungs.

Atrovent nasal spray relieves runny nose. The 0.03% spray is used for year-round runny nose due to allergies and other causes. The 0.06% spray is prescribed for hay fever and for runny nose due to colds. The spray does not relieve nasal congestion or sneezing.

AUGMENTIN
Amoxicillin with Clavulanate
Other brand name: Augmentin XR

Augmentin is used in the treatment of lower respiratory, middle ear, sinus, skin, and urinary tract infections that are caused by certain specific bacteria. These bacteria produce a chemical enzyme called beta lactamase that makes some infections particularly difficult to treat.

Augmentin ES-600, a stronger, oral-suspension form of the drug, is prescribed for certain stubborn ear infections that previous treatment has failed to clear up in children two and under, or those attending day care.

Augmentin XR is an extended-release form of the drug used to treat pneumonia and sinus infections.

Auranofin *See Ridaura*

AVALIDE
Irbesartan with Hydrochlorothiazide

Avalide is a combination medication used to treat high blood pressure. One component, irbesartan, belongs to a class of blood pressure medications that prevents the hormone angiotensin II from constricting the blood vessels, thereby allowing blood to flow more freely and keeping blood pressure down. The other component, hydrochlorothiazide, is a diuretic that increases the output of urine, removing excess fluid from the body and thus lowering blood pressure.

Combinations such as Avalide are usually prescribed only when treatment with a single medication fails to lower blood pressure sufficiently. Avalide can be combined with yet other blood pressure medicines if pressure remains too high.

AVANDAMET
Rosiglitazone with Metformin

Avandamet is an oral medication used to control blood sugar levels in people with type 2 (non-insulin-dependent) diabetes. It contains two drugs commonly used to lower blood sugar, rosiglitazone (Avandia) and metformin (Glucophage). Avandamet replaces the need to take these two drugs separately. It is also used when treatment with Glucophage alone doesn't work. Avandamet is not, however, meant to take the place of weight loss or diet and exercise.

Blood sugar levels are ordinarily controlled by the body's natural supply of insulin, which helps sugar move out of the bloodstream and into the cells to be used for energy. People who have type 2 diabetes do not make enough insulin or do not respond normally to the insulin their bodies make, causing a buildup of unused sugar in the bloodstream. Avandamet helps remedy this problem in two ways: by decreasing the body's production of sugar and making the body more sensitive to its own insulin supply. Avandamet does not increase the body's production of insulin.

AVANDARYL
Glimepiride with Rosiglitazone

Avandaryl is used for treatment of type 2 diabetes, by controlling blood sugar levels. Type 2 diabetes occurs when there is a build-up of sugar in the blood, which may lead to serious health conditions. Avandaryl is used together with proper diet and exercise.

AVANDIA
Rosiglitazone

Avandia is used to hold down blood sugar levels in people with type 2 diabetes (also known as "non-insulin dependent" or "adult onset" diabetes).

Blood sugar levels are ordinarily controlled by the body's natural supply of insulin, which helps sugar move out of the bloodstream and into the cells. In type 2 diabetes, the build-up of sugar in the blood is often due not to a lack of insulin, but to the body's inability to make proper use of it. Avandia works first by decreasing sugar production, then by helping the body make more efficient use of whatever insulin is available. It does not increase the actual amount of insulin in circulation.

Avandia can be used alone or in conjunction with insulin, metformin (Glucophage), or a member of the sulfonylurea class of diabetes drugs (Diabinese, Micronase, Orinase). It takes effect slowly. Patients may not see a reduction in blood sugar levels for the first 2 weeks of therapy, and it may take 2 to 3 months for the medication to deliver maximum results.

AVAPRO
Irbesartan

Avapro is used to treat high blood pressure. A member of the family of drugs called angiotensin II receptor antagonists, it works by preventing the hormone angiotensin II from narrowing the blood vessels, an action that tends to raise blood pressure. Avapro may be prescribed alone or with other blood pressure medications.

In people with type 2 diabetes and high blood pressure, Avapro is also prescribed to stave off damage to the kidneys, often delaying the need for dialysis and a kidney transplant.

AVELOX
Moxifloxacin

Avelox, an antibiotic, is prescribed to treat sinus and lung infections. It kills bacteria that can cause sinusitis, pneumonia, and secondary infections in chronic bronchitis. It also fights skin infections caused by staph or strep.

Avelox is a member of the quinolone family of antibiotics. Like all antibiotics, Avelox works only against bacteria. It will not cure an infection caused by a virus.

AVINZA
Morphine

Avinza is sued to treat moderate to severe pain when around-the-clock pain relief is needed for a long period of time.

Avita *See Retin-A and Renova*

AVODART
Dutasteride

Avodart is used to treat prostate enlargement, a condition that is medically known as benign prostatic hyperplasia, or BPH.

The prostate is a chestnut-shaped gland that is part of the male reproductive system. It produces a liquid that forms part of the semen. This gland completely encloses the upper part of the urethra, the tube through which urine flows out of the bladder. Many men over age 50 suffer from a benign (noncancerous) enlargement of the prostate. The enlarged gland squeezes the urethra, obstructing the normal flow of urine. Resulting problems may include difficulty in starting urination, weak flow of urine, and the need to urinate urgently or more frequently. Sometimes surgical removal of the prostate is necessary.

By shrinking the enlarged prostate, Avodart may alleviate the various urinary symptoms, making surgery unnecessary. Periodic examinations by the doctor will be necessary to assess treatment response. It may take several months to notice symptom improvement.

AXERT
Almotriptan

Axert is a migraine treatment. It relieves the type of migraine that is accompanied by an aura (a set of symptoms that includes visual disturbances, speech difficulties, tingling, numbness, and weakness), as well as the kind that lacks an aura.

Axert is a member of a family of drugs called selective serotonin receptor agonists. These medications are thought to work by stopping abnormal dilation of blood vessels in the head, fighting inflammation, and reducing pain transmissions along certain nerve pathways near the brain.

Axert relieves migraines already in progress, but it won't prevent them from starting. It has not been tested for other types of headache, such as cluster headache, and should be used only for migraine attacks.

AXID
Nizatidine

Axid is prescribed for the treatment of duodenal ulcers and noncancerous stomach ulcers. Full-dose therapy for these problems lasts no longer than 8 weeks. However, doctors sometimes prescribe Axid at a reduced dosage after a duodenal ulcer has healed. The drug is also prescribed for the heartburn and the inflammation that result when acid stomach contents flow backward into the esophagus. Axid belongs to a class of drugs known as histamine H_2 blockers.

Azelaic acid for acne *See Azelex*

Azelaic acid for rosacea *See Finacea*

Azelastine eye drops *See Optivar*

Azelastine nasal spray *See Astelin*

AZELEX
Azelaic acid for acne

Azelex helps clear up mild to moderate acne. The skin eruptions and inflammation of acne typically begin during puberty, when oily secretions increase.

Azithromycin *See Zithromax*

AZMACORT
Triamcinolone

Azmacort is a metered-dose inhaler containing the anti-inflammatory steroid medication, triamcinolone acetonide. Azmacort is used as long-term therapy to control bronchial asthma attacks.

AZOPT
Brinzolamide

Azopt is a carbonic anhydrase inhibitor that is used in the eye. It is used to treat increased pressure in the eye caused by open-angle glaucoma. It is also used to treat a condition called hypertension of the eye.

AZULFIDINE
Sulfasalazine

Azulfidine, an anti-inflammatory medicine, is prescribed for the treatment of mild to moderate ulcerative colitis (a long-term, progressive bowel disease) and as an added treatment in severe ulcerative colitis (chronic inflammation and ulceration of the lining of large bowel and rectum, the main symptom of which is bloody diarrhea).

Azulfidine EN-tabs are prescribed for people with ulcerative colitis who cannot take the regular Azulfidine tablet because of symptoms of stomach and intestinal irritation such as nausea and vomiting when taking the first few doses of the drug, or for those in whom a reduction in dosage does not lessen the stomach or intestinal side effects. The EN-tabs are also prescribed for adults and children with rheumatoid arthritis who fail to get relief from salicylates (such as aspirin) or other nonsteroidal anti-inflammatory drugs (such as ibuprofen).

Baclofen *See Lioresal*

BACTRIM
Trimethoprim with Sulfamethoxazole
Other brand name: Septra

Bactrim, an antibacterial combination drug, is prescribed for the treatment of certain urinary tract infections, severe middle ear infections in children, long-lasting or frequently recurring bronchitis in adults that has increased in seriousness, inflammation of the intestine due to a severe bacterial infection, and travelers' diarrhea in adults. Bactrim is also prescribed for the treatment of *Pneumocystis carinii* pneumonia, and for prevention of this type of pneumonia in people with weakened immune systems.

BACTROBAN
Mupirocin

Bactroban is prescribed for the treatment of impetigo, a bacterial infection of the skin. An antibiotic ointment applied to the skin, it kills the staph and strep germs responsible for the problem.

Balsalazide *See Colazal*

Benazepril *See Lotensin*

Benazepril with Hydrochlorothiazide *See Lotensin HCT*

BENICAR
Olmesartan
Other brand name: Benicar HCT (olmesartan and hydrochlorothiazide)

Benicar controls high blood pressure. It works by blocking the effect of a hormone called angiotensin II. Unopposed, this substance prompts the blood vessels to contract, an action that tends to raise blood pressure. Benicar relaxes and expands the blood vessels, allowing pressure to drop. The drug may be prescribed alone or with other blood pressure medications.

Benicar HCT contains Benicar plus hydrochlorothiazide, a common diuretic that increases the output of urine. This removes excess fluid from the body and helps lower blood pressure.

High blood pressure adds to the workload of the heart and arteries. If it continues for a long time, the heart and arteries may not function properly. This can damage the blood vessels of the brain, heart, and kidneys, resulting in a stroke, heart failure, or kidney failure. High blood pressure may also increase the risk of heart attacks. These problems may be less likely to occur if blood pressure is controlled.

BENTYL
Dicyclomine

Bentyl is prescribed for the treatment of functional bowel/irritable bowel syndrome (abdominal pain, accompanied by diarrhea and constipation associated with stress). It works by quelling the spasms associated with this condition.

BENZACLIN
Clindamycin and Benzoyl peroxide

BenzaClin is an acne treatment. Both its ingredients—the antibiotic clindamycin and the antibacterial agent benzoyl peroxide—attack the bacteria that help cause acne.

BENZAMYCIN
Erythromycin with Benzoyl peroxide

A combination of the antibiotic erythromycin and the antibacterial agent benzoyl peroxide, Benzamycin is effective in stopping the bacteria that cause acne and in reducing acne infection.

Benzonatate *See Tessalon*

Benzoyl peroxide *See Brevoxyl*

BETAGAN
Levobunolol

Betagan eyedrops are given to treat chronic open-angle glaucoma (increased pressure inside the eye). This medication is in a class called beta blockers. It works by lowering pressure within the eyeball.

Betamethasone *See Diprolene*

Betamethasone valerate *See Luxiq*

Betaxolol *See Betoptic*

BETIMOL
Timolol

Betimol is a medication that reduces internal pressure in the eye. It is used to treat glaucoma. Beta-adrenergic blocking agents like Betimol appear to work by reducing the production of fluid in the eye. This lowers the pressure in the eye.

BETOPTIC
Betaxolol

Betoptic Ophthalmic Solution and Betoptic S Ophthalmic Suspension contain a medication that lowers internal eye pressure. They are used to treat open-angle glaucoma (high pressure of the fluid in the eye).

BIAXIN

Clarithromycin
Other brand name: Biaxin XL

Biaxin, an antibiotic chemically related to erythromycin, is used to treat certain bacterial infections of the respiratory tract, including:

Strep throat
Pneumonia
Sinusitis (inflamed sinuses)
Tonsillitis (inflamed tonsils)
Acute middle ear infections
Acute flare-ups of chronic bronchitis (inflamed airways)

Biaxin is also prescribed to treat infections of the skin. Combined with Prilosec or Prevacid and amoxicillin, it is used to cure ulcers near the exit from the stomach (duodenal ulcers) caused by *H. pylori* bacteria. It can also be prescribed to combat *Mycobacterium avium* infections in people with AIDS.

Biaxin is available in tablet and suspension form, and in extended-release tablets (Biaxin XL). The extended-release form is used only for sinus inflammation and flare-ups of bronchitis.

Bicalutamide *See Casodex*

Bimatoprost *See Lumigan*

Bisoprolol *See Zebeta*

Bisoprolol with Hydrochlorothiazide *See Ziac*

BLEPHAMIDE

Prednisolone with Sulfacetamide

Blephamide is an antibiotic/anti-inflammatory combination used to treat infections of the eye and eye irritation, swelling, and redness.

Bonine *See Antivert*

BONIVA

Ibrandronate

Boniva is a prescription medicine used to treat or prevent osteoporosis in women after menopause. Boniva may reverse bone loss by stopping more loss of bone and increasing bone mass in most women who take it, even though they won't be able to see or feel a difference. Boniva may help lower the chances of breaking bones (fractures). For Boniva to treat or prevent osteoporosis, patients have to take the drug as prescribed.

Brevicon *See Oral Contraceptives*

BREVOXYL
Benzoyl peroxide

Brevoxyl is a keratolytic agent used to treat acne. It is applied topically.

Brimonidine *See Alphagan P*

Brinzolamide *See Azopt*

Bromfenac *See Xibrom*

Bromocriptine *See Parlodel*

BROVANA
Arformoterol

Brovana is used for long-term treatment of lung problems that come with having chronic obstructive pulmonary disease (COPD), which includes chronic bronchitis and emphysema.

Budesonide *See Rhinocort Aqua*

Budesonide inhalation powder *See Pulmicort Turbuhaler*

Budesonide inhalation suspension *See Pulmicort Respules*

Budesonide, oral *See Entocort EC*

Bumetanide *See Bumex*

BUMEX
Bumetanide

Bumex is used to lower the amount of excess salt and water in the body by increasing the output of urine. It is prescribed in the treatment of edema, or fluid retention, associated with congestive heart failure and liver or kidney disease. It is also occasionally prescribed, along with other drugs, to treat high blood pressure.

Buprenorphine and
 Naloxone hydrochloride dihydrate *See Suboxone*

Bupropion for smoking *See Zyban*

Butalbital, Acetaminophen, and Caffeine *See Fioricet*

Butalbital, Aspirin, and Caffeine *See Fiorinal*

Butalbital, Codeine, Aspirin, and Caffeine *See Fiorinal with Codeine*

BYETTA
Exenatide

Byetta is an injectable antidiabetic medication used to improve blood sugar control in people with type 2 diabetes whose current medications alone do not adequately control their blood sugar levels. Byetta is prescribed along with oral antidiabetic medications to enhance their effectiveness. It may be used with metformin alone or with metformin and sulfonylurea combined.

Type 2 diabetes occurs in people who are unable to produce or cannot properly utilize insulin. Insulin helps carry sugar from the bloodstream into the body's cells. In diabetes, the unused sugar causes abnormally high sugar levels in the bloodstream. Byetta is in a class of drugs known as incretin mimetics because it mimics the action of incretins—natural substances found in the body that help maintain normal blood sugar levels. Byetta stimulates cells that produce insulin in the pancreas, while also decreasing the amount of sugar the produced by the liver. In addition, it slows the passage of food from the stomach, thus slowing the rate that sugar is absorbed into the bloodstream. Byetta also decreases the appetite, which can help with weight control.

CADUET
Amlodipine and Atorvastatin

Caduet is a combination of two drugs, amlodipine and atorvastatin. Amlodipine is used to treat high blood pressure and angina. Angina is characterized by episodes of crushing chest pain that usually results from a lack of oxygen in the heart muscle due to clogged arteries. Amlodipine is a calcium channel blocker, a type of drug that dilates blood vessels and slows the heart to reduce blood pressure and the pain of angina.

High blood pressure adds to the workload of the heart and arteries. If it continues for a long time, the heart and arteries may not function properly. This can damage the blood vessels of the brain, heart, and kidneys, resulting in a stroke, heart failure, or kidney failure. High blood pressure may also increase the risk of heart attacks. These problems may be less likely to occur if blood pressure is controlled.

The exact way in which this medicine works is not known. Amlodipine is a type of medicine known as a calcium channel blocker. Calcium channel blocking agents affect the movement of calcium into the cells of the heart and blood vessels. Atorvastatin is used to lower cholesterol and triglyceride (fat-like substances) levels in the blood. The action of both medicines together is to relax blood vessels, lower blood pressure, and decrease the amount of cholesterol in the blood.

CALAN

Verapamil
Other brand names: Calan SR, Covera-HS, Isoptin SR, Verelan, Verelan PM

Verapamil-based medications can be prescribed for several heart and blood pressure problems. The fast-acting brands (Calan and Isoptin) are taken for angina (chest pain due to clogged cardiac arteries), as well as irregular heartbeat and high blood pressure. The longer-acting brands (Calan SR, Isoptin SR, Verelan, and Verelan PM) are typically used only for high blood pressure. Covera-HS is prescribed for both high blood pressure and angina.

Verapamil is a type of medication called a calcium channel blocker. It eases the heart's workload by slowing down the passage of nerve impulses through it, and hence the contractions of the heart muscle. This improves blood flow through the heart and throughout the body, reduces blood pressure, corrects irregular heartbeat, and helps prevent angina pain.

Some doctors also prescribe verapamil to prevent migraine headache and asthma and to treat manic depression and panic attacks, but the drug is not officially approved for these purposes.

Calcipotriene *See Dovonex*

Calcitonin-salmon *See Miacalcin*

Calcitriol *See Rocaltrol*

Canasa *See Rowasa*

Candesartan *See Atacand*

Candesartan with Hydrochlorothiazide *See Atacand HCT*

Capecitabine *See Xeloda*

CAPOTEN
Captopril

Capoten is used in the treatment of high blood pressure and congestive heart failure. When prescribed for high blood pressure, it is effective used alone or combined with diuretics. If it is prescribed for congestive heart failure, it is used in combination with digitalis and diuretics. Capoten is in a family of drugs known as "ACE (angiotensin converting enzyme) inhibitors." It works by preventing a chemical in the blood called angiotensin I from converting into a more potent form that increases salt and water retention in the body. Capoten also enhances blood flow throughout the blood vessels.

In addition, Capoten is used to improve survival in certain people who have suffered heart attacks and to treat kidney disease in diabetics.

Some doctors also prescribe Capoten for angina pectoris (crushing chest pain), Raynaud's phenomenon (a disorder of the blood vessels that causes the fingers to turn white when exposed to cold), and rheumatoid arthritis.

CAPOZIDE
Captopril with Hydrochlorothiazide

Capozide is used in the treatment of high blood pressure. It combines an ACE inhibitor with a thiazide diuretic. Captopril, the ACE inhibitor, works by preventing a chemical in the blood called angiotensin I from converting into a more potent form that increases salt and water retention in the body. Captopril also enhances blood flow throughout the blood vessels. Hydrochlorothiazide, the diuretic, helps the body produce and eliminate more urine, which helps in lowering blood pressure.

Captopril *See Capoten*

Captopril with Hydrochlorothiazide *See Capozide*

Carac *See Efudex*

CARAFATE
Sucralfate

Carafate Tablets and Suspension are used for the short-term treatment (up to 8 weeks) of an active duodenal ulcer (an open sore in the intestinal wall near the exit from the stomach). Carafate Tablets are also used for longer-term therapy at a reduced dosage after a duodenal ulcer has healed.

Carafate helps ulcers heal by forming a protective coating over them. Some doctors also prescribe Carafate for ulcers in the mouth and esophagus that develop during cancer therapy, for digestive tract irritation caused by drugs, for long-term treatment of stomach ulcers, and to relieve pain following tonsil removal.

Carbamazepine *See Tegretol or Carbatrol*

CARBATROL
Carbamazepine

Carbamazepine is used to control some types of seizures in the treatment of epilepsy. It is also used to relieve pain due to trigeminal neuralgia (tic douloureux). It should not be used for other more common aches or pains.

Carbidopa with Levodopa *See Sinemet CR*

Carbinoxamine or Brompheniramine and Pseudoephedrine
See Rondec

CARDENE
Nicardipine

Cardene, a type of medication called a calcium channel blocker, is prescribed for the treatment of chronic stable angina (chest pain that results when clogged arteries reduce the heart's oxygen supply, brought on by exertion) and for high blood pressure. When used to treat angina, Cardene is sometimes combined with beta-blocking medications such as Tenormin or Inderal. If it is used to treat high blood pressure, Cardene may be combined with other high blood pressure medications. Calcium channel blockers ease the workload of the heart by slowing down the passage of nerve impulses through the heart and its resulting muscle contractions. This improves blood flow through the heart and throughout the body. By expanding the blood vessels, calcium channel blockers also reduce blood pressure.

Cardene SR, a long-acting form of the drug, is prescribed only for high blood pressure.

Some doctors also prescribe Cardene to prevent migraine headache and to treat congestive heart failure. In combination with other drugs, such as Amicar, Cardene is also prescribed to manage neurological problems following certain kinds of stroke.

CARDIZEM
Diltiazem
Other brand names: Cardizem CD, Dilacor XR

Cardizem and Cardizem CD (a controlled release form of diltiazem) are used in the treatment of angina pectoris (chest pain that results when clogged arteries reduce the heart's oxygen supply) and chronic stable angina (a type brought on by exertion). Cardizem CD is also used to treat high blood pressure. Another controlled release form, Cardizem SR, is used only in the treatment of high blood pressure. Cardizem, a calcium channel blocker, dilates blood vessels and slows the heart to reduce blood pressure and the pain of angina.

Doctors sometimes prescribe Cardizem for loss of circulation in the fingers and toes (Raynaud's phenomenon), for involuntary movements (tardive dyskinesia), and to prevent heart attack.

Dilacor XR is used in the treatment of high blood pressure and chronic stable angina. It may be taken alone or combined with other blood pressure medications.

CARDURA
Doxazosin

Cardura is used in the treatment of benign prostatic hyperplasia, a condition in which the prostate gland grows larger, pressing on the urethra and threatening to block the flow of urine from the bladder. The drug relieves symptoms such as a weak stream, dribbling, incomplete emptying of the bladder, frequent urination, and burning during urination.

Cardura is also used in the treatment of high blood pressure. It is effective when used alone or in combination with other blood pressure medications, such as diuretics, beta-blocking medications, calcium channel blockers or ACE inhibitors.

Doctors also prescribe Cardura, along with other drugs such as digitalis and diuretics, for treatment of congestive heart failure.

Carisoprodol *See Soma*

Carvedilol *See Coreg*

CASODEX
Bicalutamide

Casodex is used in the treatment of advanced prostate cancer. It belongs to a class of drugs known as antiandrogens. These drugs block the effect of male hormones.

Casodex is prescribed along with a drug, such as Lupron, that mimics the effect of natural luteinizing hormone-releasing hormone (LHRH).

Cataflam *See Voltaren*

CATAPRES
Clonidine

Catapres is prescribed for high blood pressure. It is effective when used alone or with other high blood pressure medications.

Doctors also prescribe Catapres for alcohol, nicotine, or benzodiazepine (tranquilizer) withdrawal; migraine headaches; smoking cessation programs; Tourette's syndrome (tics and uncontrollable utterances); narcotic/methadone detoxification; premenstrual tension; and diabetic diarrhea.

CAVERJECT
Alprostadil
Other brand names: Edex, Muse

Caverject is used to treat male impotence. Doctors also use the drug to help diagnose the exact nature of a patient's impotence.

Caverject and the similar brand Edex are both taken by injection. A third brand, Muse, is taken as a small suppository inserted in the penis.

CECLOR
Cefaclor

Ceclor, a cephalosporin antibiotic, is used in the treatment of ear, nose, throat, respiratory tract, urinary tract, and skin infections caused by specific bacteria, including staph, strep, and *E. coli*. Uses include treatment of sore or strep throat, pneumonia, and tonsillitis. Ceclor CD, an extended release form of the drug, is also used for flare-ups of chronic bronchitis.

CEDAX
Ceftibuten

Cedax cures mild-to-moderate bacterial infections of the throat, ear, and respiratory tract. Among these infections are strep throat, tonsillitis, and acute otitis media (middle ear infection) in children and adults. Cedax is also prescribed for acute flare-ups of chronic bronchitis in adults. Cedax is a cephalosporin antibiotic.

Cefaclor *See Ceclor*

Cefadroxil *See Duricef*

Cefdinir *See Omnicef*

Cefditoren *See Spectracef*

Cefixime *See Suprax*

Cefprozil *See Cefzil*

Ceftibuten *See Cedax*

CEFTIN
Cefuroxime

Ceftin, a cephalosporin antibiotic, is prescribed for mild to moderately severe bacterial infections of the throat, lungs, ears, skin, sinuses, and urinary tract, and for gonorrhea. Ceftin tablets are also prescribed in the early stages of Lyme disease.

Ceftriaxone *See Rocephin*

Cefuroxime *See Ceftin*

CEFZIL
Cefprozil

Cefzil, a cephalosporin antibiotic, is prescribed for mild to moderately severe bacterial infections of the throat, ear, sinuses, respiratory tract, and skin. Among these infections are strep throat, tonsillitis, bronchitis, and pneumonia.

CELEBREX
Celecoxib

Celebrex is prescribed for acute pain, menstrual cramps, and the pain and inflammation of osteoarthritis and rheumatoid arthritis. It is the first of a new class of nonsteroidal anti-inflammatory drugs (NSAIDs) called "COX-2 inhibitors." Like older NSAIDs such as Motrin and Naprosyn, Celebrex is believed to fight pain and inflammation by inhibiting the effect of a natural enzyme called COX-2. Unlike the older medications, however, it does not interfere with a similar substance, called COX-1, which exerts a protective effect on the lining of the stomach. Celebrex is therefore less likely to cause the bleeding and ulcers that sometimes accompany sustained use of the older NSAIDs.

Celebrex has also been found to reduce the number of colorectal polyps (growths in the wall of the lower intestine and rectum) in people who suffer from the condition called familial adenomatous polyposis (FAP), an inherited tendency to develop large numbers of colorectal polyps that eventually become cancerous.

Celecoxib *See Celebrex*

CELLCEPT
Mycophenolate

CellCept belongs to a group of medicines known as immunosuppressive agents. It is used to lower the body's natural immunity in patients who receive organ transplants.

When a patient receives an organ transplant, the body's white blood cells will try to get rid of (reject) the transplanted organ. CellCept works by preventing the white blood cells from getting rid of the transplanted organ.

CENESTIN
Synthetic conjugated estrogens, A

Estrogens are female hormones. They are produced by the body and are necessary for the normal sexual development of the female and for the regulation of the menstrual cycle during the childbearing years.

The ovaries begin to produce less estrogen after menopause. This medicine is prescribed to make up for the lower amount of estrogen. Cenestin is used to treat symptoms of menopause, such as hot flashes (warmth or redness in the face, neck, arms, or upper chest) and dryness in the vagina.

Cephalexin *See Keflex*

Cetirizine *See Zyrtec*

Cetirizine with Pseudoephedrine *See Zyrtec-D*

CHANTIX
Varenicline

Chantix is a prescription medicine to help adults stop smoking. It is used as part of a support program. Educational materials and necessary counseling should also be provided as part of the support program.

Chlorhexidine *See Peridex*

Cholestyramine *See Questran*

CIALIS
Tadalafil

Cialis is an oral drug for male impotence, also known as erectile dysfunction (ED). It works by dilating blood vessels in the penis, allowing the inflow of blood needed for an erection.

Ciclopirox *See Loprox*

Ciclopirox nail lacquer *See Penlac*

Cilostazol *See Pletal*

CILOXAN
Ciprofloxacin, ocular

Ciloxan is an antibiotic used in the treatment of eye infections. The ointment form of the drug is prescribed for eye inflammations. The solution can also be used to treat ulcers or sores on the cornea (the transparent covering over the pupil). Ciprofloxacin, the active ingredient, is a member of the quinolone family of antibiotics.

Cimetidine *See Tagamet*

Cinacalcet *See Sensipar*

CIPRO
Ciprofloxacin
Other brand name: Cipro XR

Cipro is used to treat infections of the lower respiratory tract, the abdomen, the skin, the bones and joints, and the urinary tract, including cystitis (bladder inflammation) in women. It is also prescribed for severe sinus or bronchial infections, infectious diarrhea, typhoid fever, inhalational anthrax, infections of the prostate gland, and some sexually transmitted diseases such as gonorrhea. Additionally, some doctors prescribe Cipro for certain serious ear infections, tuberculosis, and some of the infections common in people with AIDS.

Because Cipro is effective only for certain types of bacterial infections, before beginning treatment the doctor may perform tests to identify the specific organisms causing the infection.

Cipro is available as a tablet and an oral suspension and as a suspension to be used externally in the ear.

Cipro XR, an extended-release form of the drug, is used to treat cystitis, urinary tract infection, and kidney infection.

CIPRODEX OTIC
Ciprofloxacin and Dexamethasone

Ciprodex is an ear drop medication used to treat middle ear infections in children ages 6 months or older who have tubes in their ears. It's also used to treat swimmer's ear—an inflammation, irritation, or infection of the outer ear and ear canal—in adults and children 6 months or older.

Ciprodex is a combination of two drugs. One is the antibiotic ciprofloxacin, which fights bacterial infections. The other is the steroid dexamethasone, which lessens inflammation.

Ciprofloxacin *See Cipro*

Ciprofloxacin and Dexamethasone *See Ciprodex Otic*

Ciprofloxacin, ocular *See Ciloxan*

CLARINEX
Desloratadine

Clarinex is an antihistamine used to relieve the symptoms of hay fever (seasonal and perennial allergic rhinitis). Like many of the newer members of the antihistamine family, Clarinex causes less drowsiness than do older products such as Benadryl.

Clarithromycin *See Biaxin*

CLEOCIN T
Clindamycin

Cleocin T is an antibiotic used to treat acne.

CLEOCIN VAGINAL
Clindamycin

Cleocin Vaginal products (cream and ovules) are used to treat bacterial vaginosis, an infection of the vagina. The infection, which is probably sexually transmitted, often produces a gray or yellow discharge with a fishy smell that increases if the external genitals are washed with alkaline soap.

Before prescribing Cleocin, doctors typically test the vaginal discharge in the laboratory and examine it under the microscope to make certain that the patient does not have a yeast infection or another sexually transmitted disease (STD) such as chlamydia, gonorrhea, or herpes simplex.

CLIMARA PRO
Estradiol and Levonorgestrel

Climara Pro is a medicated patch containing two hormones, estrogen and progestin. It is used to reduce the symptoms of menopause such as hot flashes.

Clindamycin *See Cleocin T, Cleocin Vaginal*

Clindamycin and Benzoyl peroxide *See BenzaClin or Duac*

CLINORIL
Sulindac

Clinoril, a nonsteroidal anti-inflammatory drug, is used to relieve the inflammation, swelling, stiffness, and joint pain associated with rheumatoid arthritis, osteoarthritis (the most common form of arthritis), and ankylosing spondylitis (stiffness and progressive arthritis of the spine). It is also used to treat bursitis, tendinitis, acute gouty arthritis, and other types of pain.

The safety and effectiveness of this medication in the treatment of people with severe, incapacitating rheumatoid arthritis have not been established.

Clobetasol *See Temovate or Olux*

Clomid *See Clomiphene Citrate*

CLOMIPHENE CITRATE
Brand names: Clomid, Serophene

Clomiphene is prescribed for the treatment of ovulatory failure in women who wish to become pregnant and whose husbands are fertile and potent.

Clonidine *See Catapres*

Clopidogrel *See Plavix*

Clotrimazole with Betamethasone *See Lotrisone*

Co-Gesic *See Vicodin*

COLAZAL
Balsalazide

Colazal is used in the treatment of mild to moderate ulcerative colitis (chronic inflammation and ulceration of the lower intestine). It is an anti-inflammatory medicine specially formulated to release the active ingredient, mesalamine, directly to the lining of the colon. Its ability to provide relief without the severe side effects found with similar drugs is believed to be due to this localized drug delivery mechanism.

Colesevelam *See WelChol*

COLESTID
Colestipol

Colestid, in conjunction with diet, is used to help lower high levels of cholesterol in the blood. This reduces the chances of developing clogged arteries and heart disease. The drug is available in plain and orange-flavored granules and in tablet form.

Colestipol *See Colestid*

COLYTE
Polyethylene glycol with Electrolytes
Other brand name: GoLYTELY

Colyte is used to clean the bowel before an examination of the upper part of the rectum (colonoscopy) or a barium enema X-ray.

COMBIPATCH
Estradiol and Norethindrone acetate

A remedy for the symptoms of menopause, CombiPatch combines the hormones estrogen (estradiol) and progestin (norethindrone acetate) in a slow-release patch that's applied to the skin. The product eases such symptoms of menopause as feelings of warmth in the face, neck, and chest, and the sudden intense episodes of heat and sweating known as "hot flashes." It is also prescribed to relieve external vaginal irritation and internal vaginal dryness.

CombiPatch can also be used as an estrogen supplement by women unable to produce sufficient amounts of estrogen on their own. Problems prompting the need for supplementation include ovarian failure, hypogonadism (impaired hormone production), and surgical removal of the ovaries.

COMBIVENT
Ipratropium with Albuterol

Combivent is prescribed for people with chronic obstructive pulmonary disease (COPD) if they are already taking one airway-opening medication and need another. The product's two active ingredients act in distinctly different ways. Ipratropium quells airway-closing spasms in the bronchial walls. Albuterol relaxes the muscles in the walls, permitting them to expand. When used together, the two ingredients provide more relief than either can do alone.

Combivent is supplied in an aerosol canister for use only with the special Combivent mouthpiece.

COMBIVIR
Lamivudine and Zidovudine

Combivir is used to fight the human immunodeficiency virus (HIV) that causes AIDS. It is a combination product containing the two AIDS drugs, lamivudine (Epivir) and zidovudine (Retrovir). It is intended for use with additional AIDS drugs.

HIV does its damage by slowly destroying the immune system, eventually leaving the body defenseless against infections. The drugs in Combivir interfere with the virus's ability to reproduce, thus staving off the decline of the immune system and preserving better health.

COMTAN
Entacapone

Comtan is used for Parkinson's disease. It is prescribed when doses of the combination drug levodopa/carbidopa (Sinemet) begin to wear off too soon. By extending the effect of each dose of Sinemet, it frees the patient from the stiffness and tremors of Parkinson's for a longer period of time.

Comtan works by inhibiting the effect of an enzyme that breaks down the levodopa in Sinemet. It has no effect on Parkinson's disease when used by itself.

Conjugated estrogens *See Premarin*

COREG
Carvedilol
Other brand name: Coreg CR

Coreg lowers blood pressure and increases the output of the heart. It is prescribed for people with congestive heart failure to increase survival and reduce the need for hospitalization. Coreg may be prescribed if the patient has survived a heart attack and now suffers from left ventricular dysfunction, a condition where the left side of the heart no longer pumps properly. It is also used to control high blood pressure. When prescribed for heart failure, it can be used alone or with other drugs such as digitalis. For hypertension , it is often prescribed along with a diuretic. Coreg is a member of the beta blocker family of drugs.

Coreg CR is an extended-release version of the drug that is taken once a day.

CORGARD
Nadolol

Corgard is used in the treatment of angina pectoris (chest pain, usually caused by lack of oxygen to the heart due to clogged arteries) and to reduce high blood pressure.

When prescribed for high blood pressure, it is effective when used alone or in combination with other high blood pressure medications. Corgard is a type of drug known as a beta blocker. It decreases the force and rate of heart contractions, reducing the heart's demand for oxygen and lowering blood pressure.

Cormax *See Temovate*

COSOPT
Dorzolamide with Timolol

Cosopt lowers high pressure in the eye, a problem typically caused by the condition known as open-angle glaucoma. Cosopt works by reducing production of the liquid that fills the eyeball.

COUMADIN
Warfarin

Coumadin is an anticoagulant (blood thinner). It is prescribed to:

Prevent and/or treat a blood clot that has formed within a blood vessel or in the lungs.

Prevent and/or treat blood clots associated with certain heart conditions or replacement of a heart valve.

Aid in the prevention of blood clots that may form in blood vessels anywhere in the body after a heart attack.

Reduce the risk of death, another heart attack, or stroke after a heart attack.

Covera-HS *See Calan*

COZAAR
Losartan

Cozaar is used in the treatment of high blood pressure. It is effective when used alone or with other high blood pressure medications, such as diuretics that help the body get rid of water.

Cozaar is also used to slow the progress of kidney disease caused by type 2 diabetes (the type of diabetes that doesn't require insulin shots). This angiotensin II receptor antagonist works, in part, by preventing the hormone angiotensin II from constricting the blood vessels, which tends to raise blood pressure.

CRESTOR
Rosuvastatin

Crestor is used to lower cholesterol levels when diet and exercise alone have failed to work. The drug can help lower the total cholesterol count as well as harmful levels of low-density lipoprotein (LDL) cholesterol. It can also lower triglycerides, a type of fat that is carried through the bloodstream and can end up being stored as body fat. Sometimes Crestor may be combined with another type of cholesterol-lowering drug such as Colestid, Questran, or WelChol.

In addition, Crestor can help increase the amount of "good" cholesterol known as high-density lipoprotein (HDL).

It's especially important to keep LDL cholesterol under control, since high levels are associated with heart disease. Federal guidelines recommend considering drug therapy when LDL levels reach 130 in people at high risk for heart disease. For people with a lower risk, the cutoff is 160. For those with little or no risk, it is 190.

CRIXIVAN
Indinavir

Crixivan is used in the treatment of human immunodeficiency virus (HIV) infection. HIV causes the immune system to break down so that it can no longer fight off other infections. This leads to the fatal disease known as acquired immune deficiency syndrome (AIDS).

HIV thrives by taking over the immune system's vital CD4 cells (white blood cells) and using their inner workings to make additional copies of itself. Crixivan belongs to a class of HIV drugs called protease inhibitors, which work by interfering with an important step in the virus's reproductive cycle. Although Crixivan cannot eliminate HIV already present in the body, it can reduce the amount of virus available to infect other cells.

Crixivan can be taken alone or in combination with other HIV drugs such as Retrovir. Because Crixivan and Retrovir attack the virus in different ways, the combination is likely to be more effective than either drug alone.

Cromolyn, inhaled *See Intal*

CUTIVATE
Fluticasone topical

Cutivate cream and ointment are prescribed for relief of inflamed, itchy rashes and other inflammatory skin conditions.

Cyclessa *See Oral Contraceptives*

Cyclobenzaprine *See Flexeril*

Cyclophosphamide *See Cytoxan*

Cyclosporine *See Sandimmune*

Cyproheptadine *See Periactin*

CYTOMEL
Liothyronine

Cytomel is used to treat hypothyroidism, a condition where the thyroid gland does not produce enough thyroid hormone. It is also used to help decrease the size of enlarged thyroid glands (known as goiter).

Cytomel is also used in some medical tests to help diagnose problems with the thyroid gland.

CYTOTEC
Misoprostol

Cytotec, a synthetic prostaglandin (hormone-like substance), reduces the production of stomach acid and protects the stomach lining. People who take nonsteroidal anti-inflammatory drugs (NSAIDs) may be given Cytotec tablets to help prevent stomach ulcers.

Aspirin and other NSAIDs such as Motrin, Naprosyn, Feldene, and others, which are widely used to control the pain and inflammation of arthritis, are generally hard on the stomach. If an NSAID is needed for a prolonged period of time and the patient is elderly or has ever had a stomach ulcer, the doctor may prescribe Cytotec for as long as the patient takes the NSAID.

CYTOXAN
Cyclophosphamide

Cytoxan, an anticancer drug, works by interfering with the growth of malignant cells. It may be used alone but is often given with other anti-cancer medications. Cytoxan is used in the treatment of the following types of cancer:

Breast cancer
Leukemias (cancers affecting the white blood cells)
Malignant lymphomas (Hodgkin's disease or cancer of the lymph nodes)
Multiple myeloma (a malignant condition or cancer of the plasma cells)
Advanced mycosis fungoides (cancer of the skin and lymph nodes)
Neuroblastoma (a malignant tumor of the adrenal gland or sympathetic
  nervous system)
Ovarian cancer (adenocarcinoma)
Retinoblastoma (a malignant tumor of the retina)

In addition, Cytoxan may sometimes be given to children who have "minimal change" nephrotic syndrome (kidney damage resulting in loss of protein in the urine) and who have not responded well to treatment with steroid medications.

Darifenacin *See Enablex*

DARVOCET-N
Propoxyphene napsylate, Acetaminophen
Other brand names: Darvon-N (propoxyphene napsylate), Darvon (propoxyphene hydrochloride), Darvon Compound-65 (propoxyphene hydrochloride, aspirin, and caffeine)

Darvocet-N and its companion products all contain propoxyphene, a mild narcotic painkiller, and all are prescribed for the relief of mild to moderate pain. In addition, Darvocet-N and Darvon Compound-65 contain extra ingredients capable of reducing fever.

Darvon *See Darvocet-N*

Darvon Compound-65 *See Darvocet-N*

Darvon-N *See Darvocet-N*

DAYPRO

Oxaprozin

Daypro is a nonsteroidal anti-inflammatory drug used to relieve the inflammation, swelling, stiffness, and joint pain associated with rheumatoid arthritis and osteoarthritis (the most common kind of arthritis).

DDAVP

Desmopressin
Other brand name: Stimate

DDAVP nasal spray, nose drops, and tablets are given to prevent or control the frequent urination and loss of water associated with diabetes insipidus (a rare condition characterized by very large quantities of diluted urine and excessive thirst). They are also used to treat frequent passage of urine and increased thirst in people with certain brain injuries, and those who have undergone surgery in the pituitary region of the brain. DDAVP nasal spray and nose drops are also prescribed to help stop some types of bedwetting.

Stimate nasal spray is used to stop bleeding in certain types of hemophilia (failure of the blood to clot).

DECADRON TABLETS

Dexamethasone

Decadron, a corticosteroid drug, is used to reduce inflammation and relieve symptoms in a variety of disorders, including rheumatoid arthritis and severe cases of asthma. It may be given to people to treat primary or secondary adrenal cortex insufficiency (lack of sufficient adrenal hormone). It is also given to help treat the following disorders:

Severe allergic conditions such as drug-induced allergies
Blood disorders such as various anemias
Certain cancers (along with other drugs)
Skin diseases such as severe psoriasis
Collagen (connective tissue) diseases such as systemic lupus
  erythematosus
Digestive tract disease such as ulcerative colitis
High serum levels of calcium associated with cancer
Fluid retention due to nephrotic syndrome (a condition in which
  damage to the kidneys causes the body to lose protein in the urine)
Eye diseases such as allergic conjunctivitis
Lung diseases such as tuberculosis (along with other drugs)

DELTASONE
Prednisone

Deltasone, a steroid drug, is used to reduce inflammation and alleviate symptoms in a variety of disorders, including rheumatoid arthritis and severe cases of asthma. It may be given to treat primary or secondary adrenal cortex insufficiency (lack of sufficient adrenal hormone in the body). It is used in treating all of the following:

Abnormal adrenal gland development
Allergic conditions (severe)
Blood disorders
Certain cancers (along with other drugs)
Diseases of the connective tissue including systemic lupus erythematosus
Eye diseases of various kinds
Flare-ups of multiple sclerosis
Fluid retention due to "nephrotic syndrome" (a condition in which damage to the kidneys causes protein to be lost in the urine)
Lung diseases, including tuberculosis
Meningitis (inflamed membranes around the brain)
Prevention of organ rejection
Rheumatoid arthritis and related disorders
Severe flare-ups of ulcerative colitis or enteritis (inflammation of the intestines)
Skin diseases
Thyroid gland inflammation
Trichinosis (with complications)

DEMADEX
Torsemide

Demadex is a diuretic drug. It flushes excess water from the body by promoting the production of urine.

Demadex is prescribed to reduce the water retention and swelling that often accompany congestive heart failure, chronic kidney failure, and cirrhosis of the liver. It is also prescribed for high blood pressure, either alone or with other medications.

DEMEROL
Meperidine

Demerol, a narcotic analgesic, is prescribed for the relief of moderate to severe pain. Like other painkillers in this category, it can lead to mental and physical dependence if taken too long.

Demulen *See Oral Contraceptives*

DENAVIR
Penciclovir

Denavir cream is used to treat recurrent cold sores on the lips and face. It works by interfering with the growth of the herpesvirus responsible for the sores.

DEPAKENE
Valproic acid

Depakene, an epilepsy medicine, is used to treat certain types of seizures and convulsions. It may be prescribed alone or with other anticonvulsant medications.

DEPO-PROVERA
Medroxyprogesterone acetate

Depo-Provera Contraceptive Injection is given in the buttock or upper arm to prevent pregnancy. It is more than 99 percent effective; the chances of becoming pregnant during the first year of use are less than 1 in 100. The injection is given every 3 months (13 weeks) by a doctor. Depo-Provera works by preventing the release of hormones called gonadotropins from the pituitary gland in the brain. Without these hormones, the monthly release of an egg from the ovary cannot occur. If no egg is released, pregnancy is impossible. Depo-Provera also causes changes in the lining of the uterus that make pregnancy less likely even if an egg is released.

In higher doses, Depo-Provera is also used in the treatment of certain cancers including cancer of the endometrium (lining of the uterus) and kidney cancer.

Desloratadine *See Clarinex*

Desmopressin *See DDAVP*

Desogen *See Oral Contraceptives*

Desoximetasone *See Topicort*

DETROL
Tolterodine
Other brand name: Detrol LA

Detrol combats symptoms of overactive bladder, including frequent urination, urgency (increased need to urinate), and urge incontinence (inability to control urination). The drug works by blocking the nerve impulses that prompt the bladder to contract.

Dexamethasone *See Decadron Tablets*

DiaBeta *See Micronase*

DIAMOX
Acetazolamide

Diamox controls fluid secretion. It is used in the treatment of glaucoma (excessive pressure in the eyes), epilepsy (for both brief and unlocalized seizures), and fluid retention due to congestive heart failure or drugs. It is also used to prevent or relieve the symptoms of acute mountain sickness in climbers attempting a rapid climb and those who feel sick even though they are making a gradual climb.

Diclofenac *See Voltaren*

Diclofenac with Misoprostol *See Arthrotec*

Dicyclomine *See Bentyl*

Didanosine *See Videx*

DIDRONEL
Etidronate

Didronel tablets are prescribed for the treatment of Paget's bone disease, which causes pain, bone fractures, and problems in the circulatory and nervous systems. Didronel can decrease pain, increase the ability to move, and slow the progression of the disease.

Didronel is also prescribed following hip replacement and spinal cord injury to prevent abnormal bone formation and inflammation.

DIFFERIN
Adapalene

Differin is prescribed for the treatment of acne. Its exact mode of action is unknown, but it appears to modulate the cellular differentiation, hardening, and inflammatory processes that contribute to acne.

Diflorasone *See Psorcon*

DIFLUCAN
Fluconazole

Diflucan is used to treat fungal infections called candidiasis (also known as thrush or yeast infections). These include vaginal infections, throat infections, and fungal infections elsewhere in the body, such as infections of the urinary tract, peritonitis (inflammation of the lining of the abdomen), and pneumonia. Diflucan is also prescribed to guard against candidiasis in some people receiving bone marrow transplants, and is used to treat meningitis (brain or spinal cord inflammation) caused by another type of fungus.

In addition, Diflucan is now being prescribed for fungal infections in kidney and liver transplant patients, and fungal infections in patients with AIDS.

Digitek *See Lanoxin*

Digoxin *See Lanoxin*

Dilacor XR *See Cardizem*

DILANTIN
Phenytoin

Dilantin is an antiepileptic drug, prescribed to control grand mal seizures (a type of seizure in which the individual experiences a sudden loss of consciousness immediately followed by generalized convulsions) and temporal lobe seizures (a type of seizure caused by disease in the cortex of the temporal [side] lobe of the brain affecting smell, taste, sight, hearing, memory, and movement).

Dilantin may also be used to prevent and treat seizures occurring during and after neurosurgery (surgery of the brain and spinal cord).

DILAUDID
Hydromorphone

Dilaudid, a narcotic analgesic, is prescribed for the relief of moderate to severe pain such as that due to:

Biliary colic (pain caused by an obstruction in the gallbladder or bile duct)
Burns
Cancer
Heart attack
Injury (soft tissue and bone)

Renal colic (sharp lower back and groin pain usually caused by the
  passage of a stone through the ureter)
Surgery

Diltiazem *See Cardizem or Tiazac*

DIOVAN
Valsartan
Other brand name: Diovan HCT

Diovan is one of a new class of blood pressure medications called
angiotensin II receptor antagonists. Diovan works by preventing the
hormone angiotensin II from narrowing the blood vessels, which tends to
raise blood pressure. Diovan may be prescribed alone or with other blood
pressure medications, such as diuretics that help the body get rid of
excess water. Diovan HCT is just such a combination. It contains Diovan
plus the common diuretic hydrochlorothiazide.

Diphenoxylate with Atropine *See Lomotil*

DIPROLENE
Betamethasone

Diprolene, a synthetic cortisone-like steroid available in cream, gel,
lotion, or ointment form, is used to treat certain itchy rashes and other
inflammatory skin conditions.

Dipyridamole *See Persantine*

Disopyramide *See Norpace*

DITROPAN
Oxybutynin
Other brand name: Ditropan XL

Ditropan relaxes the bladder muscle and reduces spasms. It is used to
treat the urgency, frequency, leakage, incontinence, and painful or difficult
urination caused by neurogenic bladder (altered bladder function due to a
nervous system abnormality).

DONNATAL
Phenobarbital, Hyoscyamine, Atropine, and Scopolamine

Donnatal is a mild antispasmodic medication; it has been used with other drugs for relief of cramps and pain associated with various stomach, intestinal, and bowel disorders, including irritable bowel syndrome, acute colitis, and duodenal ulcer.

One of its ingredients, phenobarbital, is a mild sedative.

Dornase alfa *See Pulmozyme*

DORYX
Doxycycline
Other brand names: Vibramycin, Vibra-Tabs

Doxycycline is a broad-spectrum tetracycline antibiotic used against a wide variety of bacterial infections, including Rocky Mountain spotted fever and other fevers caused by ticks, fleas, and lice; urinary tract infections; trachoma (chronic infections of the eye); and some gonococcal infections in adults. It is an approved treatment for inhalational anthrax. It is also used with other medications to treat severe acne and amoebic dysentery (diarrhea caused by severe parasitic infection of the intestines).

Doxycycline may also be taken for the prevention of malaria on foreign trips of less than 4 months' duration.

Occasionally doctors prescribe doxycycline to treat early Lyme disease and to prevent "traveler's diarrhea." These are not yet officially approved uses for this drug.

Dorzolamide *See Trusopt*

Dorzolamide with Timolol *See Cosopt*

DOVONEX
Calcipotriene

Dovonex is prescribed to help clear up the scaly skin condition known as psoriasis. A synthetic form of vitamin D, it is available in cream and ointment form, and in a liquid for the scalp.

Doxazosin *See Cardura*

Doxycycline *See Doryx*

Drospirenone and Ethinyl estradiol *See Yasmin or YAZ*

DUAC
Clindamycin and Benzoyl peroxide

Duac is a topical gel used for the treatment of inflammatory acne.

DUETACT
Pioglitazone and Glimepiride

Duetact is used, along with diet and exercise, to treat people with type 2 diabetes. It contains two medications, pioglitazone and glimepiride, that work together to help keep blood sugar levels under control. Type 2 diabetes usually stems from the body's inability to make good use of insulin, the natural hormone that helps to transfer sugar out of the blood and into the cells, where it's converted to energy. Duetact works by improving the body's response to its own natural insulin supply. It also helps increase the amount of insulin produced by the pancreas.

DUONEB
Ipratropium and Albuterol

Duoneb is a bronchodilator (medicine that opens up narrowed breathing passages). It is taken by inhalation to help control the symptoms of lung diseases, such as asthma, chronic bronchitis, and emphysema.

Ipratropium in combination with albuterol helps decrease coughing, wheezing, shortness of breath, and troubled breathing by increasing the flow of air into the lungs.

DURAGESIC
Fentanyl

Duragesic patches deliver a continuous dose of the potent narcotic painkiller fentanyl for a period of three days. The patches are prescribed for chronic pain when short-acting narcotics and other types of painkillers fail to provide relief.

DURICEF
Cefadroxil

Duricef, a cephalosporin antibiotic, is used in the treatment of nose, throat, urinary tract, and skin infections that are caused by specific bacteria, including staph, strep, and *E. coli*.

Dutasteride *See Avodart*

DYAZIDE
Hydrochlorothiazide with Triamterene

Dyazide is a combination of diuretic drugs used in the treatment of high blood pressure and other conditions that require the elimination of excess fluid from the body. When used for high blood pressure, Dyazide can be taken alone or with other high blood pressure medications. Diuretics help the body produce and eliminate more urine, which helps lower blood pressure. Triamterene, one of the ingredients of Dyazide, helps to minimize the potassium loss that can be caused by the other component, hydrochlorothiazide.

Dynacin *See Minocin*

DYNACIRC
Isradipine
Other brand name: DynaCirc CR

DynaCirc, a type of medication called a calcium channel blocker, is prescribed for the treatment of high blood pressure. It is effective when used alone or with a thiazide-type diuretic to flush excess water from the body. Calcium channel blockers ease the workload of the heart by slowing down the passage of nerve impulses through the heart muscle, thereby slowing the beat. This improves blood flow through the heart and throughout the body and reduces blood pressure. A controlled-release version of this drug (DynaCirc CR) maintains lower blood pressure for 24 hours.

EC-Naprosyn *See Naprosyn*

Econazole *See Spectazole Cream*

Edex *See Caverject*

E.E.S. *See Erythromycin, oral*

Efalizumab *See Raptiva*

Efavirenz *See Sustiva*

EFUDEX
Fluorouracil
Other brand name: Carac

Efudex and Carac are prescribed for the treatment of actinic or solar keratoses (small red horny growths or flesh-colored wartlike growths caused by overexposure to ultraviolet radiation or the sun). Such growths may develop into skin cancer. When conventional methods are impractical—as when the affected sites are hard to get at—the 5 percent strength of Efudex is useful in the treatment of superficial basal cell carcinomas, or slow-growing malignant tumors of the face usually found at the edge of the nostrils, eyelids, or lips. Efudex is available in cream and solution forms. Carac comes in cream form only.

ELDEPRYL
Selegiline

Eldepryl is prescribed along with Sinemet (levodopa/carbidopa) for people with Parkinson's disease. It is used when Sinemet no longer seems to be working well. Eldepryl has no effect when taken by itself; it works only in combination with levodopa or Sinemet.

Parkinson's disease, which causes muscle rigidity and difficulty with walking and talking, involves the progressive degeneration of a particular type of nerve cell. Early on, levodopa or Sinemet alone may alleviate the symptoms of the disease. In time, however, these medications begin to lose their effect; their action seems to switch on and off at random, and the individual may begin to experience side effects such as involuntary movements and "freezing" in mid-motion.

Eldepryl may be prescribed at this stage of the disease to help restore the effectiveness of Sinemet. When a patient begins to take Eldepryl, the dosage of Sinemet may need to be reduced.

Eletriptan *See Relpax*

ELIDEL
Pimecrolimus

Elidel is a nonsteroidal cream that relieves mild to moderate symptoms of eczema, a skin condition marked by itchy red patches that often crust, scale, and ooze. Elidel is approved for use in adults and children over 2 years old. It can be used for short-term treatment or on-and-off treatment over longer periods of time. Elidel is considered an effective alternative for people who cannot tolerate or do not respond to conventional eczema therapies.

ELMIRON
Pentosan polysulfate sodium

Elmiron is used to relieve the symptoms of the bladder condition called interstitial cystitis.

ELOCON
Mometasone furoate

Elocon is a cortisone-like steroid available in cream, ointment, and lotion form. It is used to treat certain itchy rashes and other inflammatory skin conditions.

EMEND
Aprepitant

Emend is used in combination with other antiemetics to prevent acute and delayed nausea and vomiting associated with cancer chemotherapy.

Emtricitabine and Tenofovir disoproxil fumarate *See Truvada*

E-Mycin *See Erythromycin, oral*

ENABLEX
Darifenacin

Enablex is used for the treatment of overactive bladder (OAB) in adults. Symptoms of OAB are having a strong need to go to the bathroom right away (urgency), leaking or wetting accidents (urinary incontinence), having to go to the bathroom too often (urinary frequency). This drug gives OAB symptom relief by targeting specific receptors on the bladder that cause involuntary muscle spasms. Enablex helps control the bladder muscle and helps restore control of urination.

Enalapril *See Vasotec*

Enalapril with Felodipine *See Lexxel*

Enalapril with Hydrochlorothiazide *See Vaseretic*

ENBREL
Etanercept

Enbrel is used to relieve the symptoms and slow the progress of moderate to severe rheumatoid arthritis. It's also prescribed to relieve the symptoms of psoriatic arthritis. It can be added to methotrexate (Rheumatrex) therapy when methotrexate fails to provide adequate relief. Prescribed alone, it is also used for juvenile rheumatoid arthritis when other drugs have failed.

Enbrel is the first in a class of drugs designed to block the action of tumor necrosis factor (TNF), a naturally occurring protein responsible for much of the joint inflammation that plagues the victims of rheumatoid arthritis. In clinical trials, Enbrel provided the majority of patients with significant relief.

Enbrel is also used to reduce the symptoms of active ankylosing spondylitis, an inflammatory condition that results in stiffness and immobility and can sometimes cause joints and bones to fuse together.

Endocet *See Percocet*

Enoxaprin *See Lovenox*

Entacapone *See Comtan*

ENTOCORT EC
Budesonide, oral

Entocort EC is used to treat Crohn's disease, a chronic intestinal inflammation that causes sustained diarrhea and abdominal pain. The drug contains the anti-inflammatory steroid budesonide in a special formulation that concentrates in the intestines, thereby reducing its impact on the rest of the body.

Epinephrine *See Epipen*

EPIPEN
Epinephrine

Epipen is used for the emergency treatment of allergic reactions (anaphylaxis) to insect stings or bites, foods, drugs, other allergens, and idiopathic or exercise-induced anaphylaxis.

Epitol *See Tegretol*

EPIVIR
Lamivudine

Epivir is one of the drugs used to fight infection with the human immunodeficiency virus (HIV), the deadly cause of AIDS. Doctors turn to Epivir as the infection gets worse. The drug is taken along with Retrovir, another HIV medication.

HIV does its damage by slowly destroying the immune system, eventually leaving the body defenseless against infections. Like other drugs for HIV, Epivir interferes with the virus's ability to reproduce. This staves off the collapse of the immune system.

Eplerenone *See Inspra*

Eprosartan *See Teveten*

Eprosartan with Hydrochlorothiazide *See Teveten HCT*

Eryc *See Erythromycin, oral*

Ery-Tab *See Erythromycin, oral*

Erythrocin *See Erythromycin, oral*

ERYTHROMYCIN, ORAL
Brand names: E.E.S., E-Mycin, Eryc, Ery-Tab, Erythrocin, PCE

Erythromycin is an antibiotic used to treat many kinds of infections, including:

Acute pelvic inflammatory disease
Gonorrhea
Intestinal parasitic infections
Legionnaires' disease
Listeriosis
Pinkeye
Rectal infections
Reproductive tract infections
Skin infections
Syphilis
Upper and lower respiratory tract infections
Urinary tract infections
Whooping cough

Erythromycin is also prescribed to prevent rheumatic fever in people who are allergic to penicillin and sulfa drugs. It is prescribed before colorectal surgery to prevent infection.

Erythromycin with Benzoyl peroxide *See Benzamycin*

Esgic-Plus *See Fioricet*

Esidrix *See HydroDIURIL*

Esomeprazole *See Nexium*

Esterified estrogens and Methyltestosterone *See Estratest*

ESTRACE VAGINAL CREAM
Estradiol

Estrace treats some of the symptoms of menopause. These symptoms may include hot flashes and dryness and itching in the vagina. Other symptoms of menopause include pain when urinating, or the feeling of having to urinate right away. This medicine only treats dryness and itching in the vagina.

Estradiol *See Estrace Vaginal Cream or Vivelle-Dot*

Estradiol and Levonorgestrel *See Climara Pro*

Estradiol and Norethindrone acetate *See CombiPatch*

Estradiol vaginal ring *See Estring*

Estradiol vaginal tablets *See Vagifem*

ESTRATEST
Esterified estrogens and Methyltestosterone

Estratest tablets quell the flushing, sweating, "hot flashes," and vaginal irritation that trouble three-quarters of all women when they reach menopause. Estratest works by replacing some of the estrogen that is lost when the reproductive system shuts down. Although it relieves the physical symptoms of menopause, it won't help emotional symptoms such as depression if the physical symptoms are absent. It combines supplemental estrogen with a synthetic form of the male hormone testosterone, and is prescribed when estrogen alone fails to relieve menopausal symptoms.

ESTRING
Estradiol vaginal ring

Estring is an estrogen replacement system for relief of the vaginal problems that often occur after menopause, including vaginal dryness, burning, and itching, and difficult or painful intercourse. Estring is also prescribed for postmenopausal urinary problems such as difficulty urinating or urinary urgency.

Estrogen with Progestin *See Activella and femhrt*

Estropipate *See Ogen*

ESTROSTEP FE
Norethindrone and Ethinyl estradiol

Estrostep FE is an oral contraceptive. Oral contraceptives (also known as "the pill") are highly effective means of preventing pregnancy. Oral contraceptives consist of synthetic forms of two hormones produced naturally in the body. These hormones help to regulate a woman's menstrual cycle, and the fluctuating levels of these hormones play an essential role in fertility. Estrostep FE is also used to treat acne.

Etanercept *See Enbrel*

Ethinyl estradiol and Norelgestromin *See Ortho Evra*

Etidronate *See Didronel*

Etodolac *See Lodine*

Etonogestrel and Ethinyl estradiol *See NuvaRing*

EULEXIN
Flutamide

Eulexin is used along with drugs such as Lupron to treat prostate cancer. Eulexin belongs to a class of drugs known as antiandrogens. It blocks the effect of the male hormone testosterone. Giving Eulexin with Lupron, which reduces the body's testosterone levels, is one way of treating prostate cancer. For some forms of prostate cancer, radiation therapy is administered along with the drugs.

EVISTA
Raloxifene

Evista is prescribed to treat and prevent osteoporosis, the brittle-bone disease that strikes some women after menopause. A variety of factors promote osteoporosis. The more factors that apply to an individual, the greater her chances of developing the disease. These factors include:

Caucasian or Asian descent
Slender build
Early menopause
Smoking
Drinking
A diet low in calcium
An inactive lifestyle
Osteoporosis in the family

EXELON
Rivastigmine

Exelon is used in the treatment of mild to moderate Alzheimer's disease. Alzheimer's disease causes physical changes in the brain that disrupt the flow of information and interfere with memory, thinking, and behavior. By boosting levels of the chemical messenger acetylcholine, Exelon can temporarily improve brain function in some Alzheimer's sufferers, though it does not halt the progress of the underlying disease. Exelon may become less effective as the disease progresses.

Exemestane *See Aromasin*

Exenatide *See Byetta*

Ezetimibe *See Zetia*

Ezetimibe and Simvastatin *See Vytorin*

FACTIVE
Gemifloxacin

Factive is an antibiotic that is used to treat infections of the respiratory tract, such as bronchitis and pneumonia.

Famciclovir *See Famvir*

Famotidine *See Pepcid*

FAMVIR
Famciclovir

Famvir tablets are used to treat herpes zoster, commonly referred to as "shingles," in adults. Shingles is a painful rash with raised, red pimples on the trunk of the body, usually the back. Because it is caused by the same virus that causes chickenpox, only people who have had chickenpox can get shingles. When prescribed for shingles, Famvir works best in people age 50 or over.

Famvir is also prescribed to treat attacks of genital herpes and to prevent future flare-ups. For people with HIV infections, it is used as a treatment for both genital and oral herpes.

Felbamate *See Felbatol*

FELBATOL
Felbamate

Felbatol, a relatively new epilepsy medication, is used alone or with other drugs to treat partial seizures with or without generalization (seizures in which consciousness may be retained or lost). It is also used with other medications to treat seizures associated with Lennox-Gastaut syndrome (a childhood condition characterized by brief loss of awareness and muscle tone).

Felbatol is prescribed only when other medications have failed to control severe cases of epilepsy.

FELDENE
Piroxicam

Feldene, a nonsteroidal anti-inflammatory drug, is used to relieve the inflammation, swelling, stiffness, and joint pain associated with rheumatoid arthritis and osteoarthritis (the most common form of arthritis). It is prescribed both for sudden flare-ups and for long-term treatment.

Felodipine *See Plendil*

femhrt *See Activella and femhrt*

Fenofibrate *See Tricor, Antara, or Lofibra*

Fentanyl *See Duragesic*

Fexofenadine *See Allegra*

FINACEA
Azelaic acid for rosacea

Finacea is an ointment used to treat mild to moderate rosacea (a skin condition marked by red eruptions, usually on the cheeks and nose). In advanced cases—and usually only in men—the nose becomes red and bulbous. Doctors aren't sure what causes rosacea, but the condition may be aggravated by stress, infection, vitamin deficiencies, and hormonal problems.

Finasteride for baldness *See Propecia*

Finasteride for prostate problems *See Proscar*

FIORICET
Butalbital, Acetaminophen, and Caffeine
Other brand name: Esgic-Plus

Fioricet, a strong, non-narcotic pain reliever and relaxant, is prescribed for the relief of tension headache symptoms caused by muscle contractions in the head, neck, and shoulder area. It combines a sedative barbiturate (butalbital), a non-aspirin pain reliever (acetaminophen), and caffeine.

FIORINAL
Butalbital, Aspirin, and Caffeine

Fiorinal, a strong, non-narcotic pain reliever and muscle relaxant, is prescribed for the relief of tension headache symptoms caused by stress or muscle contraction in the head, neck, and shoulder area. It combines a non-narcotic, sedative barbiturate (butalbital) with a pain reliever (aspirin) and a stimulant (caffeine).

FIORINAL WITH CODEINE
Butalbital, Codeine, Aspirin, and Caffeine

Fiorinal with Codeine, a strong narcotic pain reliever and muscle relaxant, is prescribed for the relief of tension headache caused by stress and muscle contraction in the head, neck, and shoulder area. It combines a sedative-barbiturate (butalbital), a narcotic pain reliever and cough suppressant (codeine), a non-narcotic pain and fever reliever (aspirin), and a stimulant (caffeine).

FLAGYL
Metronidazole

Flagyl is an antibacterial drug prescribed for certain vaginal and urinary tract infections in men and women; amebic dysentery and liver abscess; and infections of the abdomen, skin, bones and joints, brain, lungs, and heart caused by certain bacteria.

Flecainide *See Tambocor*

FLEXERIL
Cyclobenzaprine

Flexeril is a muscle relaxant prescribed to relieve muscle spasms resulting from injuries such as sprains, strains, or pulls. Combined with rest and physical therapy, Flexeril provides relief of muscular stiffness and pain.

FLOMAX
Tamsulosin

Flomax is used to treat the symptoms of an enlarged prostate—a condition technically known as benign prostatic hyperplasia or BPH. The walnut-sized prostate gland surrounds the urethra (the duct that drains the bladder). If the gland becomes enlarged, it can squeeze the urethra, interfering with the flow of urine. This can cause difficulty in starting urination, a weak flow of urine, and the need to urinate urgently or more frequently. Flomax doesn't shrink the prostate. Instead, it relaxes the muscle around it, freeing the flow of urine and decreasing urinary symptoms.

FLONASE
Fluticasone

Flonase belongs to the family of medicines known as corticosteroids (cortisone-like medicines). Corticosteroids belong to the family of medicines called steroids. Flonase is sprayed into the nose to help relieve the stuffy or runny nose, irritation, sneezing, and discomfort of hay fever, other nasal allergies, and these symptoms when not caused by allergies.

FLOVENT HFA
Fluticasone

Flovent HFA belongs to the family of medicines known as corticosteroids (cortisone-like medicines). It is used to help prevent the symptoms of asthma. When used regularly every day, inhaled Flovent decreases the number and severity of asthma attacks. However, it will not relieve an asthma attack that has already started.

Flovent HFA is inhaled and works by preventing certain cells in the lungs and breathing passages from releasing substances that cause asthma symptoms. This medicine may be used with other asthma medicines, such as bronchodilators (medicines that open up narrowed breathing passages) or other corticosteroids taken by mouth.

FLOXIN
Ofloxacin

Floxin is an antibiotic. Floxin tablets have been used effectively to treat lower respiratory tract infections, including chronic bronchitis and pneumonia, sexually transmitted diseases (except syphilis), pelvic inflammatory disease, and infections of the urinary tract, prostate gland, and skin. Floxin Otic solution is used to treat ear infections.

Fluconazole *See Diflucan*

Flunisolide *See AeroBid*

Fluocinonide *See Lidex or Vanos*

Fluorometholone *See FML*

Fluorouracil *See Efudex*

Flutamide *See Eulexin*

Fluticasone *See Flonase or Flovent HFA*

Fluticasone Topical *See Cutivate*

Fluticasone and Salmeterol *See Advair Diskus*

Fluvastatin *See Lescol*

FML
Fluorometholone

FML is a steroid (cortisone-like) eye ointment that is used to treat inflammation of the eyelid and the eye itself.

FOLLISTIM
Follitropin beta for injection

Follistim contains "follicle stimulating hormone" (FSH). This is the natural hormone that prompts a new egg to ripen inside a follicle (egg sac) within the ovaries each month. Follistim injections are given to stimulate production of eggs for use in Assisted Reproductive Technology (ART), a procedure in which the egg is removed from the body and fertilized in the laboratory. Follistim is also used to promote ovulation and pregnancy in infertile patients if the problem is not due to primary ovarian failure (lack of viable eggs).

A second hormone—human chorionic gonadotropin (HCG)—is needed to bring an egg to full maturity. Follistim treatments therefore end with an injection of HCG.

Follitropin beta for injection *See Follistim*

FORADIL
Formoterol

Foradil is an asthma medication. It relaxes the muscles in the walls of the airways, allowing them to expand. Taken on a twice-daily basis, it helps to control asthma in people who need regular treatment with short-acting inhalers, including people with nighttime asthma. Regular twice-daily use can also relieve tightening of the airways in people with Chronic Obstructive Pulmonary Disease, including chronic bronchitis and emphysema.

Taken on an as-needed basis, Foradil can also be used to prevent exercise-induced tightening of the airways (also called "exercise-induced asthma") in adults and children 12 years of age and older.

Formoterol *See Foradil*

FORTEO
Teriparatide

Forteo is a synthetic form of the natural human parathyroid hormone and is used by injection to treat osteoporosis. Forteo forms new bone, increases bone mineral density and bone strength, and as a result reduces the chance of getting a fracture (broken bone). This medication can be used by men or postmenopausal women with osteoporosis who are at high risk for having fractures. Forteo can be used by people who have had a fracture related to osteoporosis, or who have multiple risk factors for fracture, or who cannot use other osteoporosis treatments.

FORTOVASE
Saquinavir

Fortovase is used in the treatment of advanced human immunodeficiency virus (HIV) infection. HIV causes the immune system to break down so that it can no longer fight off other infections. This leads to the fatal disease known as acquired immune deficiency syndrome (AIDS).

Fortovase belongs to a class of HIV drugs called protease inhibitors, which work by interfering with an important step in the virus's reproductive cycle. Fortovase is used in combination with other HIV drugs called nucleoside analogues (Retrovir or Hivid, for example). The combination produces an increase in the immune system's vital CD4 cells (white blood cells) and reduces the amount of virus in the bloodstream.

FOSAMAX
Alendronate
Other brand name: Fosamax Plus D

Fosamax is prescribed for the prevention and treatment of osteoporosis, the brittle bone disease, in postmenopausal women. It is also used to increase bone mass in men with osteoporosis, and is prescribed for both men and women who have developed a form of osteoporosis sometimes caused by steroid medications such as prednisone. This drug can also be used to relieve Paget's disease of bone, a painful condition that weakens and deforms the bones.

Fosamax plus D is used to treat osteoporosis in postmenopausal women or to increase bone mass in men with osteoporosis. This medication is made up of alendronate and cholecalciferol.

Fosamprenavir *See Lexiva*

Fosinopril *See Monopril*

Fosinopril with Hydrochlorothiazide *See Monopril-HCT*

FROVA
Frovatriptan

Frova is used to relieve attacks of migraine headache. It's helpful whether or not the headache is preceded by an aura (visual disturbances such as seeing halos or flickering lights).

Experts think that migraines are caused by the expansion of blood vessels serving the brain, and that this expansion is triggered by a decline in the level of serotonin, one of the brain's chief chemical messengers. Frova works by restoring serotonin levels to normal. It belongs to a class of drugs called "serotonin agonists."

Frovatriptan *See Frova*

Furosemide *See Lasix*

Gabapentin *See Neurontin*

GARAMYCIN OPHTHALMIC
Gentamicin

Garamycin Ophthalmic, an antibiotic, is applied to the eye for treatment of infections such as conjunctivitis (pinkeye) and other eye infections.

GARDASIL
Human papillomavirus vaccine

Gardasil is a vaccination to protect against diseases caused by the human papillomavirus (HPV) such as cervical cancer, abnormal and precancerous cervical, vaginal, and vulvar lesions, as well as genital warts.

Gatifloxacin eye drops *See Zymar*

Gemfibrozil *See Lopid*

Gemifloxacin *See Factive*

Gentamicin *See Garamycin Ophthalmic*

Glimepiride *See Amaryl*

Glimepiride with Rosiglitazone *See Avandaryl*

Glipizide *See Glucotrol*

Glipizide with Metformin *See Metaglip*

GLUCOPHAGE
Metformin

Glucophage is an oral antidiabetic medication used to treat type 2 (non-insulin-dependent) diabetes. Diabetes develops when the body proves unable to burn sugar and the unused sugar builds up in the bloodstream. Glucophage lowers the amount of sugar in the blood by decreasing sugar production and absorption and helping the body respond better to its own insulin, which promotes the burning of sugar. It does not, however, increase the body's production of insulin.

Glucophage is sometimes prescribed along with insulin or certain other oral antidiabetic drugs such as Micronase or Glucotrol. It is also used alone.

Standard Glucophage tablets are taken two or three times daily. An extended-release form (Glucophage XR) is available for once-daily dosing.

Glucophage is an aid to, not a substitute for, good diet and exercise. Failure to follow a sound diet and exercise plan can lead to serious complications such as dangerously high or low blood sugar levels. Glucophage is not an oral form of insulin and cannot be used in place of insulin.

GLUCOTROL
Glipizide

Glucotrol is an oral antidiabetic medication used to treat type 2 (non-insulin-dependent) diabetes. In diabetics either the body does not make enough insulin or the insulin that is produced no longer works properly.

There are actually two forms of diabetes: type 1 (insulin-dependent) and type 2 (non-insulin-dependent). Type 1 usually requires insulin injections for life, while type 2 diabetes can usually be treated by dietary changes and/or oral antidiabetic medications such as Glucotrol. Glucotrol is thought to control diabetes by stimulating the pancreas to secrete more insulin. If the patient suffers from type 1 diabetes, he or she will need to use insulin and will not be able to use Glucotrol. Occasionally, type 2 diabetics must take insulin injections on a temporary basis, especially during stressful periods or times of illness.

GLUCOVANCE
Glyburide with Metformin

Glucovance is used in the treatment of type 2 (noninsulin dependent) diabetes. Diabetes develops when the body's ability to burn sugar declines and the unused sugar builds up in the bloodstream. Ordinarily, sugar is moved out of the blood and into the body's cells by the hormone insulin. A buildup occurs when the body either fails to make enough insulin or doesn't respond to it properly.

Glucovance is a combination of 2 drugs—glyburide (DiaBeta, Micronase) and metformin (Glucophage)—that attack high blood sugar levels in several ways. The glyburide component stimulates the pancreas to produce more insulin and helps the body use it properly. The metformin component also encourages proper insulin utilization, and in addition works to decrease sugar production and absorption.

Glucovance is prescribed when diet and exercise prove insufficient to keep sugar levels under control. Glucovance can also be combined with other diabetes drugs such as Avandia.

Glyburide *See Micronase*

Glyburide with Metformin *See Glucovance*

Glynase *See Micronase*

GoLYTELY *See Colyte*

Granisetron *See Kytril*

Griseofulvin *See Gris-PEG*

GRIS-PEG
Griseofulvin

Gris-PEG is prescribed for the treatment of the following ringworm infections:

Athlete's foot
Barber's itch (inflammation of the facial hair follicles)
Ringworm of the body
Ringworm of the groin and thigh
Ringworm of the nails
Ringworm of the scalp

Because Gris-PEG is effective for only certain types of fungal infections, before treatment the doctor may perform tests to identify the source of infection.

Halobetasol *See Ultravate*

HEPSERA
Adefovir

Hepsera is used to treat adults with chronic infections of active hepatitis B. This medication is not a cure for the hepatitis B virus, but it may lower the amount of hepatitis B virus in your body. It may also lower the ability of the virus to multiply in your body.

HIVID
Zalcitabine

Hivid is one of the drugs used against the human immunodeficiency virus (HIV)—the deadly cause of AIDS. HIV does its damage by slowly undermining the immune system, finally leaving the body without any defense against infection. Hivid staves off collapse of the immune system by interfering with the virus's ability to reproduce.

Hivid is often combined with a protease inhibitor (Crixivan, Invirase, and Norvir) as part of the "cocktail" of drugs that has proven so effective in halting or even reversing the progress of HIV. Hivid can also be combined with the HIV drug Retrovir, provided the patient has not already been taking Retrovir for more than 3 months. For people with advanced cases of HIV, Hivid is sometimes prescribed by itself when other drugs don't work or can't be tolerated.

Humalog *See Insulin*

Human/papillomavirus vaccine *See Gardasil*

Humulin *See Insulin*

Hydrochlorothiazide *See HydroDIURIL*

Hydrochlorothiazide with Triamterene *See Dyazide or Maxide*

Hydrocodone with Acetaminophen *See Vicodin or Norco*

Hydrocodone with Chlorpheniramine polistirex *See Tussionex*

Hydrocodone with Ibuprofen *See Vicoprofen*

HYDRODIURIL
Hydrochlorothiazide
Other brand name: Esidrix

HydroDIURIL is used in the treatment of high blood pressure and other conditions that require the elimination of excess fluid (water) from the body. These conditions include congestive heart failure, cirrhosis of the liver, corticosteroid and estrogen therapy, and kidney disorders. When used for high blood pressure, HydroDIURIL can be used alone or with other high blood pressure medications. HydroDIURIL contains a form of thiazide, a diuretic that prompts the body to produce and eliminate more urine, which helps lower blood pressure.

Hydromorphone *See Dilaudid*

Hydroxychloroquine *See Plaquenil*

Hyoscyamine *See Levsin*

HYTRIN
Terazosin

Hytrin is prescribed to reduce high blood pressure. It may be used alone or in combination with other blood pressure lowering drugs, such as HydroDIURIL (a diuretic) or Inderal, a beta blocker.

Hytrin is also prescribed to relieve the symptoms of benign prostatic hyperplasia or BPH. BPH is an enlargement of the prostate gland that surrounds the urinary canal. It leads to the following symptoms:

a weak or interrupted stream when urinating
a feeling that the bladder cannot be completely emptied
a delay when starting to urinate
a need to urinate often, especially at night
a feeling of urgency when urination is needed

Hytrin relaxes the tightness of a certain type of muscle in the prostate and at the opening of the bladder. This can reduce the severity of the symptoms.

HYZAAR
Losartan with Hydrochlorothiazide

Hyzaar is a combination medication used in the treatment of high blood pressure. One component, losartan, belongs to a new class of blood pressure medications that work by preventing the hormone angiotensin II from constricting the blood vessels, thus allowing blood to flow more freely and keeping the blood pressure down. The other component, hydrochlorothiazide, is a diuretic that increases the output of urine, removing excess fluid from the body and thus lowering blood pressure.

Ibrandronate *See Boniva*

Ibuprofen *See Motrin*

IMDUR
Isosorbide mononitrate
Other brand names: Ismo, Monoket

Imdur is prescribed to prevent angina pectoris (crushing chest pain that results when partially clogged arteries restrict the flow of needed oxygen-rich blood to the heart muscle). This medication does not relieve angina attacks already underway.

Imiquimod *See Aldara*

IMITREX
Sumatriptan

Imitrex is prescribed for the treatment of a migraine attack with or without the presence of an aura (visual disturbances, usually sensations of halos or flickering lights, which precede an attack). The injectable form is also used to relieve cluster headache attacks. (Cluster headaches come on in waves, then disappear for long periods of time. They are limited to one side of the head, and occur mainly in men.)

Imitrex cuts headaches short. It will not reduce the number of attacks.

Indapamide *See Lozol*

INDERAL
Propranolol
Other brand name: Inderal LA

Inderal, a type of medication known as a beta blocker, is used in the treatment of high blood pressure, angina pectoris (chest pain, usually caused by lack of oxygen to the heart due to clogged arteries), changes in heart rhythm, prevention of migraine headache, hereditary tremors, hypertrophic subaortic stenosis (a condition related to exertional angina), and tumors of the adrenal gland. It is also used to reduce the risk of death from recurring heart attack.

When used for the treatment of high blood pressure, it is effective alone or combined with other high blood pressure medications, particularly thiazide-type diuretics. Beta blockers decrease the force and rate of heart contractions, reducing the heart's demand for oxygen and lowering blood pressure.

Indinavir *See Crixivan*

INDOCIN
Indomethacin

Indocin, a nonsteroidal anti-inflammatory drug, is used to relieve the inflammation, swelling, stiffness and joint pain associated with moderate or severe rheumatoid arthritis and osteoarthritis (the most common form of arthritis), and ankylosing spondylitis (arthritis of the spine). It is also used to treat bursitis, tendinitis (acute painful shoulder), acute gouty arthritis, and other kinds of pain.

Indomethacin *See Indocin*

INSPRA
Eplerenone

Inspra is prescribed to improve survival in patients who have congestive heart failure following a heart attack. It is also used to treat high blood pressure. Inspra may be used alone or with other antihypertensive agents. Inspra lowers blood pressure by blocking the actions of the hormone aldosterone.

INSULIN
Brand names: Humalog, Humulin, Novolin, Novolog

Insulin is prescribed for diabetes mellitus when diet modifications and oral medications fail to correct the condition. Insulin is a hormone produced by the pancreas, a large gland that lies near the stomach. This hormone is necessary for the body's correct use of food, especially sugar. Insulin apparently works by helping sugar penetrate the cell wall, where it is then utilized by the cell. In people with diabetes, the body either does not make enough insulin, or the insulin that is produced cannot be used properly.

There are actually two forms of diabetes: type 1 (insulin-dependent) and type 2 (non-insulin-dependent). Type 1 usually requires insulin injections for life, while type 2 diabetes can usually be treated by dietary changes and/or oral antidiabetic medications such as Diabinese, Glucotrol, and Glucophage. Occasionally, type 2 diabetics must take insulin injections on a temporary basis, especially during stressful periods or times of illness.

The various available types of insulin differ in several ways: in the source (animal, human, or genetically engineered), in the time requirements for the insulin to take effect, and in the length of time the insulin remains working.

Regular insulin, manufactured from beef and pork pancreas, begins working within 30 to 60 minutes and lasts for 6 to 8 hours. Variations of insulin have been developed to satisfy the needs of individual patients. For example, zinc suspension insulin is an intermediate-acting insulin that starts working within 1 to 1-1/2 hours and lasts approximately 24 hours. Insulin combined with zinc and protamine is a longer-acting insulin that takes effect within 4 to 6 hours and lasts up to 36 hours. The time and course of action may vary considerably in different individuals or at different times in the same individual. The genetically engineered insulin lispro injection works faster and for a shorter length of time than human regular insulin and should be used along with a longer-acting insulin. It is available only by prescription.

Animal-based insulin is a very safe product. However, some components may cause an allergic reaction. Therefore, genetically engineered human insulin has been developed to lessen the chance of an allergic reaction. It is structurally identical to the insulin produced by the human pancreas. However, some human insulin may be produced in a semi-synthetic process that begins with animal-based ingredients, and may cause an allergic reaction.

Insulin glargine recombinant *See Lantus*

INTAL
Cromolyn, inhaled
Other brand name: Nasalcrom

Intal contains the antiasthmatic/antiallergic medication cromolyn sodium.

Different forms of the drug are used to manage bronchial asthma, to prevent asthma attacks, and to prevent and treat seasonal and chronic allergies.

The drug works by preventing certain cells in the body from releasing substances that can cause allergic reactions or prompt too much bronchial activity. It also helps prevent bronchial constriction caused by exercise, aspirin, cold air, and certain environmental pollutants such as sulfur dioxide.

Ipratropium *See Atrovent*

Ipratropium with Albuterol *See Combivent or Duoneb*

Irbesartan *See Avapro*

Irbesartan with Hydrochlorothiazide *See Avalide*

Ismo *See Imdur*

ISORDIL
Isosorbide dinitrate

Isordil is prescribed to relieve or prevent angina pectoris (suffocating chest pain). Angina pectoris occurs when the arteries and veins become constricted and sufficient oxygen does not reach the heart. Isordil dilates the blood vessels by relaxing the muscles in their walls. Oxygen flow improves as the vessels relax, and chest pain subsides.

In swallowed capsules or tablets, Isordil helps to increase the amount of exercise patients can do before chest pain begins.

In chewable or sublingual (held under the tongue) tablets, Isordil can help relieve chest pain that has already started or prevent pain expected from a strenuous activity such as walking up a hill or climbing stairs.

Isosorbide dinitrate *See Isordil*

Isosorbide mononitrate *See Imdur*

Isotretinoin *See Accutane*

Isradipine *See DynaCirc*

Itraconazole *See Sporanox*

JANUMET
Metformin and Sitagliptin

Janumet is used to treats type 2 diabetes by decreasing the amount of sugar made by the body, helping to improve insulin levels after a meal, and helping the body respond better to the insulin it makes naturally. This medication is used together with proper diet and exercise to help control blood sugar in people with type 2 diabetes who have already been treated with either Januvia or metformin and their blood sugar is not controlled well enough, or patients who are currently taking both Januvia and metformin as separate medicines.

JANUVIA
Sitagliptin

Januvia is used to lower blood sugar levels in people with type 2 diabetes. It can be taken alone or combined with certain types of other medications also used to control blood sugar. Januvia works by decreasing sugar production and increasing the levels of insulin your body produces, especially after a meal.

KADIAN
Morphine

Kadian, a controlled-release tablet containing morphine, is used to relieve moderate to severe pain. While regular morphine is usually given every 4 hours, Kadian may be taken once or twice a day. This drug is intended for people who need a morphine painkiller for more than just a few days.

KALETRA
Lopinavir and Ritonavir

Kaletra combats the human immunodeficiency virus (HIV). HIV is the deadly virus that undermines the infection-fighting capacity of the body's immune system, eventually leading to AIDS.

Kaletra is a combination of two drugs, lopinavir and ritonavir (Norvir), both of which fall into the drug category known as protease inhibitors. When taken along with other HIV drugs, Kaletra lowers the amount of the virus circulating in the bloodstream. However, it does not completely eradicate the virus, and the patient may continue to develop the rare infections that attack when the immune system weakens. It's also important to remember that Kaletra does not eliminate the danger of transmitting the virus to others.

Kaon-CL *See Micro-K*

K-Dur *See Micro-K*

KEFLEX
Cephalexin

Keflex is a cephalosporin antibiotic. It is prescribed for bacterial infections of the respiratory tract, the middle ear, the bones, the skin, and the reproductive and urinary systems. Because the drug is effective for only certain types of bacterial infections, before beginning treatment the doctor may perform tests to identify the organisms causing the infection.

Keflex is available in capsules and an oral suspension form for use in children.

KEPPRA
Levetiracetam

Keppra helps reduce the frequency of partial epileptic seizures, a form of epilepsy in which neural disturbances are limited to a specific region of the brain and the victim remains conscious throughout the attack. The drug is used along with other epilepsy medications—never by itself.

KETEK
Telithromycin

Ketek is an antibiotic used to treat adults with community-acquired pneumonia, a type of lung infection caused by certain bacteria germs. Ketek should not be used to treat other types of bacterial infections. And like all antibiotics, Ketek is not effective for treating infections caused by viruses, such as the common cold.

Ketoconazole *See Nizoral*

Ketorolac *See Toradol*

Ketorolac, ocular *See Acular*

Ketotifen *See Zaditor*

KINERET
Anakinra

Kineret is used to relieve the symptoms of rheumatoid arthritis. It is usually prescribed after other antirheumatic drugs have failed to make an improvement. Kineret can be prescribed alone or in combination with other drugs for rheumatoid arthritis.

Kineret works by blocking the effects of interleukin-1, an inflammatory compound released by the immune system. While fighting inflammation, Kineret may also affect the immune system's ability to fight infection.

KLARON
Sulfacetamide

Klaron is an antibacterial medication used to treat dandruff and skin infections like acne caused by certain types of bacteria.

KLOR-CON
Potassium chloride

Klor-con is used to treat or prevent low potassium levels in people who may face potassium loss caused by digitalis, non-potassium-sparing diuretics, and certain diseases.

Potassium plays an essential role in the proper functioning of a wide range of systems in the body, including the kidneys, muscles, and nerves. As a result, a potassium deficiency may have a wide range of effects, including dry mouth, thirst, reduced urination, weakness, fatigue, drowsiness, low blood pressure, restlessness, muscle cramps, abnormal heart rate, nausea, and vomiting.

K-Tab *See Micro-K*

KYTRIL
Granisetron

Kytril is prescribed to prevent the nausea and vomiting associated with radiation therapy and chemotherapy for cancer. It is available in tablet and liquid forms.

Labetalol *See Normodyne*

LACTULOSE

Lactulose treats constipation. In people who are chronically constipated, Lactulose increases the number and frequency of bowel movements.

LAMISIL
Terbinafine

Lamisil fights fungal infections. In tablet form, it's used for fungus of the toenail or fingernail. The cream and the solution are used for other fungal infections such as athlete's foot, jock itch, and ringworm. The solution is also used to treat tinea versicolor, a fungal infection that produces brown, tan, or white spots on the trunk of the body.

Lamivudine *See Epivir*

Lamivudine and Zidovudine *See Combivir*

LANOXIN
Digoxin
Other brand name: Digitek

Lanoxin is used in the treatment of congestive heart failure, certain types of irregular heartbeat, and other heart problems. It improves the strength and efficiency of the heart, which leads to better circulation of blood and reduction of the uncomfortable swelling that is common in people with congestive heart failure. Lanoxin is usually prescribed along with a water pill (to help relieve swelling) and a drug called an ACE inhibitor (to further improve circulation). It belongs to a class of drugs known as digitalis glycosides.

Lansoprazole *See Prevacid*

Lansoprazole and Naproxen *See Prevacid NapraPAC*

LANTUS
Insulin glargine recombinant

Insulin glargine is a type of insulin. Insulin is one of many hormones that help the body turn the food we eat into energy. This is done by using the glucose (sugar) in the blood as quick energy. Also, insulin helps us store energy that we can use later. People with type 2 diabetes mellitus do not produce enough insulin, or the insulin produced is not used properly. This causes them to have too much sugar in their blood. Like other types of insulin,

Lantus is used to keep the blood sugar level close to normal. Lantus is a long-acting insulin that works slowly over about 24 hours. Patients may have to use insulin glargine in combination with another type of insulin or with a type of oral diabetes medicine to keep their blood sugar under control.

LASIX
Furosemide

Lasix is a diuretic (water pill) used in the treatment of high blood pressure and other conditions that require the elimination of excess fluid from the body. These conditions include congestive heart failure, cirrhosis of the liver, and kidney disease. When used to treat high blood pressure, Lasix is effective alone or in combination with other high blood pressure medications. Diuretics help the body produce and eliminate more urine, which helps lower blood pressure. Lasix is classified as a "loop diuretic" because of its point of action in the kidneys.

Lasix is also used with other drugs in people with fluid accumulation in the lungs.

Latanoprost *See Xalatan*

Leflunomide *See Arava*

LESCOL
Fluvastatin
Other brand name: Lescol XL

Lescol reduces "bad" LDL cholesterol—and increases "good" HDL cholesterol—in the blood, and can lower the risk of developing clogged arteries and heart disease. It is also prescribed to slow the accumulation of plaque in the arteries of people who already have coronary heart disease, and can also be prescribed when a patient is released from the hospital after a heart attack.

Also, if you have coronary heart disease you may be prescribed Lescol to reduce the risk of undergoing coronary revascularization procedures (angioplasty, bypass surgery, or stent insertion).

Doctors prescribe Lescol only when patients have been unable to reduce their blood cholesterol level sufficiently with a low-fat, low-cholesterol diet alone. For people at high risk of heart disease, current guidelines call for considering drug therapy when LDL levels reach 130. For people at lower risk, the cut-off is 160. For those at little or no risk, it's 190.

Lescol is available in standard capsules and extended-release tablets (Lescol XL).

Leuprolide *See Lupron Depot*

Levalbuterol *See Xopenex*

LEVAQUIN
Levofloxacin

Levaquin cures a variety of bacterial infections, including several types of sinus infection and pneumonia. It is also prescribed for flare-ups of chronic bronchitis, acute kidney infections, certain urinary or chronic prostate and skin infections. Levaquin is a member of the quinolone family of antibiotics.

Levbid *See Levsin*

Levetiracetam *See Keppra*

LEVITRA
Vardenafil

Levitra is an oral drug for male impotence, also known as erectile dysfunction (ED). It works by dilating blood vessels in the penis, allowing the inflow of blood needed for an erection.

Levlen *See Oral Contraceptives*

Levlite *See Oral Contraceptives*

Levobunolol *See Betagan*

Levofloxacin *See Levaquin*

Levonorgestrel *See Plan B*

Levonorgestrel and Ethinyl estradiol *See Seasonale*

Levora *See Oral Contraceptives*

Levothroid *See Synthroid*

Levothyroxine *See Synthroid or Levoxyl*

LEVOXYL
Levothyroxine

Levoxyl is a thyroid replacement hormone. It may be given in any of the following cases: If a patient's thyroid gland is not making enough hormone; If a patient has an enlarged thyroid (a goiter) or is at risk for developing a goiter; If a patient has certain cancers of the thyroid; If a patient's thyroid production is low due to surgery, radiation, certain drugs, or disease of the pituitary gland or hypothalamus in the brain.

LEVSIN

Hyoscyamine
Other brand names: Anaspaz, Levbid, Levsinex, NuLev

Levsin is an antispasmodic medication given to help treat various stomach, intestinal, and urinary tract disorders that involve cramps, colic, or other painful muscle contractions. Because Levsin has a drying effect, it may also be used to dry a runny nose or to dry excess secretions before anesthesia is administered.

Together with morphine or other narcotics, Levsin is prescribed for the pain of gallstones or kidney stones. For inflammation of the pancreas, Levsin may be used to help control excess secretions and reduce pain. Levsin may also be taken in Parkinson's disease to help reduce muscle rigidity and tremors and to help control drooling and excess sweating. The drug is sometimes prescribed during treatment for peptic ulcer.

Doctors also give Levsin as part of the preparation for certain diagnostic x-rays (for example, of the stomach, intestines, or kidneys).

Levsin comes in several forms, including regular tablets, tablets to be dissolved under the tongue, tablets that dissolve on the tongue (NuLev), sustained-release capsules (Levsinex Timecaps), and sustained-release tablets (Levbid), as well as liquid, drops, and an injectable solution.

Levsinex *See Levsin*

LEXIVA

Fosamprenavir

Lexiva is prescribed for adults with human immunodeficiency virus (HIV) infection. HIV undermines the immune system, reducing the body's ability to fight off other infections and eventually leading to the deadly condition known as acquired immune deficiency syndrome (AIDS).

Lexiva slows the progression of HIV by interfering with an important step in the virus's reproductive cycle. The drug is a member of the group of "protease inhibitors." Lexiva is prescribed only as part of a "drug cocktail" that attacks the virus on several fronts. It is not to be used alone.

Lexiva is not a cure for HIV infection or AIDS. It does not completely eliminate HIV from the body, nor does it totally restore the immune system. There is still a danger of developing serious opportunistic infections (that is, infections that develop when the immune system falters). It is important, therefore, for the patient to continue to see a doctor for regular blood counts and tests. Notify the healthcare provider immediately of any change in the patient's general health.

LEXXEL
Enalapril with Felodipine

Lexxel is used to treat high blood pressure. It combines two blood pressure drugs: an ACE inhibitor and a calcium channel blocker. The ACE inhibitor (enalapril) lowers blood pressure by preventing a chemical in the blood called angiotensin I from converting to a more potent form that narrows the blood vessels and increases salt and water retention. The calcium channel blocker (felodipine) also works to keep the blood vessels open, and eases the heart's workload by reducing the force and rate of the heartbeat.

Lexxel can be prescribed alone or in combination with other blood pressure medicines, especially water pills (diuretics) such as HydroDIURIL or Esidrix.

LIDEX
Fluocinonide

Lidex is a steroid medication that relieves the itching and inflammation of a wide variety of skin problems, including redness and swelling.

Lidocaine *See Lidoderm Patch*

LIDODERM PATCH
Lidocaine

Lidoderm belongs to the family of medicines called local anesthetics. When lidocaine is applied to the skin, it produces pain relief by blocking the signals at the nerve endings in the skin. Lidoderm patch is used to relieve pain and discomfort associated with herpes zoster virus infection of the skin (shingles).

Linezolid *See Zyvox*

LIORESAL
Baclofen

Lioresal is a muscle relaxant that helps relieve the symptoms and pain of muscle spasms caused by multiple sclerosis (MS), particularly in muscles that control joints. It also relieves pain due to rhythmic expansion and contraction of muscles (clonus) and pain due to muscular stiffness. Lioresal may also be of some help to people with spinal cord injuries and diseases.

Liothyronine *See Cytomel*

LIPITOR
Atorvastatin

Lipitor is a cholesterol-lowering drug. Doctors may prescribe it along with a special diet if blood cholesterol or triglyceride levels are high enough to pose a risk of heart disease, and the patient has been unable to lower the readings by diet alone.

The drug works by helping to clear harmful low density lipoprotein (LDL) cholesterol out of the blood and by limiting the body's ability to form new LDL cholesterol.

For people at high risk of heart disease, the doctor may suggest a cholesterol-lowering medication if LDL readings are 130 or more. For those at low risk, a medication is considered at readings of 190 or more.

Lisinopril *See Zestril*

Lisinopril with Hydrochlorothiazide *See Zestoretic*

LODINE
Etodolac

Lodine, a nonsteroidal anti-inflammatory drug, is available in regular and extended-release forms (Lodine XL). Both forms are used to relieve the inflammation, swelling, stiffness, and joint pain of osteoarthritis (the most common form of arthritis) and rheumatoid arthritis. Regular Lodine is also used to relieve pain in other situations.

Loestrin *See Oral Contraceptives*

LOFIBRA
Fenofibrate

Lofibra is used, along with a special diet, to treat people with very high levels of triglycerides (a fatty substance in the blood). Lofibra also improves cholesterol levels by lowering total cholesterol—including "bad" LDL cholesterol—and raising "good" HDL cholesterol. It works by promoting the dissolution and elimination of fat particles in the blood.

This may help prevent the development of pancreatitis (inflammation of the pancreas) caused by high levels of triglycerides in the blood.

LOMOTIL
Diphenoxylate with Atropine

Lomotil is used, along with other drugs, in the treatment of diarrhea. It should not be used for antibiotic-induced diarrhea (pseudomembranous colitis) or diarrhea caused by enterotoxin-producing bacteria.

LO/OVRAL-28
Norgestrel and Ethinyl estradiol

Lo/Ovral is an oral contraceptive. Oral contraceptives (also known as "the pill") are highly effective means of preventing pregnancy. Oral contraceptives consist of synthetic forms of two hormones produced naturally in the body. These hormones help to regulate a woman's menstrual cycle, and the fluctuating levels of these hormones play an essential role in fertility.

LOPID
Gemfibrozil

Lopid is prescribed, along with a special diet, for treatment of people with very high levels of serum triglycerides (a fatty substance in the blood) who are at risk of developing pancreatitis (inflammation of the pancreas) and who do not respond adequately to a strict diet.

This drug can also be used to reduce the risk of coronary heart disease in people who have failed to respond to weight loss, diet, exercise, and other triglyceride- or cholesterol-lowering drugs.

Lopinavir and Ritonavir *See Kaletra*

LOPRESSOR
Metoprolol

Lopressor, a type of medication known as a beta blocker, is used in the treatment of high blood pressure, angina pectoris (chest pain, usually caused by lack of oxygen to the heart due to clogged arteries), and heart attack. When prescribed for high blood pressure, it is effective when used alone or in combination with other high blood pressure medications. Beta blockers decrease the force and rate of heart contractions, thereby reducing the demand for oxygen and lowering blood pressure.

Occasionally doctors prescribe Lopressor for the treatment of aggressive behavior, prevention of migraine headache, and relief of temporary anxiety.

LOPROX
Ciclopirox

Loprox cream, lotion, and topical solution are prescribed for the treatment of the following fungal skin infections:

Athlete's foot
Fungal infection of the groin (jock itch)
Fungal infection of non-hairy parts of the skin
Candidiasis (yeastlike fungal infection of the skin)
Tinea versicolor—infection of the skin that is characterized by brown or tan patches on the trunk.

Loprox gel is used for athlete's foot, fungal infections of the non-hairy parts of the skin, and certain scalp inflammations (seborrheic dermatitis of the scalp).

LORABID
Loracarbef

Lorabid is a carbacephem antibiotic. It is used to treat mild-to-moderate bacterial infections of the lungs, ears, throat, sinuses, skin, urinary tract, and kidneys.

Loracarbef *See Lorabid*

Lorcet *See Vicodin*

Lortab *See Vicodin*

Losartan *See Cozaar*

Losartan with Hydrochlorothiazide *See Hyzaar*

LOTEMAX
Loteprednol

Lotemax belongs to the group of medicines known as corticosteroids (cortisone-like medicines). It is used to treat inflammation (redness) of the eye, which may occur with certain eye problems or following eye surgery. This medicine is also used to temporarily treat the symptoms of the eye caused by a condition known as seasonal allergic conjunctivitis (seasonal eye allergy).

LOTENSIN
Benazepril

Lotensin is used in the treatment of high blood pressure. It is effective when used alone or in combination with thiazide diuretics. Lotensin is in a family of drugs called ACE (angiotensin-converting enzyme) inhibitors. It works by preventing a chemical in the blood called angiotensin I from converting into a more potent form that increases salt and water retention in the body. Lotensin also enhances blood flow throughout the circulatory system.

LOTENSIN HCT
Benazepril with Hydrochlorothiazide

Lotensin HCT combines two types of blood pressure medication. The first, benazepril hydrochloride, is an ACE (angiotensin-converting enzyme) inhibitor. It works by preventing a chemical in the blood called angiotensin I from converting into a more potent form (angiotensin II) that increases salt and water retention in the body and causes the blood vessels to constrict—two actions that tend to increase blood pressure.

To aid in clearing excess water from the body, Lotensin HCT also contains hydrochlorothiazide, a diuretic that promotes production of urine. Diuretics often wash too much potassium out of the body along with the water. However, the ACE inhibitor part of Lotensin HCT tends to keep potassium in the body, thereby canceling this unwanted effect.

Lotensin HCT is not used for the initial treatment of high blood pressure. It is saved for later use, when a single blood pressure medication is not sufficient for the job. In addition, some doctors are using Lotensin HCT along with other drugs to treat congestive heart failure.

Loteprednol *See Alrex or Lotemax*

Loteprednol and Tobramycin *See Zylet*

LOTREL
Amlodipine with Benazepril

Lotrel is used in the treatment of high blood pressure. It is a combination medicine that is used when treatment with a single drug has not been successful or has caused side effects.

One component, amlodipine, is a calcium channel blocker. It eases the workload of the heart by slowing down the passage of nerve impulses and hence the contractions of the heart muscle. This improves blood flow through the heart and throughout the body and reduces blood pressure. The other component, benazepril, is an angiotensin-converting enzyme (ACE) inhibitor. It works by preventing the transformation of a hormone called angiotensin I into a more potent substance that increases salt and water retention in the body.

LOTRISONE
Clotrimazole with Betamethasone

Lotrisone cream and lotion contain a combination of a steroid (betamethasone) and an antifungal drug (clotrimazole). Lotrisone is used to treat skin infections caused by fungus, such as athlete's foot, jock itch, and ringworm of the body.

Betamethasone treats symptoms (such as itching, redness, swelling, and inflammation) that result from fungus infections, while clotrimazole treats the cause of the infection by inhibiting the growth of certain yeast and fungus organisms. If the infection is not inflamed, the doctor may prescribe a different medication.

Lovastatin *See Altoprev or Mevacor*

Lovastatin and Extended-release niacin *See Advicor*

LOVENOX
Enoxaprin

Lovenox is used to prevent deep venous thrombosis, a condition in which harmful blood clots form in the blood vessels of the legs. This medicine is used for several days after hip or knee replacement surgery, and in some cases following abdominal surgery, while the patient is unable to walk. It is during this time that blood clots are most likely to form. Lovenox is also used to treat patient who are unable to get out of bed because of a serious illness. In addition, it is used to prevent blood clots from forming in the arteries of the heart during certain types of chest pain and heart attacks.

Low-Ogestrel *See Oral Contraceptives*

LOZOL
Indapamide

Lozol is used in the treatment of high blood pressure, either alone or in combination with other high blood pressure medications. Lozol is also used to relieve salt and fluid retention. During pregnancy, doctors may prescribe

Lozol to relieve fluid retention caused by a specific condition or when fluid retention causes extreme discomfort that is not relieved by rest.

Lubiprostone *See Amitiza*

LUMIGAN
Bimatoprost

Lumigan is an eye drop that combats high pressure inside the eyeball. It is prescribed for a condition called open-angle glaucoma (a gradual increase of pressure in the eye). It is typically used after other remedies have caused problems or fail to work. It lowers pressure by promoting drainage of the fluid (aqueous humor) that fills the eye.

LUPRON DEPOT
Leuprolide

Lupron is a synthetic version of the naturally occurring gonadotropin releasing hormone (GnRH). Lupron suppresses shedding of the endometrium (lining of the uterus) during menstruation and is used to treat endometriosis, a condition in which cells from the endometrium grow outside of the uterus. Endometriosis causes painful growths to form around the outside of the uterus, fallopian tubes, and ovaries.

Two forms of Lupron—Lupron Depot 3.75 and Lupron Depot 11.25—are prescribed to relieve the pain of endometriosis and shrink the growths. (The hormonal medication norethindrone acetate is often added to the regimen.) Three other forms of Lupron—Lupron Depot 7.5, Lupron Depot 22.5, and Lupron Depot 30—are prescribed to relieve the symptoms of advanced prostate cancer.

The first two forms of Lupron are also used before surgery, along with iron, to treat anemia caused by fibroids (tumors) in the uterus when iron alone is not effective. Some doctors also prescribe Lupron for infertility and for early puberty.

LUXIQ
Betamethasone valerate

Luxiq belongs to the group of medicines known as corticosteroids (cortisone-like medicines). It is used to treat swelling and itching of the skin, specifically dermatoses of the scalp that are responsive to corticosteroids.

LYRICA
Pregabalin

Lyrica is used to help control some types of seizures in the treatment of epilepsy. This medicine cannot cure epilepsy and will only work to control seizures for as long as you continue to take it.

This medicine is also used to manage a condition called post-herpetic neuralgia (pain after shingles). It is also used for pain caused by nerve damage associated with diabetes. Lyrica can also be used to treat fibromyalgia—a complex chronic painful condition.

Macrobid *See Macrodantin*

MACRODANTIN
Nitrofurantoin
Other brand name: Macrobid

Nitrofurantoin, an antibacterial drug, is prescribed for the treatment of urinary tract infections caused by certain strains of bacteria.

MAVIK
Trandolapril

Mavik controls high blood pressure. It is effective when used alone or combined with other high blood pressure medications such as diuretics that help rid the body of excess water. Mavik is also used to treat heart failure or dysfunction following a heart attack.

Mavik is in a family of drugs known as ACE (angiotensin converting enzyme) inhibitors. It works by preventing a chemical in the blood called angiotensin I from converting into a more potent form that increases salt and water retention in the body. ACE inhibitors also expand the blood vessels, further reducing blood pressure.

MAXAIR
Pirbuterol

Maxair is used to treat asthma and other lung problems such as chronic bronchitis.

MAXALT
Rizatriptan
Other brand name: Maxalt-MLT

Maxalt is prescribed for the treatment of a migraine attack with or without the presence of an aura (visual disturbances, usually sensations of halos or flickering lights, which precede an attack). Maxalt cuts headaches short, but won't prevent attacks.

Maxidone *See Vicodin*

MAXZIDE
Hydrochlorothiazide and Triamterene
Other brand name: Maxzide-25 MG

Maxzide is a combination of two diuretics (water pills). It is commonly used to help reduce the amount of water in the body.

This combination is also used to treat high blood pressure (hypertension). High blood pressure adds to the work load of the heart and arteries. If it continues for a long time, the heart and arteries may not function properly. This can damage the blood vessels of the brain, heart, and kidneys, resulting in a stroke, heart failure, or kidney failure. High blood pressure may also increase the risk of heart attacks. These problems may be less likely to occur if blood pressure is controlled.

Diuretics help to reduce the amount of water in the body by acting on the kidneys to increase the flow of urine. This also helps to lower blood pressure.

This combination is also used to treat problems caused by too little potassium in the body.

Meclizine *See Antivert*

MEDROL
Methylprednisolone

Medrol, a corticosteroid drug, is used to reduce inflammation and improve symptoms in a variety of disorders, including rheumatoid arthritis, acute gouty arthritis, and severe cases of asthma. Medrol may be prescribed to treat primary or secondary adrenal cortex insufficiency (inability of the adrenal gland to produce sufficient hormone). It is also given to help treat the following disorders:

Severe allergic conditions (including drug-induced allergic states)
Blood disorders (leukemia and various anemias)
Certain cancers (along with other drugs)
Skin diseases (including severe psoriasis)

Connective tissue diseases such as systemic lupus erythematosus
Digestive tract diseases such as ulcerative colitis
High serum levels of calcium associated with cancer
Fluid retention due to nephrotic syndrome (a condition in which
  damage to the kidney causes loss of protein in urine)
Various eye diseases
Lung diseases such as tuberculosis
Worsening of multiple sclerosis

Medroxyprogesterone acetate *See Depo-Provera*

Medroxyprogesterone and conjugated estrogens *See Prempro*

Medroxyprogesterone for contraception *See Depo-Provera*

Medroxyprogesterone for menstrual problems *See Provera*

MEGACE
Megestrol acetate

Megace is a synthetic drug that has the same effect as the female hormone
progesterone. In tablet form it is used to treat cancer of the breast and
uterus. Megace is usually prescribed when a tumor cannot be removed by
surgery or has recurred after surgery, or when other drugs or radiation
therapy are ineffective. Megace Oral Suspension is used to treat lack or
loss of appetite, malnutrition and wasting away, and unexplained, significant weight loss in people with AIDS.

Megestrol acetate *See Megace*

Meloxicam *See Mobic*

Meperidine *See Demerol*

MERIDIA
Sibutramine

Meridia helps the seriously overweight shed pounds and keep them off. It
is especially recommended for those who in addition to being overweight
have other health problems such as high blood pressure, diabetes, or high
cholesterol. It is used in conjunction with a low-calorie diet.

    Meridia works by boosting levels of certain chemical messengers in
the nervous system, including serotonin, dopamine, and norepinephrine.

Mesalamine *See Rowasa or Asacol*

METAGLIP
Glipizide with Metformin

Metaglip is an oral medication used to control blood sugar levels in people with type 2 (non-insulin-dependent) diabetes. It contains two drugs commonly used to lower blood sugar, glipizide (Glucotrol) and metformin (Glucophage). Metaglip replaces the need to take these two drugs separately. It is prescribed when diet and exercise alone do not control blood sugar levels, or when treatment with another antidiabetic medication does not work.

Blood sugar levels are ordinarily controlled by the body's natural supply of insulin, which helps sugar move out of the bloodstream and into the cells to be used for energy. People who have type 2 diabetes do not make enough insulin or do not respond normally to the insulin their bodies make, causing a buildup of unused sugar in the bloodstream. Metaglip helps remedy this problem in two ways: by causing the body to release more insulin and by helping the body use insulin more effectively.

Metaxalone *See Skelaxin*

Metformin *See Glucophage*

Metformin and Sitagliptin *See Janumet*

Methenamine *See Urised*

Methocarbamol *See Robaxin*

METHOTREXATE
Brand names: Rheumatrex, Trexall

Methotrexate is an anticancer drug used in the treatment of lymphoma (cancer of the lymph nodes) and certain forms of leukemia. It is also given to treat some forms of cancers of the uterus, breast, lung, head, neck, and ovary. Methotrexate is also given to treat rheumatoid arthritis when other treatments have proved ineffective, and is sometimes used to treat very severe and disabling psoriasis (a skin disease characterized by thickened patches of red, inflamed skin often covered by silver scales).

Methyldopa *See Aldomet*

Methylprednisolone *See Medrol*

Metoclopramide *See Reglan*

Metolazone *See Zaroxolyn*

Metoprolol *See Lopressor or Toprol-XL*

MetroCream *See MetroGel*

METROGEL
Metronidazole
Other brand names: MetroCream, MetroLotion

MetroGel is a preparation of the drug metronidazole used for the treatment of a skin condition called rosacea (red eruptions, usually on the face). The cream and lotion forms of metronidazole are used for the same problem. All are for external (topical) use only.

METROGEL-VAGINAL
Metronidazole

Metrogel-Vaginal is used to treat bacterial vaginosis, a bacteria-caused inflammation of the vagina accompanied by pain and a vaginal discharge.

MetroLotion *See MetroGel*

Metronidazole *See Flagyl*

Metronidazole cream, gel, and lotion *See MetroGel*

Metronidazole vaginal gel *See Metrogel-Vaginal*

MEVACOR
Lovastatin

Mevacor is used, along with diet, to lower cholesterol levels in people with primary hypercholesterolemia (too much cholesterol in the bloodstream). High cholesterol levels foster the buildup of artery-clogging plaque, which can be especially dangerous when it collects in the vessels serving the muscles of the heart. Mevacor is prescribed to prevent this problem—called coronary heart disease—or to slow its advance if the arteries are already clogging up.

Mexiletine *See Mexitil*

MEXITIL
Mexiletine

Mexitil is used to treat severe irregular heartbeat (arrhythmia). Irregular heart rhythms are generally divided into two main types: heartbeats that are faster than normal (tachycardia) and heartbeats that are slower than normal (bradycardia). Arrhythmias are often caused by drugs or disease but can occur in otherwise healthy people with no history of heart disease or other illness.

MIACALCIN
Calcitonin-salmon

Miacalcin is a synthetic form of calcitonin, a naturally occurring hormone produced by the thyroid gland. Miacalcin reduces the rate of calcium loss from bones. Since less calcium passes from the bones to the blood, Miacalcin also helps control blood calcium levels.

Miacalcin Nasal Spray is used to treat postmenopausal osteoporosis (bone loss occurring after menopause) in women who cannot or will not take estrogen.

MICARDIS
Telmisartan

Micardis controls high blood pressure. It works by blocking the effects of a hormone called angiotensin II. Unopposed, this substance tends to constrict the blood vessels while promoting retention of salt and water—actions that tend to raise blood pressure. Micardis prevents these effects and thus keeps blood pressure lower. It can be prescribed alone or with other high blood pressure medications, such as diuretics that help rid the body of excess water.

MICARDIS HCT
Telmisartan with Hydrochlorothiazide

Micardis HCT is a combination medication used in the treatment of high blood pressure. One component, telmisartan, belongs to a class of blood pressure medications that work by preventing the hormone angiotensin II from constricting the blood vessels. This allows the blood to flow more freely and helps keep blood pressure down. The other component of Micardis HCT, hydrochlorothiazide, is a diuretic that increases the output of urine. This removes excess fluid from the body and helps lower blood pressure. Doctors usually prescribe Micardis HCT in place of its individual components. It can also be prescribed along with other blood pressure medications.

MICRO-K
Potassium chloride
Other brand names: Kaon-CL, K-Dur, K-Tab

Micro-K is used to treat or prevent low potassium levels in people who may face potassium loss caused by digitalis (Lanoxin), non-potassium-sparing diuretics (such as Diuril and Dyazide), and certain diseases.

Potassium plays an essential role in the proper functioning of a wide range of systems in the body, including the kidneys, muscles, and nerves. As a result, a potassium deficiency may have a wide range of effects, including dry mouth, thirst, reduced urination, weakness, fatigue, drowsiness, low blood pressure, restlessness, muscle cramps, abnormal heart rate, nausea, and vomiting.

Micro-K and its sister products are slow-release potassium formulations.

MICRONASE
Glyburide
Other brand names: DiaBeta, Glynase

Micronase is an oral antidiabetic medication used to treat type 2 diabetes, the kind that occurs when the body either does not make enough insulin or fails to use insulin properly. Insulin transfers sugar from the bloodstream to the body's cells, where it is then used for energy.

There are two forms of diabetes: type 1 and type 2. Type 1 diabetes results from a complete shutdown of normal insulin production and usually requires insulin injections for life, while type 2 diabetes can usually be treated by dietary changes, exercise, and/or oral antidiabetic medications such as Micronase. This medication controls diabetes by stimulating the pancreas to produce more insulin and by helping insulin to work better. Type 2 diabetics may need insulin injections, sometimes only temporarily during stressful periods such as illness, or on a long-term basis if an oral antidiabetic medication fails to control blood sugar.

Micronase can be used alone or along with a drug called metformin (Glucophage) if diet plus either drug alone fails to control sugar levels.

Micronor *See Oral Contraceptives*

MINIPRESS
Prazosin

Minipress is used to treat high blood pressure. It is effective used alone or with other high blood pressure medications such as diuretics or beta-blocking medications (drugs that ease heart contractions) such as Tenormin.

Minipress is also prescribed for the treatment of benign prostatic hyperplasia (BPH), an abnormal enlargement of the prostate gland.

MINOCIN
Minocycline
Other brand name: Dynacin

Minocin is a form of the antibiotic tetracycline. It is given to help treat many different kinds of infection, including:

Acne
Amebic dysentery
Anthrax (when penicillin cannot be given)
Cholera
Gonorrhea (when penicillin cannot be given)
Plague
Respiratory infections such as pneumonia
Rocky Mountain spotted fever
Syphilis (when penicillin cannot be given)
Urinary tract infections, rectal infections, and infections of the cervix
    caused by certain microbes

Minocycline *See Minocin or Solodyn*

MIRALAX
Polyethylene glycol

MiraLax is a remedy for constipation. It works by retaining water in the stool, softening it and increasing the frequency of bowel movements. It may take up to 2 to 4 days to work.

Mircette *See Oral Contraceptives*

MIRAPEX
Pramipexole

Although it is not a cure, Mirapex eases the symptoms of Parkinson's disease—a progressive disorder marked by muscle rigidity, weakness, shaking, tremor, and eventually difficulty with walking and talking. Parkinson's disease results from a shortage of the chemical messenger dopamine in certain areas of the brain. Mirapex is believed to work by boosting the action of whatever dopamine is available. The drug can be used with other Parkinson's medications such as Eldepryl and Sinemet.

Misoprostol *See Cytotec*

MOBIC
Meloxicam

Mobic is a nonsteroidal anti-inflammatory drug (NSAID) in prescription form. It is used to relieve the pain and stiffness of osteoarthritis.

Modicon *See Oral Contraceptives*

MODURETIC
Amiloride with Hydrochlorothiazide

Moduretic is a diuretic combination used in the treatment of high blood pressure and congestive heart failure, conditions which require the elimination of excess fluid (water) from the body. When used for high blood pressure, Moduretic can be used alone or with other high blood pressure medications. Diuretics help the body produce and eliminate more urine, which helps lower blood pressure. Amiloride, one of the ingredients, helps minimize the potassium loss that can be caused by the other component, hydrochlorothiazide.

Moexipril *See Univasc*

Moexipril with Hydrochlorothiazide *See Uniretic*

Mometasone furoate *See Elocon or Asmanex*

Mometasone furoate monohydrate *See Nasonex*

Monoket *See Imdur*

MONOPRIL
Fosinopril

Monopril is a high blood pressure medication known as an ACE inhibitor. It is effective when used alone or in combination with other medications for the treatment of high blood pressure. Monopril is also prescribed for heart failure.

Monopril works by preventing the conversion of a chemical in the blood called angiotensin I into a more potent substance that increases salt and water retention in the body and causes blood vessels to constrict—two actions that tend to increase blood pressure. Monopril also enhances blood flow in the circulatory system.

MONOPRIL-HCT
Fosinopril with Hydrochlorothiazide

Monopril-HCT is used to treat high blood pressure. It usually is prescribed after other blood pressure medications have failed to do the job. Monopril-HCT combines two types of blood pressure medicine. The first, fosinopril sodium, is an ACE (angiotensin-converting enzyme) inhibitor. It works by preventing a chemical in the blood called angiotensin I from converting into a more potent form (angiotensin II) that increases salt and water retention in the body and causes blood vessels to constrict—two actions that tend to increase blood pressure. To aid in clearing water from the body, Monopril-HCT also contains hydrochlorothiazide, a diuretic that promotes the production of urine.

Montelukast *See Singulair*

Morphine *See MS Contin, Avinza, or Kadian*

MOTRIN
Ibuprofen
Other brand name: Advil

Motrin is a nonsteroidal anti-inflammatory drug available in both prescription and nonprescription forms. Prescription Motrin is used in adults for relief of the symptoms of rheumatoid arthritis and osteoarthritis, treatment of menstrual pain, and relief of mild to moderate pain. In children aged 6 months and older it can be given to reduce fever and relieve mild to moderate pain. It is also used to relieve the symptoms of juvenile arthritis.

Motrin IB tablets, caplets, and gelcaps; Children's Motrin Suspension; and Advil tablets and caplets are available without a prescription. Check the packages for uses, dosage, and other information on these products.

Moxifloxacin *See Avelox or Vigamox*

MS CONTIN
Morphine

MS Contin, a controlled-release tablet containing morphine, is used to relieve moderate to severe pain. While regular morphine is usually given every 4 hours, MS Contin is typically taken every 12 hours—only twice a day.

Mupirocin *See Bactroban*

Muse *See Caverject*

Mycelex *See Gyne-Lotrimin*

MYCOLOG-II
Nystatin with Triamcinolone

Mycolog-II Cream and Ointment are prescribed for the treatment of candidiasis (a yeast-like fungal infection) of the skin. The combination of an antifungal (nystatin) and a steroid (triamcinolone acetonide) provides greater benefit than nystatin alone during the first few days of treatment. Nystatin kills the fungus or prevents its growth; triamcinolone helps relieve the redness, swelling, itching, and other discomfort that can accompany a skin infection.

Mycophenolate *See CellCept*

MYSOLINE
Primidone

Mysoline is used to treat epileptic and other seizures. It can be used alone or with other anticonvulsant drugs. It is chemically similar to barbiturates.

Nabumetone *See Relafen*

Nadolol *See Corgard*

Naftifine *See Naftin*

NAFTIN
Naftifine

Naftifine is used to treat fungus infections. It works by killing the fungus or preventing its growth. Naftifine is applied to the skin to treat athlete's foot (ringworm of the foot; tinea pedis); jock itch (ringworm of the groin; tinea cruris); and ringworm of the body (tinea corporis).

Naltrexone *See ReVia*

Naprelan *See Anaprox*

NAPROSYN
Naproxen
Other brand name: EC-Naprosyn

Naprosyn, a nonsteroidal anti-inflammatory drug, is used to relieve the inflammation, swelling, stiffness, and joint pain associated with rheumatoid arthritis, osteoarthritis (the most common form of arthritis), juvenile arthritis, ankylosing spondylitis (spinal arthritis), tendinitis, bursitis, and acute gout; it is also used to relieve menstrual cramps and other types of mild to moderate pain.

Naproxen *See Naprosyn*

Naproxen sodium *See Anaprox*

Naratriptan *See Amerge*

NASACORT AQ
Triamcinolone

Nasal corticosteroids like Nasacort AQ are cortisone-like medicines. They belong to the family of medicines called steroids. These medicines are sprayed or inhaled into the nose to help relieve the stuffy nose, irritation, and discomfort of hay fever, other allergies, and other nasal problems.

Nasalcrom *See Intal*

NASONEX
Mometasone furoate monohydrate

Nasonex nasal spray prevents and relieves the runny, stuffy nose that accompanies hay fever and year-round allergies. It contains a steroid medication that fights inflammation.

Nateglinide *See Starlix*

Necon *See Oral Contraceptives*

Nedocromil *See Tilade*

Nelfinavir *See Viracept*

Neoral *See Sandimmune*

Nepafenac *See Nevanac*

NEURONTIN
Gabapentin

Neurontin has two uses. First, it may be prescribed with other medications to treat partial seizures (the type in which symptoms are limited). It can be used whether or not the seizures eventually become general and result in loss of consciousness.

Second, it can be used to relieve the burning nerve pain that sometimes persists for months or even years after an attack of shingles (herpes zoster).

NEVANAC
Nepafenac

Nevanac is an ophthalmic anti-inflammatory medicine used in the eye to relieve pain and inflammation or edema (too much fluid in the eye) that can occur during or after some kinds of eye surgery, specifically cataract surgery.

Nevirapine *See Viramune*

NEXIUM
Esomeprazole

Nexium relieves heartburn and other symptoms caused by the backflow of stomach acid into the canal to the stomach (the esophagus)—a condition known as gastroesophageal reflux disease. It is also prescribed to heal the damage (erosive esophagitis) that reflux disease can cause.

Prescribed in combination with the antibiotics Biaxin and Amoxil, Nexium is also used to treat the infection that causes most duodenal ulcers (ulcers occurring just beyond the exit from the stomach).

Like its sister drug Prilosec, Nexium works by reducing the production of stomach acid.

Niacin *See Niaspan*

NIASPAN
Niacin

Although the niacin in Niaspan is one of the B-complex vitamins, this drug isn't taken to prevent deficiencies. In large doses, niacin also lowers cholesterol, and Niaspan extended-release tablets are designed specifically for this purpose.

Excessive levels of cholesterol in the blood can lead to clogged arteries and increased risk of heart attack. Niaspan is prescribed, along with a low-fat, low cholesterol diet, to reduce blood cholesterol levels, combat clogged arteries, and lower the chance of repeated heart attacks. It is used only when diet alone fails to do the job, and is often taken along with another type of cholesterol-lowering drug known as a bile acid sequestrant (Colestid, Questran, WelChol). It can also be combined with any of the cholesterol-lowering "statin" drugs (Lescol, Lipitor, Mevacor, Pravachol, Zocor).

Niaspan is also used to reduce very high levels of the blood fats known as triglycerides, a condition that can cause painful inflammation of the pancreas.

Nicardipine *See Cardene*

Nifedipine *See Procardia or Adalat CC*

Nimodipine *See Nimotop*

NIMOTOP
Nimodipine

Nimotop is used to prevent and treat problems caused by a burst blood vessel in the head (subarachnoid hemorrhage).

It is also occasionally prescribed for certain types of migraine headaches, stroke, and age-related memory problems such as Alzheimer's disease.

Nimotop belongs to a class of drugs known as calcium channel blockers which are frequently prescribed for high blood pressure and the crushing chest pain of angina.

Nisoldipine *See Sular*

Nitro-Bid *See Nitroglycerin*

Nitro-Dur *See Nitroglycerin*

Nitrofurantoin *See Macrodantin*

NITROGLYCERIN
Brand names: Nitro-Bid, Nitro-Dur, Nitrolingual Spray, NitroQuick, Nitrostat Tablets

Nitroglycerin is prescribed to prevent and treat angina pectoris (suffocating chest pain). This condition occurs when the coronary arteries become constricted and are not able to carry sufficient oxygen to the heart muscle. Nitroglycerin is thought to improve oxygen flow by relaxing muscles in the walls of arteries and veins, thus allowing them to dilate.

Nitroglycerin is used in different forms. As a patch or ointment, nitroglycerin may be applied to the skin. The patch and the ointment are for *prevention* of chest pain.

Swallowing nitroglycerin in capsule or tablet form also helps to *prevent* chest pain from occurring.

In the form of sublingual (held under the tongue) or buccal (held in the cheek) tablets, or in oral spray (sprayed on or under the tongue), nitroglycerin helps relieve chest pain that has *already begun*. The spray can also prevent anginal pain. The type of nitroglycerin prescribed depends on the patient's condition.

Nitrolingual Spray *See Nitroglycerin*

Nitrostat Tablets *See Nitroglycerin*

Nizatidine *See Axid*

NIZORAL
Ketoconazole

Nizoral, a broad-spectrum antifungal drug available in tablet form, may be given to treat several fungal infections within the body, including oral thrush and candidiasis.

It may also be given to treat severe, hard-to-treat fungal skin infections that have not cleared up after treatment with creams, ointments, or the oral drug griseofulvin (Fulvicin, Grisactin).

NOLVADEX
Tamoxifen citrate

Nolvadex, an anticancer drug, is given to treat breast cancer. It also has proved effective when cancer has spread to other parts of the body. Nolvadex is most effective in stopping the kind of breast cancer that thrives on estrogen.

Nolvadex is also prescribed to reduce the risk of invasive breast cancer following surgery and radiation therapy for ductal carcinoma in situ (a localized cancer that can be totally removed surgically). The drug can also be used to reduce the odds of breast cancer in women at high risk of developing the disease. It does not completely eliminate the risk, but in a five-year study of over 1,500 high-risk women, it slashed the number of cases by 44 percent.

NORCO
Hydrocodone and Acetaminophen

Norco treats moderate to moderately severe pain. It contains a narcotic pain reliever.

Nordette *See Oral Contraceptives*

Norethindrone and Ethinyl estradiol *See Estrostep FE or Ovcon 35*

Norgestrel and Ethinyl estradiol *See Lo/Ovral-28, Ortho Tri-Cyclen, or Ortho-Cyclen*

Norinyl *See Oral Contraceptives*

NORMODYNE
Labetalol
Other brand name: Trandate

Normodyne is used in the treatment of high blood pressure. It is effective when used alone or in combination with other high blood pressure medications, especially thiazide diuretics such as HydroDIURIL and "loop" diuretics such as Lasix.

NORPACE
Disopyramide
Other brand name: Norpace CR

Norpace is used to treat severe irregular heartbeat. It relaxes an overactive heart and improves the efficiency of the heart's pumping action.

Nor-QD *See Oral Contraceptives*

NORVASC
Amlodipine

Norvasc is prescribed for angina, a condition characterized by episodes of crushing chest pain that usually results from a lack of oxygen in the heart muscle due to clogged arteries. Norvasc is also prescribed for high blood pressure. It is a type of medication called a calcium channel blocker. These drugs dilate blood vessels and slow the heart to reduce blood pressure and the pain of angina.

NORVIR
Ritonavir

Norvir is prescribed to slow the progress of HIV (human immunodeficiency virus) infection. HIV causes the immune system to break down so that it can no longer respond effectively to infection, leading to the fatal disease known as acquired immune deficiency syndrome (AIDS). Without treatment, HIV takes over certain human cells, especially white blood cells, and uses the inner workings of the infected cell to make additional copies of itself. Norvir belongs to a class of HIV drugs called protease inhibitors, which work by interfering with an important step in this reproduction process. Although Norvir cannot get rid of HIV already present in the body, it can reduce the amount of virus available to infect other cells.

Norvir is used in combination with other HIV drugs called nucleoside analogues (Retrovir, Hivid, and others). These two types of drugs act against HIV in different ways, thus improving the odds of success.

Novolin *See Insulin*

NuLev *See Levsin*

NUVARING
Etonogestrel and Ethinyl estradiol

NuvaRing is a contraceptive device. Like oral contraceptives ("The Pill"), it prevents pregnancy by providing a steady level of the female hormones estrogen and progestin. This eliminates the hormonal surge that ordinarily triggers the release of an egg. Hormonal contraceptives such as NuvaRing are extremely reliable when used exactly as directed.

Nystatin with Triamcinolone *See Mycolog-II*

OCUFLOX
Ofloxacin, ocular

Ocuflox is an antibiotic used in the treatment of eye infections. It is prescribed for eye inflammations and for ulcers or sores on the cornea (the transparent covering over the pupil). Ofloxacin, the active ingredient, is a member of the quinolone family of antibiotics.

Ofloxacin *See Floxin*

Ofloxacin, ocular *See Ocuflox*

OGEN
Estropipate
Other brand name: Ortho-Est

Ogen and Ortho-Est are estrogen replacement drugs. The tablets are used to reduce symptoms of menopause, including feelings of warmth in face, neck, and chest, and the sudden intense episodes of heat and sweating known as "hot flashes." They also may be prescribed for teenagers who fail to mature at the usual rate.

In addition, either the tablets or Ogen vaginal cream can be used for other conditions caused by lack of estrogen, such as dry, itchy external genitals and vaginal irritation.

Along with diet, calcium supplements, and exercise, Ogen and Ortho-Est tablets are also prescribed to prevent osteoporosis, a condition in which the bones become brittle and easily broken.

Some doctors also prescribe these drugs to treat breast cancer and cancer of the prostate.

Ogestrel *See Oral Contraceptives*

Olmesartan *See Benicar*

Olopatadine *See Patanol*

OLUX
Clobetasol

Olux belongs to the group of medicines known as corticosteroids (cortisone-like medicines). It is used to treat psoriasis, skin irritation, allergic reactions, and other types of skin problems.

Omeprazole *See Prilosec*

Omeprazole and Sodium bicarbonate *See Zegerid*

OMNICEF
Cefdinir

Omnicef is a member of the family of antibiotics known as cephalosporins. It is used to treat mild to moderate infections, including:

Acute flare-ups of chronic bronchitis
Middle ear infections (otitis media)
Throat and tonsil infections (pharyngitis/tonsillitis)
Pneumonia
Sinus infections
Skin infections

Ondansetron *See Zofran*

OPANA

Oxymorphone
Other brand name: Opana ER

Opana is indicated for the relief of moderate to severe acute pain where the use of an opioid is appropriate. Opana ER is indicated for the relief of moderate to severe pain in patients requiring continuous, around-the-clock opioid therapy for an extended period of time. These medicines are narcotic analgesics (pain medicines).

OPTIVAR

Azelastine eye drops

Optivar is taken to relieve and prevent the itchy eyes brought on by seasonal allergies. The drug usually starts to work within 3 minutes of placing the drops in the eye, and its effects usually last for about 8 hours.

ORAL CONTRACEPTIVES

Brand names: Alesse, Apri, Brevicon, Cyclessa, Demulen, Desogen, Levlen, Levlite, Levora, Loestrin, Low-Ogestrel, Micronor, Mircette, Modicon, Necon, Nordette, Norinyl, Nor-QD, Ogestrel, Ortho-Cept, Ortho-Novum, Ovral, Tri-Levlen, Tri-Norinyl, Triphasil, Trivora, Zovia

Oral contraceptives (also known as "The Pill") are highly effective means of preventing pregnancy. Oral contraceptives consist of synthetic forms of two hormones produced naturally in the body: either progestin alone or estrogen and progestin. Estrogen and progestin regulate a woman's menstrual cycle, and the fluctuating levels of these hormones play an essential role in fertility.

To reduce side effects, oral contraceptives are available in a wide range of estrogen and progestin concentrations. Progestin-only products (such as Micronor) are usually prescribed for women who should avoid estrogens; however, they may not be as effective as estrogen/progestin contraceptives.

ORAPRED

Prednisolone sodium phosphate

Orapred treats inflammation, arthritis, asthma, allergies, and other medical problems. It also treats flare-ups of ongoing illnesses such as multiple sclerosis. This medication may be used for some symptoms of cancer. Orapred is a corticosteroid (steroid).

Orlistat *See Xenical*

Ortho-Cept *See Oral Contraceptives*

ORTHO-CYCLEN
Norgestrel and Ethinyl estradiol

This medication is an oral contraceptive. Oral contraceptives (also known as "the pill") are highly effective means of preventing pregnancy. Oral contraceptives consist of synthetic forms of two hormones produced naturally in the body. These hormones help to regulate a woman's menstrual cycle, and the fluctuating levels of these hormones play an essential role in fertility.

Ortho-Est *See Ogen*

ORTHO EVRA
Ethinyl estradiol and Norelgestromin

Ortho Evra is a contraceptive skin patch. It contains estrogen and progestin, the same hormones found in many birth control pills. Fertility depends on regular fluctuations in the levels of these hormones. Contraceptives such as Ortho Evra reduce fertility by eliminating the fluctuations. Once applied to the skin, the Ortho Evra patch releases a steady supply of estrogen and progestin through the skin and into the bloodstream.

Ortho-Novum *See Oral Contraceptives*

ORTHO TRI-CYCLEN
Norgestrel and Ethinyl estradiol

This medication is an oral contraceptive. Oral contraceptives (also known as "the pill") are highly effective means of preventing pregnancy. Oral contraceptives consist of synthetic forms of two hormones produced naturally in the body. These hormones help to regulate a woman's menstrual cycle, and the fluctuating levels of these hormones play an essential role in fertility. Ortho Tri-Cyclen is also used to treat acne.

Oseltamivir *See Tamiflu*

OVCON 35
Norethindrone and Ethinyl estradiol

Ovcon 35 is an oral contraceptive. Oral contraceptives (also known as "the pill") are highly effective means of preventing pregnancy. Oral contraceptives consist of synthetic forms of two hormones produced naturally in the body. These hormones help to regulate a woman's menstrual cycle, and the fluctuating levels of these hormones play an essential role in fertility.

Ovral *See Oral Contraceptives*

Oxaprozin *See Daypro*

Oxcarbazepine *See Trileptal*

Oxybutynin *See Ditropan or Oxytrol*

Oxycodone *See OxyContin*

Oxycodone with Aspirin *See Percodan*

OXYCONTIN
Oxycodone

OxyContin is a controlled-release form of the narcotic painkiller oxycodone. It is prescribed for moderate to severe pain when continuous, around-the-clock relief is needed for an extended period of time.

Oxymorphone *See Opana*

OXYTROL
Oxybutynin

Oxytrol is indicated for the treatment of overactive bladder with symptoms of urge urinary incontinence, urgency, and frequency. It is a patch that is applied to the skin.

Paclitaxel *See Taxol*

Pantoprazole *See Protonix*

PARLODEL
Bromocriptine

Parlodel inhibits the secretion of the hormone prolactin from the pituitary gland. It also mimics the action of dopamine, a shortage of which leads to Parkinson's disease. It is used to treat a variety of medical conditions, including:

Infertility in some women

Menstrual problems such as the abnormal stoppage or absence of flow, with or without excessive production of milk

Growth hormone overproduction leading to acromegaly, a condition characterized by an abnormally large skull, jaw, hands, and feet

Parkinson's disease

Pituitary gland tumors

Some doctors also prescribe Parlodel to treat cocaine addiction, the eye condition known as glaucoma, erection problems in certain men, restless leg syndrome, and a dangerous reaction to major tranquilizers called neuroleptic malignant syndrome.

PATANOL
Olopatadine

Patanol is an antihistamine that relieves the red, itchy eyes often caused by allergies.

PCE *See Erythromycin, oral*

PEDIAPRED
Prednisolone sodium phosphate

Pediapred, a steroid drug, is used to reduce inflammation and improve symptoms in a variety of disorders, including rheumatoid arthritis, acute gouty arthritis, and severe cases of asthma. It may be given to people to treat primary or secondary adrenal cortex insufficiency (lack of or insufficient adrenal cortical hormone in the body). It is also given to help treat the following disorders:

Blood disorders such as leukemia and various anemias

Certain cancers (along with other drugs)

Connective tissue diseases such as systemic lupus erythematosus

Digestive tract diseases such as ulcerative colitis

Eye diseases of various kinds

Fluid retention due to nephrotic syndrome (a condition in which damage to the kidneys causes a loss of protein in the urine)

High blood levels of calcium associated with cancer

Lung diseases such as tuberculosis

Severe allergic conditions such as drug-induced allergic reactions

Severe skin eruptions

Studies have shown that high doses of Pediapred are effective in controlling severe symptoms of multiple sclerosis, although they do not affect the ultimate outcome or natural history of the disease.

Penciclovir *See Denavir*

Penicillin VK *See Penicillin V Potassium*

PENICILLIN V POTASSIUM
Brand names: Penicillin VK, Veetids

Penicillin V potassium is used to treat infections, including dental infection, infections in the heart, middle ear infections, rheumatic fever, scarlet fever, skin infections, and upper and lower respiratory tract infections.

Penicillin V works against only certain types of bacteria—it is ineffective against fungi, viruses, and parasites.

PENLAC
Ciclopirox nail lacquer

Penlac is a nail lacquer used in the treatment of nail infections caused by the fungus *Trichophyton rubrum* (ringworm of the nails). It is prescribed only if the pale semicircle at the base of the nail is free of infection. It is part of a comprehensive treatment plan that includes professional removal of the unattached infected nails as frequently as monthly

Pentasa *See Rowasa*

Pentosan polysulfate sodium *See Elmiron*

Pentoxifylline *See Trental*

PEPCID
Famotidine
Other brand name: Pepcid AC

Pepcid is prescribed for the short-term treatment of active duodenal ulcer (in the upper intestine) for 4 to 8 weeks and for active, benign gastric ulcer (in the stomach) for 6 to 8 weeks. It is prescribed for maintenance therapy, at reduced dosage, after a duodenal ulcer has healed. It is also used for short-term treatment of GERD, a condition in which the acid contents of the stomach flow back into the food canal (esophagus), and for the resulting inflammation of the esophagus. And it is prescribed for certain diseases that cause the stomach to produce excessive quantities of acid, such as Zollinger-Ellison syndrome. Pepcid belongs to a class of drugs known as histamine H_2 blockers.

An over-the-counter formulation, Pepcid AC, is used to relieve and prevent heartburn, acid indigestion, and sour stomach. Pepcid RPD is a preparation that dissolves rapidly in the mouth.

PERCOCET
Acetaminophen with Oxycodone
Other brand names: Endocet, Roxicet, Tylox

Percocet, a narcotic analgesic, is used to treat moderate to moderately severe pain. It contains two drugs—acetaminophen and oxycodone. Acetaminophen is used to reduce both pain and fever. Oxycodone, a narcotic analgesic, is used for its calming effect and for pain.

PERCODAN
Oxycodone with Aspirin

Percodan combines two pain-killing drugs: the narcotic analgesic oxycodone, and the common pain reliever aspirin. It is prescribed for moderate to moderately severe pain.

PERIACTIN
Cyproheptadine

Periactin is an antihistamine given to help relieve cold- and allergy-related symptoms such as hay fever, nasal inflammation, stuffy nose, red and inflamed eyes, hives, and swelling. Periactin may also be given after epinephrine to help treat anaphylaxis, a life-threatening allergic reaction.

Some doctors prescribe Periactin to treat cluster headache and to stimulate appetite in underweight people.

PERIDEX
Chlorhexidine

Peridex is an oral rinse used to treat gingivitis, a condition in which the gums become red and swollen. Peridex is also used to control gum bleeding caused by gingivitis. It is not effective for the more serious form of gum disease known as periodontitis.

Perindopril *See Aceon*

PERSANTINE
Dipyridamole

Persantine helps reduce the formation of blood clots in people who have had heart valve surgery. It is used in combination with blood thinners such as Coumadin.

Some doctors also prescribe Persantine in combination with other drugs, such as aspirin, to reduce the damage from a heart attack and prevent a recurrence, to treat angina, and to prevent complications during heart bypass surgery.

Phenazopyridine *See Pyridium*

PHENERGAN WITH CODEINE
Promethazine with Codeine

Phenergan with Codeine is used to relieve coughs and other symptoms of allergies and the common cold. Promethazine, an antihistamine, helps reduce itching and swelling and dries up secretions from the nose, eyes, and throat. It also has sedative effects and helps control nausea and vomiting. Codeine, a narcotic analgesic, helps relieve pain and stops coughing.

Phenobarbital, Hyoscyamine, Atropine, and Scopolamine
See Donnatal

Phentermine *See Adipex-P*

Phenytoin *See Dilantin*

Pimecrolimus *See Elidel*

PINDOLOL

Pindolol, a type of medication known as a beta blocker, is used in the treatment of high blood pressure. It is effective alone or combined with other high blood pressure medications, particularly with a thiazide-type diuretic (a "water pill" that increases urine output to remove excess fluid from the body). Beta blockers decrease the force and rate of heart contractions.

Pioglitazone *See Actos*

Pioglitazone and Glimepiride *See Duetact*

Pioglitazone with Metformin *See ACTOplus Met*

Pirbuterol *See Maxair*

Piroxicam *See Feldene*

PLAN B
Levonorgestrel

Plan B contains the hormone levonorgestrel, the same ingredient found in many birth control pills. The difference is that Plan B contains a larger dose of levonorgestrel than the amount found in a single birth control pill. And, unlike many birth control pills, Plan B does not contain any estrogen. Plan B is used to prevent pregnancy after known or suspected contraceptive failure or unprotected intercourse.

PLAQUENIL
Hydroxychloroquine

Plaquenil is prescribed for the prevention and treatment of certain forms of malaria. Plaquenil is also used to treat the symptoms of rheumatoid arthritis such as swelling, inflammation, stiffness, and joint pain. It is also prescribed for lupus erythematosus, a chronic inflammation of the connective tissue.

PLAVIX
Clopidogrel

Plavix keeps blood platelets slippery and discourages formation of clots, thereby improving blood flow to the heart, brain, and body. The drug is prescribed to reduce the risk of heart attack, stroke, and serious circulation problems in people with hardening of the arteries or unstable angina (dangerous chest pain), and in people who have already suffered a heart attack or stroke.

PLENDIL
Felodipine

Plendil is prescribed for the treatment of high blood pressure. It is effective alone or in combination with other high blood pressure medications. A type of medication called a calcium channel blocker, Plendil eases the workload of the heart by slowing down the passage of nerve impulses through the heart, thereby reducing the rate at which it beats. This improves blood flow through the heart and throughout the body, reduces blood pressure, and helps prevent angina pain (chest pain, often accompanied by a feeling of choking, usually caused by lack of oxygen in the heart due to clogged arteries).

PLETAL
Cilostazol

Pletal helps relieve the painful leg cramps caused by "intermittent claudication," a condition that results when arteries clogged with fatty plaque are unable to deliver an adequate blood supply to the muscles of the legs. Pletal helps the blood get through by dilating the blood vessels and preventing blood cells from clumping together.

Polyethylene glycol *See MiraLax*

Polyethylene glycol with Electrolytes *See Colyte*

Potassium chloride *See Micro-K or Klor-con*

Pramipexole *See Mirapex*

PRANDIN
Repaglinide

Prandin is used to reduce blood sugar levels in people with type 2 diabetes (the kind that does not require insulin shots). It works by promoting the production of insulin, the hormone responsible for transporting sugar out of the bloodstream and into the cells, where it supplies energy. Prandin is prescribed when diet and exercise alone fail to correct the problem. A combination of Prandin and a second diabetes drug called Glucophage can be prescribed if either drug alone proves insufficient.

PRAVACHOL
Pravastatin

Pravachol is a cholesterol-lowering drug. A doctor will prescribe it along with a cholesterol-lowering diet when blood cholesterol levels are dangerously high and the patient has not been able to lower it by diet alone.

High cholesterol can lead to heart problems. By lowering cholesterol, Pravachol improves a patient's chances of avoiding a heart attack, heart surgery, and death from heart disease. In people who already have hardening of the arteries, it slows progression of the disease and cuts the risk of acute attacks.

The drug works by helping to clear harmful low-density lipoprotein (LDL) cholesterol out of the blood and by limiting the body's ability to form new LDL cholesterol. For people at high risk of heart disease, current guidelines call for considering drug therapy when LDL levels reach 130. For people at lower risk, the cut-off is 160. For those at little or no risk, it's 190.

Pravachol can also be prescribed for children ages 8 and older when diet alone fails to lower their cholesterol levels.

Pravastatin *See Pravachol*

Prazosin *See Minipress*

PRECOSE
Acarbose

Precose is an oral medication used to treat type 2 (noninsulin-dependent) diabetes when high blood sugar levels cannot be controlled by diet alone. Precose works by slowing the body's digestion of carbohydrates so that blood sugar levels won't surge upward after a meal. Precose may be taken alone or in combination with certain other diabetes medications such as Diabinese, Micronase, Glucophage, and Insulin.

PRED FORTE
Prednisolone acetate

Pred Forte contains a steroid medication that eases redness, irritation, and swelling due to inflammation of the eye.

Prednisolone acetate *See Pred Forte*

Prednisolone sodium phosphate *See Pediapred or Orapred*

Prednisolone with sulfacetamide *See Blephamide*

Prednisolone sodium phosphate *See Pediapred*

Prednisone *See Deltasone*

Prefest *See Activella and femhrt*

Pregabalin *See Lyrica*

PREMARIN
Conjugated estrogens

Premarin is an estrogen replacement drug. The tablets are used to reduce moderate to servere symptoms of menopause, including feelings of warmth in the face, neck, and chest, and the sudden intense episodes of heat and sweating known as "hot flashes."

In addition to the symptoms of menopause, Premarin tablets are prescribed for teenagers who fail to mature at the usual rate, and to relieve the symptoms of certain types of cancer, including some forms of breast and prostate cancer.

In addition, either the tablets or Premarin vaginal cream can be used for other conditions caused by lack of estrogen, such as dry, itchy external genitals and vaginal irritation.

Along with diet, calcium supplements, and exercise, Premarin tablets are also prescribed to prevent postmenopausal osteoporosis, a condition in which the bones become brittle and easily broken. Before taking Premarin solely for this purpose, alternative, nonestrogen therapies should be carefully considered.

Premphase *See Premarin*

PREMPRO
Medroxyprogesterone and Conjugated estrogens

Prempro is used after menopause in women with a uterus to reduce moderate to severe hot flashes; to treat moderate to severe dryness, itching, and burning, in and around the vagina; and to help reduce a woman's chances of getting osteoporosis (thin weak bones). Prempro is a hormone therapy that contains a combination of estrogens and a progestin.

PREVACID
Lansoprazole

Prevacid blocks the production of stomach acid. It is prescribed for the short-term treatment (up to 4 weeks) of duodenal ulcers (ulcers in the intestinal wall near the exit from the stomach). It is also used for up to 8 weeks in the treatment of stomach ulcers, gastroesophageal reflux disease (backflow of acid into the canal to the stomach), and a condition called erosive esophagitis (severe inflammation of the canal). Once a duodenal ulcer or case of esophagitis has cleared up, the doctor may continue prescribing Prevacid to prevent a relapse. Prevacid is also prescribed to reduce the risk of stomach ulcers in people who develop this problem while taking nonsteroidal anti-inflammatory drugs such as Advil, Motrin, and Naprosyn. The drug is also used for long-term treatment of certain diseases marked by excessive acid production, such as Zollinger-Ellison syndrome.

Prevacid is also prescribed as part of a combination treatment to eliminate the *H. pylori* infection that causes most cases of duodenal ulcer.

PREVACID NAPRAPAC
Lansoprazole and Naproxen

Prevacid NapraPAC is used to treat symptoms of osteoarthritis, rheumatoid arthritis, and ankylosing spondylitis. It is also used to treat people with stomach ulcers who cannot take regular NSAIDs (non-steroidal anti-inflammatory drugs) for joint disease.

Naproxen belongs to a group of drugs called NSAIDs. Lansoprazole is in a group of drugs called proton pump inhibitors. Naproxen works by reducing substances in the body that cause inflammation, pain, and fever and lansoprazole decreases the amount of acid produced in the stomach.

PREVPAC
Amoxicillin, Clarithromycin, and Lansoprazole

Prevpac is a prepackaged combination of drugs designed to cure duodenal ulcers (ulcers in the intestinal wall near the exit from the stomach) caused by *H. pylori* bacteria, the most common source of ulcers. With two antibiotics and an acid-blocking agent, Prevpac will eradicate the *H. pylori* infection and improve the odds of remaining ulcer-free. This type of therapy is usually reserved for people with an active ulcer and those who've had one for at least a year.

PRILOSEC
Omeprazole

Prilosec is prescribed for the short-term treatment (4 to 8 weeks) of stomach ulcer, duodenal ulcer (near the exit from the stomach), and erosive esophagitis (inflammation of the esophagus), and for the treatment of heartburn and other symptoms of gastroesophageal reflux disease (backflow of acid stomach contents into the canal leading to the stomach). It is also used to maintain healing of erosive esophagitis and for the long-term treatment of conditions in which too much stomach acid is secreted, including Zollinger-Ellison syndrome, multiple endocrine adenomas (benign tumors), and systemic mastocytosis (cancerous cells).

Combined with the antibiotic clarithromycin (Biaxin) (and sometimes with the antibiotic amoxicillin as well), Prilosec is also used to cure patients whose ulcers are caused by infection with the germ *H. pylori*, the most common source of duodenal ulcers.

Primidone *See Mysoline*

Principen *See Ampicillin*

Prinivil *See Zestril*

Prinzide *See Zestoretic*

PROAIR HFA
Albuterol

Proair HFA is an inhalation aerosol used to treat asthma and other lung problems, such as exercise-induced bronchospasm. Bronchospasm is wheezing or difficulty in breathing.

Procainamide *See Procanbid*

PROCANBID
Procainamide
Other brand name: Pronestyl

Procanbid is used to treat severe irregular heartbeats (arrhythmias). Arrhythmias are generally divided into two main types: heartbeats that are faster than normal (tachycardia), and heartbeats that are slower than normal (bradycardia). Irregular heartbeats are often caused by drugs or disease but can occur in otherwise healthy people with no history of heart disease or other illness.

PROCARDIA
Nifedipine
Other brand name: Procardia XL

Procardia and Procardia XL are used to treat angina (chest pain caused by lack of oxygen to the heart due to clogged arteries or spasm of the arteries). Procardia XL is also used to treat high blood pressure. Procardia and Procardia XL are calcium channel blockers. They ease the workload of the heart by relaxing the muscles in the walls of the arteries, allowing them to dilate. This improves blood flow through the heart and through-out the body, reduces blood pressure, and helps prevent angina. Procardia XL is taken once a day and provides a steady rate of medication over a 24-hour period.

Progesterone *See Prometrium*

PROGRAF
Tacrolimus

Prograf belongs to a group of medicines known as immunosuppressive agents. It is used to lower the body's natural immunity in patients who receive organ (for example, kidney, liver, pancreas, lung, and heart) transplants.

When a patient receives an organ transplant, the body's white blood cells will try to get rid of (reject) the transplanted organ. Prograf works by preventing the white blood cells from getting rid of the transplanted organ.

Prograf is a very strong medicine. It can cause side effects that can be very serious, such as kidney problems. It may also reduce the body's ability to fight infections.

Promethazine with Codeine *See Phenergan with Codeine*

PROMETRIUM
Progesterone

Prometrium is prescribed for postmenopausal women who are taking estrogen (hormone replacement therapy); it prevents a buildup of the lining of the uterus and abnormal bleeding. Prometrium also may be prescribed to restore menstruation if a woman's menstrual periods have stopped.

Pronestyl *See Procanbid*

Propafenone *See Rythmol*

PROPECIA
Finasteride for baldness

Propecia is a remedy for baldness in men with mild to moderate hair loss on the top of the head and the front of the mid-scalp area. It increases hair growth, improves hair regrowth, and slows down hair loss. It works only on scalp hair and does not affect hair on other parts of the body.

Improvement can be seen as early as 3 months after starting therapy with Propecia, but for many men it takes longer. The improvement lasts only as long as therapy continues; when it stops, new hair growth ceases and hair loss resumes.

Propecia is a low-dose form of Proscar, a drug prescribed for prostate enlargement.

Propoxyphene *See Darvocet-N*

Propranolol *See Inderal*

PROSCAR
Finasteride for prostate problems

Proscar is prescribed to help shrink an enlarged prostate.

The prostate, a chestnut-shaped gland present in males, produces a liquid that forms part of the semen. This gland completely surrounds the upper part of the urethra, the tube through which urine flows out of the bladder. Many men over age 50 suffer from a benign (noncancerous) enlargement of the prostate. The enlarged gland squeezes the urethra, obstructing the normal flow of urine. Resulting problems may include difficulty in starting urination, weak flow of urine, and the need to urinate urgently or frequently. Sometimes surgical removal of the prostate is necessary.

By shrinking the enlarged prostate, Proscar may alleviate the various associated urinary problems, making surgery unnecessary.

Some doctors are also prescribing Proscar for baldness and as a preventive measure against prostate cancer.

PROTONIX
Pantoprazole

Protonix blocks the production of stomach acid. It is prescribed to heal a condition called erosive esophagitis (a severe inflammation of the passage to the stomach) brought on by a persistent backflow of stomach acid (gastroesophageal reflux disease). Later, it may be prescribed to maintain healing and prevent a relapse.

Protonix is a member of the "proton pump inhibitor" class of acid blockers, which includes AcipHex, Nexium, Prilosec, and Prevacid.

PROVENTIL
Albuterol
Other brand names: AccuNeb, Proventil HFA, Ventolin HFA, VoSpire Extended-Release Tablets

Drugs containing albuterol are prescribed for the prevention and relief of bronchial spasms that narrow the airway. This especially applies to the treatment of asthma. Some brands of this medication are also used for the prevention of bronchial spasm due to exercise.

PROVERA
Medroxyprogesterone acetate

Provera is derived from the female hormone progesterone. It is prescribed for problems such as failure to menstruate or abnormal menstruation. Provera is also prescribed to prevent abnormal growth of the uterine lining in women taking estrogen replacement therapy.

Other forms of medroxyprogesterone, such as Depo-Provera, are used as a contraceptive injection and are prescribed in the treatment of endometrial cancer.

Some doctors also prescribe Provera to treat endometriosis, menopausal symptoms, premenstrual tension, sexual aggressive behavior in men, and sleep apnea (temporary failure to breath while sleeping).

PSORCON
Diflorasone

Psorcon is prescribed for the relief of the inflammation and itching of skin disorders that respond to the application of steroids (hormones produced by the body that have potent anti-inflammatory effects).

Psorcon is available in ointment and cream forms, and in emollient ointment and cream.

PULMICORT RESPULES
Budesonide inhalation suspension

Budesonide, the active ingredient in Pulmicort Respules, is an anti-inflammatory steroid medication. Inhaled on a regular basis, Pulmicort helps prevent asthma attacks.

Pulmicort Respules are prescribed for children 12 months to 8 years of age. They are given by nebulizer (a device that produces a fine spray). Adults and children over 6 can use another form of budesonide, Pulmicort Turbuhaler, that's taken with an inhaler. Both types of Pulmicort are preventive medicines. They will not relieve an acute or life-threatening episode of asthma.

PULMICORT TURBUHALER
Budesonide inhalation powder

Budesonide, the active ingredient in Pulmicort Turbuhaler, is an anti-inflammatory steroid medication. Inhaled on a regular basis, Pulmicort helps prevent asthma attacks. It is sometimes prescribed in addition to oral steroids, and may reduce or eliminate the need for them.

Pulmicort Turbuhaler is used to treat asthma in adults and children over age 6. Children 12 months to 8 years of age can be treated with another form of budesonide, Pulmicort Respules, which is given by nebulizer. Both types of Pulmicort are preventive medicines. They will not relieve an acute or life-threatening episode of asthma.

PULMOZYME
Dornase alfa

Pulmozyme inhalation solution reduces the number of respiratory infections that require injectable antibiotics in people with cystic fibrosis. It is also used to make breathing easier by thinning the mucus in the lungs.

PYRIDIUM
Phenazopyridine

Pyridium is a urinary tract analgesic that helps relieve the pain, burning, urgency, frequency, and irritation caused by infection, trauma, catheters, or various surgical procedures in the lower urinary tract. Pyridium is indicated for short-term use and can only relieve symptoms; it is not a treatment for the underlying cause of the symptoms.

QUESTRAN
Cholestyramine
Other brand name: Questran Light

Questran is used to lower cholesterol levels in the blood of people with primary hypercholesterolemia (too much LDL cholesterol). Hypercholesterolemia is a genetic condition characterized by a lack of the LDL receptors that remove cholesterol from the bloodstream.

This drug can be used to lower cholesterol levels in people who also have hypertriglyceridemia, a condition in which an excess of fat is stored in the body.

This drug may also be prescribed to relieve itching associated with gallbladder obstruction.

It is available in two forms: Questran and Questran Light.

Quinapril *See Accupril*

Quinapril with Hydrochlorothiazide *See Accuretic*

Rabeprazole *See AcipHex*

Raloxifene *See Evista*

Ramipril *See Altace*

Ranitidine *See Zantac*

RAPAMUNE
Sirolimus

Rapamune belongs to a group of medicines known as immunosuppressive agents. It is used to lower the body's natural immunity in patients who receive kidney transplants.

When a patient receives an organ transplant, the body's white blood cells will try to get rid of (reject) the transplanted organ. Rapamune works by preventing the white blood cells from getting rid of the transplanted organ.

Rapamune is a very strong medicine. It can cause side effects that can be very serious, such as kidney problems. It may also reduce the body's ability to fight infections.

RAPTIVA
Efalizumab

Psoriasis is a skin disease that is caused, in part, by an overactive immune system. Raptiva belongs to a class of drugs called immunosuppressives, which decrease the activity of the immune system. It is prescribed for patients with severe plaque psoriasis who can no longer control their disease with medications applied to the skin.

REBETOL
Ribavirin

In combination with the interferon drugs Intron A or PEG-Intron, Rebetol is prescribed to treat chronic hepatitis C. Rebetol is always used with one of the other drugs. By itself, it is ineffective against hepatitis C.

REGLAN
Metoclopramide

Reglan increases the contractions of the stomach and small intestine, helping the passage of food. It is given to treat the symptoms of diabetic gastroparesis, a condition in which the stomach does not contract. These symptoms include vomiting, nausea, heartburn, feeling of indigestion, persistent fullness after meals, and appetite loss. Reglan is also used, for short periods, to treat heartburn in people with gastroesophageal reflux disease (backflow of stomach contents into the esophagus). In addition, it is given to prevent nausea and vomiting caused by cancer chemotherapy and surgery.

RELAFEN
Nabumetone

Relafen, a nonsteroidal anti-inflammatory drug, is used to relieve the inflammation, swelling, stiffness, and joint pain associated with rheumatoid arthritis and osteoarthritis (the most common form of arthritis).

RELENZA
Zanamivir

Relenza is an antiviral drug that hastens recovery from the flu. Victims who begin taking Relenza within the first 2 days of their illness typically start to feel improvement a day earlier than they would otherwise. The drug is believed to work by interfering with the spread of virus particles inside the respiratory tract.

RELPAX
Eletriptan

Relpax is used to treat migraine headaches with or without the presence of auras (visual disturbances that precede an attack, such as halos or flickering lights). It shortens the duration of the headache but will not prevent attacks.

Renova *See Retin-A and Renova*

Repaglinide *See Prandin*

REQUIP
Ropinirole

Requip helps relieve the signs and symptoms of Parkinson's disease. Caused by a deficit of dopamine (one of the brain's chief chemical messengers), this disorder is marked by progressive muscle stiffness, tremor, and fatigue. Requip works by stimulating dopamine receptors in the brain, thus promoting better, easier movement.

Requip can be taken with or without levodopa (usually prescribed as Sinemet), another drug used to treat the symptoms of Parkinson's disease.

RETIN-A AND RENOVA
Tretinoin
Other brand name: Avita

Retin-A, Avita, and Renova contain the skin medication tretinoin. Retin-A and Avita are used in the treatment of acne. Renova is prescribed to reduce fine wrinkles, discoloration, and roughness on facial skin (as part of a comprehensive program of skin care and sun avoidance).

Retin-A is available in liquid, cream, or gel form, and in a stronger gel called Retin-A Micro. Avita comes only as a gel. Renova is available in cream form only.

RETROVIR
Zidovudine

Retrovir is prescribed for adults infected with human immunodeficiency virus (HIV). HIV causes the immune system to break down so that it can no longer respond effectively to infection, leading to the fatal disease known as acquired immune deficiency syndrome (AIDS). Retrovir slows down the progress of HIV. Combining Retrovir with other drugs such as Epivir and Crixivan can further slow the progression.

Retrovir is also prescribed for HIV-infected children over 3 months of age who have symptoms of HIV or who have no symptoms but, through testing, have shown evidence of impaired immunity.

Retrovir taken during pregnancy often prevents transmission of HIV from mother to child.

Signs and symptoms of HIV disease are significant weight loss, fever, diarrhea, infections, and problems with the nervous system.

REVIA
Naltrexone

ReVia is prescribed to treat alcohol dependence and narcotic addiction. ReVia is not a cure. Patients must be ready to make a change and be willing to undertake a comprehensive treatment program that includes professional counseling, support groups, and close medical supervision.

REYATAZ
Atazanavir

Reyataz is used with other medications to treat human immunodeficiency virus (HIV) infection. HIV causes the immune system to break down so that it can no longer fight off other infections. This leads to acquired immune deficiency syndrome (AIDS).

HIV thrives by taking over the immune system's vital CD4 cells (white blood cells) and using their inner workings to make additional copies of itself. Reyataz belongs to a class of HIV drugs called protease inhibitors, which work by interfering with an important step in the virus's reproductive cycle.

Reyataz is approved for used only in combination with other anti-HIV medications.

Rheumatrex *See Methotrexate*

RHINOCORT AQUA
Budesonide

Rhinocort Aqua is an anti-inflammatory steroid nasal spray. It is prescribed to relieve the symptoms of hay fever and similar allergic nasal inflammations.

Ribavirin *See Rebetol*

RIDAURA
Auranofin

Ridaura, a gold preparation, is given to help treat rheumatoid arthritis. Ridaura is taken by mouth, unlike other gold compounds, which are given by injection. It is recommended only for people who have not been helped sufficiently by nonsteroidal anti-inflammatory drugs (Anaprox, Dolobid, Indocin, Motrin, and others). Ridaura should be part of a comprehensive arthritis treatment program that includes non-drug forms of therapy.

The patients most likely to benefit from Ridaura are those with active joint inflammation, especially in the early stages.

RIFADIN
Rifampin
Other brand name: Rimactane

Rifadin is used to treat all forms of tuberculosis. Rifadin is used in combination with two other antituberculosis drugs at the start of therapy: isoniazid and pyrazinamide. Later, streptomycin or ethambutol may be added. Rifadin is also used to eliminate a meningitis-causing bacteria in people who are carriers of the disease but have no symptoms of the illness. Rifadin is not effective as a treatment for active meningitis.

Occasionally doctors prescribe rifampin to treat leprosy or Legionnaires' disease.

Rifampin *See Rifadin*

Rifampin, Isoniazid, and Pyrazinamide *See Rifater*

RIFATER
Rifampin, Isoniazid, and Pyrazinamide

Rifater is a combination antibiotic used to treat the initial phase of tuberculosis. After a 2-month period, the doctor may prescribe another combination of antituberculosis drugs (Rifamate), which can be continued for longer periods.

Rifaximin *See Xifaxan*

Rimactane *See Rifadin*

Risedronate *See Actonel*

Ritonavir *See Norvir*

Rivastigmine *See Exelon*

Rizatriptan *See Maxalt*

ROBAXIN
Methocarbamol

Robaxin is prescribed, along with rest, physical therapy, and other measures, for the relief of pain due to severe muscular injuries, sprains, and strains.

ROCALTROL
Calcitriol

Rocaltrol is a synthetic form of vitamin D used to treat people on dialysis who have hypocalcemia (abnormally low blood calcium levels) and resulting bone damage. Rocaltrol is also prescribed to treat low blood calcium levels in people who have hypoparathyroidism (decreased functioning of the parathyroid glands). When functioning correctly, these glands help control the level of calcium in the blood.

Rocaltrol is also prescribed for hyperparathyroidism (increased functioning of the parathyroid glands) and resulting bone disorders in people with kidney disease who are not yet on dialysis.

ROCEPHIN
Ceftriaxone

Rocephin is a member of the cephalosporin family of antibiotics. It is used to treat infections of the skin, blood, bones, joints, ears, respiratory tract, abdomen, and urinary tract. It is also prescribed for gonorrhea, pelvic inflammatory disease, and meningitis (brain infection), and to protect against infection after surgery.

RONDEC
Carbinoxamine or Brompheniramine and Pseudoephedrine

Rondec is an antihistamine/decongestant that relieves nasal inflammation and runny nose, and the symptoms of hay fever and other allergies. Carbinoxamine and brompheniramine, the antihistamines, fight the effects of histamine, a chemical released by the body in response to certain irritants. Histamine narrows air passages in the lungs and contributes to inflammation. Antihistamines reduce itching and swelling and dry up secretions from the nose, eyes, and throat. Pseudoephedrine, the decongestant, reduces nasal congestion and makes breathing easier.

Ropinirole *See Requip*

Rosiglitazone *See Avandia*

Rosiglitazone with Metformin *See Avandamet*

Rosuvastatin *See Crestor*

ROWASA
Mesalamine
Other brand names: Canasa, Pentasa

Rowasa Suspension Enema, and Pentasa, are used to treat mild to moderate ulcerative colitis (inflammation of the large intestine and rectum). Rowasa Suspension Enema is also prescribed for inflammation of the lower colon, and inflammation of the rectum.

Rowasa Suppositories and Canasa Suppositories are used to treat inflammation of the rectum.

Roxicet *See Percocet*

RYTHMOL
Propafenone

Rythmol is used to help correct certain life-threatening heartbeat irregularities (ventricular arrhythmias) by reducing the excitability of the heart muscle.

Salmeterol *See Serevent Diskus*

SANCTURA
Trospium

Sanctura is used to treat bladder problems such as frequent need to urinate or loss of control of urinary function.

SANDIMMUNE
Cyclosporine
Other brand name: Neoral

Sandimmune suppresses the body's immune system. It is given after transplant surgery to help prevent rejection of organs (kidney, heart, or liver). It is also used to avoid long-term rejection in people previously treated with other immunosuppressant drugs, such as Imuran.

Neoral is a newer formulation of Sandimmune's active ingredient, cyclosporine. In addition to prevention of organ rejection, it is prescribed for certain severe cases of rheumatoid arthritis and psoriasis.

Some doctors also prescribe Sandimmune to treat alopecia areata (localized areas of hair loss), aplastic anemia (shortage of red and white blood cells and platelets), Crohn's disease (chronic inflammation of the digestive tract), and nephropathy (kidney disease). Sandimmune is sometimes used in the treatment of severe skin disorders, including psoriasis and dermatomyositis (inflammation of the skin and muscles causing weakness and rash). The drug is also used in procedures involving bone marrow, the pancreas, and the lungs.

Sandimmune is always given with prednisone or a similar steroid. It is available in capsules and liquid, or as an injection.

Saquinavir *See Fortovase*

SEASONALE
Levonorgestrel and Ethinyl estradiol

This medication is an oral contraceptive. Oral contraceptives (also known as "the pill") are highly effective means of preventing pregnancy. Oral contraceptives consist of synthetic forms of two hormones produced naturally in the body. These hormones help to regulate a woman's menstrual cycle, and the fluctuating levels of these hormones play an essential role in fertility.

SECTRAL
Acebutolol

Sectral, a type of medication known as a beta blocker, is used in the treatment of high blood pressure and abnormal heart rhythms. When used to treat high blood pressure, it is effective used alone or in combination with other high blood pressure medications, particularly with a thiazide-type diuretic. Beta blockers decrease the force and rate of heart contractions, thus reducing pressure within the circulatory system.

Selegiline *See Eldepryl*

SENSIPAR
Cinacalcet

Sensipar is a medicine used to treat hyperparathyroidism in patients with chronic kidney disease who are on dialysis. Hyperparathyroidism is a condition that is caused when the parathyroid glands located in the neck make too much parathyroid hormone (PTH). This hormone controls the concentrations of calcium and phosphorus in your blood. Sensipar helps lower the amount of PTH which lowers the calcium and phosphorus concentrations. This medication is also used to lower calcium in the blood in patients with parathyroid cancer.

Septra *See Bactrim*

SEREVENT DISKUS
Salmeterol xinafoate

Serevent relaxes the muscles in the walls of the bronchial tubes, allowing the passageways to expand and carry more air. Taken regularly (twice a day), the drug is used in the treatment of asthma and chronic obstructive pulmonary disease (COPD), including emphysema and chronic bronchitis. A relatively long-acting medication, it is recommended only for the type of asthma patient who needs shorter-acting bronchodilators such as Alupent and Ventolin on a frequent, regular basis.

Serevent is available as an inhalation powder. Serevent can be used with or without inhaled or oral steroid therapy.

Serophene *See Clomiphene Citrate*

Sibutramine *See Meridia*

Sildenafil *See Viagra*

SILVADENE CREAM 1%
Silver sulfadiazine

Silvadene Cream 1% is applied directly to the skin. The cream is used along with other medications to prevent and treat wound infections in people with second- and third-degree burns. It is effective against a variety of bacteria as well as yeast.

Silver sulfadiazine *See Silvadene Cream 1%*

Simvastatin *See Zocor*

SINEMET CR
Carbidopa with Levodopa

Sinemet CR is a controlled-release tablet that may be given to help relieve the muscle stiffness, tremor, and weakness caused by Parkinson's disease. It may also be given to relieve Parkinson-like symptoms caused by encephalitis (brain fever), carbon monoxide poisoning, or manganese poisoning.

Sinemet CR contains two drugs, carbidopa and levodopa. The drug that actually produces the anti-Parkinson's effect is levodopa. Carbidopa prevents vitamin B-6 from destroying levodopa, thus allowing levodopa to work more efficiently.

Parkinson's drugs such as Sinemet CR relieve the symptoms of the disease, but are not a permanent cure.

SINGULAIR
Montelukast

Singulair is used for long-term prevention of asthma. It reduces the swelling and inflammation that tend to close up the airways, and relaxes the walls of the bronchial tubes, expanding the airways and permitting more air to pass through.

Singulair is also used to relieve the stuffy, runny nose and sneezing caused by seasonal allergies.

Sirolimus *See Rapamune*

Sitagliptin *See Januvia*

SKELAXIN
Metaxalone

Along with rest and physical therapy, Skelaxin is prescribed for the relief of painful musculoskeletal conditions. Researchers aren't sure how the drug works, but suspect that its effectiveness stems from its sedative properties.

Solifenacin *See Vesicare*

SOLODYN
Minocycline

Solodyn treats pimples and red bumps in acne patients who are 12 years of age and older. This medicine is a tetracycline antibiotic.

SOMA
Carisoprodol

Soma is used, along with rest, physical therapy, and other measures, for the relief of acute, painful muscle strains and spasms.

SPECTAZOLE CREAM
Econazole

Spectazole cream is prescribed for fungal skin diseases commonly called ringworm (tinea). It is used to treat athlete's foot (tinea pedis), "jock itch" (tinea cruris), a fungus infection of the entire body (tinea corporis), and a skin infection that causes yellow- or brown-colored skin eruptions (tinea versicolor). It is also prescribed for yeast infections of the skin caused by candida fungus (cutaneous candidiasis).

SPECTRACEF
Cefditoren

Spectracef cures mild-to-moderate bacterial infections of the skin, throat, and respiratory tract. Among these infections are pneumonia, strep throat, and tonsillitis. Spectracef is also prescribed for acute flare-ups of chronic bronchitis. Spectracef is a cephalosporin antibiotic.

SPIRIVA
Tiotropium

Spiriva is a medicine used to treat bronchospasm (wheezing or difficulty in breathing) that is associated with chronic obstructive pulmonary disease (COPD). Chronic obstructive pulmonary disease is a long-term lung disease. COPD also includes breathing problems like chronic bronchitis (swelling of the airways or tubes leading to the lungs) and emphysema (damage to the air sacs in the lungs).

Spiriva is a bronchodilator. A bronchodilator is a medicine that opens up narrowed breathing passages. It is taken by inhalation (an inhaler) to help decrease coughing, wheezing, shortness of breath, and troubled breathing by increasing the flow of air into the lungs.

Spironolactone *See Aldactone*

Spironolactone with Hydrochlorothiazide *See Aldactazide*

SPORANOX
Itraconazole

Sporanox capsules are used to treat three types of serious fungal infections: blastomycosis, histoplasmosis, and aspergillosis. Blastomycosis can affect the lungs, bones, and skin. Histoplasmosis can affect the lungs, heart, and blood. Aspergillosis can affect the lungs, kidneys, and other organs. The drug is also prescribed for onychomycosis, which infects the toenails and fingernails. Additionally, Sporanox is used against fungal infections in people with weak immune systems, such as AIDS patients.

Sporanox oral solution is used to treat candidiasis (fungal infection) of the mouth, throat, and gullet (esophagus), and for other fungal infections in people with weakened immunity and fever.

STARLIX
Nateglinide

Starlix combats high blood sugar levels in people with type 2 diabetes (the kind that does not require insulin shots). Insulin speeds the transfer of sugar from the bloodstream to the body's cells, where it's burned to produce energy. In diabetes, the body either fails to make enough insulin, or proves unable to properly use what's available. Starlix attacks the problem from the production angle, stimulating the pancreas to secrete more insulin.

Starlix can be used alone or combined with another diabetes drug, called Glucophage, that tackles the other part of the problem, working to improve the body's response to whatever insulin it makes. Starlix is prescribed only when diet and exercise—or Glucophage alone—have failed to control blood sugar levels.

Stavudine *See Zerit*

Stimate *See DDAVP*

SUBOXONE
Buprenorphine and Naloxone hydrochloride dihydrate

Suboxone is prescribed to help treat opioid dependence, including an addiction to opioid drugs such as heroin, oxycodone, and other narcotic painkillers. It is used to help patients stay in treatment by suppressing symptoms of opioid withdrawal, decreasing cravings, reducing illicit opioid use, and blocking the effects of highly addictive opioids.

Sucralfate *See Carafate*

SULAR
Nisoldipine

Sular controls high blood pressure. A long-acting tablet, Sular may be used alone or in combination with other blood pressure medications.

Sular is a type of medication called a calcium channel blocker. It inhibits the flow of calcium through the smooth muscles of the heart, delaying the passage of nerve impulses, slowing down the heart, and expanding the blood vessels. This eases the heart's workload and reduces blood pressure.

Sulfacetamide *See Klaron*

Sulfasalazine *See Azulfidine*

Sulindac *See Clinoril*

Sumatriptan *See Imitrex*

Sumycin *See Tetracycline*

SUPRAX
Cefixime

Suprax, a cephalosporin antibiotic, is prescribed for bacterial infections of the chest, ears, urinary tract, and throat, and for uncomplicated gonorrhea.

SUSTIVA
Efavirenz

Sustiva is one of the growing number of drugs used to fight HIV infection. HIV, the human immunodeficiency virus, weakens the immune system until it can no longer fight off infections, leading to the fatal disease known as AIDS (acquired immune deficiency syndrome).

Like other drugs for HIV, Sustiva works by impairing the virus's ability to multiply. However, when taken alone it may prompt the virus to become resistant. Sustiva is therefore always taken with at least one other HIV medication, such as Retrovir or Crixivan. Even when used properly, it may remain effective for only a limited time.

SYMMETREL
Amantadine

Symmetrel is used to treat or prevent flu caused by the Influenza A virus; to treat Parkinson's disease; and to relieve tremors, jerks, or writhing caused by treatment with other drugs.

Hospital workers—and others in close contact with someone who has or is likely to get flu caused by the Influenza A virus—should have a flu shot each year. If a flu shot is impossible or contraindicated, preventive treatment with Symmetrel may be advisable. A flu shot can still be taken after starting treatment with Symmetrel. Once the body has manufactured enough anti-bodies to the Influenza A virus, Symmetrel will no longer be needed.

Synthetic conjugaated estrogens, A *See Cenestin*

SYNTHROID
Levothyroxine
Other brand names: Levothroid, Unithroid

Synthroid, a synthetic thyroid hormone may be given in any of the following cases:

If the thyroid gland is not making enough hormone
If the thyroid is enlarged (a goiter) or there is a risk for developing a goiter
If the patient has certain cancers of the thyroid

If thyroid production is low due to surgery, radiation, certain drugs, or disease of the pituitary gland or the hypothalamus in the brain.

Tacrolimus *See Prograf*

Tadalafil *See Cialis*

TAGAMET
Cimetidine
Other brand name: Tagamet HB

Tagamet is prescribed for the treatment of certain kinds of stomach and intestinal ulcers and related conditions. These include: active duodenal (upper intestinal) ulcers; active benign stomach ulcers; erosive gastro-esophageal reflux disease (backflow of acid stomach contents); prevention of upper abdominal bleeding in those who are critically ill; and excess-acid conditions such as Zollinger-Ellison syndrome (a form of peptic ulcer with too much acid). It is also used to prevent a relapse after the healing of active ulcers. Tagamet is a histamine blocker.

Some doctors also use Tagamet to treat acne and to prevent stress-induced ulcers. It may also be used to treat chronic hives, herpes virus infections (including shingles), abnormal hair growth in women, and overactivity of the parathyroid gland.

An over-the-counter version of the drug, Tagamet HB, is used to relieve heartburn, acid indigestion, and sour stomach.

TAMBOCOR
Flecainide

Tambocor is prescribed to treat certain heart rhythm disturbances, including paroxysmal atrial fibrillation (a sudden attack or worsening of irregular heartbeat in which the upper chamber of the heart beats irregularly and very rapidly) and paroxysmal supraventricular tachycardia (a sudden attack or worsening of an abnormally fast but regular heart rate that occurs in intermittent episodes).

TAMIFLU
Oseltamivir

Tamiflu speeds recovery from the flu. When started during the first 2 days of the illness, it hastens improvement by at least a day. It also can prevent the flu if treatment is started within 2 days after exposure to a flu victim. Tamiflu is one of a new class of antiviral drugs called neuraminidase inhibitors.

As the flu virus takes hold in the body, it forms new copies of itself and spreads from cell to cell. Neuraminidase inhibitors fight the virus by preventing the release of new copies from infected cells. The other drug in this class, Relenza, is taken by inhalation. Tamiflu is taken in liquid or capsule form.

Tamoxifen *See Nolvadex*

Tamsulosin *See Flomax*

TARKA
Trandolapril with Verapamil

Tarka is used to treat high blood pressure. It combines two blood pressure drugs: an ACE inhibitor and a calcium channel blocker. The ACE inhibitor (trandolapril) lowers blood pressure by preventing a chemical in the blood called angiotensin I from converting to a more potent form that narrows the blood vessels and increases salt and water retention. The calcium channel blocker (verapamil hydrochloride) also works to keep the blood vessels open, and eases the heart's workload by reducing the force and rate of the heartbeat.

TASMAR
Tolcapone

Tasmar helps to relieve the muscle stiffness, tremor, and weakness caused by Parkinson's disease. When taken with Sinemet (levodopa/carbidopa), it sustains the blood levels of dopamine needed for normal muscle function. Because Tasmar has been known to cause liver failure, it is prescribed only when other Parkinson's drugs fail to control the symptoms.

Like all Parkinson's medications, Tasmar can provide long-term relief of symptoms, but won't cure the underlying disease. If symptoms do not improve after 3 weeks of Tasmar therapy, the doctor will discontinue the drug.

TAXOL
Paclitaxel

Taxol is used to treat cancer of the ovary and breast cancer that does not respond to other drugs. An extract of the bark of the Pacific yew tree, it works by interfering with the growth of cancer cells.

Some doctors also prescribe Taxol to treat certain kinds of lung cancer.

Tazarotene *See Tazorac*

TAZORAC
Tazarotene

Tazorac gel comes in two strengths, 0.05% and 0.1%. Both strengths are used to treat the type of psoriasis that causes large plaques on the skin. The 0.1% strength is also used to treat mild to moderate facial acne. The drug is chemically related to vitamin A.

TEGRETOL
Carbamazepine
Other brand names: Epitol, Tegretol-XR

Tegretol is used in the treatment of seizure disorders, including certain types of epilepsy. It is also prescribed for trigeminal neuralgia (severe pain in the jaws) and pain in the tongue and throat.

Without official approval, Tegretol is also used to treat alcohol withdrawal, cocaine addiction, and emotional disorders such as depression and abnormally aggressive behavior. The drug is also used to treat migraine headache and "restless legs."

TEKTURNA
Aliskiren

Tekturna is used to treat high blood pressure (hypertension). It belongs to the general class of medicines called antihypertensives.

High blood pressure adds to the work load of the heart and arteries. If it continues for a long time, the heart and arteries may not function properly. This can damage the blood vessels of the brain, heart, and kidneys, resulting in a stroke, heart failure, or kidney failure. High blood pressure may also increase the risk of heart attacks. These problems may be less likely to occur if blood pressure is controlled.

Tekturna works by blocking the action of a substance in the body that causes blood vessels to tighten. As a result, blood vessels relax and widen. This lowers blood pressure.

Telithromycin *See Ketek*

Telmisartan *See Micardis*

Telmisartan with Hydrochlorothiazide *See Micardis HCT*

TEMOVATE
Clobetasol
Other brand name: Cormax

Temovate and Cormax relieve the itching and inflammation of moderate to severe skin conditions. The scalp application is used for short-term treatment of scalp conditions; the cream, ointment, emollient cream, and gel are used for short-term treatment of skin conditions on the body. The products contain a steroid medication for external use only.

Tenofovir disoproxil *See Viread*

TENORETIC
Atenolol with Chlorthalidone

Tenoretic is used in the treatment of high blood pressure. It combines a beta-blocker drug and a diuretic. Tenoretic can be used alone or in combination with other high blood pressure medications. Atenolol, the beta blocker, decreases the force and rate of heart contractions. Chlorthalidone, the diuretic, helps the body produce and eliminate more urine, which clears excess fluid from the body and tends to lower blood pressure.

TENORMIN
Atenolol

Tenormin, a type of medication known as a beta-blocker, is used in the treatment of high blood pressure, angina pectoris (chest pain, usually caused by lack of oxygen in the heart muscle due to clogged arteries), and heart attack. When used for high blood pressure it is effective alone or combined with other high blood pressure medications, particularly with a thiazide-type water pill (diuretic). Beta-blockers decrease the force and rate of heart contractions.

Without official approval, Tenormin is also used for treatment of alcohol withdrawal, prevention of migraine headache, and bouts of anxiety.

TERAZOL
Terconazole

Terazol is an antifungal medication. It is prescribed to treat candidiasis (a yeast-like fungal infection) of the vulva and vagina.

Terazosin *See Hytrin*

Terbinafine *See Lamisil*

Terconazole *See Terazol*

Teriparatide *See Forteo*

TESSALON
Benzonatate

Tessalon is taken for relief of a cough. It works by deadening certain receptors in the respiratory tract, thereby dampening the cough reflex.

TESTIM
Testosterone

Testim treats a lack of testosterone when the body does not produce enough of its own natural testosterone. Testosterone is a male hormone.

Testosterone *See Testim*

Testosterone gel *See AndroGel*

Testred *See Android*

TETRACYCLINE
Brand name: Sumycin

Tetracycline, a "broad-spectrum" antibiotic, is used to treat bacterial infections such as Rocky Mountain spotted fever, typhus fever, and tick fevers; upper respiratory infections; pneumonia; gonorrhea; amoebic infections; and urinary tract infections. It is also used to help treat severe acne and to treat trachoma (a chronic eye infection) and conjunctivitis (pinkeye). Tetracycline is often a viable alternative for people who are allergic to penicillin.

TEVETEN
Eprosartan

Teveten is used to treat high blood pressure. It is a member of the family of drugs called angiotensin II receptor blockers. The hormone angiotensin II makes the blood vessels constrict, causing blood pressure to rise. Teveten works by blocking the receptors that respond to this hormone. The drug may be prescribed alone or in combination with other medications that help lower blood pressure, such as water pills (diuretics) or calcium channel blockers.

TEVETEN HCT
Eprosartan with Hydrochlorothiazide

Teveten HCT is a combination medication used in the treatment of high blood pressure. One component, eprosartan, belongs to a class of blood pressure medications that work by preventing the hormone angiotensin II from constricting the blood vessels, thus allowing blood to flow more freely and keeping blood pressure down. The other component, hydrochlorothiazide, is a diuretic that increases the output of urine, removing excess fluid from the body and thus lowering blood pressure.

Theo-24 *See Theo-Dur*

Theochron *See Theo-Dur*

THEO-DUR
Theophylline
Other brand names: Theo-24, Theochron

Theo-Dur, an oral bronchodilator medication, is given to treat symptoms of asthma, chronic bronchitis, and emphysema. The active ingredient of Theo-Dur, theophylline, is a chemical cousin of caffeine. It opens the airways by relaxing the smooth muscle that circles the tubes and blood vessels in the lungs.

Theophylline *See Theo-Dur or Uniphyl*

Thyroid Hormones *See Armour Thyroid*

TIAZAC
Diltiazem

Tiazac is in a group of drugs called calcium channel blockers. Tiazac works by relaxing the muscles of the heart and blood vessels. Tiazac is used to treat hypertension (high blood pressure), angina (chest pain), and certain heart rhythm disorders.

TICLID
Ticlopidine

Ticlid makes the blood less likely to clot. It is prescribed to reduce the risk of stroke in people who have already suffered a stroke or had warning signs of stroke, and who either cannot take aspirin or fail to benefit from aspirin therapy.

Ticlid is also given, along with aspirin, to reduce the chances of a clot forming after a stent (a metal mesh tube) has been inserted in a coronary artery (a procedure used to keep the artery open and relieve the chest pain of angina).

Ticlopidine *See Ticlid*

TIGAN
Trimethobenzamide

Tigan is prescribed to control nausea and vomiting.

TILADE
Nedocromil

Tilade is an anti-inflammatory medication prescribed for use on a regular basis to control symptoms of mild to moderate asthma.

Timolol *See Timoptic or Betimol*

TIMOPTIC
Timolol
Other brand name: Timoptic-XE

Timoptic is an eyedrop that effectively reduces internal pressure in the eye. Timoptic is used in the treatment of open-angle glaucoma (potentially damaging chronic high pressure in the eye).

Tiotropium *See Spiriva*

Tizanidine *See Zanaflex*

TOBRADEX
Tobramycin and Dexamethasone

Tobradex combines a steroid drug, dexamethasone, and an antibiotic, tobramycin. It is prescribed to control inflammation and infection in the eye.

Tobramycin *See Tobrex*

Tobramycin and Dexamethasone *See Tobradex*

TOBREX
Tobramycin
Other brand name: Aktob

Tobrex is an antibiotic applied to the eye to treat bacterial infections.

TOLBUTAMIDE

Tolbutamide is an oral antidiabetic medication used to treat type 2 (non-insulin-dependent) diabetes. Diabetes occurs when the body does not make enough insulin, or when the insulin that is produced no longer works properly. Insulin works by helping sugar get inside the body's cells, where it is then used for energy.

There are two forms of diabetes: type 1 (insulin-dependent) and type 2 (non-insulin-dependent). Type 1 diabetes usually requires taking insulin injections for life, while type 2 diabetes can usually be treated by dietary changes, exercise, and/or oral antidiabetic medications such as tolbutamide. This drug controls diabetes by stimulating the pancreas to secrete more insulin and by helping insulin work better.

Occasionally, type 2 diabetics must take insulin injections temporarily during stressful periods or times of illness. When diet, exercise, and an oral antidiabetic medication fail to reduce symptoms and/or blood sugar levels, a person with type 2 diabetes may require long-term insulin injections.

Tolcapone *See Tasmar*

Tolterodine *See Detrol*

TOPAMAX
Topiramate

Topamax is an antiepileptic drug, prescribed to control both the mild attacks known as partial seizures and the severe tonic-clonic convulsions known as grand mal seizures. It is typically added to the treatment regimen when other drugs fail to fully control a patient's attacks.

TOPICORT
Desoximetasone

Topicort is a synthetic steroid medication in cream, gel, or ointment form that relieves the inflammation and itching caused by a variety of skin conditions.

Topiramate *See Topamax*

TOPROL-XL
Metoprolol

Toprol-XL treats high blood pressure, angina (chest pain), and heart failure. This medicine is a beta-blocker.

TORADOL
Ketorolac

Toradol, a nonsteroidal anti-inflammatory drug, is used to relieve moderately severe, acute pain. It is prescribed for a limited amount of time (no more than 5 days for adults and as a single dose for children), not for long-term therapy.

Torsemide *See Demadex*

Tramadol *See Ultram*

Tramadol and Acetaminophen *See Ultracet*

Trandate *See Normodyne*

Trandolapril *See Mavik*

Trandolapril with Verapamil *See Tarka*

TRAVATAN
Travoprost
Other brand name: Travatan Z

Travatan is an eyedrop that reduces excessive pressure in the eye (often a result of the condition called open-angle glaucoma). Travatan works by promoting drainage of the fluid that fills the eye. It is usually prescribed when other remedies cannot be used or the other drugs have not been effective.

Travoprost *See Travatan*

TRENTAL
Pentoxifylline

Trental is a medication that reduces the viscosity or "stickiness" of the blood, allowing it to flow more freely. It helps relieve the painful leg cramps caused by "intermittent claudication," a condition that results when hardening of the arteries reduces the leg muscles' blood supply.

Some doctors also prescribe Trental for dementia, strokes, circulatory and nerve problems caused by diabetes, and Raynaud's syndrome (a disorder of the blood vessels in which exposure to cold causes the fingers and toes to turn white). The drug is also used to treat impotence and to increase sperm motility in infertile men.

Tretinoin *See Retin-A and Renova*

Trexall *See Methotrexate*

Triamcinolone *See Azmacort or Nasacort AQ*

TRICOR
Fenofibrate

Tricor is used, along with a special diet, to treat people with very high levels of triglycerides (a fatty substance in the blood). Tricor also improves cholesterol levels by lowering total cholesterol—including "bad" LDL cholesterol—and raising "good" HDL cholesterol. It works by promoting the dissolution and elimination of fat particles in the blood.

Tricor is usually added to a treatment regimen only when other measures have failed to produce adequate results. Often, diet and exercise are enough to bring blood fats under control. Likewise, it's sometimes sufficient to simply treat an underlying problem such as diabetes, underactive thyroid, kidney disease, liver dysfunction, or alcoholism. In some cases, just discontinuing a medication is enough to do the job. For instance, certain water pills and "beta-blocker" heart medications are capable of causing a massive increase in triglyceride levels. Estrogen replacement therapy is another potential culprit.

Whatever the other treatment measures may be, it's important to remember that Tricor is intended to supplement them, rather than replace them outright. To get the full benefit of the medication, patients need to stick to the diet, exercise program, and other treatments the doctor prescribes. All these efforts to keep cholesterol and triglyceride levels normal are important because together they may lower the risk of heart disease.

For people at high risk of heart disease, current guidelines call for considering drug therapy when LDL levels reach 130. For people at lower risk, the cut-off is 160. For those at little or no risk, it's 190.

TRILEPTAL

Oxcarbazepine

Trileptal helps reduce the frequency of partial epileptic seizures, a form of epilepsy in which neural disturbances are limited to a specific region of the brain and the victim remains conscious throughout the attack. Trileptal may be prescribed by itself to treat the problem in adults. It can also be used in combination with other seizure medications in adults and in children as young as four years old.

Tri-Levlen *See Oral Contraceptives*

Trimethobenzamide *See Tigan*

Trimethoprim with Sulfamethoxazole *See Bactrim*

Tri-Norinyl *See Oral Contraceptives*

Triphasil *See Oral Contraceptives*

Trivora *See Oral Contraceptives*

TRIZIVIR

Abacavir, Lamivudine, and Zidovudine

Trizivir combines three drugs used to fight HIV, the deadly virus that undermines the immune system, leaving the body ever more vulnerable to infection, and eventually leading to AIDS. The components of Trizivir are all members of the category of HIV drugs known as nucleoside analogs:

Abacavir (also called Ziagen)
Lamivudine (also called Epivir or 3TC)
Zidovudine (also called Retrovir, AZT, or ZDV)

Trizivir may be prescribed alone or in combination with other HIV drugs. It reduces the amount of HIV in the bloodstream, but does not completely cure the disease. Patients may still develop the rare infections and other complications that accompany HIV. Remember, too, that Trizivir does not reduce the risk of transmitting the virus to others.

Trospium *See Sanctura*

TRUSOPT
Dorzolamide

Trusopt eye drops are prescribed for the treatment of the excessive pressure in the eyeball known as open-angle glaucoma.

TRUVADA
Emtricitabine and Tenofovir disoproxil fumarate

Truvada is used with other anti-HIV medicines in the treatment of human immunodeficiency virus (HIV) infection. HIV is the virus that causes acquired immune deficiency syndrome (AIDS).

Truvada will not cure or prevent HIV infection or the symptoms of AIDS; however, it helps keep HIV from reproducing, and appears to slow down the destruction of the immune system. This may help delay the development of serious health problems usually related to AIDS or HIV infection. Truvada will not keep you from spreading HIV to other people. People who receive this medicine may continue to have other problems usually related to AIDS or HIV infection.

TUSSIONEX
Hydrocodone with Chlorpheniramine polistirex

Tussionex Extended-Release Suspension is a cough-suppressant/antihistamine combination used to relieve coughs and the upper respiratory symptoms of colds and allergies. Hydrocodone, a mild narcotic similar to codeine, is believed to work directly on the cough center. Chlorpheniramine, an antihistamine, reduces itching and swelling and dries up secretions from the eyes, nose, and throat.

TYLENOL WITH CODEINE
Acetaminophen with Codeine

Tylenol with Codeine, a narcotic analgesic, is used to treat mild to moderately severe pain. It contains two drugs—acetaminophen and codeine. Acetaminophen, an antipyretic (fever-reducing) analgesic, is used to reduce pain and fever. Codeine, a narcotic analgesic, relieves moderate to severe pain.

People who are allergic to aspirin can take Tylenol with Codeine.

Tylox *See Percocet*

ULTRACET
Tramadol and Acetaminophen

Ultracet is used to treat moderate to severe pain for a period of five days or less. It contains two pain-relieving agents. Tramadol, known technically as an opioid analgesic, is a narcotic pain reliever. Acetaminophen is the active ingredient in the over-the-counter pain remedy Tylenol.

ULTRAM
Tramadol
Other brand name: Ultram ER

Ultram, known technically as an opioid analgesic, is a narcotic painkiller. It is prescribed to relieve moderate to moderately severe pain.

Ultram ER is the extended-release version of Ultram. It is used for the management of moderate to moderately severe chronic pain in adults who require around-the-clock treatment of their pain for an extended period of time.

ULTRAVATE
Halobetasol

Ultravate is a high-potency steroid medication that relieves the itching and inflammation caused by a wide variety of skin disorders. It is available in cream and ointment formulations.

UNIPHYL
Theophylline

Uniphyl treats symptoms of asthma and other lung problems such as emphysema and on-going bronchitis. This medicine is a bronchodilator. It works by relaxing muscles in the lungs and chest, and makes the lungs less sensitive to allergens and other causes of bronchospasm.

UNIRETIC
Moexipril with Hydrochlorothiazide

Uniretic combines two types of blood pressure medication. The first, moexipril hydrochloride, is an ACE (angiotensin-converting enzyme) inhibitor. It works by preventing a chemical in the blood called angiotensin I from converting into a more potent form (angiotensin II) that increases salt and water retention in the body and causes the blood vessels to constrict—two actions that tend to increase blood pressure.

To aid in clearing excess water from the body, Uniretic also contains hydrochlorothiazide, a diuretic that promotes production of urine.

Diuretics often wash too much potassium out of the body along with the water. However, the ACE inhibitor part of Uniretic tends to keep potassium in the body, thereby canceling this unwanted effect.

Uniretic is not used for the initial treatment of high blood pressure. It is saved for later use, when a single blood pressure medication is not sufficient for the job.

Unithroid *See Synthroid*

UNIVASC
Moexipril

Univasc is used in the treatment of high blood pressure. It is effective when used alone or with thiazide diuretics that help rid the body of excess water. Univasc belongs to a family of drugs called angiotensin-converting enzyme (ACE) inhibitors. It works by preventing the transformation of a hormone in the blood called angiotensin I into a more potent substance that increases salt and water retention in the body and causes the blood vessels to constrict—two actions that tend to increase blood pressure.

URISED
Methenamine

Urised relieves lower urinary tract discomfort caused by inflammation or diagnostic procedures. It is used to treat urinary tract infections including cystitis (inflammation of the bladder and ureters), urethritis (inflammation of the urethra), and trigonitis (inflammation of the mucous membrane of the bladder). Methenamine, the major component of this drug, acts as a mild antiseptic by changing into formaldehyde in the urinary tract when it comes in contact with acidic urine.

UROXATRAL
Alfuzosin

Uroxatral is used to treat the symptoms of an enlarged prostate—a condition technically known as benign prostatic hyperplasia or BPH. The walnut-sized prostate gland surrounds the urethra (the duct that drains the bladder). If the gland becomes enlarged, it can squeeze the urethra, interfering with the flow of urine. This can cause difficulty in starting urination, a weak flow of urine, and the need to urinate urgently or more frequently. Uroxatral doesn't shrink the prostate. Instead, it relaxes the muscle around it, freeing the flow of urine and decreasing urinary symptoms.

VAGIFEM
Estradiol vaginal tablets

As estrogen levels decline during menopause, vaginal tissues tend to shrink and lose their elasticity—sometimes producing a condition known as atrophic vaginitis. Inserted in the vagina on a regular basis, Vagifem tablets provide a local source of estrogen replacement without passing through the rest of the system. This helps relieve such symptoms of atrophic vaginitis as vaginal dryness, soreness, and itching.

Valacyclovir *See Valtrex*

VALCYTE
Valganciclovir

Valcyte tablets are used in the treatment of an eye disease called cytomegalovirus (CMV) retinitis, one of the many infections that take hold when the immune system is undermined by AIDS.

Valcyte is also used to prevent CMV disease in people who've had a kidney, heart, or kidney-pancreas transplant. Valcyte is not approved for use in liver transplant patients.

Valcyte is very similar to the CMV medication Cytovene (ganciclovir).

Valganciclovir *See Valcyte*

Valproic acid *See Depakene*

Valsartan *See Diovan*

VALTREX
Valacyclovir

Valtrex is used to treat certain herpes infections, including herpes zoster (the painful rash known as shingles), genital herpes, and herpes cold sores on the face and lips.

Vancenase *See Beclomethasone*

Vanceril *See Beclomethasone*

VANOS
Fluocinonide

Vanos belongs to the group of medicines known as corticosteroids (cortisone-like medicines). Vanos is used for the relief of the inflammatory and pruritic manifestations of corticosteroid responsive skin diseases.

Vardenafil *See Levitra*

Varenicline *See Chantix*

VASERETIC
Enalapril with Hydrochlorothiazide

Vaseretic is used in the treatment of high blood pressure. It combines an ACE inhibitor with a thiazide diuretic. Enalapril, the ACE inhibitor, works by preventing a chemical in the blood called angiotensin I from converting into a more potent form that increases salt and water retention in the body and constricts the blood vessels—actions that tend to increase blood pressure. Hydrochlorothiazide, a diuretic, rids the body of excess fluid by promoting the production of urine, which also helps in lowering blood pressure.

VASOTEC
Enalapril

Vasotec is a high blood pressure medication known as an ACE inhibitor. It works by preventing a chemical in the blood called angiotensin I from converting into a more potent form that increases salt and water retention in the body and constricts the blood vessels—actions that tend to increase blood pressure. It is effective when used alone or in combination with other medications, especially thiazide-type diuretics. It is also used in the treatment of congestive heart failure, usually in combination with diuretics and digitalis, and is prescribed as a preventive measure in certain conditions that could lead to heart failure.

Veetids *See Penicillin V Potassium*

Ventolin HFA *See Proventil*

Verapamil *See Calan*

Verelan *See Calan*

VESICARE
Solifenacin

Vesicare treats the symptoms of overactive bladder, such as urinary urgency, incontinence, and urinary frequency.

VIAGRA
Sildenafil

Viagra is an oral drug for male impotence, also known as erectile dysfunction (ED). It works by dilating blood vessels in the penis, allowing the inflow of blood needed for an erection.

Vibramycin *See Doryx*

Vibra-Tabs *See Doryx*

VICODIN
Hydrocodone with Acetaminophen
Other brand names: Anexsia, Co-Gesic, Lorcet, Lortab, Maxidone, Zydone

Vicodin combines a narcotic analgesic (painkiller) and cough reliever with a non-narcotic analgesic for the relief of moderate to moderately severe pain.

VICOPROFEN
Hydrocodone with Ibuprofen

Vicoprofen is a chemical cousin of the well-known painkiller Vicodin. Both products contain the prescription pain medication hydrocodone. However, while Vicodin also includes acetaminophen (the active ingredient in Tylenol), Vicoprofen replaces it with ibuprofen (the active ingredient in Advil).

Vicoprofen relieves acute pain. It is generally prescribed for less than 10 days, and cannot be used in the long-term treatment of osteoarthritis or rheumatoid arthritis.

VIDEX
Didanosine

Videx is one of the drugs used to fight the human immunodeficiency virus (HIV)—the deadly cause of AIDS. Over a period of years, HIV slowly destroys the immune system, leaving the body defenseless against infection. Videx disrupts reproduction of HIV, thereby staving off the immune system's collapse.

Signs and symptoms of advanced HIV infection include diarrhea, fever, headache, infections, problems with the nervous system, rash, sore throat, and significant weight loss.

VIGAMOX
Moxifloxacin

Vigamox is an antibiotic used to treat eye infections that are caused by bacteria. Vigamox is a fluoroquinolone antibiotic.

VIRACEPT
Nelfinavir

Viracept is one of the drugs prescribed to fight HIV, the human immuno-deficiency virus that causes AIDS (acquired immune deficiency syndrome). Once inside the body, HIV spreads through certain key cells in the immune system, weakening the body's ability to fight off other infections. Viracept works by interfering with an important step in the virus's reproductive cycle. This slows the spread of the virus and prolongs the strength of the immune system.

Viracept belongs to the new class of drugs that has successfully reversed the course of HIV infection in many people. Called protease inhibitors, these drugs work better when used in combination with other HIV medications called nucleoside analogues (Retrovir, Hivid, and others) that act against the virus in other ways.

VIRAMUNE
Nevirapine

Viramune is prescribed for advanced cases of HIV. HIV—the human immunodeficiency virus that causes AIDS—undermines the immune system over a period of years, eventually leaving the body defenseless against infection. Viramune is generally prescribed only after the immune system has declined and infections have begun to appear. It is always taken with at least one other HIV medication such as Retrovir or Videx. If taken alone, it can cause the virus to become resistant. Even if used properly, it may be effective for only a limited time.

Like other drugs for HIV, Viramune works by impairing the virus's ability to multiply.

VIREAD
Tenofovir disoproxil

Viread is one of the drugs prescribed to fight HIV, the human immuno-deficiency virus that causes AIDS (acquired immune deficiency syndrome). HIV attacks the immune system, slowly destroying the body's ability to fight off infection. Viread staves off the attack by interfering with HIV reverse transcriptase, an enzyme the virus needs to reproduce.

Viread lowers the amount of HIV in the blood and may help increase the number of T cells, important agents of the immune system that kill microscopic foreign invaders. It is used in combination with other anti-HIV drugs when these drugs are not effective by themselves.

VIVELLE-DOT
Estradiol

The Vivelle-Dot patch is a small translucent estrogen patch that is applied directly to the abdomen. The Vivelle-Dot patch delivers estrogen through the skin and directly into the bloodstream, for relief of moderate to severe menopausal symptoms and prevention of postmenopausal osteoporosis. Menopausal symptoms include hot flashes, night sweats and associated sleep disturbances, and dryness, itching and burning in and around the vagina.

VOLTAREN
Diclofenac
Other brand name: Cataflam (Diclofenac potassium)

Voltaren and Cataflam are nonsteroidal anti-inflammatory drugs used to relieve the inflammation, swelling, stiffness, and joint pain associated with rheumatoid arthritis, osteoarthritis (the most common form of arthritis), and ankylosing spondylitis (arthritis and stiffness of the spine). Voltaren-XR, the extended-release form of Voltaren, is used only for long-term treatment. Cataflam is also prescribed for immediate relief of pain and menstrual discomfort.

VoSpire *See Proventil*

VYTORIN
Ezetimibe and Simvastatin

Vytorin is used to lower cholesterol and triglyceride (fat-like substances) levels in the blood. Using this medicine may help prevent medical problems caused by such substances clogging the blood vessels.

Warfarin *See Coumadin*

WELCHOL
Colesevelam

WelChol is used to lower blood cholesterol levels when diet and exercise prove insufficient. It works by binding with cholesterol-based bile acids to take them out of circulation. This prompts the liver to produce a replacement supply of bile acids, drawing the extra cholesterol it needs out of the bloodstream.

WelChol is sometimes prescribed along with one of the popular "statin" drugs that fight cholesterol in a different way. Among these drugs are Lescol, Lipitor, Mevacor, Pravachol, and Zocor.

XALATAN
Latanoprost

Xalatan is used to relieve high pressure within the eye (a hallmark of the condition known as open-angle glaucoma). It can be prescribed alone or with other glaucoma medications.

XELODA
Capecitabine

Xeloda belongs to the group of medicines called antimetabolites. It is used to treat breast cancer and colorectal cancer.

Xeloda interferes with the growth of cancer cells, which are eventually destroyed. Since the growth of normal cells may also be affected by the medicine, other effects will also occur. Some of these may be serious and must be reported to your doctor. Other effects may not be serious but may cause concern.

XENICAL
Orlistat

Xenical blocks absorption of dietary fat into the bloodstream, thereby reducing the number of calories obtained from a meal. At the usual dosage level, it cuts fat absorption by almost one-third. Combined with a low-calorie diet, it is used to promote weight loss and discourage the return of unwanted pounds.

The drug is prescribed for the frankly obese and for merely overweight people who have other health problems such as high blood pressure, diabetes, or high cholesterol levels. Weight status is determined by the body mass index (BMI), a comparison of height to weight.

XIBROM
Bromfenac

Xibrom is a drug used to treat inflammation of the eye following cataract surgery. This medicine is a nonsteroidal anti-inflammatory drug (NSAID).

XIFAXAN
Rifaximin

Xifaxan treats traveler's diarrhea caused by bacteria called *E coli.*

XOPENEX
Levalbuterol
Other brand name: Xopenex HFA (Levalbuterol tartrate)

Xopenex is a "bronchodilator." It works by relaxing the muscles in the walls of the lungs' many tiny airways (bronchioles), allowing them to expand so patients can get more air. It is prescribed for asthma.

While Xopenex contains levalbuterol hydrochloride, Xopenex HFA contains levalbuterol tartrate and is an inhalation aerosol. Xopenex HFA is a short-acting beta-agonist and has been approved by the FDA for the treatment or prevention of bronchospasm in patients 4 years of age and older.

YASMIN
Drospirenone and Ethinyl estradiol

Yasmin is used as an oral contraceptive. Oral contraceptives are also known as the Pill, OCs, BCs, BC tablets, or birth control pills. This medicine usually contains two types of hormones, estrogens and progestins and, when taken properly, prevents pregnancy. It works by stopping a woman's egg from fully developing each month. The egg can no longer accept a sperm and fertilization is prevented. Although oral contraceptives have other effects that help prevent a pregnancy from occurring, this is the main action.

YAZ
Drospirenone and Ethinyl estradiol

YAZ is used as an oral contraceptive. Oral contraceptives are also known as the Pill, OCs, BCs, BC tablets, or birth control pills. This medicine usually contains two types of hormones, estrogens and progestins and, when taken properly, prevents pregnancy. It works by stopping a woman's egg from fully developing each month. The egg can no longer accept a sperm and fertilization is prevented. Although oral contraceptives have other effects that help prevent a pregnancy from occurring, this is the main action.

This medicine is also used to treat premenstrual dysphoric disorder (PMDD). PMDD is a severe form of premenstrual syndrome (PMS). Patients with PMDD may experience severe emotional and physical symptoms 10 to 14 days before their menstrual flow starts.

YAZ is also used to treat acne in women at least 14 years of age, who have already started menstruating and choose to use a birth control pill to prevent pregnancy.

ZADITOR
Ketotifen

Zaditor combats the release of chemicals that trigger allergic reactions. Available in eyedrop form, it works within minutes to relieve the itchy eyes brought on by allergies.

Zafirlukast *See Accolate*

Zalcitabine *See Hivid*

ZANAFLEX
Tizanidine

Zanaflex relaxes the tense, rigid muscles caused by spasticity. It is prescribed for people with multiple sclerosis, spinal cord injuries, and other disorders that produce protracted muscle spasms. The effect of the drug peaks 1 to 2 hours after each dose and is gone within 3 to 6 hours, so it's best to schedule doses for shortly before the daily activities when relief of spasticity is most important.

Zanamivir *See Relenza*

ZANTAC
Ranitidine

Zantac is prescribed for the short-term treatment (4 to 8 weeks) of active duodenal ulcer (near the exit from the stomach) and active benign gastric ulcer (in the stomach itself), and as maintenance therapy for gastric or duodenal ulcer, at a reduced dosage, after the ulcer has healed. It is also used for the treatment of conditions in which the stomach produces too much acid, such as Zollinger-Ellison syndrome and systemic mastocytosis, for gastroesophageal reflux disease (backflow of acid stomach contents into the entry to the stomach) and for healing—and maintaining healing of— erosive esophagitis (severe inflammation of the esophagus).

Some doctors prescribe Zantac to prevent damage to the stomach and duodenum from long-term use of nonsteroidal anti-inflammatory drugs such as Indocin and Motrin, and to treat bleeding of the stomach and intestine. Zantac is also sometimes prescribed for stress-induced ulcers.

ZAROXOLYN
Metolazone

Zaroxolyn is a diuretic used in the treatment of high blood pressure and other conditions that require the elimination of excess fluid from the body. These conditions include congestive heart failure and kidney disease. When used for high blood pressure, Zaroxolyn can be used alone or with other high blood pressure medications. Diuretics prompt the body to produce and eliminate more urine, which helps lower blood pressure.

ZEBETA
Bisoprolol

Zebeta, a type of medication known as a beta-blocker, is used to treat high blood pressure. Beta-blockers lower blood pressure by decreasing the force and rate of heart contractions, which reduces the heart's demand for oxygen. Zebeta can be used alone or in combination with other high blood pressure medications.

ZEGERID
Omeprazole and Sodium bicarbonate

Zegerid treats stomach ulcers (such as duodenal ulcer or gastric ulcer) and gastroesophageal reflux disease (GERD), and aids in healing damage to the esophagus that is caused by stomach acid. This medicine also helps prevent gastrointestinal bleeding in patients with a serious illness.

ZERIT
Stavudine

Zerit is one of the drugs used to fight the human immunodeficiency virus (HIV)—the deadly cause of AIDS. It is usually prescribed for people who have already been taking the HIV drug Retrovir for an extended period. HIV attacks the immune system, slowly destroying the body's ability to fight off infection. Zerit helps stave off the attack by disrupting the virus's ability to reproduce.

Signs and symptoms of HIV infection include diarrhea, fever, headache, infections, problems with the nervous system, rash, sore throat, and significant weight loss.

ZESTORETIC

Lisinopril with Hydrochlorothiazide
Other brand name: Prinzide

Zestoretic is used in the treatment of high blood pressure. It combines an ACE inhibitor drug with a diuretic. Lisinopril, the ACE inhibitor, works by limiting production of a substance that promotes salt and water retention in the body. Hydrochlorothiazide, a diuretic, prompts the body to produce and eliminate more urine, which helps in lowering blood pressure. Combination products such as Zestoretic are usually not prescribed until therapy is already under way.

ZESTRIL

Lisinopril
Other brand name: Prinivil

Lisinopril is used in the treatment of high blood pressure. It is effective when used alone or when combined with other high blood pressure medications. It may also be used with other medications in the treatment of heart failure, and may be given within 24 hours of a heart attack to improve chances of survival.

Lisinopril is a type of drug called an ACE inhibitor. It works by reducing production of a substance that increases salt and water retention in the body.

ZETIA

Ezetimibe

Zetia is a new kind of cholesterol-lowering drug. The older cholesterol-lowering drugs, called "statins," reduce cholesterol by interfering with its production in the body. Zetia acts by diminishing the absorption of dietary cholesterol through the intestines.

Zetia may be taken alone or with a statin drug. Because the two drugs fight cholesterol in different ways, the Zetia/statin combination has a greater impact than either drug alone.

Cholesterol—especially "bad" LDL cholesterol—promotes clogged arteries, increasing the risk of heart attack and stroke. "Good" HDL cholesterol helps to prevent clogged arteries. Zetia lowers the bad cholesterol and raises the good. It also lowers total cholesterol readings and reduces levels of triglycerides (fats in the blood).

Cholesterol-lowering drugs are typically prescribed for people who either have heart disease or are in danger of developing it. For people at high risk of heart disease, current guidelines call for considering drug therapy when LDL levels reach 130. For people at lower risk, the cut-off is 160. For those at little or no risk, it is 190.

ZIAC
Bisoprolol with Hydrochlorothiazide

Ziac is used to treat high blood pressure. It combines a beta-blocker (bisoprolol, which is the ingredient in the drug Zebeta) with a thiazide diuretic (hydrochlorothiazide). Beta-blockers decrease the force and rate of heart contractions, thus lowering blood pressure. Diuretics help the body produce and eliminate more urine, which also helps lower blood pressure.

ZIAGEN
Abacavir

Ziagen helps to halt the inroads of the human immunodeficiency virus (HIV). Without treatment, HIV gradually undermines the body's immune system, encouraging other infections to take hold until the body succumbs to full-blown acquired immune deficiency syndrome (AIDS).

Like other anti-HIV drugs, Ziagen holds back the advance of the virus by disrupting its reproductive cycle. This medication is used only as part of a "drug cocktail" that attacks the virus on several fronts. It is not prescribed alone.

Zidovudine *See Retrovir*

Zileuton *See Zyflo*

ZITHROMAX
Azithromycin
Other brand name: Zmax

Zithromax is an antibiotic related to erythromycin. For adults, it is pre-scribed to treat certain mild to moderate skin infections; upper and lower respiratory tract infections, including pharyngitis (strep throat), tonsillitis, worsening of chronic obstructive pulmonary disease, and pneumonia; sexually transmitted infections of the cervix or urinary tract; and genital ulcer disease in men. In children, Zithromax is used to treat middle ear infection, pneumonia, tonsillitis, and strep throat.

Zmax is used for the treatment of certain types of bacterial infections in sinusitis and pneumonia. Zmax works only for infections caused by certain types of bacteria. It does not work against infections not caused by bacteria, like the common cold.

ZOCOR
Simvastatin

Zocor is a cholesterol-lowering drug. Doctors prescribe Zocor in addition to a cholesterol-lowering diet when blood cholesterol levels are too high and a patient has been unable to lower it by diet alone. For people at high risk of heart disease, current guidelines call for considering drug therapy when LDL levels reach 130. For people at lower risk, the cut-off is 160. For those at little or no risk, it's 190.

In people with high cholesterol and heart disease, Zocor reduces the risk of heart attack, stroke, and "mini-stroke" (transient ischemic attack) and can stave off the need for bypass surgery or angioplasty to clear clogged arteries. Zocor can also reduce these risks in people with diabetes, peripheral vascular disease, and a history of stroke.

ZOFRAN
Ondansetron
Other brand name: Zofran ODT

Zofran is used for the prevention of nausea and vomiting caused by radiation therapy and chemotherapy for cancer. In some cases, it is also used to prevent these problems following surgery.

Zolmitriptan *See Zomig*

ZOMIG
Zolmitriptan

Zomig relieves migraine headaches. It's effective whether or not the headache is preceded by an aura (visual disturbances such as halos and flickering lights). For most people Zomig provides relief within 2 hours, but it will not abort an attack or reduce the number of headaches experienced.

Migraines are thought to be caused by expansion and inflammation of blood vessels in the head. Zomig ends a migraine attack by constricting these blood vessels and reducing inflammation.

ZONEGRAN
Zonisamide

Zonegran helps reduce the frequency of partial epileptic seizures, a form of epilepsy in which neural disturbances are limited to a specific region of the brain and the victim remains conscious throughout the attack. The drug is used in combination with other antiseizure medications, not by itself.

Zonisamide *See Zonegran*

Zovia *See Oral Contraceptives*

ZOVIRAX
Acyclovir

Zovirax liquid, capsules, and tablets are used in the treatment of certain infections with herpesviruses. These include genital herpes, shingles, and chickenpox. This drug may not be appropriate for everyone, and its use should be thoroughly discussed with the doctor. Zovirax ointment is used to treat initial episodes of genital herpes and certain herpes simplex infections of the skin and mucous membranes. Zovirax cream is used for herpes cold sores on the lips and face only.

Some doctors use Zovirax, along with other drugs, in the treatment of AIDS, and for unusual herpes infections such as those following kidney and bone marrow transplants.

ZYBAN
Bupropion

Zyban is a nicotine-free quit-smoking aid. Instead of nicotine, it contains the same active ingredient as the antidepressant medication Wellbutrin. It works by boosting the levels of several chemical messengers in the brain. With more of these chemicals at work, patients experience a reduction in nicotine withdrawal symptoms and a weakening of the urge to smoke. More than a third of the people who take Zyban while participating in a support program are able to quit smoking for at least 1 month. Zyban can also prove helpful when people with conditions such as chronic bronchitis and emphysema decide it's time to quit.

Zydone *See Vicodin*

ZYFLO
Zileuton
Other brand name: Zyflo CR

Zyflo tablets prevent and relieve the symptoms of chronic asthma. The drug works by relaxing the muscles in the walls of the airways, allowing them to open wider, and by reducing inflammation, swelling, and mucus secretion in the lungs.

Zyflo CR is the extended-release version of Zyflo.

ZYLET
Loteprednol and Tobramycin

Zylet is a combination of an antibiotic and a corticosteroid. It is used in the eye to prevent permanent damage, which may occur with certain eye problems.

ZYLOPRIM
Allopurinol

Zyloprim is used in the treatment of many symptoms of gout, including acute attacks, tophi (collection of uric acid crystals in the tissues, especially around joints), joint destruction, and uric acid stones. Gout is a form of arthritis characterized by increased blood levels of uric acid. Zyloprim works by reducing uric acid production in the body, thus preventing crystals from forming.

Zyloprim is also used to manage increased uric acid levels in the blood of people with certain cancers, such as leukemia. It is also prescribed to manage some types of kidney stones.

ZYMAR
Gatifloxacin eye drops

Zymar is an antibiotic used in the treatment of eye infections such as conjunctivitis (pinkeye) and other bacterial infections. Gatifloxacin, the active ingredient, is a member of the quinolone family of antibiotics.

ZYRTEC
Cetirizine

Zyrtec is an antihistamine. It is prescribed to treat the sneezing; itchy, runny nose; and itchy, red, watery eyes caused by seasonal allergies such as hay fever. Zyrtec also relieves the symptoms of year-round allergies due to dust, mold, and animal dander. This medication is also used in the treatment of chronic itchy skin and hives.

ZYRTEC-D

Cetirizine with Pseudoephedrine

Zyrtec-D contains the same antihistamine found in regular Zyrtec, plus the decongestant pseudoephedrine. The drug is prescribed to relieve the symptoms of hay fever and similar allergies, whether seasonal or year-round.

ZYVOX

Linezolid

Zyvox is a member of a new class of antibiotics called oxazolidinones. It is used to treat certain types of pneumonia, some forms of skin infection, and infections involving certain strains of a germ called *Enterococcus faecium.*

Mental and Emotional Side Effects

Psychological symptoms are sometimes the result of medications prescribed for an entirely unrelated purpose. These unwanted side effects can confound diagnosis and complicate therapy, leading to additional and perhaps unnecessary medication. Part 1 of this section lists about 175 mental and emotional symptoms and the drugs that can cause them. (For example, you will see here a list of drugs that can trigger or exacerbate depression.) Part 2 lists the potential psychological side effects of each drug (for example, the symptoms that can be caused by the antibiotic Cipro). Both parts are organized alphabetically.

The information in this section is extracted from the Side Effects Index of *Physicians' Desk Reference*®, a compilation of adverse events reported in official product labeling as published in *PDR*. The reported incidence of a particular side effect for some drugs is shown in parentheses following the entry. Side effects known to occur in 3% of patients or more are marked with a ▲ symbol. Entries are limited to reactions that may be expected to occur at recommended dosage levels in the general patient population. In addition, it is important to keep in mind that this is not a comprehensive list of all possible drugs that can cause these side effects. Effects of overdose are not included.

Part 1.
Side Effects by Symptom

Aggression

Accutane Capsules
Adderall XR Capsules
Advair Diskus 100/50
Advair Diskus 250/50
Advair Diskus 500/50
Advair HFA Inhalation Aerosol
Ambien Tablets (Rare)
Amerge Tablets (Rare)
Aricept ODT Tablets (Frequent)
Aricept Tablets (Frequent)
Celexa Oral Solution (Infrequent)
Celexa Tablets (Infrequent)
Chantix Tablets (Infrequent)
Concerta Extended-Release Tablets
Copegus Tablets (Less than 1%)
Depacon Injection
Depakene Capsules
Depakene Oral Solution
Depakote ER Tablets
Depakote Sprinkle Capsules
Depakote Tablets
DextroStat Tablets
Effexor Tablets
Effexor XR Capsules
Evoxac Capsules
▲ Exelon Capsules (3%)
▲ Exelon Oral Solution (3%)
Flovent Diskus 100 mcg
Flovent Diskus 250 mcg
Flovent Diskus 50 mcg
Flovent HFA 110 mcg
  Inhalation Aerosol
Flovent HFA 220 mcg
  Inhalation Aerosol
Flovent HFA 44 mcg
  Inhalation Aerosol
Genotropin Lyophilized Powder
Imitrex Injection
Imitrex Tablets (Rare)
▲ Intron A for Injection (Less than 5%)
Keppra Oral Solution
Keppra Tablets
Klonopin Tablets (Infrequent)
Klonopin Wafers (Infrequent)
Levaquin in 5% Dextrose Injection
  (0.1% to 0.9%)
Levaquin Injection (0.1% to 0.9%)
Levaquin Oral Solution (0.1% to 0.9%)
Levaquin Tablets (0.1% to 0.9%)

Lexapro Oral Suspension (Infrequent)
Lexapro Tablets (Infrequent)
Mirapex Tablets
Neurontin Capsules
Neurontin Oral Solution
Neurontin Tablets
Nexium Delayed-Release Capsules
Nexium Delayed-Release
  Oral Suspension
Nexium I.V.
Niravam Orally Disintegrating
  Tablets (Rare)
Parnate Tablets
Paxil CR Controlled-Release Tablets
Paxil Oral Suspension
Paxil Tablets
Pegasys (Less than 1%)
PegIntron Powder for Injection (1%)
Prochieve 4% Gel
Prochieve 8% Gel
Prozac Pulvules and Liquid
Pulmicort Respules (Less than 1%)
Razadyne ER Extended-Release
  Capsules
Razadyne Oral Solution
Razadyne Tablets
Requip Tablets (Infrequent)
▲ Risperdal M-Tab Orally Disintegrating
  Tablets (1% to 3%)
▲ Risperdal Oral Solution (1% to 3%)
▲ Risperdal Tablets (1% to 3%)
Ritalin Hydrochloride Tablets
Ritalin LA Capsules
Ritalin-SR Tablets
Seromycin Capsules
Seroquel Tablets
Singulair Chewable Tablets
Singulair Oral Granules
Singulair Tablets
Soriatane Capsules
Strattera Capsules (0.5%)
Sustiva Capsules (0.4%)
Sustiva Tablets (0.4%)
Symbyax Capsules
Symmetrel Tablets
▲ Topamax Sprinkle Capsules
  (2% to 9%)
▲ Topamax Tablets (2% to 9%)
Trileptal Oral Suspension
Trileptal Tablets

Wellbutrin SR Sustained-Release
Tablets
Wellbutrin Tablets
Wellbutrin XL Extended-Release
Tablets
Zegerid Capsules (Less than 1%)
Zegerid Powder for Oral Solution
(Less than 1%)
Zoloft Oral Concentrate
(Infrequent to 2%)
Zoloft Tablets (Infrequent to 2%)
Zyban Sustained-Release Tablets

Agitation
▲ Abilify Discmelt Orally Disintegrating
Tablets (25%)
▲ Abilify Oral Solution (25%)
▲ Abilify Tablets (25%)
AcipHex Tablets (Rare)
Actiq (Less than 1%)
▲ Adderall XR Capsules (8%)
Advair Diskus 100/50
Advair Diskus 250/50
Advair Diskus 500/50
Advair HFA Inhalation Aerosol
Aggrenox Capsules (Less than 1%)
Aldara Cream, 5%
Allegra-D 12 Hour Extended-Release
Tablets (1.9%)
Allegra-D 24 Hour Extended-Release
Tablets (1.9%)
Aloprim for Injection (Less than 1%)
Ambien CR Tablets (Infrequent)
Ambien Tablets (Infrequent)
AmBisome for Injection
(Less common)
Amerge Tablets (Rare)
Amoxil Capsules (Rare)
Amoxil Chewable Tablets (Rare)
Amoxil Pediatric Drops for
Oral Suspension (Rare)
Amoxil Powder for
Oral Suspension (Rare)
Amoxil Tablets (Rare)
Anzemet Injection (Infrequently)
Anzemet Tablets (Infrequently)
Aricept ODT Tablets (Frequent)
Aricept Tablets (Frequent)
Atripla Tablets
Augmentin Chewable Tablets (Rare)
Augmentin ES-600 Powder for
Oral Suspension (Rare)
Augmentin Powder for
Oral Suspension (Rare)
Augmentin Tablets (Rare)

Augmentin XR Extended-Release
Tablets (Rare)
Avelox I.V. (Less than 0.1%)
Avelox Tablets (Less than 0.1%)
▲ Avinza Capsules (Less than 5%)
Azilect Tablets (Infrequent)
Bayer Aspirin
Bicillin C-R Injectable Suspension
Brovana Inhalation Solution
(Less than 2%)
Buprenex Injectable (Rare)
Caduet Tablets (Less than or
equal to 0.1%)
Campral Tablets (Infrequent)
Carbatrol Capsules
Cardura XL Tablets
Catapres Tablets (About 3 in
100 patients)
Catapres-TTS (0.5% or less)
▲ Celexa Oral Solution (3%)
▲ Celexa Tablets (3%)
▲ CellCept Capsules
(3% to less than 20%)
▲ CellCept Intravenous
(3% to less than 20%)
▲ CellCept Oral Suspension
(3% to less than 20%)
▲ CellCept Tablets
(3% to less than 20%)
Chantix Tablets (Infrequent)
Cipro I.V.
Cipro Oral Suspension
Cipro Tablets
Cipro XR Tablets
▲ Clorpres Tablets (About 3%)
▲ Clozaril Tablets (4%)
Comtan Tablets (1%)
Comvax
▲ Copaxone for Injection (4%)
Cuprimine Capsules
Depacon Injection (1% or more)
Depakene Capsules (1% or more)
Depakene Oral Solution (1% or more)
Depakote ER Tablets
(Greater than 1%)
Depakote Sprinkle Capsules
▲ Depakote Tablets (1% to 5%)
Dexedrine Spansule Capsules
Dexedrine Tablets
Diastat Rectal Delivery System
(Greater than or equal to 1%)
Dilaudid Ampules
Dilaudid Multiple Dose Vials
Dilaudid Non-Sterile Powder
Dilaudid Oral Liquid (Less frequent)

Dilaudid Rectal Suppositories
Dilaudid Tablets
Dilaudid Tablets - 8 mg
  (Less frequent)
Dilaudid-HP Injection (Less frequent)
Dilaudid-HP Lyophilized Powder
  250 mg (Less frequent)
Donnatal Extentabs
▲ Doxil Injection (1% to 10%)
Duragesic Transdermal System
  (1% or greater)
▲ Effexor Tablets (2% to 4.5%)
▲ Effexor XR Capsules (4%)
Eldepryl Capsules
Elspar for Injection
Engerix-B Vaccine (Less than 1%)
▲ Entocort EC Capsules (Less than 5%)
Equetro Extended-Release Capsules
Evoxac Capsules (Less than 1%)
Exelon Capsules (2% or more)
Exelon Oral Solution (2% or more)
▲ FazaClo Orally Disintegrating
  Tablets (4%)
Ferrlecit Injection
Flovent Diskus 100 mcg
Flovent Diskus 250 mcg
Flovent Diskus 50 mcg
Flovent HFA 110 mcg
  Inhalation Aerosol
Flovent HFA 220 mcg
  Inhalation Aerosol
Flovent HFA 44 mcg
  Inhalation Aerosol
Flumadine Syrup (0.3% to 1%)
Flumadine Tablets (0.3% to 1%)
Frova Tablets (Infrequent)
Gabitril Tablets (1%)
Geodon Capsules (Frequent)
I.V. Busulfex (2%)
Imitrex Injection (Infrequent)
Imitrex Nasal Spray (Infrequent)
Imitrex Tablets (Up to 2%)
▲ Indapamide Tablets
  (Greater than or equal to 5%)
▲ Infergen (4% to 6%)
▲ Intron A for Injection (Less than 5%)
▲ Invanz for Injection (3.3% to 5.1%)
Invega Extended-Release Tablets
Invirase Capsules (Less than 2%)
Invirase Tablets (Less than 2%)
Ionsys Transdermal System
  (.1% to less than 1%)
Kadian Capsules (Less than 3%)
Kaletra Oral Solution (Less than 2%)
Kaletra Tablets (Less than 2%)

Keflex Capsules
▲ Keppra Oral Solution (6%)
▲ Keppra Tablets (6%)
Klonopin Tablets
Klonopin Wafers
Kytril Injection (Less than 2%)
▲ Lamictal Chewable Dispersible Tablets
  (Greater than 1% to less than 5%)
▲ Lamictal Tablets (Greater than 1% to
  less than 5%)
Lariam Tablets (Occasional)
Leukeran Tablets (Rare)
Levaquin in 5% Dextrose Injection
  (0.1% to 0.9%)
Levaquin Injection (0.1% to 0.9%)
Levaquin Oral Solution
  (0.1% to 0.9%)
Levaquin Tablets (0.1% to 0.9%)
Lexapro Oral Suspension (Infrequent)
Lexapro Tablets (Infrequent)
Lunesta Tablets (Infrequent)
▲ Lupron Depot 7.5 mg (Less than 5%)
Lupron Depot-3 Month 11.25 mg
Lyrica Capsules (0.1% to 1%)
Maxalt Tablets (Infrequent)
Maxalt-MLT Orally Disintegrating
  Tablets (Infrequent)
Meridia Capsules
  (Greater than or equal to 1%)
Merrem I.V. (Greater than 0.1% to 1%)
Miacalcin Nasal Spray (Less than 1%)
Mirapex Tablets (Less than 1%)
MS Contin Tablets (Less frequent)
Myozyme for Intravenous Infusion
Namenda Oral Solution
  (Greater than or equal to 2%)
Namenda Tablets
  (Greater than or equal to 2%)
Nembutal Sodium Solution, USP
  (Less than 1%)
Neurontin Capsules (Infrequent)
Neurontin Oral Solution (Infrequent)
Neurontin Tablets (Infrequent)
Nexium Delayed-Release Capsules
Nexium Delayed-Release
  Oral Suspension
Nexium I.V.
Niravam Orally Disintegrating Tablets
  (2.9%)
Norflex Injection
Norvasc Tablets (Less than 0.1%)
Norvir Oral Solution (Less than 2%)
Norvir Soft Gelatin Capsules
  (Less than 2%)

Opana ER Tablets (Less than 1%)
Opana Tablets (Less than 1%)
Oramorph SR Tablets (Less frequent)
Orthoclone OKT3 Sterile Solution
OxyContin Tablets (Less than 1%)
Parcopa Orally Disintegrating Tablets
Parnate Tablets
▲ Paxil CR Controlled-Release Tablets
   (1.1% to 5%)
▲ Paxil Oral Suspension (1.1% to 5%)
▲ Paxil Tablets (1.1% to 5%)
PegIntron Powder for Injection (2%)
Pepcid for Oral Suspension
   (Infrequent)
Pepcid Injection (Infrequent)
Pepcid Injection Premixed
   (Infrequent)
Pepcid Tablets (Infrequent)
Percodan Tablets
Permax Tablets (Infrequent)
▲ Pexeva Tablets (1.1% to 5%)
Phenergan Tablets and Suppositories
Prevacid Delayed-Release Capsules
   (Less than 1%)
Prevacid for Delayed-Release
   Oral Suspension (Less than 1%)
Prevacid NapraPAC 375
   (Less than 1%)
Prevacid NapraPAC 500
   (Less than 1%)
Prevacid SoluTab Delayed-Release
   Orally Disintegrating Tablets
   (Less than 1%)
PREVPAC (Less than 1%)
▲ Prograf Capsules and Injection
   (3% to 15%)
Proleukin for Injection
ProQuad
Proquin XR Tablets
ProSom Tablets (Infrequent)
Provigil Tablets (1%)
Prozac Pulvules and Liquid
   (At least 2%)
Raniclor Tablets, Chewable (Rare)
Razadyne ER Extended-Release
   Capsules (Greater than or
   equal to 2%)
Razadyne Oral Solution (Greater than
   or equal to 2%)
Razadyne Tablets (Greater than or
   equal to 2%)
▲ Rebetol Capsules (5% to 8%)
▲ Rebetol Oral Solution (5% to 8%)
Recombivax HB

Relpax Tablets (Infrequent)
ReoPro Vials (0.7%)
Requip Tablets (Infrequent)
Rescriptor Tablets
Restoril Capsules (Less than 0.5%)
Reyataz Capsules (Less than 3%)
▲ Ribavirin, USP Capsules (5% to 8%)
Rilutek Tablets (Frequent)
Risperdal Consta Long-Acting
   Injection (Frequent)
▲ Risperdal M-Tab Orally Disintegrating
   Tablets (8% to 26%)
▲ Risperdal Oral Solution (8% to 26%)
▲ Risperdal Tablets (8% to 26%)
▲ Romazicon Injection (3% to 9%)
▲ Seroquel Tablets (6% to 20%)
▲ Simulect for Injection (3% to 10%)
Singulair Chewable Tablets
Singulair Oral Granules
Singulair Tablets
Sonata Capsules (Infrequent)
St. Joseph 81 mg Aspirin Chewable
   and Enteric Coated Tablets
Stalevo Tablets (1%)
Sustiva Capsules (Less than 2%)
Sustiva Tablets (Less than 2%)
Symbyax Capsules
▲ Symmetrel Tablets (1% to 5%)
Targretin Capsules
Tasmar Tablets (1%)
Tegretol Chewable Tablets
Tegretol Suspension
Tegretol Tablets
Tegretol-XR Tablets
Thalomid Capsules
Thioridazine Hydrochloride Tablets
Thiothixene Capsules
▲ Topamax Sprinkle Capsules
   (1% to 3%)
▲ Topamax Tablets (1% to 3%)
Trasylol Injection (1% to 2%)
Trileptal Oral Suspension (1% to 2%)
Trileptal Tablets (1% to 2%)
▲ Trisenox Injection (5%)
Twinrix Vaccine (Less than 1%)
▲ Ultane Liquid for Inhalation
   (7% to 15%)
Ultram ER Tablets (0.5% to less
   than 1%)
▲ Valcyte Tablets (Less than 5%)
Valtrex Caplets
▲ Vesanoid Capsules (9%)
VFEND I.V. (Less than 2%)
VFEND Oral Suspension
   (Less than 2%)

VFEND Tablets (Less than 2%)
Vicoprofen Tablets (Less than 1%)
▲ Vivitrol (8% to 12%)
▲ Wellbutrin SR Sustained-Release
  Tablets (3% to 9%)
▲ Wellbutrin Tablets (31.9%)
▲ Wellbutrin XL Extended-Release
  Tablets (2% to 9%)
Zantac 150 EFFERdose Tablets (Rare)
Zantac 150 Tablets (Rare)
Zantac 25 EFFERdose Tablets (Rare)
Zantac 300 Tablets (Rare)
Zantac Injection
Zantac Injection Pharmacy Bulk
  Package (Rare)
Zantac Injection Premixed
Zantac Syrup (Rare)
Zelapar Tablets
Zmax for Oral Suspension
▲ Zofran Injection (2% to 6%)
▲ Zofran Injection Premixed (2% to 6%)
▲ Zofran ODT Orally Disintegrating
  Tablets (6%)
▲ Zofran Oral Solution (6%)
▲ Zofran Tablets (6%)
▲ Zoloft Oral Concentrate (1% to 6%)
▲ Zoloft Tablets (1% to 6%)
▲ Zometa for Intravenous Infusion
  (12.8%)
Zomig Nasal Spray (Infrequent to
  less than 2%)
Zomig Tablets (Infrequent)
Zomig-ZMT Tablets (Infrequent)
▲ Zonegran Capsules (9%)
▲ Zosyn (2.1% to 7.1%)
Zovirax Capsules
Zovirax Suspension
Zovirax Tablets
Zyban Sustained-Release Tablets
  (Frequent)
▲ Zyprexa Tablets (23%)
▲ Zyprexa ZYDIS Orally Disintegrating
  Tablets (23%)
Zyrtec Chewable Tablets
  (Less than 2%)
Zyrtec Syrup (Less than 2%)
Zyrtec Tablets (Less than 2%)
Zyrtec-D 12 Hour Extended Release
  Tablets (Less than 2%)

Alcohol abuse

Effexor Tablets (Rare)
Effexor XR Capsules (Rare)
Paxil CR Controlled-Release Tablets
  (Infrequent)

Paxil Oral Suspension (Infrequent)
Paxil Tablets (Infrequent)
Pexeva Tablets (Infrequent)
Zyprexa Tablets (Infrequent)
Zyprexa ZYDIS Orally Disintegrating
  Tablets (Infrequent)

Antisocial reaction

Pexeva Tablets (Rare)
Prozac Pulvules and Liquid (Rare)
Zyprexa Tablets (Infrequent)
Zyprexa ZYDIS Orally Disintegrating
  Tablets (Infrequent)

Anxiety

▲ Abilify Discmelt Orally Disintegrating
  Tablets (20%)
▲ Abilify Oral Solution (20%)
▲ Abilify Tablets (20%)
Aceon Tablets (2 mg, 4 mg, 8 mg)
  (0.3% to 1%)
AcipHex Tablets
▲ Actonel Tablets (0.6% to 4.3%)
▲ Actonel with Calcium Tablets (0.6%
  to 4.7%)
Adalat CC Tablets (Less than 1%)
▲ Adderall XR Capsules (8%)
Advair HFA Inhalation Aerosol
Advicor Tablets
▲ Aerobid Inhaler System (1% to 3%)
▲ Aerobid-M Inhaler System
  (1% to 3%)
Allegra-D 12 Hour
  Extended-Release Tablets (1.4%)
Allegra-D 24 Hour
  Extended-Release Tablets (1.4%)
Aloxi Injection (1%)
Altace Capsules (Less than 1%)
Altoprev Extended-Release Tablets
▲ Ambien CR Tablets (2% to 3%)
Ambien Tablets (1%)
▲ AmBisome for Injection (7.4% to
  13.7%)
Amerge Tablets (Infrequent)
Amitiza Capsules (0% to 1.4%)
Amoxil Capsules (Rare)
Amoxil Chewable Tablets (Rare)
Amoxil Pediatric Drops for
  Oral Suspension (Rare)
Amoxil Powder for Oral Suspension
  (Rare)
Amoxil Tablets (Rare)
Anaprox DS Tablets (Less than 1%)
Anaprox Tablets (Less than 1%)
AndroGel (Fewer than 1%)

Androxy Tablets
Anzemet Injection (Infrequently)
Anzemet Tablets (Infrequently)
▲ Aredia for Injection (14.3%)
Aricept ODT Tablets (Frequent)
Aricept Tablets (Frequent)
▲ Arimidex Tablets (2% to 6%)
Arixtra Injection (0.8%)
▲ Aromasin Tablets (4.1% to 10%)
Arthrotec Tablets (Rare)
Asacol Delayed-Release Tablets
  (2% or greater)
Astelin Nasal Spray (Infrequent)
Atacand HCT 16-12.5 Tablets
  (0.5% or greater)
Atacand HCT 32-12.5 Tablets
  (0.5% or greater)
Atacand Tablets (0.5% or greater)
Atripla Tablets (Greater than or
  equal to 2%)
Augmentin Chewable Tablets (Rare)
Augmentin ES-600 Powder for
  Oral Suspension (Rare)
Augmentin Powder for
  Oral Suspension (Rare)
Augmentin Tablets (Rare)
Augmentin XR Extended-Release
  Tablets (Rare)
Avalide Tablets (1% or greater)
Avapro Tablets (Less than 1%)
Avelox I.V. (0.1% to less than 2%)
Avelox Tablets (0.1% to less than 2%)
▲ Avinza Capsules (Less than 5%)
Axert Tablets (Infrequent)
Axid Oral Solution (1.8%)
Azilect Tablets (Frequent)
▲ Betaseron for SC Injection (10%)
Biaxin Filmtab Tablets
Biaxin Granules
Biaxin XL Filmtab Tablets
Bicillin C-R Injectable Suspension
▲ BOTOX Purified Neurotoxin Complex
  (3% to 10%)
Caduet Tablets (Greater than 0.1% to
  less than or equal to 1%)
▲ Campral Tablets (5% to 8%)
Cardene SR Capsules (Rare)
Carnitor Injection (1% to 2%)
Catapres Tablets
Catapres-TTS (0.5% or less)
Celebrex Capsules (0.1% to 1.9%)
▲ Celexa Oral Solution (4%)
▲ Celexa Tablets (4%)
▲ CellCept Capsules (3% to 28.4%)
▲ CellCept Intravenous (3% to 28.4%)

▲ CellCept Oral Suspension
  (3% to 28.4%)
▲ CellCept Tablets (3% to 28.4%)
Cesamet Capsules
Chantix Tablets (Frequent)
Cipro I.V. (1% or less)
Cipro Oral Suspension
Cipro Tablets
Cipro XR Tablets
▲ Clolar for Intravenous Infusion (22%)
Clorpres Tablets
Clozaril Tablets (1%)
Colazal Capsules
Comtan Tablets (2%)
▲ Copaxone for Injection (23%)
▲ Copegus Tablets (33%)
Cosopt Sterile Ophthalmic Solution
Cozaar Tablets (Less than 1%)
Crestor Tablets (Greater than or
  equal to 1%)
Crixivan Capsules (Less than 2%)
▲ Cubicin for Injection (1% to 5%)
Cuprimine Capsules
▲ Cymbalta Delayed-Release Capsules
  (3%)
▲ Dacogen Injection (11%)
▲ DAPTACEL Vaccine
  (23.6% to 39.6%)
Demser Capsules
▲ Depacon Injection (1% to 5%)
▲ Depakene Capsules (1% to 5%)
▲ Depakene Oral Solution (1% to 5%)
▲ Depakote ER Tablets (1% to 5%)
▲ Depakote Sprinkle Capsules
  (1% to 5%)
▲ Depakote Tablets (1% to 5%)
▲ DepoDur Extended-Release Injection
  (2% to 5%)
▲ depo-subQ provera 104 Injectable
  Suspension (1% to less than 5%)
Detrol LA Capsules (1%)
Dilaudid Ampules
Dilaudid Multiple Dose Vials
Dilaudid Non-Sterile Powder
Dilaudid Rectal Suppositories
Dilaudid Tablets
Diovan HCT Tablets (Greater
  than 0.2%)
Diovan Tablets
▲ Doxil Injection (Less than 1% to 10%)
▲ Duragesic Transdermal System
  (3% to 10%)
EC-Naprosyn Delayed-Release Tablets
  (Less than 1%)
▲ Effexor Tablets (2% to 11.2%)

Effexor XR Capsules (1%)
Eldepryl Capsules (1 of 49 patients)
▲ Eloxatin for Injection (2% to 5%)
Emcyt Capsules (1%)
Emend Capsules (Greater than 0.5%)
Emsam Transdermal System
EpiPen Auto-Injector
EpiPen Jr. Auto-Injector
▲ Epogen for Injection (2% to 7%)
▲ Epzicom Tablets (3% to 5%)
▲ Equetro Extended-Release
  Capsules (7%)
Estratest H.S. Tablets
Estratest Tablets
▲ Estring Vaginal Ring (1% to 3%)
Eulexin Capsules (1%)
Evoxac Capsules (1.3%)
▲ Exelon Capsules (4% to 5%)
▲ Exelon Oral Solution (4% to 5%)
▲ Fabrazyme for Intravenous
  Infusion (8%)
▲ Faslodex Injection (5%)
FazaClo Orally Disintegrating
  Tablets (1%)
Femara Tablets (Less frequent)
Flebogamma 5%, Immune Globulin
  Intravenous (Human)
▲ Focalin XR Capsules (5% to 11%)
Foradil Aerolizer (1.5%)
Frova Tablets (Frequent)
Fuzeon Injection
Gabitril Tablets (1% or more)
Gantrisin Pediatric Suspension
Gengraf Capsules
  (1% to less than 3%)
▲ Geodon Capsules (5%)
Geodon for Injection (Up to 2%)
▲ Gleevec Tablets (0% to 12%)
Hycodan Syrup
Hycodan Tablets
Hycotuss Expectorant Syrup
Hyperstat I.V.
Hytrin Capsules (At least 1%)
Hyzaar 100-12.5 Tablets
Hyzaar 100-25 Tablets
Hyzaar 50-12.5 Tablets
▲ I.V. Busulfex (72% to 75%)
▲ Imdur Tablets (Less than or
  equal to 5%)
Imitrex Injection (Frequent)
Imitrex Nasal Spray (Infrequent)
Imitrex Tablets
▲ Indapamide Tablets (Greater than or
  equal to 5%)
Indocin Capsules (Less than 1%)

Indocin Oral Suspension
  (Less than 1%)
Indocin Suppositories (Less than 1%)
▲ Infanrix Vaccine (3.3% to 9.2%)
▲ Infergen (10% to 19%)
▲ Intron A for Injection (Up to 5%)
Invanz for Injection (0.8% to 1.1%)
▲ Invega Extended-Release Tablets (5%
  to 9%)
Invirase Capsules (Greater than or
  equal to 2%)
Invirase Tablets (Greater than or
  equal to 2%)
▲ Ionsys Transdermal System
  (1% to less than 10%)
▲ Kadian Capsules
  (Less than 3% to 6%)
Kaletra Oral Solution (Less than 2%)
Kaletra Tablets (Less than 2%)
Keppra Injection (2%)
Keppra Oral Solution (2%)
Keppra Tablets (2%)
Ketek Tablets (Less than 0.2%)
Klonopin Tablets (Infrequent)
Klonopin Wafers (Infrequent)
▲ Kytril Injection (Less than 2%
  to 3.4%)
Kytril Oral Solution (2%)
Kytril Tablets (2%)
▲ Lamictal Chewable Dispersible Tablets
  (4% to 5%)
▲ Lamictal Tablets (4% to 5%)
Lanoxicaps Capsules
Lanoxin Injection
Lanoxin Injection Pediatric
Lanoxin Tablets
Lariam Tablets (Occasional)
Lescol Capsules
Lescol XL Tablets
▲ Leukine (11%)
Levaquin in 5% Dextrose
  Injection (1.2%)
Levaquin Injection (1.2%)
Levaquin Oral Solution (1.2%)
Levaquin Tablets (1.2%)
Levothroid Tablets
Levoxyl Tablets
Lexapro Oral Suspension
  (At least 2%)
Lexapro Tablets (At least 2%)
▲ Lithostat Tablets (20%)
Lotensin Tablets (Less than 1%)
Lotrel Capsules
Lotronex Tablets (Infrequent)
Lunesta Tablets (Infrequent)

▲ Lupron Depot 3.75 mg (3%)
▲ Lupron Depot-3 Month 11.25 mg
   (Less than 5%)
Lyrica Capsules (Greater than or equal
   to 1%)
Malarone Pediatric Tablets
   (Less than 1%)
Malarone Tablets (Less than 1%)
Marinol Capsules (Greater than 1%)
Mavik Tablets (0.3% to 1.0%)
Maxair Autohaler
Maxalt Tablets (Infrequent)
Maxalt-MLT Orally Disintegrating
   Tablets (Infrequent)
▲ Mepron Suspension (7%)
▲ Meridia Capsules (4.5%)
Merrem I.V. (0.1% to 1%)
Mevacor Tablets (0.5% to 1.0%)
Miacalcin Nasal Spray (Less than 1%)
Micardis HCT Tablets
Micardis Tablets (More than 0.3%)
Migranal Nasal Spray (Rare)
Mirapex Tablets (1% or more)
Mobic Oral Suspension
   (Less than 2%)
Mobic Tablets (Less than 2%)
▲ Myfortic Tablets (3% to less than 20%)
▲ Mylotarg for Injection (7% to 10%)
Myobloc Injection (Greater than 2%)
Namenda Oral Solution (Greater than
   or equal to 2%)
Namenda Tablets (Greater than or
   equal to 2%)
Naprosyn Suspension (Less than 1%)
Naprosyn Tablets (Less than 1%)
▲ Natrecor for Injection (2% to 3%)
Nembutal Sodium Solution, USP
   (Less than 1%)
Neoral Oral Solution (1% to less
   than 3%)
Neoral Soft Gelatin Capsules
   (1% to less than 3%)
Neurontin Capsules (Frequent)
Neurontin Oral Solution (Frequent)
Neurontin Tablets (Frequent)
▲ Nipent for Injection (3% to 10%)
▲ Niravam Orally Disintegrating Tablets
   (16.6% to 19.2%)
Noroxin Tablets (Less frequent)
Norvasc Tablets (More than 0.1%
   to 1%)
Norvir Oral Solution (0% to 1.7%)
Norvir Soft Gelatin Capsules
   (0 to 1.7%)

▲ Noxafil Oral Suspension (9%)
▲ Opana ER Tablets (1% to less
   than 10%)
▲ Opana Tablets (1% to less than 10%)
Oracea Capsules (1.5%)
▲ OxyContin Tablets (Between 1%
   and 5%)
Parcopa Orally Disintegrating Tablets
Parnate Tablets
▲ Paxil CR Controlled-Release Tablets
   (1% to 5.9%)
▲ Paxil Oral Suspension (1% to 5.9%)
▲ Paxil Tablets (1% to 5.9%)
▲ Pegasys (19%)
▲ PegIntron Powder for Injection (28%)
Pepcid for Oral Suspension
   (Infrequent)
Pepcid Injection (Infrequent)
Pepcid Injection Premixed
   (Infrequent)
Pepcid Tablets (Infrequent)
Percodan Tablets
▲ Permax Tablets (6.4%)
▲ Pexeva Tablets (2% to 5.9%)
▲ Photofrin for Injection (3% to 7%)
Plavix Tablets (1% to 2.5%)
Pletal Tablets (Less than 2%)
▲ Premphase Tablets (2% to 5%)
▲ Prempro Tablets (2% to 5%)
Prevacid Delayed-Release Capsules
   (Less than 1%)
Prevacid for Delayed-Release
   Oral Suspension (Less than 1%)
Prevacid NapraPAC 375
   (Less than 1%)
Prevacid NapraPAC 500
   (Less than 1%)
Prevacid SoluTab Delayed-Release
   Orally Disintegrating Tablets
   (Less than 1%)
PREVPAC (Less than 1%)
Prezista Tablets (Less than 2%)
ProAir HFA Inhalation Aerosol
   (Less than 3%)
ProAmatine Tablets (Less frequent)
▲ Procrit for Injection (2% to 11%)
▲ Prograf Capsules and Injection
   (3% to 15%)
▲ Proleukin for Injection (12%)
▲ Prometrium Capsules (100 mg,
   200 mg) (Less than 5%)
Proquin XR Tablets
ProSom Tablets (Frequent)
Protonix I.V. (Greater than or
   equal to 1%)

Protonix Tablets (Greater than or equal to 1%)

Proventil HFA Inhalation Aerosol (Less than 3%)

▲ Provigil Tablets (5%)

▲ Prozac Pulvules and Liquid (4% to 17%)

Pulmicort Respules (Less than 1%)

▲ Rapamune Oral Solution and Tablets (3% to 20%)

Razadyne ER Extended-Release Capsules (Greater than or equal to 2%)

Razadyne Oral Solution (Greater than or equal to 2%)

Razadyne Tablets (Greater than or equal to 2%)

▲ Rebetol Capsules (47%)

▲ Rebetol Oral Solution (47%)

Relpax Tablets (Infrequent)

ReoPro Vials (1.7%)

Requip Tablets (1% or more)

▲ Rescriptor Tablets (2.4% to 6.7%)

Restoril Capsules (2%)

Retrovir Capsules

Retrovir IV Infusion

Retrovir Syrup

Retrovir Tablets

Reyataz Capsules (Less than 3%)

▲ Ribavirin, USP Capsules (47%)

Risperdal Consta Long-Acting Injection (Frequent)

▲ Risperdal M-Tab Orally Disintegrating Tablets (4% to 20%)

▲ Risperdal Oral Solution (4% to 20%)

▲ Risperdal Tablets (4% to 20%)

▲ Rituxan I.V. (1% to 5%)

▲ Romazicon Injection (3% to 9%)

▲ Rythmol SR Capsules (10% to 13%)

Sandimmune I.V. Ampuls for Infusion (Rare)

Sandimmune Oral Solution (Rare)

Sandimmune Soft Gelatin Capsules (Rare)

Sandostatin Injection (Less than 1%)

▲ Sandostatin LAR Depot (5% to 15%)

Serevent Diskus (1% to less than 3%)

▲ Seroquel Tablets (4%)

▲ Simulect for Injection (3% to 10%)

Sonata Capsules (Frequent)

Soriatane Capsules (Less than 1%)

Stalevo Tablets (2%)

Striant Mucoadhesive

▲ Suboxone Tablets (12%)

▲ Subutex Tablets (12%)

Sular Tablets (Less than or equal to 1%)

▲ Sustiva Capsules (2% to 13%)

▲ Sustiva Tablets (2% to 13%)

Symbyax Capsules

▲ Symmetrel Tablets (1% to 5%)

▲ Tambocor Tablets (1% to 3%)

▲ Tarceva Tablets (0% to 13%)

Tarka Tablets (0.3% or more)

Tasmar Tablets (1% or more)

▲ Temodar Capsules (7%)

Teveten HCT Tablets (Less than 1%)

Teveten Tablets (Less than 1%)

Thalomid Capsules

Thyrolar Tablets

Timoptic in Ocudose (Less frequent)

Timoptic Sterile Ophthalmic Solution (Less frequent)

Timoptic-XE Sterile Ophthalmic Gel Forming Solution

▲ Topamax Sprinkle Capsules (4% to 24%)

▲ Topamax Tablets (4% to 24%)

Toprol-XL Tablets

Trasylol Injection (1% to 2%)

▲ Travatan Ophthalmic Solution (1% to 5%)

▲ Travatan Z Ophthalmic Solution (1% to 5%)

Tricor Tablets

▲ Trileptal Oral Suspension (5% to 7%)

▲ Trileptal Tablets (5% to 7%)

▲ Trisenox Injection (30%)

Truvada Tablets

Tussionex Pennkinetic Extended-Release Suspension

Twinject 0.15

Twinject 0.3

▲ Ultram ER Tablets (1% to less than 5%)

Uniretic Tablets (Less than 1%)

Univasc Tablets (Less than 1%)

Vantin Tablets and Oral Suspension (Less than 1%)

▲ Velcade for Injection (14%)

▲ Vesanoid Capsules (17%)

VFEND I.V. (Less than 2%)

VFEND Oral Suspension (Less than 2%)

VFEND Tablets (Less than 2%)

Viadur Implant (Less than 2%)

Viagra Tablets

Vicodin ES Tablets

Vicodin HP Tablets

Vicodin Tablets

▲ Vicoprofen Tablets (3% to 9%)
  Viracept Oral Powder (Less than 2%)
  Viracept Tablets (Less than 2%)
▲ Viread Tablets (6%)
▲ Vivitrol (8% to 12%)
  Voltaren Tablets (Occasionally)
  Voltaren-XR Tablets (Occasionally)
  Vytorin 10/10 Tablets
  Vytorin 10/20 Tablets
  Vytorin 10/40 Tablets
  Vytorin 10/80 Tablets
▲ Wellbutrin SR Sustained-Release
  Tablets (5% to 6%)
▲ Wellbutrin Tablets (3.1%)
▲ Wellbutrin XL Extended-Release
  Tablets (5% to 7%)
▲ Xenical Capsules (2.8% to 4.4%)
  Xopenex HFA Inhalation Aerosol
  (2.7%)
  Xopenex Inhalation Solution (2.7%)
  Xopenex Inhalation Solution
  Concentrate (2.7%)
  Zegerid Capsules (Less than 1%)
  Zegerid Powder for Oral Solution
  (Less than 1%)
▲ Ziagen Oral Solution (5%)
▲ Ziagen Tablets (5%)
  Zmax for Oral Suspension
  Zocor Tablets
▲ Zofran Injection (2% to 6%)
▲ Zofran Injection Premixed (2% to 6%)
▲ Zofran ODT Orally Disintegrating
  Tablets (6%)
▲ Zofran Oral Solution (6%)
▲ Zofran Tablets (6%)
▲ Zoloft Oral Concentrate (4%)
▲ Zoloft Tablets (4%)
▲ Zometa for Intravenous Infusion (11%
  to 14%)
  Zomig Nasal Spray (Infrequent)
  Zomig Tablets (Infrequent)
  Zomig-ZMT Tablets (Infrequent)
▲ Zonegran Capsules (3%)
▲ Zosyn (1.2% to 3.2%)
▲ Zyban Sustained-Release Tablets (8%)
  Zydone Tablets
▲ Zyprexa Tablets (9%)
▲ Zyprexa ZYDIS Orally Disintegrating
  Tablets (9%)
  Zyrtec Chewable Tablets (Less
  than 2%)
  Zyrtec Syrup (Less than 2%)
  Zyrtec Tablets (Less than 2%)
  Zyrtec-D 12 Hour Extended Release
  Tablets (Less than 2%)

Anxiety, paradoxical
  Diastat Rectal Delivery System
  Valium Tablets

Apathy
  Abilify Discmelt Orally Disintegrating
  Tablets (Infrequent)
  Abilify Oral Solution (Infrequent)
  Abilify Tablets (Infrequent)
  Ambien CR Tablets (Rare)
  Ambien Tablets (Rare)
  Aricept ODT Tablets (Infrequent)
  Aricept Tablets (Infrequent)
  Azilect Tablets (Rare)
  Caduet Tablets (Less than or equal
  to 0.1%)
  Campath Ampules
  Campral Tablets (Infrequent)
  Celexa Oral Solution (Infrequent)
  Celexa Tablets (Infrequent)
  Cesamet Capsules
  Effexor Tablets (Infrequent)
  Effexor XR Capsules (Infrequent)
  Eldepryl Capsules
  Evoxac Capsules
  Exelon Capsules (Infrequent)
  Exelon Oral Solution (Infrequent)
  Fansidar Tablets
  Gabitril Tablets (Infrequent)
  Gantrisin Pediatric Suspension
  Hectorol Capsules
  Hectorol Injection
  Imitrex Injection
  Imitrex Nasal Spray (Rare)
  Imitrex Tablets (Rare)
▲ Intron A for Injection (Less than 5%)
  Kadian Capsules (Less than 3%)
  Keppra Oral Solution
  Keppra Tablets
  Klonopin Tablets (Infrequent)
  Klonopin Wafers (Infrequent)
  Lamictal Chewable Dispersible
  Tablets (Infrequent)
  Lamictal Tablets (Infrequent)
  Lanoxicaps Capsules
  Lanoxin Injection
  Lanoxin Injection Pediatric
  Lanoxin Tablets
  Lexapro Oral Suspension (Infrequent)
  Lexapro Tablets (Infrequent)
  Lunesta Tablets
  Lyrica Capsules (0.1% to 1%)
  Mirapex Tablets (1% or more)
  Namenda Oral Solution (Infrequent)

Namenda Tablets (Infrequent)
Neurontin Capsules (Infrequent)
Neurontin Oral Solution (Infrequent)
Neurontin Tablets (Infrequent)
Nexium Delayed-Release Capsules (Less than 1%)
Nexium Delayed-Release Oral Suspension (Less than 1%)
Nexium I.V. (Less than 1%)
Norvasc Tablets (Less than 0.1%)
Permax Tablets (Infrequent)
Prevacid Delayed-Release Capsules (Less than 1%)
Prevacid for Delayed-Release Oral Suspension (Less than 1%)
Prevacid NapraPAC 375 (Less than 1%)
Prevacid NapraPAC 500 (Less than 1%)
Prevacid SoluTab Delayed-Release Orally Disintegrating Tablets (Less than 1%)
PREVPAC (Less than 1%)
ProQuad
ProSom Tablets (Infrequent)
Prozac Pulvules and Liquid (Infrequent)
Razadyne ER Extended-Release Capsules (Infrequent)
Razadyne Oral Solution (Infrequent)
Razadyne Tablets (Infrequent)
Relpax Tablets (Infrequent)
Requip Tablets (Infrequent)
Rilutek Tablets (Infrequent)
Risperdal Consta Long-Acting Injection (Frequent)
Risperdal M-Tab Orally Disintegrating Tablets (Infrequent)
Risperdal Oral Solution (Infrequent)
Risperdal Tablets (Infrequent)
Rocaltrol Capsules
Rocaltrol Oral Solution
Seroquel Tablets (Infrequent)
Sonata Capsules (Frequent)
Sustiva Capsules (Less than 2%)
Sustiva Tablets (Less than 2%)
Tambocor Tablets (Less than 1%)
Tasmar Tablets (Infrequent)
▲ Topamax Sprinkle Capsules (1% to 3%)
▲ Topamax Tablets (1% to 3%)
Trileptal Oral Suspension
Trileptal Tablets
Zegerid Capsules (Less than 1%)
Zegerid Powder for Oral Solution (Less than 1%)
Zoloft Oral Concentrate (Infrequent)
Zoloft Tablets (Infrequent)
Zomig Nasal Spray (Rare)
Zomig Tablets (Rare)
Zomig-ZMT Tablets (Rare)
▲ Zyprexa Tablets (4%)
▲ Zyprexa ZYDIS Orally Disintegrating Tablets (4%)

Awareness, heightened

Demser Capsules
Imitrex Tablets (Rare)
▲ Marinol Capsules (8% to 24%)

Behavioral changes

Advair HFA Inhalation Aerosol (Very Rare)
Ambien Tablets
Amoxil Capsules (Rare)
Amoxil Chewable Tablets (Rare)
Amoxil Pediatric Drops for Oral Suspension (Rare)
Amoxil Powder for Oral Suspension (Rare)
Amoxil Tablets (Rare)
Augmentin Chewable Tablets (Rare)
Augmentin ES-600 Powder for Oral Suspension (Rare)
Augmentin Powder for Oral Suspension (Rare)
Augmentin Tablets (Rare)
Augmentin XR Extended-Release Tablets (Rare)
Biaxin Filmtab Tablets
Biaxin Granules
Biaxin XL Filmtab Tablets
Catapres Tablets
Catapres-TTS (0.5% or less)
Celexa Oral Solution
Celexa Tablets
Clorpres Tablets
Cosopt Sterile Ophthalmic Solution
Effexor Tablets
Effexor XR Capsules
Eldepryl Capsules
▲ Keppra Oral Solution (38%)
▲ Keppra Tablets (38%)
▲ Klonopin Tablets (5% to 25%)
▲ Klonopin Wafers (5% to 25%)
Lexapro Oral Suspension
Lexapro Tablets
Nadolol Tablets (6 of 1000 patients)
Neurontin Capsules

Neurontin Oral Solution
Neurontin Tablets
Paxil CR Controlled-Release Tablets
Paxil Oral Suspension
Paxil Tablets
PREVPAC
Seroquel Tablets
Thioridazine Hydrochloride Tablets
Timoptic in Ocudose (Less frequent)
Timoptic Sterile Ophthalmic Solution
  (Less frequent)
Timoptic-XE Sterile Ophthalmic Gel
  Forming Solution
Uniphyl Tablets
Valtrex Caplets
Wellbutrin SR Sustained-Release
  Tablets
Wellbutrin Tablets
Wellbutrin XL Extended-Release
  Tablets
Zoloft Oral Concentrate
Zoloft Tablets
Zyban Sustained-Release Tablets
Zyprexa Tablets
Zyprexa ZYDIS Orally Disintegrating
  Tablets

Bulimia
Paxil CR Controlled-Release Tablets
  (Rare)
Paxil Oral Suspension (Rare)
Paxil Tablets (Rare)
Pexeva Tablets (Rare)

Catatonia
Celexa Oral Solution (Rare)
Celexa Tablets (Rare)
Cosopt Sterile Ophthalmic Solution
Depacon Injection (1% or more)
Depakene Capsules (1% or more)
Depakene Oral Solution (1% or more)
Depakote ER Tablets (Greater than 1%)
Depakote Sprinkle Capsules
▲ Depakote Tablets (1% to 5%)
Effexor Tablets
Effexor XR Capsules
Inderal LA Long-Acting Capsules
InnoPran XL Capsules
Lopressor HCT 100/25 Tablets
Lopressor HCT 100/50 Tablets
Lopressor HCT 50/25 Tablets
Lopressor Injection
Lopressor Tablets
Nadolol Tablets
Phenergan Tablets and Suppositories

Relpax Tablets (Rare)
Risperdal M-Tab Orally Disintegrating
  Tablets (Infrequent)
Risperdal Oral Solution (Infrequent)
Risperdal Tablets (Infrequent)
Seroquel Tablets (Infrequent)
Timolide Tablets
Timoptic in Ocudose
Timoptic Sterile Ophthalmic Solution
Timoptic-XE Sterile Ophthalmic Gel
  Forming Solution
Toprol-XL Tablets

CNS depression
Anaprox DS Tablets (Less than 1%)
Anaprox Tablets (Less than 1%)
Cesamet Capsules
Depacon Injection
Depakene Capsules
Depakene Oral Solution
Depakote ER Tablets
Depakote Tablets
Diastat Rectal Delivery System
EC-Naprosyn Delayed-Release Tablets
  (Less than 1%)
▲ Klonopin Tablets (Most frequent)
▲ Klonopin Wafers (Most frequent)
Lamictal Chewable Dispersible
  Tablets (Infrequent)
Lamictal Tablets (Infrequent)
Lidoderm Patch
Naprosyn Suspension (Less than 1%)
Naprosyn Tablets (Less than 1%)
Nembutal Sodium Solution, USP
  (Less than 1%)
Neurontin Capsules
Neurontin Oral Solution
Neurontin Tablets
Opana ER Tablets (Less than 1%)
Opana Tablets (Less than 1%)
Prozac Pulvules and Liquid
  (Infrequent)
Rilutek Tablets (Rare)
Skelaxin Tablets
Synera Topical Patch
▲ Vesanoid Capsules (3%)

CNS reactions
Attenuvax
Clozaril Tablets
▲ Intron A for Injection (Less than 5%)
Lanoxicaps Capsules (Rare)
Lanoxin Injection
Lanoxin Injection Pediatric
Lanoxin Tablets

Lariam Tablets
▲ Leukine (11%)
▲ Nipent for Injection (1% to 11%)
Noroxin Tablets
Orthoclone OKT3 Sterile Solution
Stalevo Tablets

CNS stimulation

Adipex-P Capsules
Adipex-P Tablets
Avelox I.V.
Avelox Tablets
Axert Tablets (Infrequent)
Cafcit Injection
Cafcit Oral Solution
Cesamet Capsules
Cipro I.V.
Cipro Oral Suspension
Cipro Tablets
Cipro XR Tablets
Clarinex-D 24-Hour Extended-
  Release Tablets
Combivent Inhalation Aerosol
Effexor Tablets (Infrequent)
Effexor XR Capsules (Infrequent)
Kytril Injection (Less than 2%)
Lamictal Chewable Dispersible
  Tablets (Rare)
Lamictal Tablets (Rare)
Lidoderm Patch
Meridia Capsules (1.5%)
Noroxin Tablets
Paxil CR Controlled-Release Tablets
  (Frequent)
Paxil Oral Suspension (Frequent)
Paxil Tablets (Frequent)
Proventil HFA Inhalation Aerosol
Proventil Inhalation Aerosol
Prozac Pulvules and Liquid
  (Infrequent)
Synera Topical Patch
Ventolin HFA Inhalation Aerosol
VoSpire ER Tablets
Wellbutrin SR Sustained-Release
  Tablets (1% to 2%)
Wellbutrin XL Extended-Release
  Tablets (1% to 2%)
Zyban Sustained-Release Tablets
  (Infrequent)
Zyprexa Tablets (Infrequent)
Zyprexa ZYDIS Orally Disintegrating
  Tablets (Infrequent)
Zyrtec-D 12 Hour Extended Release
  Tablets

CNS stimulation, paradoxical

Diastat Rectal Delivery System
Niravam Orally Disintegrating Tablets
  (Rare)
Numorphan Injection

Cognitive dysfunction

Ambien Tablets (Infrequent)
Amerge Tablets (Infrequent)
Anaprox DS Tablets (Rare)
Anaprox Tablets (Rare)
EC-Naprosyn Delayed-Release Tablets
  (Rare)
Mirapex Tablets
Naprosyn Suspension (Rare)
Naprosyn Tablets (Rare)
▲ Niravam Orally Disintegrating Tablets
  (10.3% to 28.8%)
Orthoclone OKT3 Sterile Solution
Prevacid NapraPAC 375 (Less
  than 1%)
Prevacid NapraPAC 500 (Less
  than 1%)
Rescriptor Tablets
Risperdal M-Tab Orally Disintegrating
  Tablets
Risperdal Oral Solution
Risperdal Tablets
▲ Topamax Sprinkle Capsules (0%
  to 7%)
▲ Topamax Tablets (0% to 7%)
Zyvox for Oral Suspension
Zyvox Injection
Zyvox Tablets

Coma

AmBisome for Injection (Less
  common)
Anaprox DS Tablets (Less than 1%)
Anaprox Tablets (Less than 1%)
Arranon Injection (1%)
Arthrotec Tablets (Rare)
▲ Avinza Capsules (Less than 5%)
Bayer Aspirin
Bicillin C-R Injectable Suspension
Buprenex Injectable (Infrequent)
Campath Ampules
Carimune NF
Celexa Oral Solution
Celexa Tablets
Copaxone for Injection (Infrequent)
Copegus Tablets (Less than 1%)
Dalmane Capsules
Depacon Injection (Rare)
▲ Depakene Capsules (Rare)

Depakene Oral Solution (Rare)
Depakote ER Tablets (Rare)
Depakote Sprinkle Capsules (Rare)
Depakote Tablets (Rare)
EC-Naprosyn Delayed-Release Tablets (Less than 1%)
Elspar for Injection
Evoxac Capsules (Less than 1%)
Flebogamma 5%, Immune Globulin Intravenous (Human)
Fortaz Injection
Gabitril Tablets (Infrequent)
Gammagard Liquid
Gammagard S/D (Rare)
Gamunex Immune Globulin I.V., 10% (Rare)
I.V. Busulfex (One patient)
Indocin Capsules (Less than 1%)
Indocin I.V. (Less than 1%)
Indocin Oral Suspension (Less than 1%)
Indocin Suppositories (Less than 1%)
▲ Intron A for Injection (Less than 5%)
Klonopin Tablets
Klonopin Wafers
Levaquin in 5% Dextrose Injection (0.1% to 0.9%)
Levaquin Injection (0.1% to 0.9%)
Levaquin Oral Solution (0.1% to 0.9%)
Levaquin Tablets (0.1% to 0.9%)
Lexapro Oral Suspension
Lexapro Tablets
Lithobid Tablets
Lyrica Capsules (Rare)
Matulane Capsules
Maxipime for Injection
Mirapex Tablets
Namenda Oral Solution
Namenda Tablets
Naprosyn Suspension (Less than 1%)
Naprosyn Tablets (Less than 1%)
Orthoclone OKT3 Sterile Solution
Pegasys (Less than 1%)
Percodan Tablets
Permax Tablets (Infrequent)
PhosLo GelCaps
Podocon-25 Liquid
Prograf Capsules and Injection
Proleukin for Injection (1%)
Prozac Pulvules and Liquid (Rare)
ReoPro Vials (0.4%)
Requip Tablets (Infrequent)
Rilutek Tablets (Infrequent)

Risperdal M-Tab Orally Disintegrating Tablets (Rare)
Risperdal Oral Solution (Rare)
Risperdal Tablets (Rare)
Seromycin Capsules
St. Joseph 81 mg Aspirin Chewable and Enteric Coated Tablets
Stromectol Tablets
Symbyax Capsules (Infrequent)
Symmetrel Tablets
Tindamax Tablets (Rare)
▲ Trisenox Injection (5%)
Valtrex Caplets
▲ Vesanoid Capsules (3%)
VFEND I.V. (Less than 2%)
VFEND Oral Suspension (Less than 2%)
VFEND Tablets (Less than 2%)
Voltaren Tablets (Rarely)
Voltaren-XR Tablets (Rarely)
Wellbutrin SR Sustained-Release Tablets
Wellbutrin Tablets
Wellbutrin XL Extended-Release Tablets
Zoloft Oral Concentrate (Rare)
Zoloft Tablets (Rare)
Zomig Nasal Spray
Zovirax Capsules
Zovirax Suspension
Zovirax Tablets
Zyban Sustained-Release Tablets
Zyprexa Tablets (Rare)
Zyprexa ZYDIS Orally Disintegrating Tablets (Rare)

Combativeness

Orthoclone OKT3 Sterile Solution

Confusion

Abilify Discmelt Orally Disintegrating Tablets (Frequent)
Abilify Oral Solution (Frequent)
Abilify Tablets (Frequent)
AcipHex Tablets (Rare)
Actimmune (Rare)
▲ Actiq (1% to 6%)
Adalat CC Tablets (Less than 1%)
Aggrenox Capsules (1.1%)
▲ Agrylin Capsules (1% to 5%)
Aldoril Tablets
▲ Alferon N Injection (One patient to 3%)
Ambien CR Tablets (Frequent)
Ambien Tablets (Frequent)

▲ AmBisome for Injection (8.6% to 12.9%)

Amerge Tablets (Rare)

Amoxil Capsules (Rare)

Amoxil Chewable Tablets (Rare)

Amoxil Pediatric Drops for Oral Suspension (Rare)

Amoxil Powder for Oral Suspension (Rare)

Amoxil Tablets (Rare)

Anaprox DS Tablets (Less than 1%)

Anaprox Tablets (Less than 1%)

Anzemet Injection (Infrequently)

Anzemet Tablets (Infrequently)

Aricept ODT Tablets (2%)

Aricept Tablets (2%)

▲ Arimidex Tablets (2% to 5%)

▲ Arixtra Injection (1.2% to 3.1%)

▲ Aromasin Tablets (2% to 5%)

▲ Arranon Injection (0% to 8%)

Arthrotec Tablets (Rare)

Asacol Delayed-Release Tablets

Astelin Nasal Spray

Augmentin Chewable Tablets (Rare)

Augmentin ES-600 Powder for Oral Suspension (Rare)

Augmentin Powder for Oral Suspension (Rare)

Augmentin Tablets (Rare)

Augmentin XR Extended-Release Tablets (Rare)

Avalide Tablets

▲ Avastin IV (1% to 6%)

Avelox I.V. (Less than 0.1%)

Avelox Tablets (Less than 0.1%)

▲ Avinza Capsules (Less than 5%)

Axid Oral Solution (Rare)

Bayer Aspirin

Bentyl Capsules

Bentyl Injection

Bentyl Syrup

Bentyl Tablets

Betaseron for SC Injection

Biaxin Filmtab Tablets

Biaxin Granules

Biaxin XL Filmtab Tablets

Bicillin C-R Injectable Suspension

Campath Ampules

Campral Tablets (Infrequent)

Camptosar Injection (0% to 2.7%)

Captopril Tablets

Carbatrol Capsules

Cardene I.V. (Rare)

Cardene SR Capsules (Rare)

Celexa Oral Solution (Frequent)

Celexa Tablets (Frequent)

▲ CellCept Capsules (3% to less than 20%)

▲ CellCept Intravenous (3% to less than 20%)

▲ CellCept Oral Suspension (3% to less than 20%)

▲ CellCept Tablets (3% to less than 20%)

Cesamet Capsules

Cipro I.V. (1% or less)

Cipro Oral Suspension

Cipro Tablets

Cipro XR Tablets

▲ Clozaril Tablets (3%)

Copaxone for Injection (2%)

Cosopt Sterile Ophthalmic Solution

Covera-HS Tablets (Less than 2%)

Cozaar Tablets (Less than 1%)

Cubicin for Injection (1% to 2%)

▲ Dacogen Injection (12%)

Dalmane Capsules (Rare)

Dantrium Capsules (Less frequent)

Daytrana Transdermal Patch

Demser Capsules

▲ Depacon Injection (1% to 5%)

▲ Depakene Capsules (1% to 5%)

▲ Depakene Oral Solution (1% to 5%)

▲ Depakote ER Tablets (1% to 5%)

▲ Depakote Sprinkle Capsules (1% to 5%)

▲ Depakote Tablets (1% to 5%)

▲ DepoCyt Injection (4% to 14%)

Detrol LA Capsules

Diastat Rectal Delivery System (Greater than or equal to 1%)

Didronel Tablets

Diovan HCT Tablets

▲ Ditropan XL Extended-Release Tablets (2% to less than 5%)

Diuril Oral Suspension

Diuril Sodium Intravenous

Dolobid Tablets (Less than 1 in 100)

▲ Doxil Injection (1% to 10%)

▲ Duragesic Transdermal System (10% or more)

Dyazide Capsules

EC-Naprosyn Delayed-Release Tablets (Less than 1%)

Edecrin Sodium Intravenous

Edecrin Tablets

Effexor Tablets (2%)

Effexor XR Capsules (Frequent)

▲ Eldepryl Capsules (3 of 49 patients)

Elspar for Injection

Emend Capsules (Greater than 0.5%)

▲ Entocort EC Capsules (Less than 5%)
Equetro Extended-Release Capsules
Erbitux (2%)
Ery-Tab Tablets (Isolated reports)
Erythrocin Stearate Filmtab Tablets
  (Isolated reports)
Erythromycin Base Filmtab Tablets
  (Isolated reports)
Erythromycin Delayed-Release
  Capsules, USP (Isolated reports)
Eulexin Capsules (1%)
Evoxac Capsules (Less than 1%)
▲ Exelon Capsules (8%)
▲ Exelon Oral Solution (8%)
Famvir Tablets (Infrequent)
▲ FazaClo Orally Disintegrating Tablets
  (3%)
▲ Fentora Tablets (1% to 16%)
Flovent HFA 110 mcg Inhalation
  Aerosol
Flovent HFA 220 mcg Inhalation
  Aerosol
Flovent HFA 44 mcg Inhalation
  Aerosol
Flumadine Syrup (Less than 0.3%)
Flumadine Tablets (Less than 0.3%)
Frova Tablets (Infrequent)
▲ Gabitril Tablets (5%)
Garamycin Injectable
Gengraf Capsules (1% to less
  than 3%)
Geodon Capsules (Frequent)
Gleevec Tablets (Rare)
Gris-PEG Tablets (Occasional)
Guanidine Hydrochloride Tablets
Herceptin I.V. (At least one of the 958
  patients)
▲ Humira Injection (Less than 5%)
Hyperstat I.V.
Hyzaar 100-12.5 Tablets
Hyzaar 100-25 Tablets
Hyzaar 50-12.5 Tablets
▲ I.V. Busulfex (11%)
▲ Imdur Tablets (Less than or equal
  to 5%)
Imitrex Injection (Infrequent)
Imitrex Nasal Spray (Infrequent)
Imitrex Tablets (Infrequent)
Indocin Capsules (Less than 1%)
Indocin Oral Suspension (Less
  than 1%)
Indocin Suppositories (Less than 1%)
▲ Infergen (4%)
▲ Intron A for Injection (Up to 12%)
▲ Invanz for Injection (3.3% to 5.1%)

Invega Extended-Release Tablets
  (Infrequent)
Invirase Capsules (Less than 2%)
Invirase Tablets (Less than 2%)
Ionsys Transdermal System (.1% to
  less than 1%)
Kadian Capsules (Less than 3%)
Kaletra Oral Solution (Less than 2%)
Kaletra Tablets (Less than 2%)
Keflex Capsules
Keppra Injection
Keppra Oral Solution (1% to 2%)
Keppra Tablets (1% to 2%)
Klonopin Tablets (1%)
Klonopin Wafers (1%)
K-Phos Neutral Tablets
K-Phos Original (Sodium Free)
  Tablets (Less frequent)
Lamictal Chewable Dispersible
  Tablets (Frequent)
Lamictal Tablets (Frequent)
Lanoxicaps Capsules
Lanoxin Injection
Lanoxin Injection Pediatric
Lanoxin Tablets
Lariam Tablets (Occasional)
Leukeran Tablets (Rare)
Levaquin in 5% Dextrose Injection
  (0.1% to 0.9%)
Levaquin Injection (0.1% to 0.9%)
Levaquin Oral Solution (0.1% to 0.9%)
Levaquin Tablets (0.1% to 0.9%)
Lexapro Oral Suspension (Infrequent)
Lexapro Tablets (Infrequent)
Librium Capsules
Lidoderm Patch
Lithobid Tablets
Lopressor HCT 100/25 Tablets
Lopressor HCT 100/50 Tablets
Lopressor HCT 50/25 Tablets
Lopressor Injection
Lopressor Tablets
Lotronex Tablets (Rare)
Lovenox Injection (2.2%)
▲ Lunesta Tablets (0% to 3%)
Lupron Depot 3.75 mg
▲ Lyrica Capsules (1% to 7%)
Marinol Capsules (Greater than 1%)
Matulane Capsules
Maxair Autohaler
Maxalt Tablets (Infrequent)
Maxalt-MLT Orally Disintegrating
  Tablets (Infrequent)
Maxipime for Injection

▲ Megace ES Oral Suspension (1% to 3%)
Meridia Capsules
Merrem I.V. (Greater than 0.1% to 1%)
Midamor Tablets (Less than or equal to 1%)
Migranal Nasal Spray (Infrequent)
Mintezol Chewable Tablets
Mintezol Suspension
▲ Mirapex Tablets (4% to 10%)
Mobic Oral Suspension (Less than 2%)
Mobic Tablets (Less than 2%)
Moduretic Tablets (Less than or equal to 1%)
Myobloc Injection (Greater than 2%)
Nalfon Capsules (1.4%)
▲ Namenda Oral Solution (6%)
▲ Namenda Tablets (6%)
Naprosyn Suspension (Less than 1%)
Naprosyn Tablets (Less than 1%)
Natrecor for Injection (Greater than or equal to 1%)
Nembutal Sodium Solution, USP (Less than 1%)
Neoral Oral Solution (1% to less than 3%)
Neoral Soft Gelatin Capsules (1% to less than 3%)
Neumega for Injection
Neurontin Capsules
Neurontin Oral Solution
Neurontin Tablets
Nexium Delayed-Release Capsules (Less than 1%)
Nexium Delayed-Release Oral Suspension (Less than 1%)
Nexium I.V. (Less than 1%)
▲ Niravam Orally Disintegrating Tablets (5% to 10.4%)
Norflex Injection (Infrequent)
Noroxin Tablets
Norvir Oral Solution (0.6% to 0.9%)
Norvir Soft Gelatin Capsules (0.6% to 0.9%)
Numorphan Injection
▲ Ontak Vials (8%)
Opana Tablets (2.7%)
Orthoclone OKT3 Sterile Solution
▲ OxyContin Tablets (Between 1% and 5%)
Parcopa Orally Disintegrating Tablets
Parnate Tablets
Paxil CR Controlled-Release Tablets (1%)

Paxil Oral Suspension (1%)
Paxil Tablets (1%)
Pepcid for Oral Suspension (Infrequent)
Pepcid Injection (Infrequent)
Pepcid Injection Premixed (Infrequent)
Pepcid Tablets (Infrequent)
Percodan Tablets
▲ Permax Tablets (11.1%)
Pexeva Tablets (1%)
Phenergan Tablets and Suppositories
▲ Phenytek Capsules (Among most common)
PhosLo GelCaps
▲ Photofrin for Injection (8%)
Plavix Tablets
Prevacid Delayed-Release Capsules (Less than 1%)
Prevacid for Delayed-Release Oral Suspension (Less than 1%)
Prevacid NapraPAC 375 (Less than 1%)
Prevacid NapraPAC 500 (Less than 1%)
Prevacid SoluTab Delayed-Release Orally Disintegrating Tablets (Less than 1%)
▲ PREVPAC (Less than 1% to 3%)
Prezista Tablets (Less than 2%)
Primaxin I.M.
Primaxin I.V. (Less than 0.2%)
Prinivil Tablets (0.3% to 1.0%)
Prinzide Tablets
ProAmatine Tablets (Less frequent)
▲ Prograf Capsules and Injection (3% to 15%)
▲ Proleukin for Injection (34%)
▲ Prometrium Capsules (100 mg, 200 mg) (Less than 5%)
Proquin XR Tablets
ProSom Tablets (2%)
Protonix I.V. (Less than 1%)
Protonix Tablets (Less than 1%)
Provigil Tablets (1%)
Prozac Pulvules and Liquid (Frequent)
Raniclor Tablets, Chewable (Rare)
▲ Rapamune Oral Solution and Tablets (3% to 20%)
Razadyne ER Extended-Release Capsules (Greater than or equal to 2%)
Razadyne Oral Solution (Greater than or equal to 2%)
Razadyne Tablets (Greater than or equal to 2%)
Relpax Tablets (Infrequent)

Remicade for IV Injection (Greater than or equal to 0.2%)
ReoPro Vials (0.6%)
▲ Requip Tablets (5%)
Rescriptor Tablets
Restoril Capsules (1.3%)
Retrovir Capsules
Retrovir IV Infusion
Retrovir Syrup
Retrovir Tablets
Revlimid Capsules (1.7% to 2.3%)
Reyataz Capsules (Less than 3%)
Rilutek Tablets (Infrequent)
Risperdal Consta Long-Acting Injection (Infrequent)
Risperdal M-Tab Orally Disintegrating Tablets (Infrequent)
Risperdal Oral Solution (Infrequent)
Risperdal Tablets (Infrequent)
Romazicon Injection (Less than 1%)
Sandimmune I.V. Ampuls for Infusion (2% or less)
Sandimmune Oral Solution (2% or less)
Sandimmune Soft Gelatin Capsules (2% or less)
▲ Sandostatin LAR Depot (5% to 15%)
Seromycin Capsules
Seroquel Tablets (Infrequent)
Sonata Capsules (1% or less)
St. Joseph 81 mg Aspirin Chewable and Enteric Coated Tablets
Stalevo Tablets
Stromectol Tablets
Sular Tablets (Less than or equal to 1%)
Sustiva Capsules (Less than 2%)
Sustiva Tablets (Less than 2%)
Symbyax Capsules (Infrequent)
▲ Symmetrel Tablets (0.1% to 5%)
Synera Topical Patch
Tambocor Tablets (Less than 1%)
Tamiflu Capsules
Tamiflu Oral Suspension
Targretin Capsules
Tarka Tablets
▲ Tasmar Tablets (10% to 11%)
Taxotere Injection Concentrate
Tegretol Chewable Tablets
Tegretol Suspension
Tegretol Tablets
Tegretol-XR Tablets
▲ Temodar Capsules (1% to 5%)
Tessalon Capsules

Tessalon Perles
Thalomid Capsules
Timolide Tablets (Less than 1%)
Timoptic in Ocudose (Less frequent)
Timoptic Sterile Ophthalmic Solution (Less frequent)
Timoptic-XE Sterile Ophthalmic Gel Forming Solution
Tindamax Tablets (Rare)
▲ Topamax Sprinkle Capsules (2% to 14%)
▲ Topamax Tablets (2% to 14%)
Toprol-XL Tablets
Transderm Scop Transdermal Therapeutic System (Infrequent)
Tranxene T-TAB Tablets (Less common)
Tranxene-SD Half Strength Tablets (Less common)
Tranxene-SD Tablets (Less common)
▲ Trasylol Injection (4%)
Tricor Tablets
Trileptal Oral Suspension (1% to 2%)
Trileptal Tablets (1% to 2%)
▲ Trisenox Injection (5%)
Ultane Liquid for Inhalation (Less than 1%)
▲ Ultram ER Tablets (1% to greater than 5%)
Uroqid-Acid No. 2 Tablets
▲ Valcyte Tablets (Less than 5%)
Valium Tablets (Infrequent)
Valtrex Caplets
Vantin Tablets and Oral Suspension (Less than 1%)
▲ Vaprisol (3.8%)
Verelan PM Extended-Release Capsules, Controlled-Onset (2% or less)
▲ Vesanoid Capsules (14%)
VFEND I.V. (Less than 2%)
VFEND Oral Suspension (Less than 2%)
VFEND Tablets (Less than 2%)
Vicoprofen Tablets (Less than 3%)
Voltaren Tablets (Occasionally)
Voltaren-XR Tablets (Occasionally)
Wellbutrin SR Sustained-Release Tablets
▲ Wellbutrin Tablets (8.4%)
▲ Wellbutrin XL Extended-Release Tablets (8%)
▲ Xeloda Tablets (Less than 5%)
▲ Xyrem Oral Solution (Less than 1% to 5.9%)

Zantac 150 EFFERdose Tablets (Rare)
Zantac 150 Tablets (Rare)
Zantac 25 EFFERdose Tablets (Rare)
Zantac 300 Tablets (Rare)
Zantac Injection (Rare)
Zantac Injection Pharmacy Bulk
  Package (Rare)
Zantac Injection Premixed (Rare)
Zantac Syrup (Rare)
Zegerid Capsules (Less than 1%)
Zegerid Powder for Oral Solution
  (Less than 1%)
Zoloft Oral Concentrate (Infrequent)
Zoloft Tablets (Infrequent)
▲ Zometa for Intravenous Infusion (7%
  to 12.8%)
Zomig Nasal Spray (Infrequent)
▲ Zonegran Capsules (6%)
Zosyn (1.0% or less)
Zovirax Capsules
Zovirax Suspension
Zovirax Tablets
Zyban Sustained-Release Tablets
  (Infrequent)
Zyprexa IntraMuscular (Infrequent)
▲ Zyprexa Tablets (4%)
▲ Zyprexa ZYDIS Orally Disintegrating
  Tablets (4%)
Zyrtec Chewable Tablets
  (Less than 2%)
Zyrtec Syrup (Less than 2%)
Zyrtec Tablets (Less than 2%)
Zyrtec-D 12 Hour Extended Release
  Tablets (Less than 2%)

Confusion, nocturnal

Thioridazine Hydrochloride Tablets
  (Extremely rare)

Consciousness, disorders of

Amerge Tablets (Rare)
Comtan Tablets
▲ Intron A for Injection (Less than 5%)
Neoral Oral Solution
Neoral Soft Gelatin Capsules
Permax Tablets
Sandimmune I.V. Ampuls for Infusion
Sandimmune Oral Solution
Sandimmune Soft Gelatin Capsules
Symmetrel Tablets (Uncommon)
Tasmar Tablets (Four cases)
Valtrex Caplets
Zovirax Capsules
Zovirax Suspension
Zovirax Tablets

Delirium

Abilify Discmelt Orally Disintegrating
  Tablets (Infrequent)
Abilify Oral Solution (Infrequent)
Abilify Tablets (Infrequent)
AcipHex Tablets
▲ Avinza Capsules (Less than 5%)
Azilect Tablets (Rare)
Catapres Tablets
Catapres-TTS (0.5% or less)
Celexa Oral Solution
Celexa Tablets
▲ CellCept Capsules (3% to less
  than 20%)
▲ CellCept Intravenous (3% to less
  than 20%)
▲ CellCept Oral Suspension (3% to less
  than 20%)
▲ CellCept Tablets (3% to less
  than 20%)
Cipro I.V.
Cipro Oral Suspension
Cipro Tablets
Cipro XR Tablets
Clorpres Tablets
Clozaril Tablets
Effexor Tablets
Effexor XR Capsules
Evoxac Capsules
Exelon Capsules (Infrequent)
Exelon Oral Solution (Infrequent)
Famvir Tablets (Infrequent)
FazaClo Orally Disintegrating Tablets
Geodon Capsules (Frequent)
I.V. Busulfex (2%)
Lamictal Chewable Dispersible
  Tablets (Rare)
Lamictal Tablets (Rare)
Lanoxicaps Capsules
Lanoxin Injection
Lanoxin Injection Pediatric
Lanoxin Tablets
Levaquin in 5% Dextrose Injection
  (0.1% to 0.9%)
Levaquin Injection (0.1% to 0.9%)
Levaquin Oral Solution (0.1% to 0.9%)
Levaquin Tablets (0.1% to 0.9%)
Lexapro Oral Suspension
Lexapro Tablets
Lyrica Capsules (Rare)
Merrem I.V. (Greater than
  0.1% to 1%)
Mirapex Tablets
Mycamine for Injection (0.8%)

Namenda Oral Solution
(Infrequent)
Namenda Tablets (Infrequent)
Orthoclone OKT3 Sterile Solution
(Less than 1%)
Paxil CR Controlled-Release Tablets
(Rare)
Paxil Oral Suspension (Rare)
Paxil Tablets (Rare)
Pexeva Tablets (Rare)
Phenergan Tablets and Suppositories
PhosLo GelCaps
Prograf Capsules and Injection
Proquin XR Tablets
Razadyne ER Extended-Release
Capsules (Infrequent)
Razadyne Oral Solution (Infrequent)
Razadyne Tablets (Infrequent)
Requip Tablets (Infrequent)
Revlimid Capsules
Rilutek Tablets (Infrequent)
Risperdal Consta Long-Acting
Injection (Infrequent)
Risperdal M-Tab Orally Disintegrating
Tablets (Rare)
Risperdal Oral Solution (Rare)
Risperdal Tablets (Rare)
Romazicon Injection (Less than 1%)
Sanctura Tablets
Seroquel Tablets (Rare)
Symmetrel Tablets
Tamiflu Capsules
Tamiflu Oral Suspension
Tasmar Tablets (Rare)
Topamax Sprinkle Capsules
(Infrequent)
Topamax Tablets (Infrequent)
Trileptal Oral Suspension
Trileptal Tablets
VFEND I.V. (Less than 2%)
VFEND Oral Suspension
(Less than 2%)
VFEND Tablets (Less than 2%)
Vivitrol
Wellbutrin SR Sustained-Release
Tablets
Wellbutrin Tablets
Wellbutrin XL Extended-Release
Tablets
Zovirax Capsules
Zovirax Suspension
Zovirax Tablets
Zyban Sustained-Release Tablets
Zyprexa Tablets (Infrequent)

Zyprexa ZYDIS Orally Disintegrating
Tablets (Infrequent)

Delusions

Abilify Discmelt Orally Disintegrating
Tablets (Frequent)
Abilify Oral Solution (Frequent)
Abilify Tablets (Frequent)
Adderall Tablets
Ambien CR Tablets (Rare)
Ambien Tablets (Rare)
Aricept ODT Tablets (Infrequent)
Aricept Tablets (Infrequent)
Atripla Tablets
Azilect Tablets (Infrequent)
Celexa Oral Solution (Rare)
Celexa Tablets (Rare)
Clozaril Tablets (Less than 1%)
Detrol LA Capsules
Effexor Tablets (Rare)
Effexor XR Capsules (Rare)
Eldepryl Capsules
Evoxac Capsules
Exelon Capsules (2% or more)
Exelon Oral Solution (2% or more)
FazaClo Orally Disintegrating Tablets
(Less than 1%)
Gabitril Tablets (Infrequent)
Lamictal Chewable Dispersible
Tablets (Rare)
Lamictal Tablets (Rare)
Lexapro Oral Suspension
Lexapro Tablets
▲ Lupron Depot 3.75 mg (Among most
frequent)
▲ Lupron Depot-3 Month 11.25 mg
(Less than 5%)
Lyrica Capsules (Rare)
Mirapex Tablets (1%)
Namenda Oral Solution (Infrequent)
Namenda Tablets (Infrequent)
Parcopa Orally Disintegrating Tablets
Paxil CR Controlled-Release Tablets
(Rare)
Paxil Oral Suspension (Rare)
Paxil Tablets (Rare)
Permax Tablets (Infrequent)
Pexeva Tablets (Rare)
Prozac Pulvules and Liquid (Rare)
Requip Tablets (Infrequent)
Revlimid Capsules
Rilutek Tablets (Infrequent)
Risperdal Consta Long-Acting
Injection (Frequent)
Seroquel Tablets (Infrequent)

Sonata Capsules (Rare)
Stalevo Tablets
Sustiva Capsules
Sustiva Tablets
Symmetrel Tablets
Tasmar Tablets (Infrequent)
Topamax Sprinkle Capsules
   (Infrequent)
Topamax Tablets (Infrequent)
Trileptal Oral Suspension
Trileptal Tablets
Vyvanse Capsules
Wellbutrin SR Sustained-Release
   Tablets
Wellbutrin Tablets (1.2%)
Wellbutrin XL Extended-Release
   Tablets
Zoloft Oral Concentrate (Infrequent)
Zoloft Tablets (Infrequent)
Zyban Sustained-Release Tablets
Zyprexa Tablets (Frequent)

Dementia
Ambien CR Tablets (Rare)
Ambien Tablets (Rare)
Angeliq Tablets
Aricept ODT Tablets (Infrequent)
Aricept Tablets (Infrequent)
Azilect Tablets (Infrequent)
Depacon Injection (Several reports)
Depakene Capsules (Several reports)
Depakene Oral Solution
   (Several reports)
Depakote ER Tablets (Several reports)
Depakote Sprinkle Capsules
   (Several reports)
Depakote Tablets (Several reports)
Effexor Tablets (Rare)
Effexor XR Capsules (Rare)
Enjuvia Tablets
Estrasorb Topical Emulsion
Estratest H.S. Tablets (1.8%)
Estratest Tablets (1.8%)
Evoxac Capsules
Exelon Capsules (Infrequent)
Exelon Oral Solution (Infrequent)
Menostar Transdermal System
Mirapex Tablets
Parcopa Orally Disintegrating Tablets
Premarin Intravenous
Premarin Tablets
Premarin Vaginal Cream
Premphase Tablets
Prempro Tablets

Relpax Tablets (Rare)
Requip Tablets (Infrequent)
Rilutek Tablets (Rare)
Risperdal Consta Long-Acting
   Injection (Infrequent)
Rythmol SR Capsules
Stalevo Tablets
▲ Vesanoid Capsules (3%)
VFEND I.V. (Less than 2%)
VFEND Oral Suspension
   (Less than 2%)
VFEND Tablets (Less than 2%)
Zelapar Tablets
Zyprexa Tablets (Infrequent)
Zyprexa ZYDIS Orally Disintegrating
   Tablets (Infrequent)

Depersonalization
Abilify Discmelt Orally Disintegrating
   Tablets (Infrequent)
Abilify Oral Solution (Infrequent)
Abilify Tablets (Infrequent)
Ambien CR Tablets (Rare to 1%)
Ambien Tablets (Rare)
Anzemet Injection (Infrequently)
Anzemet Tablets (Infrequently)
Astelin Nasal Spray (Infrequent)
Avelox I.V. (Less than 0.1%)
Avelox Tablets (Less than 0.1%)
Betaseron for SC Injection
Biaxin Filmtab Tablets
Biaxin Granules
Biaxin XL Filmtab Tablets
Buprenex Injectable (Infrequent)
Caduet Tablets (Greater than
   0.1% to 1%)
Campral Tablets (Rare)
Celexa Oral Solution (Infrequent)
Celexa Tablets (Infrequent)
Cesamet Capsules (2%)
Cipro I.V. (1% or less)
Cipro Oral Suspension (Less than 1%)
Cipro Tablets (Less than 1%)
Cipro XR Tablets (Less than 1%)
Copaxone for Injection (Infrequent)
Duragesic Transdermal System (Less
   than 1%)
Effexor Tablets (1%)
Effexor XR Capsules (Frequent)
▲ Equetro Extended-Release Capsules
   (Less than 5%)
Evoxac Capsules (Less than 1%)
Exelon Capsules (Infrequent)
Exelon Oral Solution (Infrequent)

Frova Tablets (Infrequent)
Gabitril Tablets (Frequent)
Indocin Capsules (Less than 1%)
Indocin Oral Suspension
  (Less than 1%)
Indocin Suppositories (Less than 1%)
Keppra Oral Solution
Keppra Tablets
Klonopin Tablets (Infrequent)
Klonopin Wafers (Infrequent)
Kogenate FS
Kogenate FS with Bio-Set (1 case)
Lamictal Chewable Dispersible
  Tablets (Infrequent)
Lamictal Tablets (Infrequent)
Lexapro Oral Suspension (Infrequent)
Lexapro Tablets (Infrequent)
Lyrica Capsules (Greather than or
  equal to 1%)
Marinol Capsules (Greater than 1%)
Maxalt Tablets (Rare)
Maxalt-MLT Orally Disintegrating
  Tablets (Rare)
Namenda Oral Solution (Infrequent)
Namenda Tablets (Infrequent)
Neurontin Capsules (Infrequent)
Neurontin Oral Solution (Infrequent)
Neurontin Tablets (Infrequent)
Niravam Orally Disintegrating Tablets
Norvasc Tablets (More than
  0.1% to 1%)
OxyContin Tablets (Less than 1%)
Paxil CR Controlled-Release Tablets
  (Infrequent)
Paxil Oral Suspension (Infrequent)
Paxil Tablets (Infrequent)
▲ Pexeva Tablets (3%)
Prevacid Delayed-Release Capsules
  (Less than 1%)
Prevacid for Delayed-Release Oral
  Suspension (Less than 1%)
Prevacid NapraPAC 375 (Less
  than 1%)
Prevacid NapraPAC 500 (Less than 1%)
Prevacid SoluTab Delayed-Release
  Orally Disintegrating Tablets (Less
  than 1%)
PREVPAC
Prozac Pulvules and Liquid
  (Infrequent)
Relpax Tablets (Infrequent)
Requip Tablets (Infrequent)
Rilutek Tablets (Infrequent)
Risperdal Consta Long-Acting

Injection (Infrequent)
▲ Romazicon Injection (1% to 3%)
Seroquel Tablets (Infrequent)
Sonata Capsules (Less than
  1% to 2%)
Symbyax Capsules (Infrequent)
Tambocor Tablets (Less than 1%)
Topamax Sprinkle Capsules
  (1% to 2%)
Topamax Tablets (1% to 2%)
VFEND I.V. (Less than 2%)
VFEND Oral Suspension
  (Less than 2%)
VFEND Tablets (Less than 2%)
Wellbutrin SR Sustained-Release
  Tablets (Infrequent)
Wellbutrin Tablets (Infrequent)
Wellbutrin XL Extended-Release
  Tablets (Infrequent)
Zoloft Oral Concentrate (Infrequent)
Zoloft Tablets (Infrequent)
Zomig Nasal Spray (Infrequent)
Zyban Sustained-Release Tablets
  (Infrequent)
Zyprexa Tablets (Infrequent)
Zyprexa ZYDIS Orally Disintegrating
  Tablets (Infrequent)
Zyrtec Chewable Tablets (Less
  than 2%)
Zyrtec Syrup (Less than 2%)
Zyrtec Tablets (Less than 2%)
Zyrtec-D 12 Hour Extended Release
  Tablets (Less than 2%)

Depression
Abilify Discmelt Orally Disintegrating
  Tablets (Frequent)
Abilify Oral Solution (Frequent)
Abilify Tablets (Frequent)
Accutane Capsules
Aceon Tablets (2 mg, 4 mg, 8 mg)
  (2%)
AcipHex Tablets
▲ Actimmune (3%)
▲ Actonel Tablets (2.3% to 6.8%)
▲ Actonel with Calcium Tablets (2.3%
  to 6.8%)
Adalat CC Tablets (Less than 1%)
Adderall Tablets
Adderall XR Capsules (0.7%)
Advair Diskus 100/50
Advair Diskus 250/50
Advair Diskus 500/50
Advair HFA Inhalation Aerosol
▲ Aerobid Inhaler System (1% to 3%)

▲ Aerobid-M Inhaler System
  (1% to 3%)
▲ Agenerase Capsules (4% to 16%)
▲ Agenerase Oral Solution (4% to 16%)
▲ Agrylin Capsules (1% to 5%)
  Aldara Cream, 5%
  Aldoril Tablets
▲ Alferon N Injection (One patient
  to 3%)
▲ Alimta for Injection (Up to 14%)
  Alphagan P Ophthalmic Solution
  Altace Capsules (Less than 1%)
  Altoprev Extended-Release Tablets
  Ambien CR Tablets (1%)
  Ambien Tablets (2%)
  AmBisome for Injection (Less
  common)
  Amerge Tablets (Infrequent)
  Amitiza Capsules (0% to 1.4%)
  AndroGel (Up to 1%)
  Androxy Tablets
  Angeliq Tablets
  Aptivus Capsules (2%)
  Aricept ODT Tablets (2%)
  Aricept Tablets (2%)
▲ Arimidex Tablets (2% to 13%)
▲ Aromasin Tablets (6.2% to 13%)
▲ Arranon Injection (0% to 6%)
  Arthrotec Tablets (Rare)
  Asacol Delayed-Release Tablets
▲ Asmanex Twisthaler (11%)
  Astelin Nasal Spray (Infrequent)
  Atacand HCT 16-12.5 Tablets (0.5%
  or greater)
  Atacand HCT 32-12.5 Tablets (0.5%
  or greater)
  Atacand Tablets (0.5% or greater)
▲ Atripla Tablets (4%)
  Avalide Tablets
  Avapro Tablets (Less than 1%)
  Avelox I.V.
  Avelox Tablets
  Axert Tablets (Rare)
▲ Azilect Tablets (5%)
  Azmacort Inhalation Aerosol
  Beconase AQ Nasal Spray
▲ Betaseron for SC Injection (34%)
  Betimol Ophthalmic Solution
  Betoptic S Ophthalmic Suspension
  (Rare)
  Bravelle for Intramuscular or
  Subcutaneous Injection (2.7%)
  Caduet Tablets (Greater than 0.1% to
  less than 2%)
▲ Campath Ampules (1% to 7%)

▲ Campral Tablets (4% to 8%)
  Captopril Tablets
  Carbatrol Capsules
  Cardene SR Capsules (Rare)
  Cardizem LA Extended Release
  Tablets (Less than 2%)
▲ Carnitor Injection (5% to 6%)
  Catapres Tablets (About 1 in 100
  patients)
  Catapres-TTS (0.5% or less)
  Celebrex Capsules (0.1% to 1.9%)
  Celexa Oral Solution (Frequent)
  Celexa Tablets (Frequent)
▲ CellCept Capsules (3% to less
  than 20%)
▲ CellCept Intravenous (3% to less
  than 20%)
▲ CellCept Oral Suspension (3% to less
  than 20%)
▲ CellCept Tablets (3% to less than 20%)
▲ Cesamet Capsules (14%)
  Chantix Tablets (Frequent)
  Cipro I.V. (1% or less)
  Cipro Oral Suspension (Less than 1%)
  Cipro Tablets (Less than 1%)
  Cipro XR Tablets (Less than 1%)
▲ Climara Pro Transdermal System
  (5.7%)
▲ Climara Transdermal System
  (1% to 8%)
  Clinoril Tablets (Less than 1%)
▲ Clolar for Intravenous Infusion (11%)
  Clorpres Tablets (About 1%)
  Clozaril Tablets (1%)
  Colazal Capsules
  Concerta Extended-Release Tablets
  Copaxone for Injection (At least 2%)
▲ Copegus Tablets (20%)
  Coreg CR Extended-Release Capsules
  (1% to 3%)
▲ Coreg Tablets (Greater than
  1% to 3%)
  Cosopt Sterile Ophthalmic Solution
  (Less than 1%)
  Cozaar Tablets (Less than 1%)
  Crestor Tablets (Greater than or equal
  to 2%)
  Crixivan Capsules
  Dacogen Injection (Greater than or
  equal to 1%)
  Dalmane Capsules (Rare)
  Dantrium Capsules (Less frequent)
  Daytrana Transdermal Patch
  Decadron Tablets
  Demser Capsules

▲ Depacon Injection (4% to 5%)
▲ Depakene Capsules (5%)
▲ Depakene Oral Solution (5%)
▲ Depakote ER Tablets (4% to 5%)
▲ Depakote Sprinkle Capsules
  (4% to 5%)
▲ Depakote Tablets (1% to 5%)
▲ Depo-Provera Contraceptive Injection
  (1% to 5%)
▲ depo-subQ provera 104 Injectable
  Suspension (1% to less than 5%)
  Diastat Rectal Delivery System
  (Infrequent)
  Didronel Tablets
  Dilaudid Oral Liquid (Less frequent)
  Dilaudid Tablets - 8 mg (Less frequent)
  Dilaudid-HP Injection (Less frequent)
  Dilaudid-HP Lyophilized Powder
  250 mg (Less frequent)
  Diovan HCT Tablets (Less frequent)
  Dolobid Tablets (Less than 1 in 100)
▲ Doxil Injection (Less than 1% to 10%)
▲ Duragesic Transdermal System
  (3% to 10%)
  DynaCirc CR Tablets (0.5% to 1%)
  Effexor Tablets (1%)
▲ Effexor XR Capsules (3%)
  Eldepryl Capsules
  Eligard 30 mg (1.1%)
  Eligard 7.5 mg (Less than 2%)
  Elmiron Capsules
▲ Eloxatin for Injection (2% to 5%)
  Elspar for Injection
  Emend Capsules (Greater than 0.5%)
▲ Emtriva Capsules (6% to 9%)
▲ Emtriva Oral Solution (6% to 9%)
  Enbrel for Injection (Infrequent)
  Enjuvia Tablets
▲ Epzicom Tablets (7%)
▲ Equetro Extended-Release Capsules
  (7%)
▲ Erbitux (7% to 10%)
  Estrasorb Topical Emulsion
  Estratest H.S. Tablets
  Estratest Tablets
  Estring Vaginal Ring
  Eulexin Capsules (1%)
▲ Evista Tablets (6.4%)
▲ Evoxac Capsules (1% to 3%)
▲ Exelon Capsules (6%)
▲ Exelon Oral Solution (6%)
▲ Fabrazyme for Intravenous Infusion
  (3%)
  Fansidar Tablets
▲ Faslodex Injection (5.7%)

FazaClo Orally Disintegrating Tablets
  (1%)
Femara Tablets (Less frequent)
▲ Fentora Tablets (3% to 11%)
  Flovent Diskus 100 mcg
  Flovent Diskus 250 mcg
  Flovent Diskus 50 mcg
  Flovent HFA 110 mcg Inhalation
    Aerosol
  Flovent HFA 220 mcg Inhalation
    Aerosol
  Flovent HFA 44 mcg Inhalation
    Aerosol
  Flumadine Syrup (0.3% to 1%)
  Flumadine Tablets (0.3% to 1%)
  Focalin Tablets
  Focalin XR Capsules
▲ Forteo for Injection (4.1%)
  Frova Tablets (Infrequent)
  Fuzeon Injection
▲ Gabitril Tablets (3%)
  Gantrisin Pediatric Suspension
  Garamycin Injectable
  Gengraf Capsules (Rare)
  Geodon Capsules
▲ Gleevec Tablets (0.5% to 12.7%)
▲ Hectorol Capsules (Greater than or
    equal to 5%)
▲ Herceptin I.V. (6%)
  Hydrocortone Tablets
  Hytrin Tablets (0.3%)
  Hyzaar 100-12.5 Tablets
  Hyzaar 100-25 Tablets
  Hyzaar 50-12.5 Tablets
▲ I.V. Busulfex (23%)
▲ Imdur Tablets (Less than
    or equal to 5%)
  Imitrex Injection (Rare)
  Imitrex Nasal Spray (Infrequent)
  Imitrex Tablets (Infrequent)
▲ Indapamide Tablets (Less than 5%)
  Inderal LA Long-Acting Capsules
  Indocin Capsules (Greater than 1%)
  Indocin Oral Suspension (Greater
    than 1%)
  Indocin Suppositories (Greater
    than 1%)
▲ Infergen (18% to 26%)
  InnoPran XL Capsules
▲ Intron A for Injection (2% to 40%)
  Invanz for Injection (Greater than 0.1%)
  Invirase Capsules (Greater than or
    equal to 2%)
  Invirase Tablets (Greater than or equal
    to 2%)

Kadian Capsules (Less than 3%)
Kaletra Oral Solution (Up to 2%)
Kaletra Tablets (0% to 2%)
▲ Keppra Injection (4%)
▲ Keppra Oral Solution (3% to 5%)
▲ Keppra Tablets (3% to 5%)
▲ Klonopin Tablets (4% to 7%)
▲ Klonopin Wafers (4% to 7%)
▲ Lamictal Chewable Dispersible Tablets (Greater than 1% to less than 5%)
▲ Lamictal Tablets (Greater than 1% to less than 5%)
Lanoxicaps Capsules
Lanoxin Injection
Lanoxin Injection Pediatric
Lanoxin Tablets
Lariam Tablets (Occasional)
Lescol Capsules
Lescol XL Tablets
Levaquin in 5% Dextrose Injection (0.1% to 0.9%)
Levaquin Injection (0.1% to 0.9%)
Levaquin Oral Solution (0.1% to 0.9%)
Levaquin Tablets (0.1% to 0.9%)
Lexapro Oral Suspension (Infrequent)
Lexapro Tablets (Infrequent)
▲ Lexiva Tablets (Less than 1% to 11%)
Lipitor Tablets (Less than 2%)
▲ Lithostat Tablets (20%)
▲ Lopressor HCT 100/25 Tablets (5%)
▲ Lopressor HCT 100/50 Tablets (5%)
▲ Lopressor HCT 50/25 Tablets (5%)
▲ Lopressor Injection (5%)
▲ Lopressor Tablets (5%)
Lotronex Tablets (2%)
▲ Lunesta Tablets (1% to 4%)
▲ Lupron Depot 3.75 mg (16%)
▲ Lupron Depot-3 Month 11.25 mg (16%)
Malarone Pediatric Tablets (Less than 1%)
Malarone Tablets (Less than 1%)
Marinol Capsules (Less than 1%)
Matulane Capsules
Maxair Autohaler
Maxalt Tablets (Infrequent)
Maxalt-MLT Orally Disintegrating Tablets (Infrequent)
▲ Megace ES Oral Suspension (1% to 3%)
Menostar Transdermal System
▲ Meridia Capsules (4.3%)
Merrem I.V. (Greater than 0.1% to 1%)
Metadate CD Capsules

MetroGel-Vaginal Gel (Less than 1%)
Mevacor Tablets (0.5% to 1.0%)
▲ Miacalcin Nasal Spray (1% to 3%)
Micardis HCT Tablets
Micardis Tablets (More than 0.3%)
Midamor Tablets (Less than or equal to 1%)
Migranal Nasal Spray (Rare)
Mintezol Chewable Tablets
Mintezol Suspension
Mirapex Tablets (1% or more)
Mircette Tablets
▲ Mirena Intrauterine System (5% or more)
Moban Tablets (Less frequent)
Mobic Oral Suspension (Less than 2%)
Mobic Tablets (Less than 2%)
Moduretic Tablets (Less than or equal to 1%)
MS Contin Tablets (Less frequent)
▲ Myfortic Tablets (3% to less than 20%)
▲ Mylotarg for Injection (8% to 10%)
Nadolol Tablets
Nalfon Capsules (Less than 1%)
Namenda Oral Solution (Greater than or equal to 2%)
Namenda Tablets (Greater than or equal to 2%)
Neoral Oral Solution (1%)
Neoral Soft Gelatin Capsules (1%)
Neurontin Capsules (1.8%)
Neurontin Oral Solution (1.8%)
Neurontin Tablets (1.8%)
▲ Nexavar Tablets (Common)
Nexium Delayed-Release Capsules
Nexium Delayed-Release Oral Suspension
Nexium I.V. (Rare)
Nimotop Capsules (Up to 1.4%)
▲ Nipent for Injection (3% to 10%)
▲ Niravam Orally Disintegrating Tablets (5.1% to 13.9%)
Noroxin Tablets (Less frequent)
Norvasc Tablets (0.1% to 1%)
Norvir Oral Solution (1.7%)
Norvir Soft Gelatin Capsules (1.7%)
Numorphan Injection
NuvaRing
Omacor Capsules
Opana ER Tablets (Less than 1%)
Opana Tablets (Less than 1%)

Oramorph SR Tablets
(Less frequent)
Ortho Evra Transdermal System
Ortho Tri-Cyclen Lo Tablets
Ortho Tri-Cyclen Tablets
Ortho-Cyclen Tablets
Oxandrin Tablets
Oxsoralen-Ultra Capsules
OxyContin Tablets (Less than 1%)
Parcopa Orally Disintegrating Tablets
Paxil CR Controlled-Release Tablets
(Frequent)
Paxil Oral Suspension (Frequent)
Paxil Tablets (Frequent)
▲ Pegasys (18%)
▲ PegIntron Powder for Injection
(1% to 29%)
Pentasa Capsules (Less than 1%)
Pepcid for Oral Suspension
(Infrequent)
Pepcid Injection (Infrequent)
Pepcid Injection Premixed
(Infrequent)
Pepcid Tablets (Infrequent)
Percodan Tablets
▲ Permax Tablets (3.2%)
▲ Plavix Tablets (3.6%)
Premarin Intravenous
▲ Premarin Tablets (5% to 8%)
Premarin Vaginal Cream
▲ Premphase Tablets (6% to 11%)
▲ Prempro Tablets (6% to 11%)
Prevacid Delayed-Release Capsules
(Less than 1%)
Prevacid for Delayed-Release Oral
Suspension (Less than 1%)
Prevacid NapraPAC 375
(Less than 1%)
Prevacid NapraPAC 500
(Less than 1%)
Prevacid SoluTab Delayed-Release
Orally Disintegrating Tablets (Less
than 1%)
PREVPAC (Less than 1%)
Prinivil Tablets (Greater than 1%)
Prinzide Tablets (0.3% to 1%)
▲ Prochieve 4% Gel (8% to 11%)
▲ Prochieve 8% Gel (8% to 11%)
▲ Prograf Capsules and Injection
(3% to 15%)
Proleukin for Injection (Less than 1%)
▲ Prometrium Capsules (100 mg, 200 mg)
(5% to 19%)
Proquin XR Tablets
ProSom Tablets (2%)

Protonix I.V. (Less than 1%)
Protonix Tablets (Less than 1%)
Protopic Ointment (Greater than or
equal to 1% to 2%)
Proventil HFA Inhalation Aerosol
(Less than 3%)
Provigil Tablets (2%)
Prozac Pulvules and Liquid
Pulmicort Respules (Less than 1%)
▲ Rapamune Oral Solution and Tablets
(3% to 20%)
▲ Razadyne ER Extended-Release
Capsules (7%)
▲ Razadyne Oral Solution (7%)
▲ Razadyne Tablets (7%)
▲ Rebetol Capsules (13% to 36%)
▲ Rebetol Oral Solution (13% to 36%)
▲ Rebetron Combination Therapy (23%
to 36%)
▲ Rebif Prefilled Syringe for Injection
(25%)
Relpax Tablets (Infrequent)
Requip Tablets (1% or more)
Restoril Capsules (1.7%)
Retrovir Capsules
Retrovir IV Infusion
Retrovir Syrup
Retrovir Tablets
▲ Revlimid Capsules (0.3% to 5.4%)
▲ Reyataz Capsules (3% to 8%)
▲ Ribavirin, USP Capsules
(13% to 36%)
▲ Rilutek Tablets (4.2% to 6.1%)
Risperdal Consta Long-Acting
Injection (Frequent)
Risperdal M-Tab Orally Disintegrating
Tablets (Infrequent)
Risperdal Oral Solution (Infrequent)
Risperdal Tablets (Infrequent)
Ritalin Hydrochloride Tablets
Ritalin LA Capsules
Ritalin-SR Tablets
▲ Romazicon Injection (1% to 3%)
Rozerem Tablets (2%)
▲ Rythmol SR Capsules (1% to 3%)
Sandimmune I.V. Ampuls for Infusion
(Rare)
Sandimmune Oral Solution (Rare)
Sandimmune Soft Gelatin Capsules
(Rare)
▲ Sandostatin Injection (1% to 4%)
▲ Sandostatin LAR Depot (5% to 15%)
Seasonique Tablets
▲ Simulect for Injection (3% to 10%)
Singulair Chewable Tablets

Singulair Oral Granules
Singulair Tablets
Soltamox Oral Solution (2%)
Sonata Capsules (Frequent)
▲ Soriatane Capsules (1% to 10%)
▲ Spiriva HandiHaler (1% to 3%)
Stalevo Tablets
▲ Strattera Capsules (2% to 6%)
Striant Mucoadhesive
▲ Suboxone Tablets (11%)
▲ Subutex Tablets (11%)
Sular Tablets (Less than or
equal to 1%)
▲ Sustiva Capsules (2% to 19%)
▲ Sustiva Tablets (2% to 19%)
▲ Symmetrel Tablets (1% to 5%)
▲ Tambocor Tablets (1% to 3%)
▲ Tarceva Tablets (0% to 19%)
Targretin Capsules
Tasmar Tablets (Frequent)
Tegretol Chewable Tablets
Tegretol Suspension
Tegretol Tablets
▲ Temodar Capsules (6%)
Testim 1% Gel
Teveten HCT Tablets (Less than 1%)
Teveten Tablets (1%)
Thalomid Capsules
Thyrolar Tablets
Tiazac Capsules (Less than 2%)
Timolide Tablets
Timoptic in Ocudose (Less frequent)
Timoptic Sterile Ophthalmic Solution
(Less frequent)
Timoptic-XE Sterile Ophthalmic Gel
Forming Solution
Tindamax Tablets (Rare)
▲ Topamax Sprinkle Capsules
(1% to 13%)
▲ Topamax Tablets (1% to 13%)
▲ Toprol-XL Tablets (About 5 of 100
patients)
Tranxene T-TAB Tablets
Tranxene-SD Half Strength Tablets
Tranxene-SD Tablets
▲ Travatan Ophthalmic Solution
(1% to 5%)
▲ Travatan Z Ophthalmic Solution
(1% to 5%)
Trecator Tablets
Tricor Tablets
▲ Trisenox Injection (20%)
▲ Trizivir Tablets (9%)
▲ Truvada Tablets (4%)
▲ Ultram ER Tablets (1% to less than 5%)

Uniretic Tablets (Less than 1%)
▲ Valcyte Tablets (Less than 5%)
Valium Tablets (Infrequent)
▲ Valtrex Caplets (Less than 1% to 7%)
Vantas (Less than 2%)
Veramyst Nasal Spray
▲ Vesanoid Capsules (14%)
VESIcare Tablets (0.8% to 1.2%)
VFEND I.V. (Less than 2%)
VFEND Oral Suspension
(Less than 2%)
VFEND Tablets (Less than 2%)
▲ Viadur Implant (5.3%)
Viagra Tablets (Less than 2%)
Vicoprofen Tablets (Less than 1%)
Viracept Oral Powder (Less than 2%)
Viracept Tablets (Less than 2%)
▲ Viread Tablets (4% to 11%)
▲ Vivitrol (3% to 8%)
Voltaren Tablets (Occasionally)
Voltaren-XR Tablets (Occasionally)
Vytorin 10/10 Tablets
Vytorin 10/20 Tablets
Vytorin 10/40 Tablets
Vytorin 10/80 Tablets
Vyvanse Capsules
Wellbutrin SR Sustained-Release
Tablets
Wellbutrin Tablets (Frequent)
Wellbutrin XL Extended-Release
Tablets
▲ Xeloda Tablets (Less than 5%)
▲ Xenical Capsules (3.4%)
▲ Xyrem Oral Solution (5.9%)
Yasmin 28 Tablets (Greater than 1%)
YAZ Tablets (Greater than 1%)
Zantac 150 EFFERdose Tablets
(Rare)
Zantac 150 Tablets (Rare)
Zantac 25 EFFERdose Tablets (Rare)
Zantac 300 Tablets (Rare)
Zantac Injection (Rare)
Zantac Injection Pharmacy Bulk
Package (Rare)
Zantac Injection Premixed (Rare)
Zantac Syrup (Rare)
Zegerid Capsules (Less than 1%)
Zegerid Powder for Oral Solution
(Less than 1%)
Zelapar Tablets (2%)
Zocor Tablets
Zoloft Oral Concentrate (Infrequent)
Zoloft Tablets (Infrequent)
▲ Zometa for Intravenous Infusion (14%)

Zomig Nasal Spray (Infrequent)
Zomig Tablets (Infrequent)
Zomig-ZMT Tablets (Infrequent)
▲ Zonegran Capsules (6%)
Zostavax Injection (9%)
Zosyn (1.0% or less)
Zyban Sustained-Release Tablets
(Frequent)
▲ Zyprexa Tablets (18%)
▲ Zyprexa ZYDIS Orally Disintegrating
Tablets (18%)
Zyrtec Chewable Tablets
(Less than 2%)
Zyrtec Syrup (Less than 2%)
Zyrtec Tablets (Less than 2%)
Zyrtec-D 12 Hour Extended Release
Tablets (Less than 2%)

Depression, aggravation of

Celexa Oral Solution (Frequent)
Celexa Tablets (Frequent)
Coreg CR Extended-Release Capsules
(0.1% to less than or equal to 1%)
Coreg Tablets (0.1% to 1%)
Evoxac Capsules (Less than 1%)
Frova Tablets (Rare)
▲ Intron A for Injection (Less than 5%)
Lexapro Oral Suspension (Infrequent)
Lexapro Tablets (Infrequent)
Lupron Depot 3.75 mg
Lupron Depot-3 Month 11.25 mg
(Possible)
Meridia Capsules
Nexium Delayed-Release Capsules
(Less than 1%)
Nexium Delayed-Release Oral
Suspension (Less than 1%)
Nexium I.V. (Less than 1%)
Sustiva Capsules (Less than 2%)
Sustiva Tablets (Less than 2%)
Tegretol-XR Tablets
Wellbutrin SR Sustained-Release
Tablets
Wellbutrin Tablets
Wellbutrin XL Extended-Release
Tablets
Ziagen Oral Solution (5 patients)
Ziagen Tablets (5 patients)
Zoloft Oral Concentrate (Infrequent)
Zoloft Tablets (Infrequent)

Depression, psychotic

Azilect Tablets (Rare)
Celexa Oral Solution (Infrequent)
Celexa Tablets (Infrequent)

Copaxone for Injection (Infrequent)
Effexor Tablets (Rare)
Effexor XR Capsules (Infrequent)
Lyrica Capsules (Rare)
Paxil CR Controlled-Release Tablets
(Rare)
Paxil Oral Suspension (Rare)
Paxil Tablets (Rare)
Pexeva Tablets (Rare)
Relpax Tablets (Rare)
Rilutek Tablets (Rare)
Risperdal Consta Long-Acting
Injection (Infrequent)

Depressive reactions

▲ Combivir Tablets (9%)
▲ Epivir Oral Solution (9%)
▲ Epivir Tablets (9%)
▲ Rescriptor Tablets (4.9% to 12.6%)
Truvada Tablets
▲ Ziagen Oral Solution (6%)
▲ Ziagen Tablets (6%)

Diplopia

Abelcet Injection
Abilify Discmelt Orally Disintegrating
Tablets (Rare)
Abilify Oral Solution (Rare)
Abilify Tablets (Rare)
AcipHex Tablets
Adalat CC Tablets (Less than 1%)
▲ Agrylin Capsules (1% to 5%)
Ambien CR Tablets (Frequent)
Ambien Tablets (Frequent)
Arthrotec Tablets (Rare)
Axert Tablets (Rare)
Azopt Ophthalmic Suspension (Less
than 1%)
Bentyl Capsules
Bentyl Injection
Bentyl Syrup
Bentyl Tablets
Betimol Ophthalmic Solution
BOTOX Purified Neurotoxin
Complex (Rare)
Buprenex Injectable (Less than 1%)
Caduet Tablets (Greater than 0.1% to
less than or equal to 1%)
Campral Tablets (Rare)
Carbatrol Capsules
Celexa Oral Solution (Rare)
Celexa Tablets (Rare)
Cipro I.V. (1% or less)
Cipro Oral Suspension (Less than 1%)
Cipro Tablets (Less than 1%)

Cipro XR Tablets (Less than 1%)
Copaxone for Injection (At least 2%)
Cosopt Sterile Ophthalmic Solution
Cymbalta Delayed-Release Capsules
 (Infrequent)
Dantrium Capsules (Less frequent)
▲ Depacon Injection (16%)
▲ Depakene Capsules (16%)
▲ Depakene Oral Solution (16%)
▲ Depakote ER Tablets (16%)
▲ Depakote Sprinkle Capsules (16%)
▲ Depakote Tablets (1% to 16%)
Dilaudid Ampules
Dilaudid Multiple Dose Vials
Dilaudid Non-Sterile Powder
Dilaudid Oral Liquid (Less frequent)
Dilaudid Rectal Suppositories
Dilaudid Tablets
Dilaudid Tablets - 8 mg (Less
 frequent)
Dilaudid-HP Injection (Less frequent)
Dilaudid-HP Lyophilized Powder
 250 mg (Less frequent)
Effexor Tablets (Infrequent)
Effexor XR Capsules (Infrequent)
Eldepryl Capsules
▲ Equetro Extended-Release Capsules
 (Less than 5%)
Evoxac Capsules (Less than 1%)
Exelon Capsules (Infrequent)
Exelon Oral Solution (Infrequent)
Gabitril Tablets (1% or more)
Geodon Capsules (Frequent)
Indocin Capsules (Less than 1%)
Indocin Oral Suspension (Less than 1%)
Indocin Suppositories (Less than 1%)
▲ Intron A for Injection (Less than 5%)
Kadian Capsules (Less than 3%)
Keppra Injection (2%)
Keppra Oral Solution (2%)
Keppra Tablets (2%)
Ketek Tablets (0.2% to less than 2%)
Klonopin Tablets (Infrequent)
Klonopin Wafers (Infrequent)
▲ Lamictal Chewable Dispersible Tablets
 (5% to 49%)
▲ Lamictal Tablets (5% to 49%)
Levaquin in 5% Dextrose Injection
Levaquin Injection
Levaquin Oral Solution
Levaquin Tablets
Lexapro Oral Suspension
Lexapro Tablets
Lidoderm Patch
▲ Lyrica Capsules (2% to 12%)

Matulane Capsules
Mirapex Tablets (1% or more)
MS Contin Tablets (Less frequent)
Nalfon Capsules (Less than 1%)
Namenda Oral Solution (Infrequent)
Namenda Tablets (Infrequent)
▲ Neurontin Capsules (1.2% to 5.9%)
▲ Neurontin Oral Solution (1.2 to 5.9%)
▲ Neurontin Tablets (1.2% to 5.9%)
Niravam Orally Disintegrating Tablets
Noroxin Tablets
Norvasc Tablets (0.1% to 1%)
Norvir Oral Solution (Less than 2%)
Norvir Soft Gelatin Capsules (Less
 than 2%)
Numorphan Injection
Oramorph SR Tablets (Less frequent)
Ortho Tri-Cyclen Lo Tablets
Ortho Tri-Cyclen Tablets (Rare)
Orthoclone OKT3 Sterile Solution
Ortho-Cyclen Tablets (Rare)
Parcopa Orally Disintegrating Tablets
Paxil CR Controlled-Release Tablets
 (Rare)
Paxil Oral Suspension (Rare)
Paxil Tablets (Rare)
Permax Tablets (2.1%)
Pexeva Tablets (Rare)
Phenergan Tablets and Suppositories
Photofrin for Injection
Pletal Tablets (Less than 2%)
Premphase Tablets
Prempro Tablets
Prevacid Delayed-Release Capsules
 (Less than 1%)
Prevacid for Delayed-Release Oral
 Suspension (Less than 1%)
Prevacid NapraPAC 375
 (Less than 1%)
Prevacid NapraPAC 500
 (Less than 1%)
Prevacid SoluTab Delayed-Release
 Orally Disintegrating Tablets
 (Less than 1%)
PREVPAC (Less than 1%)
Prinivil Tablets (0.3% to 1.0%)
Prinzide Tablets
Proquin XR Tablets
ProSom Tablets (Rare)
Protonix I.V. (Less than 1%)
Protonix Tablets (Less than 1%)
Prozac Pulvules and Liquid (Rare)
Relpax Tablets (Rare)
ReoPro Vials (0.1%)

Requip Tablets (2%)
Rescriptor Tablets
Rilutek Tablets (Rare)
Risperdal M-Tab Orally Disintegrating
  Tablets (Rare)
Risperdal Oral Solution (Rare)
Risperdal Tablets (Rare)
▲ Romazicon Injection (1% to 3%)
Sonata Capsules (Infrequent)
▲ Soriatane Capsules (1% to 5%)
Stalevo Tablets
Sustiva Capsules (Less than 2%)
Sustiva Tablets (Less than 2%)
Symbyax Capsules (Infrequent)
Synera Topical Patch
▲ Tambocor Tablets (1% to 3%)
Tasmar Tablets (Infrequent)
Tegretol Chewable Tablets
Tegretol Suspension
Tegretol Tablets
Tegretol-XR Tablets
▲ Temodar Capsules (5%)
Thalomid Capsules
Timolide Tablets
Timoptic in Ocudose (Less frequent)
Timoptic Sterile Ophthalmic Solution
  (Less frequent)
Timoptic-XE Sterile Ophthalmic Gel
  Forming Solution
▲ Topamax Sprinkle Capsules (1% to 10%)
▲ Topamax Tablets (1% to 10%)
Tranxene T-TAB Tablets
Tranxene-SD Half Strength Tablets
Tranxene-SD Tablets
Trecator Tablets
▲ Trileptal Oral Suspension
  (5% to 40%)
▲ Trileptal Tablets (5% to 40%)
Valium Tablets (Infrequent)
VFEND I.V. (Less than 2%)
VFEND Oral Suspension
  (Less than 2%)
VFEND Tablets (Less than 2%)
Viagra Tablets
▲ Visudyne for Injection (1% to 10%)
▲ Wellbutrin SR Sustained-Release
  Tablets (2% to 3%)
Wellbutrin Tablets (Rare)
▲ Wellbutrin XL Extended-Release
  Tablets (2% to 3%)
Xalatan Sterile Ophthalmic Solution
  (Less than 1%)
Zegerid Capsules (Less than 1%)
Zegerid Powder for Oral Solution
  (Less than 1%)

Zelapar Tablets
Zoloft Oral Concentrate (Rare)
Zoloft Tablets (Rare)
Zomig Tablets (Rare)
Zomig-ZMT Tablets (Rare)
▲ Zonegran Capsules (6%)
Zyban Sustained-Release Tablets
  (Frequent)
Zyprexa Tablets (Infrequent)
Zyprexa ZYDIS Orally Disintegrating
  Tablets (Infrequent)

Disorientation
AcipHex Tablets
Actimmune (Rare)
Alferon N Injection (1%)
▲ Ambien CR Tablets (3%)
Arthrotec Tablets (Rare)
Asacol Delayed-Release Tablets
Biaxin Filmtab Tablets
Biaxin Granules
Biaxin XL Filmtab Tablets
BiDil Tablets
BOTOX Purified Neurotoxin
  Complex
Cesamet Capsules (2%)
Chantix Tablets (Infrequent)
Cosopt Sterile Ophthalmic Solution
Dalmane Capsules
Demser Capsules
Detrol LA Capsules
Dilaudid Ampules
Dilaudid Multiple Dose Vials
Dilaudid Non-Sterile Powder
Dilaudid Oral Liquid (Less frequent)
Dilaudid Rectal Suppositories
Dilaudid Tablets
Dilaudid Tablets - 8 mg (Less frequent)
Dilaudid-HP Injection (Less frequent)
Dilaudid-HP Lyophilized Powder
  250 mg (Less frequent)
Dolobid Tablets (Less than 1 in 100)
Eldepryl Capsules
Emend Capsules (Isolated cases)
Famvir Tablets (Infrequent)
Fentora Tablets (Greater than 1%)
Gantrisin Pediatric Suspension
Infed Injection
▲ Invanz for Injection (3.3% to 5.1%)
Lexapro Oral Suspension (Infrequent)
Lexapro Tablets (Infrequent)
Lidoderm Patch
Lopressor HCT 100/25 Tablets
Lopressor HCT 100/50 Tablets

Lopressor HCT 50/25 Tablets
Lopressor Injection
Lopressor Tablets
Maxalt Tablets (Infrequent)
Maxalt-MLT Orally Disintegrating
  Tablets (Infrequent)
Mirapex Tablets
MS Contin Tablets (Less frequent)
Nalfon Capsules (Less than 1%)
Opana ER Tablets (Less than 1%)
Opana Tablets (Less than 1%)
Oramorph SR Tablets (Less frequent)
Orthoclone OKT3 Sterile Solution
Parcopa Orally Disintegrating Tablets
Parnate Tablets
Phenergan Tablets and Suppositories
PREVPAC
Prezista Tablets (Less than 2%)
Rescriptor Tablets
Seromycin Capsules
Stalevo Tablets
Timoptic in Ocudose (Less frequent)
Timoptic Sterile Ophthalmic Solution
  (Less frequent)
Timoptic-XE Sterile Ophthalmic Gel
  Forming Solution
Transderm Scop Transdermal
  Therapeutic System (Infrequent)
▲ Ultram ER Tablets (0.5% to
  less than 1%)
▲ Xyrem Oral Solution (2.9% to 8.6%)

Disorientation, place

Cosopt Sterile Ophthalmic Solution
Inderal LA Long-Acting Capsules
InnoPran XL Capsules
Nadolol Tablets
Timolide Tablets
Timoptic in Ocudose
Timoptic Sterile Ophthalmic Solution
Timoptic-XE Sterile Ophthalmic Gel
  Forming Solution
Toprol-XL Tablets

Disorientation, time

Cosopt Sterile Ophthalmic Solution
Inderal LA Long-Acting Capsules
InnoPran XL Capsules
Nadolol Tablets
Timolide Tablets
Timoptic in Ocudose
Timoptic Sterile Ophthalmic Solution
Timoptic-XE Sterile Ophthalmic Gel
  Forming Solution
Toprol-XL Tablets

Dreaming

Amerge Tablets (Rare)
Dilaudid Oral Liquid (Less frequent)
Dilaudid Tablets - 8 mg (Less
  frequent)
▲ Malarone Pediatric Tablets (2% to 7%)
▲ Malarone Tablets (2% to 7%)
MS Contin Tablets (Less frequent)
Oramorph SR Tablets (Less frequent)

Dreaming abnormalities

Abilify Discmelt Orally Disintegrating
  Tablets (Frequent)
Abilify Oral Solution (Frequent)
Abilify Tablets (Frequent)
AcipHex Tablets
Actiq (Less than 1%)
Ambien CR Tablets (Infrequent)
Ambien Tablets (1%)
Anaprox DS Tablets (Less than 1%)
Anaprox Tablets (Less than 1%)
Anzemet Injection (Infrequently)
Anzemet Tablets (Infrequently)
Aricept ODT Tablets (Infrequent)
Aricept Tablets (Infrequent)
Arthrotec Tablets (Rare)
▲ Atripla Tablets (4%)
Avelox I.V. (Less than 0.1%)
Avelox Tablets (Less than 0.1%)
▲ Avinza Capsules (Less than 5%)
Axert Tablets (Rare)
Axid Oral Solution (1.9%)
▲ Azilect Tablets (4%)
Buprenex Injectable (Less than 1%)
Caduet Tablets (Greater than 0.1% to
  less than 2%)
Campral Tablets (Infrequent)
Cardizem LA Extended Release
  Tablets (Less than 2%)
Catapres Tablets
Catapres-TTS (0.5% or less)
Cesamet Capsules
▲ Chantix Tablets (9% to 13%)
Cipro XR Tablets (Less than 1%)
Clorpres Tablets
Copaxone for Injection (Frequent)
Cozaar Tablets (Less than 1%)
▲ Depacon Injection (1% to 5%)
▲ Depakene Capsules (1% to 5%)
▲ Depakene Oral Solution (1% to 5%)
▲ Depakote ER Tablets (1% to 5%)
▲ Depakote Sprinkle Capsules
  (1% to 5%)
▲ Depakote Tablets (1% to 5%)
Dilaudid-HP Injection (Less frequent)

Dilaudid-HP Lyophilized Powder 250 mg (Less frequent)

Duragesic Transdermal System (1% or greater)

EC-Naprosyn Delayed-Release Tablets (Less than 1%)

▲ Effexor Tablets (4%)

▲ Effexor XR Capsules (3% to 7%)

▲ Eldepryl Capsules (2 of 49 patients)

▲ Emtriva Capsules (2% to 11%)

▲ Emtriva Oral Solution (2% to 11%)

▲ Epzicom Tablets (4% to 5%)

Evoxac Capsules (Less than 1%)

Exelon Capsules (Infrequent)

Exelon Oral Solution (Infrequent)

Frova Tablets (Rare)

Gabitril Tablets (Infrequent)

Hyzaar 100-12.5 Tablets

Hyzaar 100-25 Tablets

Hyzaar 50-12.5 Tablets

Inderal LA Long-Acting Capsules

▲ Intron A for Injection (Less than 5%)

Invirase Capsules (Less than 2%)

Invirase Tablets (Less than 2%)

Ionsys Transdermal System (.1% to less than 1%)

Kadian Capsules (Less than 3%)

Kaletra Oral Solution (Less than 2%)

Kaletra Tablets (Less than 2%)

Klonopin Tablets (Infrequent)

Klonopin Wafers (Infrequent)

Lamictal Chewable Dispersible Tablets (Infrequent)

Lamictal Tablets (Infrequent)

▲ Lariam Tablets (Among most frequent)

Levaquin in 5% Dextrose Injection (0.1% to 0.9%)

Levaquin Injection (0.1% to 0.9%)

Levaquin Oral Solution (0.1% to 0.9%)

Levaquin Tablets (0.1% to 0.9%)

▲ Lexapro Oral Suspension (3%)

▲ Lexapro Tablets (3%)

Lipitor Tablets (Less than 2%)

Lotensin HCT Tablets (0.3% or more)

Lotronex Tablets (Rare)

▲ Lunesta Tablets (1% to 3%)

Lyrica Capsules (0.1% to 1%)

Maxalt Tablets (Infrequent)

Maxalt-MLT Orally Disintegrating Tablets (Infrequent)

Meridia Capsules

▲ Mirapex Tablets (11%)

Mobic Oral Suspension (Less than 2%)

Mobic Tablets (Less than 2%)

Naprosyn Suspension (Less than 1%)

Naprosyn Tablets (Less than 1%)

Neurontin Capsules (Infrequent)

Neurontin Oral Solution (Infrequent)

Neurontin Tablets (Infrequent)

Nipent for Injection (Less than 3%)

Niravam Orally Disintegrating Tablets (1.8%)

Norvasc Tablets (0.1% to 1%)

Norvir Oral Solution (Less than 2%)

Norvir Soft Gelatin Capsules (Less than 2%)

▲ OxyContin Tablets (Between 1% and 5%)

Parcopa Orally Disintegrating Tablets

▲ Paxil CR Controlled-Release Tablets (3% to 4%)

▲ Paxil Oral Suspension (3% to 4%)

▲ Paxil Tablets (3% to 4%)

Permax Tablets (2.7%)

▲ Pexeva Tablets (4%)

Prevacid Delayed-Release Capsules (Less than 1%)

Prevacid for Delayed-Release Oral Suspension (Less than 1%)

Prevacid NapraPAC 375 (Less than 1%)

Prevacid NapraPAC 500 (Less than 1%)

Prevacid SoluTab Delayed-Release Orally Disintegrating Tablets (Less than 1%)

PREVPAC (Less than 1%)

▲ Prograf Capsules and Injection (3% to 15%)

ProQuad

ProSom Tablets (2%)

Protonix I.V. (Less than 1%)

Protonix Tablets (Less than 1%)

▲ Prozac Pulvules and Liquid (1% to 5%)

Relpax Tablets (Infrequent)

▲ Requip Tablets (11%)

Rescriptor Tablets

Reyataz Capsules (Less than 3%)

Rilutek Tablets (Rare)

Risperdal Consta Long-Acting Injection (Up to 2%)

Risperdal M-Tab Orally Disintegrating Tablets (Frequent)

Risperdal Oral Solution (Frequent)

Risperdal Tablets (Frequent)

Seroquel Tablets (Infrequent)

Singulair Chewable Tablets (Very rare)

Singulair Oral Granules (Very rare)
Singulair Tablets (Very rare)
Stalevo Tablets
▲ Strattera Capsules (4%)
Sular Tablets (Less than or
  equal to 1%)
Sustiva Capsules (1% to 4%)
Sustiva Tablets (1% to 4%)
▲ Symmetrel Tablets (1% to 5%)
Tambocor Tablets (Less than 1%)
▲ Tasmar Tablets (16% to 21%)
Thioridazine Hydrochloride Tablets
Tiazac Capsules (Less than 2%)
Topamax Sprinkle Capsules
  (Infrequent)
Topamax Tablets (Infrequent)
▲ Truvada Tablets (4%)
Ultram ER Tablets (0.5% to less
  than 1%)
Vantin Tablets and Oral Suspension
  (Less than 1%)
VFEND I.V. (Less than 2%)
VFEND Oral Suspension (Less
  than 2%)
VFEND Tablets (Less than 2%)
Viagra Tablets (Less than 2%)
Vicoprofen Tablets (Less than 1%)
Vivitrol
Voltaren Tablets (Occasionally)
Voltaren-XR Tablets (Occasionally)
Wellbutrin SR Sustained-Release
  Tablets (At least 1%)
Wellbutrin Tablets
▲ Wellbutrin XL Extended-Release
  Tablets (At least 1% to 3%)
Xifaxan Tablets (Less than 2%)
Xyrem Oral Solution (Frequent)
Zegerid Capsules (Less than 1%)
Zegerid Powder for Oral Solution
  (Less than 1%)
Zoloft Oral Concentrate (Infrequent)
Zoloft Tablets (Infrequent)
Zomig Nasal Spray (Rare)
Zonegran Capsules (Infrequent)
▲ Zyban Sustained-Release Tablets
  (5%)
Zyprexa Tablets
Zyprexa ZYDIS Orally Disintegrating
  Tablets

Emotional disturbances

Accutane Capsules
Avalide Tablets
Avapro Tablets (Less than 1%)
Cesamet Capsules

Chantix Tablets (Frequent)
Decadron Tablets
Depacon Injection
Depakene Capsules
Depakene Oral Solution
Depakote ER Tablets
Depakote Sprinkle Capsules
Depakote Tablets
Efudex Topical Cream (Infrequent)
Efudex Topical Solutions (Infrequent)
Imitrex Nasal Spray (Rare)
Lariam Tablets (Less than 1%)
Paxil CR Controlled-Release Tablets
  (Infrequent)
Paxil Oral Suspension (Infrequent)
Paxil Tablets (Infrequent)
Pexeva Tablets (Infrequent)
Rythmol SR Capsules
Xyrem Oral Solution (Infrequent)

Emotional lability

Abilify Discmelt Orally Disintegrating
  Tablets (Infrequent)
Abilify Oral Solution (Infrequent)
Abilify Tablets (Infrequent)
Accutane Capsules
Actiq (Less than 1%)
▲ Adderall XR Capsules (1% to 9%)
Adenoscan (Less than 1%)
Ambien CR Tablets (Infrequent)
Ambien Tablets (Infrequent)
▲ AndroGel (Up to 3%)
Aricept ODT Tablets (2%)
Aricept Tablets (2%)
Asacol Delayed-Release Tablets
Atripla Tablets
Avelox I.V. (Less than 0.1%)
Avelox Tablets (Less than 0.1%)
Azilect Tablets (Infrequent)
Betaseron for SC Injection
Bravelle for Intramuscular or
  Subcutaneous Injection (2% to 2.7%)
Caduet Tablets (Less than 2%)
Celexa Oral Solution (Infrequent)
Celexa Tablets (Infrequent)
▲ CellCept Capsules (3% to less
  than 20%)
▲ CellCept Intravenous (3% to less
  than 20%)
▲ CellCept Oral Suspension (3% to less
  than 20%)
▲ CellCept Tablets (3% to less
  than 20%)
Cesamet Capsules
▲ Clarinex Syrup (3.1%)

Concerta Extended-Release Tablets
(0.7%)

Copaxone for Injection (At least 2%)

Coreg CR Extended-Release Capsules
(0.1% to less than or equal to 1%)

Coreg Tablets (0.1% to 1%)

Cosopt Sterile Ophthalmic Solution

▲ Depacon Injection (6%)

▲ Depakene Capsules (6%)

▲ Depakene Oral Solution (6%)

▲ Depakote ER Tablets (6%)

▲ Depakote Sprinkle Capsules (6%)

▲ Depakote Tablets (1% to 6%)

Diastat Rectal Delivery System
(Greater than or equal to 1%)

▲ Doxil Injection (1% to 5%)

Effexor Tablets (Infrequent)

Effexor XR Capsules (Infrequent)

Elmiron Capsules

Emcyt Capsules (2%)

Evoxac Capsules (Less than 1%)

Exelon Capsules (Infrequent)

Exelon Oral Solution (Infrequent)

Frova Tablets (Infrequent)

▲ Gabitril Tablets (3%)

Gengraf Capsules (1% to less than 3%)

Guanidine Hydrochloride Tablets

Inderal LA Long-Acting Capsules

▲ Infergen (6% to 12%)

InnoPran XL Capsules

▲ Intron A for Injection (Less than 5%)

Kaletra Oral Solution (Less than 2%)

Kaletra Tablets (Less than 2%)

Keppra Injection (2%)

▲ Keppra Oral Solution (2% to 6%)

▲ Keppra Tablets (2% to 6%)

Klonopin Tablets (1%)

Klonopin Wafers (1%)

▲ Lamictal Chewable Dispersible Tablets
(Greater than 1% to 5%)

▲ Lamictal Tablets (1% to 5%)

Levaquin in 5% Dextrose Injection
(0.1% to 0.9%)

Levaquin Injection (0.1% to 0.9%)

Levaquin Oral Solution
(0.1% to 0.9%)

Levaquin Tablets (0.1% to 0.9%)

Levothroid Tablets

Levoxyl Tablets

Lexapro Oral Suspension
(Infrequent)

Lexapro Tablets (Infrequent)

Lipitor Tablets (Less than 2%)

Lopressor HCT 100/25 Tablets

Lopressor HCT 100/50 Tablets

Lopressor HCT 50/25 Tablets

Lopressor Injection

Lopressor Tablets

Lunesta Tablets (Infrequent)

▲ Lupron Depot 3.75 mg (16%)

▲ Lupron Depot-3 Month 11.25 mg
(16%)

Lupron Depot-PED 7.5 mg, 11.25 mg
and 15 mg (Less than 2%)

Lupron Injection Pediatric (Less
than 2%)

Meridia Capsules (1.3%)

Nadolol Tablets

Namenda Oral Solution (Infrequent)

Namenda Tablets (Infrequent)

Neoral Oral Solution (1% to less
than 3%)

Neoral Soft Gelatin Capsules (1% to
less than 3%)

▲ Neurontin Capsules (4.2% to 6%)

▲ Neurontin Oral Solution (4.2% to 6%)

▲ Neurontin Tablets (4.2% to 6%)

Nipent for Injection (Less than 3%)

Norvir Oral Solution (Less than 2%)

Norvir Soft Gelatin Capsules (Less
than 2%)

Omacor Capsules

Ortho Evra Transdermal System (1%
to 2.4%)

OxyContin Tablets (Less than 1%)

Paxil CR Controlled-Release Tablets
(Frequent)

Paxil Oral Suspension (Frequent)

Paxil Tablets (Frequent)

▲ PegIntron Powder for Injection (28%)

Permax Tablets (Infrequent)

Pexeva Tablets (Frequent)

Prevacid Delayed-Release Capsules
(Less than 1%)

Prevacid for Delayed-Release Oral
Suspension (Less than 1%)

Prevacid NapraPAC 375
(Less than 1%)

Prevacid NapraPAC 500
(Less than 1%)

Prevacid SoluTab Delayed-Release
Orally Disintegrating Tablets (Less
than 1%)

PREVPAC (Less than 1%)

Prochieve 4% Gel

Prochieve 8% Gel

▲ Prograf Capsules and Injection
(3% to 15%)

▲ Prometrium Capsules (100 mg,
200 mg) (6%)

ProSom Tablets (Infrequent)
Protonix I.V. (Less than 1%)
Protonix Tablets (Less than 1%)
Provigil Tablets (1%)
Prozac Pulvules and Liquid (Frequent)
▲ Pulmicort Respules (1% to 3%)
▲ Rapamune Oral Solution and Tablets (3% to 20%)
▲ Rebetol Capsules (7% to 47%)
▲ Rebetol Oral Solution (7% to 47%)
▲ Rebetron Combination Therapy (7% to 12%)
Relpax Tablets (Infrequent)
Requip Tablets (Infrequent)
Rescriptor Tablets
Retrovir Capsules
Retrovir IV Infusion
Retrovir Syrup
Retrovir Tablets
Reyataz Capsules (Less than 3%)
▲ Ribavirin, USP Capsules (7% to 47%)
Rilutek Tablets (Infrequent)
Risperdal Consta Long-Acting Injection (Infrequent)
Risperdal M-Tab Orally Disintegrating Tablets (Rare)
Risperdal Oral Solution (Rare)
Risperdal Tablets (Rare)
Romazicon Injection (1% to 3%)
Seroquel Tablets (Rare)
Sonata Capsules (Frequent)
Striant Mucoadhesive
Sustiva Capsules (Less than 2%)
Sustiva Tablets (Less than 2%)
Symbyax Capsules (Infrequent)
Tasmar Tablets (Frequent)
Thalomid Capsules
Timolide Tablets
Timoptic in Ocudose
Timoptic Sterile Ophthalmic Solution
Timoptic-XE Sterile Ophthalmic Gel Forming Solution
▲ Topamax Sprinkle Capsules (3%)
▲ Topamax Tablets (3%)
Toprol-XL Tablets
Trelstar Depot (1.4%)
▲ Trileptal Oral Suspension (2% to 3%)
▲ Trileptal Tablets (2% to 3%)
Uniretic Tablets (Less than 1%)
Viracept Oral Powder (Less than 2%)
Viracept Tablets (Less than 2%)
Wellbutrin SR Sustained-Release Tablets (Infrequent)
Wellbutrin XL Extended-Release Tablets (Infrequent)

Yasmin 28 Tablets
YAZ Tablets (Greater than 1%)
Zelapar Tablets
Zoloft Oral Concentrate (Infrequent)
Zoloft Tablets (Infrequent)
Zomig Tablets (Infrequent)
Zomig-ZMT Tablets (Infrequent)
Zyban Sustained-Release Tablets (Infrequent)
Zyprexa IntraMuscular (Infrequent)
Zyprexa Tablets
Zyprexa ZYDIS Orally Disintegrating Tablets
Zyrtec Chewable Tablets (Less than 2%)
Zyrtec Syrup (Less than 2%)
Zyrtec Tablets (Less than 2%)
Zyrtec-D 12 Hour Extended Release Tablets (Less than 2%)

Euphoria

Abilify Discmelt Orally Disintegrating Tablets (Rare)
Abilify Oral Solution (Rare)
Abilify Tablets (Rare)
Actiq (Less than 1%)
Adderall Tablets
Adderall XR Capsules
Adipex-P Capsules
Adipex-P Tablets
Ambien CR Tablets (1% to frequent)
Ambien Tablets (Frequent)
Aricept ODT Tablets (Infrequent)
Aricept Tablets (Infrequent)
▲ Avinza Capsules (Less than 5%)
Axert Tablets (Rare)
Bicillin C-R Injectable Suspension
Celexa Oral Solution (Infrequent)
Celexa Tablets (Infrequent)
▲ Cesamet Capsules (11% to 38%)
Chantix Tablets (Rare)
Copaxone for Injection (At least 2%)
Dalmane Capsules (Rare)
Decadron Tablets
Depacon Injection (0.9%)
Desoxyn Tablets, USP
Dexedrine Spansule Capsules
Dexedrine Tablets
DextroStat Tablets
▲ Diastat Rectal Delivery System (3%)
Dilaudid Ampules
Dilaudid Multiple Dose Vials
Dilaudid Non-Sterile Powder
Dilaudid Oral Liquid

Dilaudid Rectal Suppositories
Dilaudid Tablets
Dilaudid Tablets - 8 mg
Dilaudid-HP Injection (Less frequent)
Dilaudid-HP Lyophilized Powder
  250 mg (Less frequent)
▲ Duragesic Transdermal System
  (3% to 10%)
Effexor Tablets (Infrequent)
Effexor XR Capsules (Infrequent)
Eldepryl Capsules
Flumadine Syrup (Less than 0.3%)
Flumadine Tablets (Less than 0.3%)
Frova Tablets (Infrequent)
Gabitril Tablets (Frequent)
Hydrocortone Tablets
Hyperstat I.V.
Imitrex Injection (Infrequent)
Imitrex Nasal Spray (Infrequent)
Imitrex Tablets (Infrequent)
Invirase Capsules (Less than 2%)
Invirase Tablets (Less than 2%)
Kadian Capsules (Less than 3%)
Lamictal Chewable Dispersible
  Tablets (Infrequent)
Lamictal Tablets (Infrequent)
Lidoderm Patch
Lunesta Tablets (Rare)
▲ Lyrica Capsules (2% to 3%)
▲ Marinol Capsules (3% to 10%)
Maxalt Tablets (Frequent)
Maxalt-MLT Orally Disintegrating
  Tablets (Frequent)
Migranal Nasal Spray (Infrequent)
Moban Tablets (Less frequent)
▲ MS Contin Tablets (Among most
  frequent)
Neurontin Capsules (Infrequent)
Neurontin Oral Solution (Infrequent)
Neurontin Tablets (Infrequent)
Norvir Oral Solution (Less than 2%)
Norvir Soft Gelatin Capsules (Less
  than 2%)
Numorphan Injection
Opana ER Tablets (Less than 1%)
Opana Tablets (Less than 1%)
Oramorph SR Tablets (Most frequent)
▲ OxyContin Tablets (Between
  1% and 5%)
OxyFast Oral Concentrate Solution
OxyIR Capsules
Parcopa Orally Disintegrating Tablets
Paxil CR Controlled-Release Tablets
  (Rare)

Paxil Oral Suspension (Rare)
Paxil Tablets (Rare)
Percocet Tablets
Percodan Tablets
Permax Tablets (Infrequent)
Pexeva Tablets (Infrequent)
Phenergan Tablets and Suppositories
ProSom Tablets (Infrequent)
Prozac Pulvules and Liquid
  (Infrequent)
Relpax Tablets (Infrequent)
Requip Tablets (Infrequent)
Rescriptor Tablets
Restoril Capsules (1.5%)
Rilutek Tablets (Rare)
Risperdal Consta Long-Acting
  Injection (Infrequent)
Risperdal M-Tab Orally Disintegrating
  Tablets (Infrequent)
Risperdal Oral Solution
  (Infrequent)
Risperdal Tablets (Infrequent)
▲ Romazicon Injection (1% to 3%)
Seroquel Tablets (Rare)
Sonata Capsules (Frequent)
Stalevo Tablets
Sustiva Capsules (Less than 2%)
Sustiva Capsules (Less than 2%)
Symbyax Capsules (Infrequent)
Symmetrel Tablets (0.1% to 1%)
Synera Topical Patch
Tambocor Tablets (Less than 1%)
Tasmar Tablets (1%)
Thalomid Capsules
Topamax Sprinkle Capsules
  (Infrequent)
Topamax Tablets (Infrequent)
Trileptal Oral Suspension
Trileptal Tablets
Tussionex Pennkinetic Extended-
  Release Suspension
Tylenol with Codeine Tablets
Ultram ER Tablets (0.5% to less
  than 1%)
VFEND I.V. (Less than 2%)
VFEND Oral Suspension (Less
  than 2%)
VFEND Tablets (Less than 2%)
Vicoprofen Tablets (Less than 1%)
Vivitrol
Vyvanse Capsules
Wellbutrin SR Sustained-Release
  Tablets
Wellbutrin Tablets (1.2%)

Wellbutrin XL Extended-Release
Tablets
Xyrem Oral Solution (Infrequent)
Zoloft Oral Concentrate (Infrequent)
Zoloft Tablets (Infrequent)
Zomig Nasal Spray (Rare)
Zomig Tablets (Rare)
Zomig-ZMT Tablets (Rare)
Zonegran Capsules (Infrequent)
Zyban Sustained-Release Tablets
▲ Zyprexa Tablets (2% to 3%)
▲ Zyprexa ZYDIS Orally Disintegrating
Tablets (2% to 3%)
Zyrtec Chewable Tablets (Less than 2%)
Zyrtec Syrup (Less than 2%)
Zyrtec Tablets (Less than 2%)
Zyrtec-D 12 Hour Extended Release
Tablets (Less than 2%)

Excitability
Bentyl Capsules
Bentyl Injection
Bentyl Syrup
Bentyl Tablets
Children's Tylenol Plus Cold &
Allergy Suspension Liquid
Children's Tylenol Plus Cold
Suspension Liquid
Children's Tylenol Plus Cough &
Runny Nose Suspension Liquid
Children's Tylenol Plus Flu
Suspension Liquid
Children's Tylenol Plus Multi-
Symptom Cold Suspension Liquid
Children's Vicks NyQuil Cold/Cough
Relief Liquid
Donnatal Extentabs
Klonopin Tablets (Infrequent)
Klonopin Wafers (Infrequent)
Lexapro Oral Suspension (Infrequent)
Lexapro Tablets (Infrequent)
Oxandrin Tablets
Pediatric Vicks Formula 44m Cough
& Cold Relief Liquid
Phenergan Tablets and Suppositories
Tylenol Allergy Multi-Symptom
Caplets with Cool Burst and Gelcaps
Tylenol Allergy Multi-Symptom
Nighttime Caplets with Cool Burst
Tylenol Cold Head Congestion
Nighttime Caplets with Cool Burst
Tylenol Cold Multi-Symptom
Nighttime Caplets with Cool Burst
Tylenol Cold Multi-Symptom
Nighttime Liquid with Cool Burst

Tylenol Cough & Sore Throat
Nighttime Liquid with Cool Burst
Tylenol Severe Allergy Caplets
Tylenol Sinus Congestion & Pain
Nighttime Caplets with Cool Burst
Tylenol Sore Throat Nighttime Liquid
with Cool Burst
Vicks NyQuil Multi-Symptom
Cold/Flu Relief LiquiCaps
Vicks NyQuil Multi-Symptom
Cold/Flu Relief Liquid
Zyrtec-D 12 Hour Extended Release
Tablets

Excitement, paradoxical
ProSom Tablets
Valium Tablets

Fear
Dilaudid Ampules
Dilaudid Multiple Dose Vials
Dilaudid Non-Sterile Powder
Dilaudid Rectal Suppositories
Dilaudid Tablets
Hycodan Syrup
Hycodan Tablets
Hycotuss Expectorant Syrup
Niravam Orally Disintegrating Tablets
(1.4%)
Romazicon Injection
Tussionex Pennkinetic Extended-
Release Suspension
Vicodin ES Tablets
Vicodin HP Tablets
Vicodin Tablets
Xyrem Oral Solution (Infrequent)
Zydone Tablets
Zyrtec-D 12 Hour Extended Release
Tablets

Feeling, drugged
Ambien CR Tablets (Frequent)
▲ Ambien Tablets (3%)
Neurontin Capsules (Infrequent)
Neurontin Oral Solution (Infrequent)
Neurontin Tablets (Infrequent)
Paxil CR Controlled-Release Tablets
(2%)
Paxil Oral Suspension (2%)
Paxil Tablets (2%)
Pexeva Tablets (2%)

Feeling, high
Neurontin Capsules (Rare)
Neurontin Oral Solution (Rare)
Neurontin Tablets (Rare)

Feeling, intoxicated
Ambien CR Tablets (Rare)
Ambien Tablets (Rare)
Effexor XR Capsules (Rare)
Imitrex Injection (Rare)
Trileptal Oral Suspension
Trileptal Tablets
Feeling, strange
Ambien CR Tablets (Rare)
Ambien Tablets (Rare)
Amerge Tablets (Infrequent)
Imitrex Injection (2%)
Imitrex Nasal Spray (Infrequent)
Imitrex Tablets
Lexapro Oral Suspension (Infrequent)
Lexapro Tablets (Infrequent)
MS Contin Tablets (Less frequent)
Neurontin Capsules (Rare)
Neurontin Oral Solution (Rare)
Neurontin Tablets (Rare)
Trileptal Oral Suspension (1% to 2%)
Trileptal Tablets (1% to 2%)

Floating feeling
Dilaudid Oral Liquid (Less frequent)
Dilaudid Tablets - 8 mg (Less frequent)
Dilaudid-HP Injection (Less frequent)
Dilaudid-HP Lyophilized Powder
  250 mg (Less frequent)
Mintezol Chewable Tablets
Mintezol Suspension
MS Contin Tablets (Less frequent)
Oramorph SR Tablets (Less frequent)

Hallucinations
Abilify Discmelt Orally Disintegrating
  Tablets (Infrequent to frequent)
Abilify Oral Solution (Infrequent to
  frequent)
Abilify Tablets (Infrequent to frequent)
Actimmune (Rare)
Actiq (1% to 2%)
Adderall Tablets
Allegra-D 12 Hour Extended-Release
  Tablets
Allegra-D 24 Hour Extended-Release
  Tablets
▲ Ambien CR Tablets (Infrequent to 4%)
Ambien Tablets (Infrequent)
AmBisome for Injection
  (Less common)
Amerge Tablets (Rare)
Anaprox DS Tablets (Less than 1%)
Anaprox Tablets (Less than 1%)
▲ Aricept ODT Tablets (3%)

▲ Aricept Tablets (3%)
Arthrotec Tablets (Rare)
Avelox I.V. (Less than 0.1%)
Avelox Tablets (Less than 0.1%)
▲ Avinza Capsules (Less than 5%)
▲ Azilect Tablets (4%)
Biaxin Filmtab Tablets
Biaxin Granules
Biaxin XL Filmtab Tablets
Buprenex Injectable (Infrequent)
Campath Ampules
Campral Tablets (Infrequent)
Cardizem LA Extended Release
  Tablets (Less than 2%)
Catapres Tablets
Celexa Oral Solution (Infrequent)
Celexa Tablets (Infrequent)
▲ CellCept Capsules (3% to less
  than 20%)
▲ CellCept Intravenous (3% to less
  than 20%)
▲ CellCept Oral Suspension (3% to less
  than 20%)
▲ CellCept Tablets (3% to less
  than 20%)
Cesamet Capsules
Chantix Tablets (Rare)
Cipro I.V. (1% or less)
Cipro Oral Suspension (Less than 1%)
Cipro Tablets (Less than 1%)
Cipro XR Tablets
Clozaril Tablets (Less than 1%)
Comtan Tablets
Copaxone for Injection (Infrequent)
Cosopt Sterile Ophthalmic Solution
Cubicin for Injection (Less than 1%)
Cymbalta Delayed-Release Capsules
Dalmane Capsules (Rare)
Demser Capsules
Depacon Injection
Depakene Capsules
Depakene Oral Solution
Depakote ER Tablets (Greater
  than 1%)
Depakote Sprinkle Capsules
▲ Depakote Tablets (1% to 5%)
Detrol LA Capsules
Detrol Tablets
Didronel Tablets
Dilaudid Ampules
Dilaudid Multiple Dose Vials
Dilaudid Non-Sterile Powder
Dilaudid Oral Liquid (Less frequent)
Dilaudid Rectal Suppositories
Dilaudid Tablets

Dilaudid Tablets - 8 mg (Less frequent)
Dilaudid-HP Injection (Less frequent)
Dilaudid-HP Lyophilized Powder 250 mg (Less frequent)
Ditropan XL Extended-Release Tablets (Rare)
Dolobid Tablets (Less than 1 in 100)
▲ Duragesic Transdermal System (3% to 10%)
EC-Naprosyn Delayed-Release Tablets (Less than 1%)
Effexor Tablets (Infrequent)
Effexor XR Capsules (Infrequent)
▲ Eldepryl Capsules (3 of 49 patients)
Elspar for Injection
Equetro Extended-Release Capsules
Ery-Tab Tablets (Isolated reports)
Erythrocin Stearate Filmtab Tablets (Isolated reports)
Erythromycin Base Filmtab Tablets (Isolated reports)
Erythromycin Delayed-Release Capsules, USP (Isolated reports)
Evoxac Capsules (Less than 1%)
▲ Exelon Capsules (4%)
▲ Exelon Oral Solution (4%)
Famvir Tablets (Infrequent)
Fansidar Tablets
FazaClo Orally Disintegrating Tablets (Less than 1%)
Fentora Tablets (Greater than 1%)
Flumadine Syrup (Less than 0.3%)
Flumadine Tablets (Less than 0.3%)
Focalin Tablets
Gabitril Tablets (Frequent)
Gantrisin Pediatric Suspension
Guanidine Hydrochloride Tablets
▲ I.V. Busulfex (5%)
Imitrex Injection
Imitrex Tablets (Rare)
Inderal LA Long-Acting Capsules
InnoPran XL Capsules
Invanz for Injection (Very rare)
Invirase Capsules (Less than 2%)
Invirase Tablets (Less than 2%)
Kadian Capsules (Less than 3%)
Keflex Capsules
Klonopin Tablets
Klonopin Wafers
Lamictal Chewable Dispersible Tablets (Infrequent)
Lamictal Tablets (Infrequent)
Lanoxicaps Capsules

Lanoxin Injection
Lanoxin Injection Pediatric
Lanoxin Tablets
Lariam Tablets (Occasional)
Leukeran Tablets (Rare)
Levaquin in 5% Dextrose Injection (0.1% to 0.9%)
Levaquin Injection (0.1% to 0.9%)
Levaquin Oral Solution (0.1% to 0.9%)
Levaquin Tablets (0.1% to 0.9%)
Lithobid Tablets
Lopressor HCT 100/25 Tablets
Lopressor HCT 100/50 Tablets
Lopressor HCT 50/25 Tablets
Lopressor Injection
Lopressor Tablets
▲ Lunesta Tablets (1% to 3%)
Lyrica Capsules (0.1% to 1%)
Marinol Capsules (Greater than 1%)
Matulane Capsules
Maxipime for Injection
Merrem I.V. (0.1% to 1%)
▲ Mirapex Tablets (9% to 17%)
MS Contin Tablets (Less frequent)
Nadolol Tablets
Namenda Oral Solution
Namenda Tablets
Naprosyn Suspension (Less than 1%)
Naprosyn Tablets (Less than 1%)
Nembutal Sodium Solution, USP (Less than 1%)
Neurontin Capsules (Infrequent)
Neurontin Oral Solution (Infrequent)
Neurontin Tablets (Infrequent)
Nexium Delayed-Release Capsules
Nexium Delayed-Release Oral Suspension
Nexium I.V.
Nipent for Injection (Less than 3%)
Niravam Orally Disintegrating Tablets
Norflex Injection
Noroxin Tablets
Norvir Oral Solution (Less than 2%)
Norvir Soft Gelatin Capsules (Less than 2%)
Numorphan Injection
Opana ER Tablets (Less than 1%)
Opana Tablets (Less than 1%)
OxyContin Tablets (Less than 1%)
Parcopa Orally Disintegrating Tablets
Paxil CR Controlled-Release Tablets (Infrequent)
Paxil Oral Suspension (Infrequent)

Paxil Tablets (Infrequent)
Pepcid for Oral Suspension (Infrequent)
Pepcid Injection (Infrequent)
Pepcid Injection Premixed (Infrequent)
Pepcid Tablets (Infrequent)
Percodan Tablets
▲ Permax Tablets (13.8%)
Pexeva Tablets (Infrequent)
Phenergan Tablets and Suppositories
Plavix Tablets
Prevacid Delayed-Release Capsules
  (Less than 1%)
Prevacid for Delayed-Release Oral
  Suspension (Less than 1%)
Prevacid NapraPAC 375 (Less than 1%)
Prevacid NapraPAC 500 (Less than 1%)
Prevacid SoluTab Delayed-Release
  Orally Disintegrating Tablets
  (Less than 1%)
PREVPAC (Less than 1%)
Primaxin I.M.
Primaxin I.V.
▲ Prograf Capsules and Injection
  (3% to 15%)
Proquin XR Tablets
ProSom Tablets (Rare)
Protonix I.V. (Less than 1%)
Protonix Tablets (Less than 1%)
Provigil Tablets (At least 1%)
Prozac Pulvules and Liquid
  (Infrequent)
Raniclor Tablets, Chewable (Rare)
Razadyne ER Extended-Release
  Capsules (Greater than
  or equal to 2%)
Razadyne Oral Solution (Greater than
  or equal to 2%)
Razadyne Tablets (Greater than or
  equal to 2%)
Relpax Tablets (Rare)
▲ Requip Tablets (5% to 10%)
Rescriptor Tablets
Restoril Capsules (Less than 0.5%)
Reyataz Capsules (Less than 3%)
Rilutek Tablets (Infrequent)
▲ Risperdal Consta Long-Acting
  Injection (6% to 7%)
Ritalin Hydrochloride Tablets
Ritalin LA Capsules
Ritalin-SR Tablets
Sanctura Tablets
▲ Sandostatin LAR Depot (1% to 4%)
Seroquel Tablets (Infrequent)
Singulair Chewable Tablets

Singulair Oral Granules
Singulair Tablets
Sonata Capsules (Less than 1%)
▲ Stalevo Tablets (4%)
Sustiva Capsules (Less than 2%)
Sustiva Tablets (Less than 2%)
▲ Symmetrel Tablets (1% to 5%)
▲ Tasmar Tablets (8% to 10%)
Tiazac Capsules (Less than 2%)
Timolide Tablets
Timoptic in Ocudose (Less frequent)
Timoptic Sterile Ophthalmic Solution
  (Less frequent)
Timoptic-XE Sterile Ophthalmic Gel
  Forming Solution
Topamax Sprinkle Capsules
  (Frequent)
Topamax Tablets (Frequent)
Toprol-XL Tablets
Transderm Scop Transdermal
  Therapeutic System (Infrequent)
▲ Valcyte Tablets (Less than 5%)
Valium Tablets
Vantin Tablets and Oral Suspension
  (Less than 1%)
▲ Vesanoid Capsules (6%)
VFEND I.V. (0% to 2.8%)
VFEND Oral Suspension (0% to 2.8%)
VFEND Tablets (0% to 2.8%)
Voltaren Tablets (Rarely)
Voltaren-XR Tablets (Rarely)
Vyvanse Capsules
Wellbutrin SR Sustained-Release
  Tablets
Wellbutrin Tablets (Frequent)
Wellbutrin XL Extended-Release
  Tablets
Zantac 150 EFFERdose Tablets (Rare)
Zantac 150 Tablets (Rare)
Zantac 25 EFFERdose Tablets (Rare)
Zantac 300 Tablets (Rare)
Zantac Injection
Zantac Injection Pharmacy Bulk
  Package (Rare)
Zantac Injection Premixed
Zantac Syrup (Rare)
Zegerid Capsules (Less than 1%)
Zegerid Powder for Oral Solution
  (Less than 1%)
▲ Zelapar Tablets (4%)
Zoloft Oral Concentrate (Infrequent)
Zoloft Tablets (Infrequent)
Zomig Nasal Spray
Zomig Tablets (Rare)

Zomig-ZMT Tablets (Rare)
Zosyn (1.0% or less)
Zovirax Capsules
Zovirax Suspension
Zovirax Tablets
Zyban Sustained-Release Tablets
Zyprexa Tablets
Zyprexa ZYDIS Orally Disintegrating
  Tablets
Zyrtec Chewable Tablets (Rare)
Zyrtec Syrup (Rare)
Zyrtec Tablets (Rare)
Zyrtec-D 12 Hour Extended Release
  Tablets

Hallucinations, auditory

Bicillin C-R Injectable Suspension
Catapres Tablets (Rare)
Catapres-TTS (0.5% or less)
Clorpres Tablets
Lexapro Oral Suspension (Infrequent)
Lexapro Tablets (Infrequent)
Mirapex Tablets
Namenda Oral Solution
Namenda Tablets
Orthoclone OKT3 Sterile Solution
Valtrex Caplets
Xyrem Oral Solution (Infrequent)
Hallucinations, visual
Bicillin C-R Injectable Suspension
Carbatrol Capsules
Catapres Tablets (Rare)
Catapres-TTS (0.5% or less)
Clorpres Tablets
Lexapro Oral Suspension
Lexapro Tablets
Mirapex Tablets
Namenda Oral Solution
Namenda Tablets
Orthoclone OKT3 Sterile Solution
Tegretol Chewable Tablets
Tegretol Suspension
Tegretol Tablets
Tegretol-XR Tablets
Tessalon Capsules
Tessalon Perles
Valtrex Caplets

Hangover

AcipHex Tablets (Rare)
▲ Advair HFA Inhalation Aerosol
  (0% to 3%)
Effexor Tablets (Infrequent)
Effexor XR Capsules (Infrequent)
Lyrica Capsules (Rare)

Maxalt Tablets (Infrequent)
Maxalt-MLT Orally Disintegrating
  Tablets (Infrequent)
Neurontin Capsules (Rare)
Neurontin Oral Solution (Rare)
Neurontin Tablets (Rare)
Nipent for Injection (Less than 3%)
▲ ProSom Tablets (3%)
Restoril Capsules (2.5%)
Sonata Capsules (Infrequent)
Thalomid Capsules
Xyrem Oral Solution (Infrequent)
Zyprexa Tablets (Infrequent)
Zyprexa ZYDIS Orally Disintegrating
  Tablets (Infrequent)

Hostility

Abilify Discmelt Orally Disintegrating
  Tablets (Frequent)
Abilify Oral Solution (Frequent)
Abilify Tablets (Frequent)
Adderall XR Capsules
Amerge Tablets (Rare)
▲ Aricept ODT Tablets (3%)
▲ Aricept Tablets (3%)
Azilect Tablets (Rare)
Campral Tablets (Infrequent)
Copaxone for Injection (Infrequent)
Depacon Injection
Depakene Capsules
Depakene Oral Solution
Depakote ER Tablets
Depakote Sprinkle Capsules
Depakote Tablets
Duragesic Transdermal System (Less
  than 1%)
Effexor Tablets (Infrequent)
Effexor XR Capsules (Infrequent)
Gabitril Tablets (0.02)
Geodon Capsules (Frequent)
Keppra Injection (2%)
▲ Keppra Oral Solution (2% to 12%)
▲ Keppra Tablets (2% to 12%)
Klonopin Tablets
Klonopin Wafers
Lamictal Chewable Dispersible
  Tablets (Infrequent)
Lamictal Tablets (Infrequent)
Lunesta Tablets (Infrequent)
Lyrica Capsules (0.1% to 1%)
▲ Neurontin Capsules (5.2% to 7.6%)
▲ Neurontin Oral Solution (5.2% to 7.6%)
▲ Neurontin Tablets (5.2% to 7.6%)
Nipent for Injection (Less than 3%)
Paxil CR Controlled-Release Tablets
  (Infrequent)

Paxil Oral Suspension (Infrequent)
Paxil Tablets (Infrequent)
Permax Tablets (Infrequent)
Pexeva Tablets (Infrequent)
Prevacid Delayed-Release Capsules
(Less than 1%)
Prevacid for Delayed-Release Oral
Suspension (Less than 1%)
Prevacid NapraPAC 375
(Less than 1%)
Prevacid NapraPAC 500
(Less than 1%)
Prevacid SoluTab Delayed-Release
Orally Disintegrating Tablets
(Less than 1%)
PREVPAC (Less than 1%)
ProSom Tablets (Infrequent)
Prozac Pulvules and Liquid
(Infrequent)
Reyataz Capsules (Less than 3%)
Rilutek Tablets (Frequent)
Ritalin LA Capsules
Seroquel Tablets
Sonata Capsules (Rare)
Strattera Capsules
Symbyax Capsules (Infrequent)
Tasmar Tablets (Infrequent)
Thalomid Capsules
Wellbutrin SR Sustained-Release
Tablets (Infrequent)
▲ Wellbutrin Tablets (5.6%)
Wellbutrin XL Extended-Release
Tablets (Infrequent)
Zoloft Oral Concentrate
Zoloft Tablets
Zyban Sustained-Release Tablets
(Infrequent)
▲ Zyprexa Tablets (15%)
▲ Zyprexa ZYDIS Orally Disintegrating
Tablets (15%)

Hyperactivity

Abilify Discmelt Orally Disintegrating
Tablets (Infrequent)
Abilify Oral Solution (Infrequent)
Abilify Tablets (Infrequent)
Advair HFA Inhalation Aerosol
(Very Rare)
▲ Aerobid Inhaler System (1% to 3%)
▲ Aerobid-M Inhaler System
(1% to 3%)
Amerge Tablets (Rare)
Amoxil Capsules (Rare)
Amoxil Chewable Tablets (Rare)

Amoxil Pediatric Drops for Oral
Suspension (Rare)
Amoxil Powder for Oral Suspension
(Rare)
Amoxil Tablets (Rare)
Augmentin Chewable Tablets (Rare)
Augmentin ES-600 Powder for Oral
Suspension (Rare)
Augmentin Powder for Oral
Suspension (Rare)
Augmentin Tablets (Rare)
Augmentin XR Extended-Release
Tablets (Rare)
Ceftin for Oral Suspension
(0.1% to 1%)
Cesamet Capsules
Clarinex-D 24-Hour Extended-
Release Tablets (2%)
Dalmane Capsules (Rare)
Depacon Injection
Depakene Capsules
Depakene Oral Solution
Depakote ER Tablets
Depakote Sprinkle Capsules
Depakote Tablets
Klonopin Tablets (Infrequent)
Klonopin Wafers (Infrequent)
Levothroid Tablets
Levoxyl Tablets
Moban Tablets (Less frequent)
Neurontin Capsules
Neurontin Oral Solution
Neurontin Tablets
PREVPAC
Raniclor Tablets, Chewable (Rare)
Tasmar Tablets (1%)
Thioridazine Hydrochloride Tablets
(Extremely rare)
Zmax for Oral Suspension

Hysteria

Ambien Tablets (Rare)
Imitrex Injection (Rare)
Imitrex Tablets (Rare)
Klonopin Tablets
Klonopin Wafers
Neurontin Capsules (Rare)
Neurontin Oral Solution (Rare)
Neurontin Tablets (Rare)
Paxil CR Controlled-Release Tablets
(Rare)
Paxil Oral Suspension (Rare)
Paxil Tablets (Rare)
Pexeva Tablets (Rare)

Phenergan Tablets and Suppositories
Propofol Injectable Emulsion 1%
(Less than 1%)
Relpax Tablets (Rare)
Trileptal Oral Suspension
Trileptal Tablets

Illusion, unspecified

Ambien CR Tablets (Infrequent)
Ambien Tablets (Infrequent)
Evoxac Capsules
Klonopin Tablets (Infrequent)
Klonopin Wafers (Infrequent)
Zoloft Oral Concentrate (Rare)
Zoloft Tablets (Rare)

Inebriated feeling

Cesamet Capsules
Klonopin Tablets (Infrequent)
Klonopin Wafers (Infrequent)
▲ Xyrem Oral Solution (8.6%)

Insomnia

▲ Abilify Tablets (20%)
Accolate Tablets
Accutane Capsules
AcipHex Tablets
Actigall Capsules (1.9%)
Actiq (1% to 2%)
▲ Actonel Tablets (4.7%)
▲ Actonel with Calcium Tablets (4.3%)
Adalat CC Tablets (Less than 1%)
Adderall Tablets
▲ Adderall XR Capsules (1.5% to 27%)
Adipex-P Capsules
Adipex-P Tablets
Advicor Tablets
▲ Aerobid Inhaler System (1% to 3%)
▲ Aerobid-M Inhaler System (1% to 3%)
▲ Agrylin Capsules (1% to 5%)
Aldara Cream, 5%
Alferon N Injection (2%)
Alinia for Oral Suspension
(Less than 1%)
Alinia Tablets (Less than 1%)
Allegra Capsules (Less than 1%)
Allegra Oral Solution (Less than 1%)
Allegra Tablets (Less than 1%)
▲ Allegra-D 12 Hour Extended-Release
Tablets (12.6%)
▲ Allegra-D 24 Hour Extended-Release
Tablets (12.6%)
▲ Alora ETS Patch (1% to 8%)
Aloxi Injection (Less than 1%)
▲ Alphagan P Ophthalmic Solution
(1% to 4%)

Altace Capsules (Less than 1%)
Altoprev Extended-Release Tablets
Ambien CR Tablets (Frequent)
Ambien Tablets (Frequent)
Amitiza Capsules (0% to 1.4%)
Amoxil Capsules (Rare)
Amoxil Chewable Tablets (Rare)
Amoxil Pediatric Drops for Oral
Suspension (Rare)
Amoxil Powder for Oral Suspension
(Rare)
Amoxil Tablets (Rare)
Anaprox DS Tablets (Less than 1%)
Anaprox Tablets (Less than 1%)
Aptivus Capsules (1.2% to
less than 2%)
▲ Aredia for Injection (22.2%)
▲ Aricept ODT Tablets (5%)
▲ Aricept Tablets (5%)
▲ Arimidex Tablets (2% to 10%)
▲ Arixtra Injection (0.9% to 5%)
▲ Aromasin Tablets (11% to 13.7%)
▲ Arranon Injection (0% to 7%)
Arthrotec Tablets (Rare)
Asacol Delayed-Release Tablets (2%)
Asmanex Twisthaler (1% to
less than 3%)
Atacand HCT 16-12.5 Tablets (0.5%
or greater)
Atacand HCT 32-12.5 Tablets (0.5%
or greater)
▲ Atripla Tablets (4%)
Atrovent Inhalation Solution (0.9%)
Augmentin Chewable Tablets (Rare)
Augmentin ES-600 Powder for Oral
Suspension (Rare)
Augmentin Powder for Oral
Suspension (Rare)
Augmentin Tablets (Rare)
Augmentin XR Extended-Release
Tablets (Rare)
Avelox I.V. (0.1% to less than 2%)
Avelox Tablets (0.1% to less than 2%)
▲ Avinza Capsules (5% to 10%)
Axert Tablets (Infrequent)
Axid Oral Solution (2.7%)
Baraclude Oral Solution (Less than 1%)
Baraclude Tablets (Less than 1%)
Benicar Tablets (Greater than 0.5%)
Bentyl Capsules
Bentyl Injection
Bentyl Syrup
Bentyl Tablets
▲ Betaseron for SC Injection (24%)

Betoptic S Ophthalmic Suspension (Rare)
Biaxin Filmtab Tablets
Biaxin Granules
Biaxin XL Filmtab Tablets
Boniva Injection (0.8% to 2%)
Boniva Tablets (0.8% to 2%)
Brovana Inhalation Solution
Caduet Tablets (Greater than 0.1%)
▲ Campath Ampules (10%)
▲ Campral Tablets (6% to 9%)
▲ Camptosar Injection (0% to 19%)
Cancidas for Injection (0% to 1.2%)
Captopril Tablets (About 0.5 to 2%)
Carafate Suspension (Less than 0.5%)
Carafate Tablets (Less than 0.5%)
Cardizem LA Extended Release Tablets (Less than 2%)
▲ Carnitor Injection (1% to 3%)
Catapres Tablets (About 5 in 1,000 patients)
Catapres-TTS (2 of 101 patients)
Celebrex Capsules (2.3%)
▲ Celexa Oral Solution (15%)
▲ Celexa Tablets (15%)
▲ CellCept Capsules (40.8%)
▲ CellCept Intravenous (40.8%)
▲ CellCept Oral Suspension (40.8%)
▲ CellCept Tablets (40.8%)
Cesamet Capsules
▲ Chantix Tablets (18% to 19%)
Children's Tylenol Plus Cold Suspension Liquid
Children's Tylenol Plus Flu Suspension Liquid
Children's Tylenol Plus Multi-Symptom Cold Suspension Liquid
Children's Vicks NyQuil Cold/Cough Relief Liquid
Cialis Tablets (Less than 2%)
Cipro I.V. (1% or less)
Cipro Oral Suspension (Less than 1%)
Cipro Tablets (Less than 1%)
Cipro XR Tablets (Less than 1%)
▲ Clarinex Syrup (4.5%)
▲ Clarinex-D 12-Hour Extended-Release Tablets (10%)
▲ Clarinex-D 24-Hour Extended-Release Tablets (5%)
Clinoril Tablets (Less than 1%)
Clorpres Tablets (About 5 in 1,000)
▲ Clozaril Tablets (2% to 20%)
Colazal Capsules (2%)
Combivent Inhalation Aerosol (Less than 2%)

▲ Combivir Tablets (11%)
Concentrated Tylenol Infants' Drops Plus Cold
Concentrated Tylenol Infants' Drops Plus Cold and Cough
▲ Concerta Extended-Release Tablets (1.5% to 5%)
▲ Condylox Topical Solution (Less than 5%)
Copaxone for Injection (At least 2%)
▲ Copegus Tablets (30%)
Coreg CR Extended-Release Capsules (1% to 2%)
Coreg Tablets (2%)
Cortifoam Rectal Foam
Cosopt Sterile Ophthalmic Solution
Covera-HS Tablets (Less than 2%)
Cozaar Tablets (1% or greater)
Crestor Tablets (Greater than or equal to 2%)
▲ Cubicin for Injection (4.5% to 11.2%)
▲ Cymbalta Delayed-Release Capsules (8% to 13%)
▲ Dacogen Injection (28%)
Dantrium Capsules (Less frequent)
Dapsone Tablets USP
▲ Daytrana Transdermal Patch (4% to 30%)
Decadron Tablets
Demadex Injection (1.2%)
Demadex Tablets (1.2%)
Demser Capsules
▲ Depacon Injection (9% to 15%)
▲ Depade Tablets (3%)
▲ Depakene Capsules (15%)
▲ Depakene Oral Solution (15%)
▲ Depakote ER Tablets (Greater than 1% to 15%)
▲ Depakote Sprinkle Capsules (9% to 15%)
▲ Depakote Tablets (1% to 15%)
▲ DepoDur Extended-Release Injection (5% to 10%)
▲ Depo-Provera Contraceptive Injection (1% to 5%)
▲ depo-subQ provera 104 Injectable Suspension (1% to less than 5%)
Desoxyn Tablets, USP
Dexedrine Spansule Capsules
Dexedrine Tablets
DextroStat Tablets
Dilacor XR Capsules (1%)
Dilaudid Ampules
Dilaudid Multiple Dose Vials
Dilaudid Non-Sterile Powder

Dilaudid Oral Liquid (Less frequent)
Dilaudid Rectal Suppositories
Dilaudid Tablets
Dilaudid Tablets, 8 mg (Less frequent)
Dilaudid-HP Injection (Less frequent)
Dilaudid-HP Lyophilized Powder
  250 mg (Less frequent)
Diovan HCT Tablets (Greater than 0.2%)
Diovan Tablets
▲ Ditropan XL Extended-Release
  Tablets (2% to less than 5%)
Dolobid Tablets (Greater than 1 in 100)
Donnatal Extentabs
▲ Doxil Injection (Less than 1% to 10%)
▲ Duragesic Transdermal System
  (3% to 10%)
DynaCirc CR Tablets (0.5% to 1%)
EC-Naprosyn Delayed-Release Tablets
  (Less than 1%)
▲ Effexor Tablets (3% to 22.5%)
▲ Effexor XR Capsules (3% to 23%)
Efudex Topical Cream
Efudex Topical Solutions
Eldepryl Capsules (1 of 49 patients)
Eligard 30 mg (1.1%)
Eligard 7.5 mg (Less than 2%)
Elmiron Capsules
▲ Eloxatin for Injection (9% to 11%)
▲ Emcyt Capsules (3%)
▲ Emend Capsules (2.1% to 4.1 %)
▲ Emsam Transdermal System (12%)
▲ Emtriva Capsules (7% to 16%)
▲ Emtriva Oral Solution (7% to 16%)
Engerix-B Vaccine (Less than 1%)
▲ Entocort EC Capsules (Less than 5%)
▲ Epivir Oral Solution (11%)
▲ Epivir Tablets (11%)
▲ Epogen for Injection (13% to 21%)
▲ Epzicom Tablets (7% to 9%)
▲ Equetro Extended-Release Capsules
  (Less than 5%)
▲ Erbitux (Less than 1% to 12%)
▲ Estring Vaginal Ring (4%)
▲ Evista Tablets (5.5%)
Evoxac Capsules (2.4%)
▲ Exelon Capsules (3% to 9%)
▲ Exelon Oral Solution (3% to 9%)
Extra Strength Tylenol PM Caplets,
  Vanilla Caplets, Geltabs, Gelcaps
  and Liquid
Famvir Tablets (1.5% to 2.5%)
Fansidar Tablets
▲ Faslodex Injection (6.9%)
▲ FazaClo Orally Disintegrating Tablets
  (2% to 20%)

▲ Femara Tablets (Less than 0.1%
  to 7%)
Femhrt Tablets
▲ Fentora Tablets (1% to 11%)
Flomax Capsules (1.4% to 2.4%)
Floxin Otic Solution (Single report)
Flulaval Injection
Flumadine Syrup (2.1% to 3.4%)
Flumadine Tablets (2.1% to 3.4%)
▲ Focalin Tablets (Among most
  common)
Focalin XR Capsules
Foradil Aerolizer (1.5%)
▲ Forteo for Injection (4.3%)
Fortical Nasal Spray (Less than 1%)
▲ Foscavir Injection (Between 1%
  and 5%)
Frova Tablets (Frequent)
Fuzeon Injection
▲ Gabitril Tablets (6%)
Gantrisin Pediatric Suspension
Gardasil Injection (1.2%)
Gemzar for Injection (Infrequent)
Gengraf Capsules (1% to less
  than 3%)
Geodon Capsules (Rare)
Geodon for Injection (Rare)
▲ Gleevec Tablets (0% to 19%)
Gris-PEG Tablets (Occasional)
Havrix Vaccine (Less than 1%)
▲ Hectorol Capsules (Greater than
  or equal to 5%)
▲ Herceptin I.V. (14%)
Hydrocortone Tablets
Hytrin Capsules (At least 1%)
Hyzaar 100-12.5 Tablets
Hyzaar 100-25 Tablets
Hyzaar 50-12.5 Tablets
▲ I.V. Busulfex (84%)
▲ Imdur Tablets (Less than or equal to
  5%)
▲ Indapamide Tablets (Less than 5%)
Inderal LA Long-Acting Capsules
Indocin Capsules (Less than 1%)
Indocin Oral Suspension (Less than 1%)
Indocin Suppositories (Less than 1%)
▲ Infergen (24% to 39%)
InnoPran XL Capsules
▲ Intron A for Injection (Up to 12%)
▲ Invanz for Injection (3% to 3.2%)
Invega Extended-Release Tablets
Invirase Capsules (Greater than or
  equal to 2%)
Invirase Tablets (Greater than or
  equal to 2%)

▲ Ionsys Transdermal System (3%)
Kadian Capsules (Less than 3%)
Kaletra Oral Solution (Up to 2%)
Kaletra Tablets (0% to 2%)
Keppra Injection
Keppra Oral Solution (1% to 2%)
Keppra Tablets (1% to 2%)
Ketek Tablets (Greater than or equal to 0.2% to less than 2%)
Klonopin Tablets (Infrequent)
Klonopin Wafers (Infrequent)
▲ Kytril Injection (Less than 2% to 4.9%)
▲ Kytril Oral Solution (3% to 5%)
▲ Kytril Tablets (3% to 5%)
▲ Lamictal Chewable Dispersible Tablets (5% to 10%)
▲ Lamictal Tablets (5% to 10%)
▲ Lariam Tablets (Among most frequent)
Lescol Capsules (2.7%)
Lescol XL Tablets (0.8%)
▲ Leukine (11%)
▲ Leustatin Injection (7%)
▲ Levaquin in 5% Dextrose Injection (0.4% to 4.6%)
▲ Levaquin Injection (0.4% to 4.6%)
▲ Levaquin Oral Solution (0.4% to 4.6%)
▲ Levaquin Tablets (0.4% to 4.6%)
Levbid Extended-Release Tablets
Levitra Tablets (Less than 2%)
Levothroid Tablets
Levoxyl Tablets
Levsin Drops
Levsin Elixir
Levsin Injection
Levsin Tablets
Levsin/SL Tablets
Levsinex Timecaps
▲ Lexapro Oral Suspension (5% to 14%)
▲ Lexapro Tablets (5% to 14%)
Lipitor Tablets (Greater than or equal to 2%)
Lopressor HCT 100/25 Tablets
Lopressor HCT 100/50 Tablets
Lopressor HCT 50/25 Tablets
Lopressor Injection
Lopressor Tablets
Lotensin HCT Tablets (0.3% to 1%)
Lotensin Tablets (Less than 1%)
Lotrel Capsules
Lunesta Tablets (Infrequent)
▲ Lupron Depot 3.75 mg (16%)
▲ Lupron Depot 7.5 mg (Less than 5%)
▲ Lupron Depot-3 Month 11.25 mg (16%)

▲ Malarone Pediatric Tablets (2% to 3%)
▲ Malarone Tablets (2% to 3%)
Matulane Capsules
Mavik Tablets (0.3% to 1.0%)
Maxair Autohaler
Maxalt Tablets (Infrequent)
Maxalt-MLT Orally Disintegrating Tablets (Infrequent)
▲ Megace ES Oral Suspension (0% to 6%)
▲ Mepron Suspension (10% to 19%)
▲ Meridia Capsules (10.7%)
Merrem I.V. (Greater than 0.1% to 1%)
▲ Metadate CD Capsules (5%)
Mevacor Tablets (0.5% to 1.0%)
Miacalcin Nasal Spray (Less than 1%)
Micardis HCT Tablets
Micardis Tablets (More than 0.3%)
Midamor Tablets (Less than or equal to 1%)
Migranal Nasal Spray (Infrequent)
▲ Mirapex Tablets (13% to 27%)
▲ Mobic Oral Suspension (0% to 3.6%)
▲ Mobic Tablets (0% to 3.6%)
Moduretic Tablets (Less than or equal to 1%)
MS Contin Tablets (Less frequent)
▲ Myfortic Tablets (23.5%)
▲ Mylotarg for Injection (11% to 13%)
Nalfon Capsules (Less than 1%)
Namenda Oral Solution (Greater than or equal to 2%)
Namenda Tablets (Greater than or equal to 2%)
Naprosyn Suspension (Less than 1%)
Naprosyn Tablets (Less than 1%)
▲ Natrecor for Injection (2% to 6%)
Nembutal Sodium Solution, USP (Less than 1%)
Neoral Oral Solution (1% to 3%)
▲ Neoral Soft Gelatin Capsules (1% to 3%)
▲ Neulasta Injection (15% to 72%)
▲ Neumega for Injection (33%)
Neurontin Capsules
Neurontin Oral Solution
Neurontin Tablets
Nexium Delayed-Release Capsules (Less than 1%)
Nexium Delayed-Release Oral Suspension (Less than 1%)
Nexium I.V. (Less than 1%)
Niaspan Extended-Release Tablets
▲ Nipent for Injection (3% to 10%)

▲ Niravam Orally Disintegrating Tablets (8.9% to 29.5%)

Noroxin Tablets (Less frequent)

Norvasc Tablets (More than 0.1% to 1%)

Norvir Oral Solution (2% to 2.6%)

Norvir Soft Gelatin Capsules (2% to 2.6%)

▲ Noxafil Oral Suspension (1% to 17%)

NuLev Orally Disintegrating Tablets

Omacor Capsules

Omnicef Capsules (0.2%)

Omnicef for Oral Suspension (0.2%)

▲ Ontak Vials (9%)

▲ Opana ER Tablets (4%)

Opana Tablets (Less than 1%)

Oramorph SR Tablets (Less frequent)

Ortho Tri-Cyclen Lo Tablets

Ortho Tri-Cyclen Tablets

Ortho-Cyclen Tablets

Ovidrel Prefilled Syringe for Injection (Less than 2%)

Oxandrin Tablets

Oxsoralen-Ultra Capsules

▲ OxyContin Tablets (Between 1% and 5%)

Parcopa Orally Disintegrating Tablets

Parnate Tablets

▲ Paxil CR Controlled-Release Tablets (1.3% to 24%)

▲ Paxil Oral Suspension (1.3% to 24%)

▲ Paxil Tablets (1.3% to 24%)

▲ Pegasys (19%)

▲ PegIntron Powder for Injection (23%)

Pentasa Capsules (Less than 1%)

Pepcid for Oral Suspension (Infrequent)

Pepcid Injection (Infrequent)

Pepcid Injection Premixed (Infrequent)

Pepcid Tablets (Infrequent)

▲ Permax Tablets (7.9%)

▲ Pexeva Tablets (1.3% to 24%)

Phenergan Tablets and Suppositories

Phenytek Capsules

▲ Photofrin for Injection (4% to 14%)

Plavix Tablets (1% to 2.5%)

Pletal Tablets (Less than 2%)

▲ Premarin Tablets (6% to 7%)

▲ Premphase Tablets (6% to 7%)

▲ Prempro Tablets (6% to 7%)

Prevacid NapraPAC 375 (Less than 1%)

Prevacid NapraPAC 500 (Less than 1%)

PREVPAC

Prinivil Tablets (0.3% to 1.0%)

Prinzide Tablets

ProAmatine Tablets (Rare)

Prochieve 4% Gel

Prochieve 8% Gel

▲ Procrit for Injection (13% to 21%)

▲ Prograf Capsules and Injection (32% to 64%)

Proleukin for Injection

▲ Prometrium Capsules (100 mg, 200 mg) (Less than 5%)

Propofol Injectable Emulsion 1% (Less than 1%)

ProQuad (Greater than or equal to 0.2% to less than 1%)

Proquin XR Tablets

Protonix I.V. (Greater than or equal to 1%)

Protonix Tablets (Less than or equal to 1%)

▲ Protopic Ointment (Up to 4%)

Proventil HFA Inhalation Aerosol

Proventil Inhalation Aerosol

▲ Proventil Inhalation Solution 0.083% (1% to 3.1%)

▲ Provigil Tablets (5%)

▲ Prozac Pulvules and Liquid (10% to 33%)

▲ Pulmicort Turbuhaler Inhalation Powder (1% to 3%)

Raniclor Tablets, Chewable (Rare)

▲ Rapamune Oral Solution and Tablets (13% to 22%)

▲ Razadyne ER Extended-Release Capsules (5%)

▲ Razadyne Oral Solution (5%)

▲ Razadyne Tablets (5%)

▲ Rebetol Capsules (14% to 41%)

▲ Rebetol Oral Solution (14% to 41%)

▲ Rebetron Combination Therapy (26% to 39%)

Recombivax HB (Less to greater than 1%)

ReFacto Vials

Relpax Tablets (Infrequent)

ReoPro Vials (0.3%)

Requip Tablets (1% or more)

▲ Rescriptor Tablets (1.2% to 5%)

▲ Retrovir Capsules (2.4% to 5%)

▲ Retrovir IV Infusion (3% to 5%)

▲ Retrovir Syrup (2.4% to 5%)

▲ Retrovir Tablets (2.4% to 5%)

▲ Revatio Tablets (7%)

▲ Revlimid Capsules (10.1% to 32.1%)

▲ Reyataz Capsules (Less than 1% to 5%)

▲ Ribavirin, USP Capsules (14% to 41%)
Rilutek Tablets (2.1% to 2.9%)
▲ Risperdal Consta Long-Acting
Injection (13% to 16%)
▲ Risperdal M-Tab Orally Disintegrating
Tablets (23% to 26%)
▲ Risperdal Oral Solution (23% to 26%)
▲ Risperdal Tablets (23% to 26%)
▲ Ritalin Hydrochloride Tablets (One of
the two most common)
▲ Ritalin LA Capsules (3.1%)
▲ Ritalin-SR Tablets (One of the two
most common)
▲ Romazicon Injection (3% to 9%)
▲ Rozerem Tablets (3%)
Rythmol SR Capsules
▲ Sandostatin LAR Depot (5% to 15%)
Septra Tablets
Seroquel Tablets
▲ Serostim for Injection (3.9% to 5.9%)
▲ Simulect for Injection (Greater than or
equal to 10%)
Singulair Chewable Tablets
Singulair Oral Granules
Singulair Tablets
Sonata Capsules (Infrequent)
▲ Soriatane Capsules (1% to 10%)
Stalevo Tablets
▲ Strattera Capsules (5% to 16%)
▲ Suboxone Tablets (14% to 25%)
▲ Subutex Tablets (21.4% to 25%)
Sular Tablets (Less than or
equal to 1%)
▲ Sustiva Capsules (1% to 7%)
▲ Sustiva Tablets (1% to 7%)
Symbyax Capsules
▲ Symmetrel Tablets (5% to 10%)
▲ Tambocor Tablets (1% to 3%)
Tamiflu Capsules (1%)
Tamiflu Oral Suspension (1.1%
to 1.2%)
▲ Tarceva Tablets (0% to 15%)
▲ Targretin Capsules (4.8% to 11.3%)
▲ Targretin Gel (4.8% to 11.3%)
Tarka Tablets (Less frequent)
▲ Temodar Capsules (10%)
Testim 1% Gel (1% or less)
Teveten HCT Tablets (Less than 1%)
Teveten Tablets (Less than 1%)
Thalomid Capsules
Thiothixene Capsules
Thyrolar Tablets
Tiazac Capsules (Less than 2%)
Timolide Tablets (Less than 1%)
Timoptic in Ocudose (Less frequent)
Timoptic Sterile Ophthalmic Solution

Timoptic-XE Sterile Ophthalmic Gel
Forming Solution
Tindamax Tablets
▲ Topamax Sprinkle Capsules (6% to
9%)
▲ Topamax Tablets (6% to 9%)
Toprol-XL Tablets
Tranxene T-TAB Tablets
Tranxene-SD Half Strength Tablets
Tranxene-SD Tablets
▲ Trasylol Injection (3%)
Trelstar Depot (2.1%)
Trelstar LA Suspension (1.7%)
Tricor Tablets
▲ Trileptal Oral Suspension (2% to 4%)
▲ Trileptal Tablets (2% to 4%)
▲ Trisenox Injection (43%)
▲ Trizivir Tablets (7% to 13%)
▲ Truvada Tablets (4%)
Twinrix Vaccine (Less than 1%)
Tygacil for Injection (2.3%)
▲ Tykerb Tablets (0% to 10%)
Tylenol Allergy Multi-Symptom
Caplets with Cool Burst and Gelcaps
Tylenol Allergy Multi-Symptom
Nighttime Caplets with Cool Burst
Tylenol Cold Head Congestion
Daytime Caplets with Cool Burst
Tylenol Cold Head Congestion
Nighttime Caplets with Cool Burst
Tylenol Cold Head Congestion Severe
Caplets with Cool Burst
Tylenol Cold Multi-Symptom Daytime
Caplets with Cool Burst and Gelcaps
Tylenol Cold Multi-Symptom Daytime
Liquid with Citrus Burst
Tylenol Cold Multi-Symptom
Nighttime Caplets with Cool Burst
Tylenol Cold Multi-Symptom
Nighttime Liquid with Cool Burst
Tylenol Cold Multi-Symptom Severe
Caplets with Cool Burst
Tylenol Cold Multi-Symptom Severe
Daytime Liquid with Citrus Burst
Tylenol Cold Severe Congestion Non-
Drowsy Caplets with Cool Burst
Tylenol Sinus Congestion & Pain
Daytime Caplets with Cool Burst
and Gelcaps
Tylenol Sinus Congestion & Pain
Nighttime Caplets with Cool Burst
Tylenol Sinus Congestion & Pain
Severe Caplets with Cool Burst
Tylenol Sinus Severe Congestion
Caplets with Cool Burst

▲ Tyzeka Tablets (3%)
Ultane Liquid for Inhalation (Less than 1%)
▲ Ultram ER Tablets (6.5% to 10.9%)
Uniphyl Tablets
Uniretic Tablets (Less than 1%)
▲ Vagifem Tablets (3% to 5%)
▲ Valcyte Tablets (16%)
Valium Tablets
Vandazole Vaginal Gel (Less than 1%)
Vantas (2.9%)
Vantin Tablets and Oral Suspension (Less than 1%)
▲ Vaprisol (3.3%)
▲ Velcade for Injection (18%)
▲ Ventavis Inhalation Solution (8%)
Ventolin HFA Inhalation Aerosol
Verelan PM Extended-Release Capsules, Controlled-Onset (2% or less)
Verelan Sustained-Release Capsules (1% or less)
▲ Vesanoid Capsules (14%)
VFEND I.V. (Less than 2%)
VFEND Oral Suspension (Less than 2%)
VFEND Tablets (Less than 2%)
Viagra Tablets (Less than 2%)
Vicks 44D Cough & Head Congestion Relief Liquid
Vicks DayQuil Multi-Symptom Cold/Flu Relief LiquiCaps
Vicks DayQuil Multi-Symptom Cold/Flu Relief Liquid
▲ Vicoprofen Tablets (3% to 9%)
Viracept Oral Powder (Less than 2%)
Viracept Tablets (Less than 2%)
▲ Viread Tablets (3% to 4%)
▲ Vivitrol (8% to 14%)
▲ Voltaren Ophthalmic Solution (Less than or equal to 3%)
Voltaren Tablets (Occasionally)
Voltaren-XR Tablets (Occasionally)
VoSpire ER Tablets (2.4%)
Vytorin 10/10 Tablets
Vytorin 10/20 Tablets
Vytorin 10/40 Tablets
Vytorin 10/80 Tablets
▲ Vyvanse Capsules (10% to 19%)
▲ Wellbutrin SR Sustained-Release Tablets (5% to 16%)
▲ Wellbutrin Tablets (18.6%)
▲ Wellbutrin XL Extended-Release Tablets (11% to 20%)
▲ Xeloda Tablets (Less than 5%)

Xifaxan Tablets (Less than 2%)
Xopenex HFA Inhalation Aerosol
Xopenex Inhalation Solution
Xopenex Inhalation Solution Concentrate
Xyrem Oral Solution (Frequent)
Zantac 150 EFFERdose Tablets (Rare)
Zantac 150 Tablets (Rare)
Zantac 25 EFFERdose Tablets (Rare)
Zantac 300 Tablets (Rare)
Zantac Injection
Zantac Injection Pharmacy Bulk Package (Rare)
Zantac Injection Premixed
Zantac Syrup (Rare)
Zegerid Capsules (Less than 1%)
Zegerid Powder for Oral Solution (Less than 1%)
▲ Zelapar Tablets (7%)
Zocor Tablets
▲ Zoloft Oral Concentrate (12% to 28%)
▲ Zoloft Tablets (12% to 28%)
▲ Zometa for Intravenous Infusion (15.1% to 16%)
Zomig Nasal Spray (Infrequent to less than 2%)
Zomig Tablets (Infrequent)
Zomig-ZMT Tablets (Infrequent)
▲ Zonegran Capsules (6%)
▲ Zosyn (4.5% to 6.6%)
▲ Zyban Sustained-Release Tablets (31% to 40%)
Zyflo Tablets (Greater than 1%)
▲ Zyprexa Tablets (12% to 20%)
▲ Zyprexa ZYDIS Orally Disintegrating Tablets (12% to 20%)
▲ Zyrtec Chewable Tablets (Less than 2% to 9%)
▲ Zyrtec Syrup (Less than 2% to 9%)
▲ Zyrtec Tablets (Less than 2% to 9%)
▲ Zyrtec-D 12 Hour Extended Release Tablets (4%)
Zyvox for Oral Suspension (2.5%)
Zyvox Injection (2.5%)
Zyvox Tablets (2.5%)

Irritability

Advair HFA Inhalation Aerosol (Very Rare)
▲ Aerobid Inhaler System (3% to 9%)
▲ Aerobid-M Inhaler System (3% to 9%)
Angeliq Tablets
Aricept ODT Tablets (Frequent)
Aricept Tablets (Frequent)

Arthrotec Tablets (Rare)
Attenuvax
Cafcit Injection
Cafcit Oral Solution
Catapres-TTS (0.5% or less)
Ceftin for Oral Suspension (0.1% to 1%)
Cesamet Capsules
Chantix Tablets (Frequent)
Cipro I.V. (1% or less)
Cipro Oral Suspension (Less than 1%)
Cipro Tablets (Less than 1%)
Cipro XR Tablets
Ciprodex Otic Suspension (0.5%)
▲ Clarinex Syrup (12.1%)
Climara Pro Transdermal System
Climara Transdermal System
▲ Clolar for Intravenous Infusion (11%)
Clozaril Tablets (Less than 1%)
▲ Comvax (32.2% to 57.0%)
▲ Copegus Tablets (33%)
Cymbalta Delayed-Release Capsules (Frequent)
Dalmane Capsules
▲ DAPTACEL Vaccine (36.9% to 41.4%)
Daytrana Transdermal Patch
▲ Depade Tablets (Less than 10%)
▲ depo-subQ provera 104 Injectable Suspension (1% to less than 5%)
Effexor Tablets
Effexor XR Capsules
Efudex Topical Cream
Efudex Topical Solutions
Eldepryl Capsules
Elspar for Injection
Engerix-B Vaccine (Less than 1%)
Enjuvia Tablets
Estrasorb Topical Emulsion
Estratest H.S. Tablets
Estratest Tablets
FazaClo Orally Disintegrating Tablets (Less than 1%)
Femring Vaginal Ring
Femtrace Tablets
▲ Flumist Vaccine (9.9% to 17.8%)
▲ Gabitril Tablets (10%)
Guanidine Hydrochloride Tablets
▲ Havrix Vaccine (24% to 36%)
HibTITER (133 of 1,118 vaccinations)
▲ Indapamide Tablets (Greater than or equal to 5%)
▲ Infanrix Vaccine (28.8% to 61.5%)
▲ Intron A for Injection (Up to 16%)
Invirase Capsules (Less than 2%)
Invirase Tablets (Less than 2%)

▲ Keppra Oral Solution (6%)
▲ Keppra Tablets (6%)
▲ Lamictal Chewable Dispersible Tablets (3%)
▲ Lamictal Tablets (3%)
Levothroid Tablets
Levoxyl Tablets
Lexapro Oral Suspension (Frequent)
Lexapro Tablets (Frequent)
Liquid PedvaxHIB
Maxalt Tablets (Infrequent)
Maxalt-MLT Orally Disintegrating Tablets (Infrequent)
Menostar Transdermal System
Meruvax II
M-M-R II
Mumpsvax
Myozyme for Intravenous Infusion
▲ Niravam Orally Disintegrating Tablets (10.5% to 33.1%)
Paxil CR Controlled-Release Tablets
Paxil Tablets
▲ Pediarix Vaccine (1.7% to 63.8%)
▲ Pegasys (19%)
▲ PegIntron Powder for Injection (28%)
Premarin Tablets
Premarin Vaginal Cream
Premphase Tablets
Prempro Tablets
▲ Prevnar for Injection (44.2% to 58.7%)
Prezista Tablets (Less than 2%)
Prinivil Tablets (0.3% to 1.0%)
Prinzide Tablets
Proleukin for Injection
▲ Prometrium Capsules (100 mg, 200 mg) (5% to 8%)
▲ ProQuad (6.7%)
Prozac Pulvules and Liquid
Pulmicort Respules (Less than 1%)
Pulmicort Turbuhaler Inhalation Powder (Rare)
▲ Rebetol Capsules (10% to 47%)
▲ Rebetol Oral Solution (10% to 47%)
▲ Rebetron Combination Therapy (23% to 32%)
Recombivax HB (Greater than 1%)
Retrovir Capsules (1.6%)
Retrovir IV Infusion (2%)
Retrovir Syrup (1.6%)
Retrovir Tablets (1.6%)
▲ Ribavirin, USP Capsules (10% to 47%)
▲ RotaTeq (2.9% to 8.1%)
Seroquel Tablets
Singulair Chewable Tablets (Very rare)
Singulair Oral Granules (Very rare)

Singulair Tablets (Very rare)
▲ Skelaxin Tablets (Most frequent)
▲ Strattera Capsules (0.5% to 8%)
Symbyax Capsules
▲ Symmetrel Tablets (1% to 5%)
Tasmar Tablets (1%)
Tranxene T-TAB Tablets
Tranxene-SD Half Strength Tablets
Tranxene-SD Tablets
Twinrix Vaccine (Less than 1%)
Ultram ER Tablets (0.5% to less than 1%)
Uniphyl Tablets
Vantas (Less than 2%)
▲ Vaqta (10.8%)
Varivax (Greater than or equal to 1%)
Verdeso Foam (0% to 1%)
Vivitrol
VoSpire ER Tablets (Less frequent)
▲ Vyvanse Capsules (10%)
▲ Wellbutrin SR Sustained-Release Tablets (2% to 3%)
▲ Wellbutrin XL Extended-Release Tablets (2% to 3%)
▲ Xeloda Tablets (Less than 5%)
Zoloft Oral Concentrate
Zoloft Tablets
Zomig Nasal Spray (Rare)
Zomig Tablets (Rare)
Zomig-ZMT Tablets (Rare)
▲ Zonegran Capsules (9%)
Zyban Sustained-Release Tablets (Frequent)
Zyrtec Chewable Tablets
Zyrtec Syrup
Zyrtec Tablets

Jitteriness
▲ Byetta Injection (9%)
Cafcit Injection
Cafcit Oral Solution
Cubicin for Injection (Less than 1%)
Cymbalta Delayed-Release Capsules (Infrequent)
▲ Focalin XR Capsules (12%)
Guanidine Hydrochloride Tablets
Lexapro Oral Suspension (Infrequent)
Lexapro Tablets (Infrequent)
Opana ER Tablets (Less than 1%)
Opana Tablets (Less than 1%)
Prograf Capsules and Injection
Ultram ER Tablets (0.5% to less than 1%)
▲ Wellbutrin XL Extended-Release Tablets (3%)
Xyrem Oral Solution (Infrequent)

Libido, changes
Adderall Tablets
Adderall XR Capsules
Adipex-P Capsules
Adipex-P Tablets
Alora ETS Patch
Avalide Tablets
Avapro Tablets (Less than 1%)
Brevicon Tablets
Climara Pro Transdermal System
Climara Transdermal System
Desoxyn Tablets, USP
Dexedrine Spansule Capsules
Dexedrine Tablets
DextroStat Tablets
Diastat Rectal Delivery System (Infrequent)
Enjuvia Tablets
Estrace Tablets
Estrace Vaginal Cream
Estrasorb Topical Emulsion
Estratest H.S. Tablets
Estratest Tablets
Femhrt Tablets
Femring Vaginal Ring
Femtrace Tablets
Invirase Capsules (Greater than or equal to 2%)
Invirase Tablets (Greater than or equal to 2%)
Levora Tablets
Low-Ogestrel Tablets
▲ Lupron Depot 3.75 mg (16%)
▲ Lupron Depot-3 Month 11.25 mg (16%)
Menostar Transdermal System
Microgestin 1.5/30 Tablets
Microgestin 1/20 Tablets
Microgestin Fe 1.5/30 Tablets
Microgestin Fe 1/20 Tablets
Mircette Tablets
Necon 0.5/35 Tablets
Necon 1/35 Tablets
Necon 1/50 Tablets
Necon 10/11 Tablets
Neurontin Capsules (Infrequent)
Neurontin Oral Solution (Infrequent)
Neurontin Tablets (Infrequent)
Nipent for Injection (Less than 3%)
▲ Niravam Orally Disintegrating Tablets (7.1%)
Norinyl 1 + 35 Tablets
Norinyl 1 + 50 Tablets

Ortho Evra Transdermal System
Ortho Tri-Cyclen Lo Tablets
Ortho Tri-Cyclen Tablets
Ortho-Cyclen Tablets
Ovcon 50 Tablets
Oxandrin Tablets
Premarin Intravenous
Premarin Tablets
Premarin Vaginal Cream
Premphase Tablets
Prempro Tablets
Seasonique Tablets
Thioridazine Hydrochloride Tablets
Tri-Norinyl Tablets
Trivora-28 Tablets
Valium Tablets (Infrequent)
Vyvanse Capsules
Yasmin 28 Tablets
YAZ Tablets
Zovia 1/35E Tablets
Zovia 1/50E Tablets

Libido, decreased

Abilify Discmelt Orally Disintegrating
  Tablets (Infrequent)
Abilify Oral Solution (Infrequent)
Abilify Tablets (Infrequent)
AcipHex Tablets
Actiq (Less than 1%)
Adalat CC Tablets (Less than 1%)
▲ Adderall XR Capsules (2% to 4%)
Aldoril Tablets
Ambien CR Tablets (Rare)
Ambien Tablets (Rare)
Amerge Tablets (Rare)
▲ AndroGel (Up to 3%)
Androxy Tablets
Aricept ODT Tablets (Infrequent)
Aricept Tablets (Infrequent)
Asacol Delayed-Release Tablets
▲ Avinza Capsules (Less than 5%)
▲ Avodart Soft Gelatin Capsules (0.3%
  to 3%)
Axid Oral Solution
Azilect Tablets (Greater than 1%)
Caduet Tablets (Less than 2%)
Calcijex Injection
Campral Tablets (Frequent)
Cardura XL Tablets (Less than 1%)
Celexa Oral Solution (2%)
Celexa Tablets (2%)
Chantix Tablets (Infrequent)
Clozaril Tablets (Less than 1%)
Copaxone for Injection
  (Infrequent)

Coreg CR Extended-Release Capsules
  (0.1% to less than or equal to 1%)
Coreg Tablets (Greater than 0.1% to
  1%)
Corzide 40/5 Tablets (1 to 5 of 1000
  patients)
Cosopt Sterile Ophthalmic Solution
Cozaar Tablets (Less than 1%)
▲ Cymbalta Delayed-Release Capsules
  (1% to 6%)
▲ Depo-Provera Contraceptive Injection
  (1% to 5%)
▲ depo-subQ provera 104 Injectable
  Suspension (1% to less than 5%)
Diovan HCT Tablets (Less frequent)
Duragesic Transdermal System (Less
  than 1%)
DynaCirc CR Tablets (0.5% to 1%)
▲ Effexor Tablets (2% to 5.7%)
▲ Effexor XR Capsules (3% to 9%)
▲ Eligard 30 mg (3.3%)
Eligard 45 mg (1%)
Eligard 7.5 mg (Less than 2%)
Emsam Transdermal System (0.7%)
Estring Vaginal Ring
Exelon Capsules (Infrequent)
Exelon Oral Solution (Infrequent)
FazaClo Orally Disintegrating Tablets
  (Less than 1%)
Flomax Capsules (1.0% to 2.0%)
Gabitril Tablets (Infrequent)
Gengraf Capsules (1% to less
  than 3%)
Hectorol Capsules
Hectorol Injection
Hyperstat I.V.
Hytrin Capsules (0.6%)
Hyzaar 100-12.5 Tablets
Hyzaar 100-25 Tablets
Hyzaar 50-12.5 Tablets
▲ Imdur Tablets (Less than or
  equal to 5%)
▲ Indapamide Tablets (Less than 5%)
▲ Infergen (5%)
▲ Intron A for Injection (Up to 5%)
Kadian Capsules (Less than 3%)
Kaletra Oral Solution (Up to 2%)
Kaletra Tablets (0% to 2%)
Klonopin Tablets (1%)
Klonopin Wafers (1%)
Lamictal Chewable Dispersible
  Tablets (Infrequent)
Lamictal Tablets (Infrequent)
▲ Lexapro Oral Suspension (3% to 7%)
▲ Lexapro Tablets (3% to 7%)

Librium Capsules
Lipitor Tablets (Less than 2%)
Lopressor Injection
Lopressor Tablets
Lotensin HCT Tablets (0.3% to 1%)
Lotrel Capsules
▲ Lunesta Tablets (0% to 3%)
▲ Lupron Depot 3.75 mg (Less than 5%)
▲ Lupron Depot 7.5 mg (5.4%)
▲ Lupron Depot-3 Month 11.25 mg (1.8% to 11%)
Lyrica Capsules (Greater than or equal to 1%)
Mavik Tablets (0.3% to 1.0%)
▲ Megace ES Oral Suspension (0% to 5%)
Meridia Capsules
Midamor Tablets (Less than or equal to 1%)
Mirapex Tablets (1%)
▲ Mirena Intrauterine System (5% or more)
Moduretic Tablets
MS Contin Tablets (Less frequent)
Nadolol Tablets (1 to 5 of 1000 patients)
Neoral Oral Solution (1% to less than 3%)
Neoral Soft Gelatin Capsules (1% to less than 3%)
Neurontin Capsules (Infrequent)
Neurontin Oral Solution (Infrequent)
Neurontin Tablets (Infrequent)
▲ Niravam Orally Disintegrating Tablets (14.4%)
Norvir Oral Solution (Less than 2%)
Norvir Soft Gelatin Capsules (Less than 2%)
Oramorph SR Tablets (Less frequent)
OxyContin Tablets
▲ Paxil CR Controlled-Release Tablets (3% to 9%)
▲ Paxil Oral Suspension (3% to 9%)
▲ Paxil Tablets (3% to 9%)
Pepcid for Oral Suspension (Infrequent)
Pepcid Injection (Infrequent)
Pepcid Injection Premixed (Infrequent)
Pepcid Tablets (Infrequent)
Permax Tablets (Infrequent)
▲ Pexeva Tablets (1% to 14%)
Prevacid Delayed-Release Capsules (Less than 1%)
Prevacid for Delayed-Release Oral Suspension (Less than 1%)

Prevacid NapraPAC 375 (Less than 1%)
Prevacid NapraPAC 500 (Less than 1%)
Prevacid SoluTab Delayed-Release Orally Disintegrating Tablets (Less than 1%)
PREVPAC (Less than 1%)
Prinivil Tablets (0.4%)
Prinzide Tablets (0.3% to 1%)
▲ Prochieve 4% Gel (10%)
▲ Prochieve 8% Gel (10%)
▲ Propecia Tablets (1.8% - 6.4%)
▲ Proscar Tablets (2.6% to 6.4%)
ProSom Tablets (Rare)
Protonix I.V. (Less than 1%)
Protonix Tablets (Less than 1%)
Provigil Tablets (At least 1%)
▲ Prozac Pulvules and Liquid (1% to 11%)
Requip Tablets (Infrequent)
Rescriptor Tablets
Reyataz Capsules (Less than 3%)
Rilutek Tablets (Infrequent)
Risperdal Consta Long-Acting Injection (Infrequent)
Rocaltrol Capsules
Rocaltrol Oral Solution
Rythmol SR Capsules
Sandostatin Injection (Less than 1%)
Sandostatin LAR Depot (Rare)
Seroquel Tablets (Rare)
Sonata Capsules (Infrequent)
Soriatane Capsules (Less than 1%)
▲ Strattera Capsules (5% or greater)
Sular Tablets (Less than or equal to 1%)
▲ Symbyax Capsules (2% to 4%)
Symmetrel Tablets (0.1% to 1%)
Tambocor Tablets (Less than 1%)
Tarka Tablets
Tasmar Tablets (Infrequent)
Thalomid Capsules
Timolide Tablets (Less than 1%)
Timoptic in Ocudose
Timoptic Sterile Ophthalmic Solution
Timoptic-XE Sterile Ophthalmic Gel Forming Solution
▲ Topamax Sprinkle Capsules (0% to 3%)
▲ Topamax Tablets (0% to 3%)
Toprol-XL Tablets
Trelstar LA Suspension (2.3%)
Tricor Tablets
Trileptal Oral Suspension
Trileptal Tablets

Ultram ER Tablets (0.5% to less than 1%)
Uniretic Tablets (Less than 1%)
Vantas (2.3%)
VFEND I.V. (Less than 2%)
VFEND Oral Suspension (Less than 2%)
VFEND Tablets (Less than 2%)
Vicoprofen Tablets (Less than 1%)
Vivitrol
Wellbutrin SR Sustained-Release Tablets (Infrequent)
▲ Wellbutrin Tablets (3.1%)
▲ Wellbutrin XL Extended-Release Tablets (3%)
YAZ Tablets (Greater than 1%)
Zantac Injection
Zantac Injection Pharmacy Bulk Package (Infrequent)
Zantac Injection Premixed
▲ Zoloft Oral Concentrate (1% to 11%)
▲ Zoloft Tablets (1% to 11%)
Zonegran Capsules (Infrequent)
Zyban Sustained-Release Tablets (Infrequent)
Zyprexa Tablets (Infrequent)
Zyprexa ZYDIS Orally Disintegrating Tablets (Infrequent)
Zyrtec Chewable Tablets (Less than 2%)
Zyrtec Syrup (Less than 2%)
Zyrtec Tablets (Less than 2%)
Zyrtec-D 12 Hour Extended Release Tablets (Less than 2%)

Libido, increased

Abilify Discmelt Orally Disintegrating Tablets (Infrequent)
Abilify Oral Solution (Infrequent)
Abilify Tablets (Infrequent)
AndroGel (One patient)
Androxy Tablets
Aricept ODT Tablets (Frequent)
Aricept Tablets (Frequent)
Campral Tablets (Infrequent)
Celexa Oral Solution (Infrequent)
Celexa Tablets (Infrequent)
Clozaril Tablets (Less than 1%)
Depo-Provera Contraceptive Injection (Less than 1%)
depo-subQ provera 104 Injectable Suspension
Effexor Tablets (Infrequent)
Effexor XR Capsules (Infrequent)
Exelon Capsules (Infrequent)

Exelon Oral Solution (Infrequent)
FazaClo Orally Disintegrating Tablets (Less than 1%)
Gabitril Tablets (Infrequent)
Gengraf Capsules (1% to less than 3%)
Klonopin Tablets (Infrequent)
Klonopin Wafers (Infrequent)
Lamictal Chewable Dispersible Tablets (Rare)
Lamictal Tablets (Rare)
Librium Capsules
Lotensin Tablets (Less than 1%)
Lyrica Capsules (0.1% to 1%)
Meridia Capsules
Mirapex Tablets
Moban Tablets
Namenda Oral Solution (Infrequent)
Namenda Tablets (Infrequent)
Neoral Oral Solution (1% to less than 3%)
Neoral Soft Gelatin Capsules (1% to less than 3%)
Neurontin Capsules (Rare)
Neurontin Oral Solution (Rare)
Neurontin Tablets (Rare)
▲ Niravam Orally Disintegrating Tablets (7.7%)
Parcopa Orally Disintegrating Tablets
Paxil CR Controlled-Release Tablets (Rare)
Paxil Oral Suspension (Rare)
Paxil Tablets (Rare)
Permax Tablets (Infrequent)
Pexeva Tablets (Infrequent)
Prevacid Delayed-Release Capsules (Less than 1%)
Prevacid for Delayed-Release Oral Suspension (Less than 1%)
Prevacid NapraPAC 375 (Less than 1%)
Prevacid NapraPAC 500 (Less than 1%)
Prevacid SoluTab Delayed-Release Orally Disintegrating Tablets (Less than 1%)
PREVPAC (Less than 1%)
Prozac Pulvules and Liquid (Infrequent)
Razadyne ER Extended-Release Capsules (Infrequent)
Razadyne Oral Solution (Infrequent)
Razadyne Tablets (Infrequent)

Requip Tablets (Infrequent)
Rilutek Tablets (Infrequent)
Risperdal M-Tab Orally Disintegrating
  Tablets (Infrequent)
Risperdal Oral Solution
  (Infrequent)
Risperdal Tablets (Infrequent)
Seroquel Tablets (Infrequent)
Stalevo Tablets
Symbyax Capsules (Rare)
Tasmar Tablets (Infrequent)
Topamax Sprinkle Capsules (Rare)
Topamax Tablets (Rare)
Trileptal Oral Suspension
Trileptal Tablets
Wellbutrin SR Sustained-Release
  Tablets
Wellbutrin Tablets (Frequent)
Wellbutrin XL Extended-Release
  Tablets
Xyrem Oral Solution (Infrequent)
Zoloft Oral Concentrate (Rare)
Zoloft Tablets (Rare)
Zyban Sustained-Release Tablets
Zyprexa Tablets
Zyprexa ZYDIS Orally Disintegrating
  Tablets

Libido, loss of

Advicor Tablets
Altoprev Extended-Release Tablets
Catapres Tablets (About 3 in 100
  patients)
Catapres-TTS (0.5% or less)
▲ Clorpres Tablets (About 3%)
▲ Eulexin Capsules (36%)
Klonopin Tablets (Infrequent)
Klonopin Wafers (Infrequent)
Lescol Capsules
Lescol XL Tablets
Mevacor Tablets (0.5% to 1.0%)
Soltamox Oral Solution
Vytorin 10/10 Tablets
Vytorin 10/20 Tablets
Vytorin 10/40 Tablets
Vytorin 10/80 Tablets
Zantac 150 EFFERdose Tablets
  (Occasional)
Zantac 150 Tablets (Occasional)
Zantac 25 EFFERdose Tablets
  (Occasional)
Zantac 300 Tablets (Occasional)
Zantac Syrup (Occasional)
Zocor Tablets

Listlessness

Aricept ODT Tablets (Infrequent)
Aricept Tablets (Infrequent)
Indocin Capsules (Greater than 1%)
Indocin Oral Suspension (Greater
  than 1%)
Indocin Suppositories (Greater than 1%)

Manic behavior

Abilify Discmelt Orally Disintegrating
  Tablets (Frequent)
Abilify Oral Solution (Frequent)
Abilify Tablets (Frequent)
Ambien Tablets (Rare)
Campral Tablets (Rare)
Celexa Oral Solution
Celexa Tablets
Cipro I.V. (1% or less)
Cipro Oral Suspension (Less than 1%)
Cipro Tablets (Less than 1%)
Cipro XR Tablets
Concerta Extended-Release Tablets
Copaxone for Injection (Infrequent)
Effexor Tablets (0.5%)
Effexor XR Capsules (0.5%)
Evoxac Capsules (Less than 1%)
Herceptin I.V. (At least one of the
  958 patients)
▲ Intron A for Injection (Less than 5%)
▲ Lamictal Chewable Dispersible Tablets
  (5%)
▲ Lamictal Tablets (5%)
Levaquin in 5% Dextrose Injection
  (0.1% to 0.9%)
Levaquin Injection (0.1% to 0.9%)
Levaquin Oral Solution (0.1% to 0.9%)
Levaquin Tablets (0.1% to 0.9%)
Levbid Extended-Release Tablets
Levsin Drops
Levsin Elixir
Levsin Injection
Levsin Tablets
Levsin/SL Tablets
Levsinex Timecaps
Neurontin Capsules (Rare)
Neurontin Oral Solution (Rare)
Neurontin Tablets (Rare)
Orthoclone OKT3 Sterile Solution
  (Less than 1%)
Parnate Tablets
Paxil CR Controlled-Release Tablets
  (Infrequent)
Paxil Oral Suspension (Infrequent)
Paxil Tablets (Infrequent)

Permax Tablets (Infrequent)
Protopam Chloride for Injection, USP (Several cases)
Provigil Tablets
Relpax Tablets (Rare)
Requip Tablets (Infrequent)
Rescriptor Tablets
Retrovir IV Infusion
Rilutek Tablets (Infrequent)
Risperdal Consta Long-Acting Injection (Infrequent)
▲ Risperdal M-Tab Orally Disintegrating Tablets (8%)
▲ Risperdal Oral Solution (8%)
▲ Risperdal Tablets (8%)
Seroquel Tablets (Infrequent)
Sustiva Capsules (0.2%)
Sustiva Tablets (0.2%)
Symmetrel Tablets
Tasmar Tablets (Infrequent)
Topamax Sprinkle Capsules (Rare)
Topamax Tablets (Rare)
Trileptal Oral Suspension
Trileptal Tablets
Valtrex Caplets
Wellbutrin SR Sustained-Release Tablets
Wellbutrin Tablets (Frequent)
Wellbutrin XL Extended-Release Tablets
Zomig Nasal Spray (Rare)
Zyban Sustained-Release Tablets
Zyprexa Tablets (Frequent)
Zyprexa ZYDIS Orally Disintegrating Tablets (Frequent)

Memory impairment

Abilify Discmelt Orally Disintegrating Tablets (Infrequent)
Abilify Oral Solution (Infrequent)
Abilify Tablets (Infrequent)
Copaxone for Injection (Infrequent)
▲ Copegus Tablets (6%)
Cozaar Tablets (Less than 1%)
Cyanokit
Detrol LA Capsules
Eldepryl Capsules
Gleevec Tablets (Infrequent)
Hyzaar 100-12.5 Tablets
Hyzaar 100-25 Tablets
Hyzaar 50-12.5 Tablets
Imitrex Nasal Spray (Rare)
Imitrex Tablets (Rare)
▲ Klonopin Tablets (4%)
▲ Klonopin Wafers (4%)

Lamictal Chewable Dispersible Tablets (2.4%)
Lamictal Tablets (2.4%)
Lithobid Tablets
Lunesta Tablets (Infrequent)
▲ Lupron Depot 3.75 mg (Among most frequent)
▲ Lupron Depot-3 Month 11.25 mg (Less than 5%)
Maxalt Tablets (Infrequent)
Maxalt-MLT Orally Disintegrating Tablets (Infrequent)
Mirapex Tablets
▲ Niravam Orally Disintegrating Tablets (5.5% to 33.1%)
Parcopa Orally Disintegrating Tablets
▲ Pegasys (5%)
Prezista Tablets (Less than 2%)
Prinivil Tablets (0.3% to 1.0%)
Prinzide Tablets
Revlimid Capsules
Seromycin Capsules
Stalevo Tablets
▲ Temodar Capsules (7%)
Timolide Tablets
▲ Topamax Sprinkle Capsules (2% to 14%)
▲ Topamax Tablets (2% to 14%)
Transderm Scop Transdermal Therapeutic System (Infrequent)
▲ Vesanoid Capsules (3%)
▲ Wellbutrin SR Sustained-Release Tablets (Up to 3%)
Wellbutrin Tablets (Infrequent)
▲ Wellbutrin XL Extended-Release Tablets (3%)
Xyrem Oral Solution (Frequent)
▲ Zonegran Capsules (6%)
Zyban Sustained-Release Tablets (Infrequent)

Memory loss, short-term

Altoprev Extended-Release Tablets
Clozaril Tablets (Less than 1%)
Corzide 40/5 Tablets
Cosopt Sterile Ophthalmic Solution
Inderal LA Long-Acting Capsules
InnoPran XL Capsules
Lescol Capsules
Lescol XL Tablets
Levbid Extended-Release Tablets
Levsin Drops
Levsin Elixir
Levsin Injection
Levsin Tablets
Levsin/SL Tablets

Levsinex Timecaps
Lopressor HCT 100/25 Tablets
Lopressor HCT 100/50 Tablets
Lopressor HCT 50/25 Tablets
Lopressor Injection
Lopressor Tablets
Meridia Capsules
Mevacor Tablets (0.5% to 1.0%)
Nadolol Tablets
Parnate Tablets
PegIntron Powder for Injection
Timoptic in Ocudose
Timoptic Sterile Ophthalmic Solution
Timoptic-XE Sterile Ophthalmic Gel
  Forming Solution
Toprol-XL Tablets
Zocor Tablets

Mental acuity, loss of

Retrovir IV Infusion
Retrovir Syrup
Retrovir Tablets
Stalevo Tablets
Tasmar Tablets (0.01)

Mental clouding

Dilaudid Ampules
Dilaudid Non-Sterile Powder
Dilaudid Rectal Suppositories
Dilaudid Tablets
Hycodan Syrup
Hycodan Tablets
Hycotuss Expectorant Syrup
Maxidone Tablets C-III
Norco Tablets C-III
Numorphan Injection
Tussionex Pennkinetic Extended-
  Release Suspension
Vicodin ES Tablets
Vicodin HP Tablets
Vicodin Tablets
Zydone Tablets

Mental performance, impairment

Aldoril Tablets
Alferon N Injection (0.01)
Ambien Tablets (Infrequent)
Amerge Tablets (Infrequent)
Anaprox DS Tablets (Less than 1%)
Anaprox Tablets (Less than 1%)
Arranon Injection (1%)
Arthrotec Tablets (Rare)
Celexa Oral Solution (Frequent)
Celexa Tablets (Frequent)

Chantix Tablets (Rare)
Clozaril Tablets
Copaxone for Injection (Infrequent)
Cosopt Sterile Ophthalmic Solution
Dilaudid Ampules
Dilaudid Multiple Dose Vials
Dilaudid Non-Sterile Powder
Dilaudid Rectal Suppositories
Dilaudid Tablets
EC-Naprosyn Delayed-Release Tablets
  (Less than 1%)
Exelon Capsules (Infrequent)
Exelon Oral Solution (Infrequent)
Flumadine Syrup (0.3% to 2.1%)
Flumadine Tablets (0.3% to 2.1%)
Frova Tablets (Infrequent)
▲ Gabitril Tablets (6%)
Gengraf Capsules (1% to less
  than 3%)
Hycodan Syrup
Hycodan Tablets
Hycotuss Expectorant Syrup
Imitrex Injection (Rare)
Imitrex Nasal Spray (Rare)
Imitrex Tablets (Infrequent)
▲ Intron A for Injection (Up to 14%)
Invirase Capsules (Less than 2%)
Invirase Tablets (Less than 2%)
Kadian Capsules (Less than 3%)
Klonopin Tablets (1% to 2%)
Klonopin Wafers (1% to 2%)
Lamictal Chewable Dispersible
  Tablets (1.7%)
Lamictal Tablets (1.7%)
Levaquin in 5% Dextrose Injection
  (0.1% to 0.9%)
Levaquin Injection (0.1% to 0.9%)
Levaquin Oral Solution
  (0.1% to 0.9%)
Levaquin Tablets (0.1% to 0.9%)
Levbid Extended-Release Tablets
Levsin Drops
Levsin Elixir
Levsin Injection
Levsin Tablets
Levsin/SL Tablets
Levsinex Timecaps
Lexapro Oral Suspension (Frequent)
Lexapro Tablets (Frequent)
Maxalt Tablets (Frequent)
Maxalt-MLT Orally Disintegrating
  Tablets (Infrequent)
Maxidone Tablets C-III
Meridia Capsules

Migranal Nasal Spray (Infrequent)
MS Contin Tablets
Naprosyn Suspension (Less than 1%)
Naprosyn Tablets (Less than 1%)
Neoral Oral Solution (1% to less than 3%)
Neoral Soft Gelatin Capsules (1% to less than 3%)
Norco Tablets C-III
Opana ER Tablets (Less than 1%)
Opana Tablets (Less than 1%)
Paxil CR Controlled-Release Tablets (Frequent)
Paxil Oral Suspension (Frequent)
Paxil Tablets (Frequent)
Percocet Tablets
Percodan Tablets
Phenergan Tablets and Suppositories
▲ Prometrium Capsules (100 mg, 200 mg) (Less than 5%)
ProSom Tablets
Rebetron Combination Therapy
Requip Tablets (Infrequent)
Risperdal M-Tab Orally Disintegrating Tablets (Infrequent)
Risperdal Oral Solution (Infrequent)
Risperdal Tablets (Infrequent)
Seroquel Tablets
▲ Sustiva Capsules (1% to 9%)
▲ Sustiva Tablets (1% to 9%)
Sutent Capsules
Tarka Tablets (Less frequent)
Timolide Tablets
Timoptic in Ocudose
Timoptic Sterile Ophthalmic Solution
Timoptic-XE Sterile Ophthalmic Gel Forming Solution
▲ Topamax Sprinkle Capsules (5% to 14%)
▲ Topamax Tablets (5% to 14%)
Tussionex Pennkinetic Extended-Release Suspension
Tylenol with Codeine Elixir
Tylenol with Codeine Tablets
Vicodin ES Tablets
Vicodin HP Tablets
Vicodin Tablets
Vivitrol
Xyrem Oral Solution (Infrequent)
Zoloft Oral Concentrate (1.3% to 2%)
Zoloft Tablets (1.3% to 2%)
▲ Zonegran Capsules (6%)
▲ Zyban Sustained-Release Tablets (9%)
Zydone Tablets

Zyrtec Chewable Tablets (Less than 2%)
Zyrtec Syrup (Less than 2%)
Zyrtec Tablets (Less than 2%)
Zyrtec-D 12 Hour Extended Release Tablets (Less than 2%)

Mental slowness
▲ Topamax Sprinkle Capsules (8% to 15.4%)
▲ Topamax Tablets (8% to 15.4%)
▲ Zonegran Capsules (4%)

Mental status, altered
Celexa Oral Solution
Celexa Tablets
Clozaril Tablets
Cubicin for Injection (Less than 1%)
Cuprimine Capsules
Dacogen Injection
Eldepryl Capsules
▲ Invanz for Injection (3.3% to 5.1%)
Lanoxicaps Capsules
Lanoxin Injection
Lanoxin Injection Pediatric
Lanoxin Tablets
Moban Tablets
Neumega for Injection
Opana ER Tablets (Less than 1%)
Opana Tablets (Less than 1%)
Orthoclone OKT3 Sterile Solution (Less than 1%)
▲ Prograf Capsules and Injection (Approximately 55%)
▲ Proleukin for Injection (73%)
Revlimid Capsules
Risperdal M-Tab Orally Disintegrating Tablets
Risperdal Oral Solution
Risperdal Tablets
Seroquel Tablets
Stalevo Tablets
Stromectol Tablets

Mood changes
Adalat CC Tablets (Rare)
▲ Aerobid Inhaler System (1% to 3%)
▲ Aerobid-M Inhaler System (1% to 3%)
▲ Agenerase Oral Solution (4% to 16%)
▲ Alimta for Injection (Up to 14%)
Aloxi Injection (Less than 1%)
Ambien CR Tablets (1%)
Angeliq Tablets
▲ Arimidex Tablets (17% to 19%)
Cesamet Capsules
Chantix Tablets (Infrequent)

Climara Pro Transdermal System
Climara Transdermal System
▲ Copegus Tablets (5% to 9%)
Cymbalta Delayed-Release Capsules
  (Infrequent)
Decadron Tablets
Dilaudid Ampules
Dilaudid Multiple Dose Vials
Dilaudid Non-Sterile Powder
Dilaudid Oral Liquid (Less frequent)
Dilaudid Rectal Suppositories
Dilaudid Tablets
Dilaudid Tablets-8 mg (Less frequent)
Dilaudid-HP Injection (Less frequent)
Dilaudid-HP Lyophilized Powder
  250 mg (Less frequent)
Eldepryl Capsules
Enbrel for Injection
Enjuvia Tablets
Estrasorb Topical Emulsion
Estratest H.S. Tablets
Estratest Tablets
Femring Vaginal Ring
Femtrace Tablets
Guanidine Hydrochloride Tablets
Hycodan Syrup
Hycodan Tablets
Hycotuss Expectorant Syrup
Hydrocortone Tablets
▲ Keppra Oral Solution (5%)
▲ Keppra Tablets (5%)
Lariam Tablets (Occasional)
▲ Lexiva Tablets (Less than 1% to 11%)
Lupron Depot 3.75 mg
Marinol Capsules
Maxidone Tablets C-III
Meridia Capsules
Mirapex Tablets
MS Contin Tablets (Less frequent)
Norco Tablets C-III
Oramorph SR Tablets (Less frequent)
Ortho Evra Transdermal System
Ortho Tri-Cyclen Lo Tablets
Ortho Tri-Cyclen Tablets
Orthoclone OKT3 Sterile Solution
Ortho-Cyclen Tablets
Paxil CR Controlled-Release Tablets
Paxil Oral Suspension
Paxil Tablets
▲ Pegasys (3%)
Premarin Tablets
Premarin Vaginal Cream
Premphase Tablets
Prempro Tablets

Prezista Tablets (Less than 2%)
Seasonique Tablets
▲ Solodyn Extended Release Tablets
  (3%)
▲ Soltamox Oral Solution (11.6%)
▲ Strattera Capsules (Greater than 5%)
Supprelin LA Implant
Testim 1% Gel (1% or less)
▲ Topamax Sprinkle Capsules
  (2% to 11%)
▲ Topamax Tablets (2% to 11%)
Tussionex Pennkinetic Extended-
  Release Suspension
Univasc Tablets (Less than 1%)
Vicodin ES Tablets
Vicodin HP Tablets
Vicodin Tablets
Vicoprofen Tablets (Less than 1%)
Wellbutrin Tablets (Infrequent)
▲ Xeloda Tablets (5%)
Xyrem Oral Solution (Infrequent)
Zydone Tablets

Nervousness

Abilify Discmelt Orally Disintegrating
  Tablets (Frequent)
Abilify Oral Solution (Frequent)
Abilify Tablets (Frequent)
Accutane Capsules
Aceon Tablets (2 mg, 4 mg, 8 mg)
  (1.1%)
AcipHex Tablets
Actiq (1% to 2%)
Adalat CC Tablets (Rare)
▲ Adderall XR Capsules (6%)
Adenoscan (2%)
▲ Aerobid Inhaler System (3% to 9%)
▲ Aerobid-M Inhaler System
  (3% to 9%)
▲ Agrylin Capsules (1% to 5%)
Alferon N Injection (1%)
Allegra Capsules (Less than 1%)
Allegra Oral Solution (Less than 1%)
Allegra Tablets (Less than 1%)
Allegra-D 12 Hour Extended-Release
  Tablets (1.4%)
Allegra-D 24 Hour Extended-Release
  Tablets (1.4%)
Altace Capsules (Less than 1%)
▲ Alupent Inhalation Aerosol (14.1%)
Ambien CR Tablets (Infrequent)
Ambien Tablets (1%)
AmBisome for Injection
  (Less common)
Amitiza Capsules (Less than 0.2%)

Anaprox DS Tablets (Less than 1%)
Anaprox Tablets (Less than 1%)
AndroGel (Up to 3%)
Angeliq Tablets
▲ Aricept ODT Tablets (3%)
▲ Aricept Tablets (3%)
▲ Arimidex Tablets (2% to 5%)
Arthrotec Tablets (Rare)
Asacol Delayed-Release Tablets (2% or greater)
Astelin Nasal Spray (Infrequent)
Atripla Tablets (Greater than or equal to 2%)
Atrovent Inhalation Solution (0.5%)
Avalide Tablets (1% or greater)
Avapro Tablets (1% or greater)
Avelox I.V. (0.1% to less than 2%)
Avelox Tablets (0.1% to less than 2%)
▲ Avinza Capsules (Less than 5%)
Axert Tablets (Rare)
Axid Oral Solution (1.1%)
▲ Bentyl Capsules (6%)
▲ Bentyl Injection (6%)
▲ Bentyl Syrup (6%)
▲ Bentyl Tablets (6%)
▲ Betaseron for SC Injection (7%)
Bicillin C-R Injectable Suspension
Brevicon Tablets
Brovana Inhalation Solution
Caduet Tablets (Greater than 0.1% to less than or equal to 1%)
Campath Ampules
Captopril Tablets
Cardizem LA Extended Release Tablets (Less than 2%)
Cardura XL Tablets
▲ Catapres Tablets (About 3 in 100 patients)
Catapres-TTS (1 of 101 patients)
Celebrex Capsules (0.1% to 1.9%)
▲ CellCept Capsules (3% to less than 20%)
▲ CellCept Intravenous (3% to less than 20%)
▲ CellCept Oral Suspension (3% to less than 20%)
▲ CellCept Tablets (3% to less than 20%)
Cesamet Capsules
Children's Tylenol Plus Cold Suspension Liquid
Children's Tylenol Plus Flu Suspension Liquid
Children's Tylenol Plus Multi-Symptom Cold Suspension Liquid
Children's Vicks NyQuil Cold/Cough Relief Liquid

Cipro I.V.
Cipro Oral Suspension
Cipro Tablets
Cipro XR Tablets
Clarinex-D 24-Hour Extended-Release Tablets (2%)
Climara Pro Transdermal System
Climara Transdermal System
Clinoril Tablets (Greater than 1%)
▲ Clorpres Tablets (About 3%)
Colazal Capsules
Combivent Inhalation Aerosol (Less than 2%)
Concentrated Tylenol Infants' Drops Plus Cold
Concentrated Tylenol Infants' Drops Plus Cold and Cough
▲ Concerta Extended-Release Tablets (Greater than 0.7%)
Copaxone for Injection (2%)
▲ Copegus Tablets (33%)
Coreg CR Extended-Release Capsules (0.1% to less than or equal to 1%)
Coreg Tablets (Greater than 0.1% to 1%)
Cosopt Sterile Ophthalmic Solution
▲ Cozaar Tablets (Less than 1% to 4%)
Cymbalta Delayed-Release Capsules (Frequent)
Dalmane Capsules
Dantrium Capsules (Less frequent)
Daytrana Transdermal Patch
Demadex Injection (1.1%)
Demadex Tablets (1.1%)
▲ Depacon Injection (0.9% to 11%)
▲ Depade Tablets (More than 10%)
▲ Depakene Capsules (11%)
▲ Depakene Oral Solution (11%)
▲ Depakote ER Tablets (Greater than 1% to 11%)
▲ Depakote Sprinkle Capsules (7% to 11%)
▲ Depakote Tablets (1% to 11%)
▲ Depo-Provera Contraceptive Injection (Greater than 5%)
depo-subQ provera 104 Injectable Suspension
Detrol Tablets (1.1%)
Diastat Rectal Delivery System (Greater than or equal to 1%)
Dilaudid Oral Liquid (Less frequent)
Dilaudid Tablets-8 mg (Less frequent)
Dilaudid-HP Injection

Dilaudid-HP Lyophilized Powder 250 mg
▲ Ditropan XL Extended-Release Tablets (2% to less than 5%)
Dolobid Tablets (Less than 1 in 100)
Donnatal Extentabs
Doxil Injection (Less than 1%)
▲ Duragesic Transdermal System (3% to 10%)
DynaCirc CR Tablets (0.5% to 1%)
EC-Naprosyn Delayed-Release Tablets (Less than 1%)
▲ Effexor Tablets (2% to 21.3%)
▲ Effexor XR Capsules (5% to 11%)
Eldepryl Capsules
▲ Eloxatin for Injection (2% to 5%)
Emsam Transdermal System
Enjuvia Tablets
▲ Entocort EC Capsules (Less than 5%)
EpiPen Jr. Auto-Injector
▲ Equetro Extended-Release Capsules (Less than 5%)
Estrasorb Topical Emulsion
Estratest H.S. Tablets
Estratest Tablets
Estring Vaginal Ring
Eulexin Capsules (1%)
Exelon Capsules (2% or more)
Exelon Oral Solution (2% or more)
Fansidar Tablets
▲ Femhrt Tablets (5.4%)
Femring Vaginal Ring
Femtrace Tablets
Fentora Tablets (Greater than 1%)
Ferrlecit Injection (Two or more patients)
Flumadine Syrup (1.3% to 2.1%)
Flumadine Tablets (1.3% to 2.1%)
▲ Focalin Tablets (Among most common)
Focalin XR Capsules
Foradil Aerolizer
▲ Foscavir Injection (Between 1% and 5%)
Frova Tablets (Infrequent)
▲ Gabitril Tablets (10%)
Gengraf Capsules (1% to less than 3%)
Hytrin Capsules (2.3%)
Hyzaar 100-12.5 Tablets
Hyzaar 100-25 Tablets
Hyzaar 50-12.5 Tablets
▲ Imdur Tablets (Less than or equal to 5%)
▲ Indapamide Tablets (Less than 5%)

Indocin Capsules (Less than 1%)
Indocin Oral Suspension (Less than 1%)
Indocin Suppositories (Less than 1%)
▲ Infergen (16% to 31%)
▲ Intron A for Injection (Up to 3%)
Invanz for Injection (Greater than 0.1%)
Ionsys Transdermal System (.1% to less than 1%)
Kaletra Oral Solution (Less than 2%)
Kaletra Tablets (Less than 2%)
▲ Keppra Injection (4%)
▲ Keppra Oral Solution (4% to 10%)
▲ Keppra Tablets (4% to 10%)
Klonopin Tablets (1% to 3%)
Klonopin Wafers (1% to 3%)
Lamictal Chewable Dispersible Tablets (2%)
Lamictal Tablets (2%)
Levaquin in 5% Dextrose Injection (0.1% to 0.9%)
Levaquin Injection (0.1% to 0.9%)
Levaquin Oral Solution (0.1% to 0.9%)
Levaquin Tablets (0.1% to 0.9%)
Levbid Extended-Release Tablets
Levora Tablets
Levothroid Tablets
Levoxyl Tablets
Levsin Drops
Levsin Elixir
Levsin Injection
Levsin Tablets
Levsin/SL Tablets
Levsinex Timecaps
Lexapro Oral Suspension (Infrequent)
Lexapro Tablets (Infrequent)
Lidoderm Patch
▲ Lithostat Tablets (20%)
Lotensin HCT Tablets (0.3% to 1%)
Lotensin Tablets (Less than 1%)
Lotrel Capsules
Low-Ogestrel Tablets
▲ Lunesta Tablets (0% to 5%)
▲ Lupron Depot 3.75 mg (4%)
▲ Lupron Depot-3 Month 11.25 mg (4%)
Lupron Depot-PED 7.5 mg, 11.25 mg and 15 mg (Less than 2%)
Lupron Injection Pediatric (Less than 2%)
Lyrica Capsules (1% to greater than or equal to 2%)
Marinol Capsules (Greater than 1%)
Matulane Capsules

▲ Maxair Autohaler (4.5% to 6.9%)
Maxalt Tablets (Infrequent)
Maxalt-MLT Orally Disintegrating
Tablets (Infrequent)
Menostar Transdermal System
▲ Meridia Capsules (5.2%)
Merrem I.V. (Greater than 0.1%
to 1%)
▲ Metadate CD Capsules (Among most
common)
Micardis HCT Tablets
Microgestin 1.5/30 Tablets
Microgestin 1/20 Tablets
Microgestin Fe 1.5/30 Tablets
Microgestin Fe 1/20 Tablets
Midamor Tablets (Less than or equal
to 1%)
Migranal Nasal Spray (Infrequent)
Mirapex Tablets (1% or more)
Mircette Tablets
▲ Mirena Intrauterine System
(5% or more)
Mobic Oral Suspension (Less than 2%)
Mobic Tablets (Less than 2%)
Moduretic Tablets (Less than or equal
to 1%)
MS Contin Tablets (Less frequent)
▲ Nalfon Capsules (5.7%)
Namenda Oral Solution (Infrequent)
Namenda Tablets (Infrequent)
Naprosyn Suspension (Less than 1%)
Naprosyn Tablets (Less than 1%)
Necon 0.5/35 Tablets
Necon 1/35 Tablets
Necon 1/50 Tablets
Necon 10/11 Tablets
Nembutal Sodium Solution, USP
(Less than 1%)
Neoral Soft Gelatin Capsules (1% to
less than 3%)
▲ Neumega for Injection (Greater than
or equal to 10%)
Neurontin Capsules (2.4%)
Neurontin Oral Solution (2.4%)
Neurontin Tablets (2.4%)
Nexium Delayed-Release Capsules
(Less than 1%)
Nexium Delayed-Release Oral
Suspension (Less than 1%)
Nexium I.V. (Less than 1%)
Niaspan Extended-Release Tablets
▲ Nipent for Injection (3% to 10%)
▲ Niravam Orally Disintegrating Tablets
(4.1%)
Norinyl 1 + 35 Tablets

Norinyl 1 + 50 Tablets
Norvasc Tablets (More than 0.1%
to 1%)
Norvir Oral Solution (Less than 2%)
Norvir Soft Gelatin Capsules (Less
than 2%)
NuLev Orally Disintegrating Tablets
Numorphan Injection
NuvaRing
▲ Ontak Vials (11%)
Opana ER Tablets (Less than 1%)
Opana Tablets (Less than 1%)
Oramorph SR Tablets (Less frequent)
Ortho Evra Transdermal System
Ortho Tri-Cyclen Lo Tablets
Ortho Tri-Cyclen Tablets
Ortho-Cyclen Tablets
Ovcon 50 Tablets
Oxsoralen-Ultra Capsules
▲ OxyContin Tablets (Between 1%
and 5%)
Parcopa Orally Disintegrating Tablets
▲ Paxil CR Controlled-Release Tablets
(4% to 9%)
▲ Paxil Oral Suspension (4% to 9%)
▲ Paxil Tablets (4% to 9%)
▲ Pegasys (19%)
▲ PegIntron Powder for Injection (4%)
Percodan Tablets
Permax Tablets (Frequent)
▲ Pexeva Tablets (2.9% to 9%)
Phenergan Tablets and Suppositories
Phenytek Capsules
Premarin Intravenous
▲ Premarin Tablets (2% to 5%)
Premarin Vaginal Cream
▲ Premphase Tablets (2% to 3%)
▲ Prempro Tablets (2% to 3%)
Prevacid Delayed-Release Capsules
(Less than 1%)
Prevacid for Delayed-Release Oral
Suspension (Less than 1%)
Prevacid NapraPAC 375
(Less than 1%)
Prevacid NapraPAC 500
(Less than 1%)
Prevacid SoluTab Delayed-Release
Orally Disintegrating Tablets
(Less than 1%)
PREVPAC (Less than 1%)
Prinivil Tablets (0.3% to 1.0%)
Prinzide Tablets
ProAir HFA Inhalation Aerosol
(Frequent)
ProAmatine Tablets (Less frequent)

▲ Prochieve 4% Gel (16%)
▲ Prochieve 8% Gel (16%)
▲ Prograf Capsules and Injection (3%)
Prometrium Capsules (100 mg, 200 mg)
ProQuad
▲ ProSom Tablets (8%)
Protonix I.V. (Less than 1%)
Protonix Tablets (Less than 1%)
▲ Proventil HFA Inhalation Aerosol (7%)
▲ Proventil Inhalation Aerosol (Less than 10%)
▲ Proventil Inhalation Solution 0.083% (4%)
▲ Provigil Tablets (7%)
▲ Prozac Pulvules and Liquid (8% to 16%)
Raniclor Tablets, Chewable (Rare)
▲ Rebetol Capsules (3% to 6%)
▲ Rebetol Oral Solution (3% to 6%)
▲ Rebetron Combination Therapy (4% to 5%)
Relpax Tablets (Infrequent)
Requip Tablets (1% or more)
Rescriptor Tablets
▲ Restoril Capsules (4.6)
Retrovir Capsules (1.6%)
Retrovir IV Infusion (2%)
Retrovir Syrup (1.6%)
Retrovir Tablets (1.6%)
Reyataz Capsules (Less than 3%)
▲ Ribavirin, USP Capsules (3% to 6%)
Risperdal Consta Long-Acting Injection (Frequent)
Risperdal M-Tab Orally Disintegrating Tablets (Frequent)
Risperdal Oral Solution (Frequent)
Risperdal Tablets (Frequent)
▲ Ritalin Hydrochloride Tablets (One of the two most common)
▲ Ritalin LA Capsules (Among most common)
▲ Ritalin-SR Tablets (One of the two most common)
▲ Romazicon Injection (3% to 9%)
▲ Sandostatin LAR Depot (1% to 4%)
Seasonique Tablets
Septra Tablets
▲ Skelaxin Tablets (Most frequent)
Sonata Capsules (Frequent)
Stalevo Tablets
▲ Suboxone Tablets (6%)
▲ Subutex Tablets (6%)
Sular Tablets (Less than or equal to 1%)
▲ Sustiva Capsules (1% to 7%)

▲ Sustiva Tablets (1% to 7%)
▲ Symmetrel Tablets (1% to 5%)
Synagis Intramuscular Powder (More than 1%)
Synagis Intramuscular Solution (More than 1%)
Synera Topical Patch
Tasmar Tablets (Infrequent)
Teveten HCT Tablets (Less than 1%)
Teveten Tablets (Less than 1%)
▲ Thalomid Capsules (2.8% to 9.4%)
Tiazac Capsules (Less than 2%)
Timolide Tablets (Less than 1%)
Timoptic in Ocudose (Less frequent)
Timoptic Sterile Ophthalmic Solution (Less frequent)
Timoptic-XE Sterile Ophthalmic Gel Forming Solution
▲ Topamax Sprinkle Capsules (4% to 19%)
▲ Topamax Tablets (4% to 19%)
Toprol-XL Tablets
Tranxene T-TAB Tablets (Less common)
Tranxene-SD Half Strength Tablets (Less common)
Tranxene-SD Tablets (Less common)
Tricor Tablets
▲ Trileptal Oral Suspension (2% to 4%)
▲ Trileptal Tablets (2% to 4%)
Tri-Norinyl Tablets
Trivora-28 Tablets
▲ Trizivir Tablets (Greater than or equal to 5%)
Tylenol Allergy Multi-Symptom Caplets with Cool Burst and Gelcaps
Tylenol Allergy Multi-Symptom Nighttime Caplets with Cool Burst
Tylenol Cold Head Congestion Daytime Caplets with Cool Burst
Tylenol Cold Head Congestion Nighttime Caplets with Cool Burst
Tylenol Cold Head Congestion Severe Caplets with Cool Burst
Tylenol Cold Multi-Symptom Daytime Caplets with Cool Burst and Gelcaps
Tylenol Cold Multi-Symptom Daytime Liquid with Citrus Burst
Tylenol Cold Multi-Symptom Nighttime Caplets with Cool Burst
Tylenol Cold Multi-Symptom Nighttime Liquid with Cool Burst
Tylenol Cold Multi-Symptom Severe Caplets with Cool Burst

Tylenol Cold Multi-Symptom Severe
  Daytime Liquid with Citrus Burst
Tylenol Cold Severe Congestion Non-
  Drowsy Caplets with Cool Burst
Tylenol Sinus Congestion & Pain
  Daytime Caplets with Cool Burst
  and Gelcaps
Tylenol Sinus Congestion & Pain
  Nighttime Caplets with Cool Burst
Tylenol Sinus Congestion & Pain
  Severe Caplets with Cool Burst
Tylenol Sinus Severe Congestion
  Caplets with Cool Burst
Ultane Liquid for Inhalation (Less
  than 1%)
▲ Ultram ER Tablets (1% to less than 5%)
Uniretic Tablets (Less than 1%)
Univasc Tablets (Less than 1%)
Vantin Tablets and Oral Suspension
  (Less than 1%)
Varivax (Greater than or equal to 1%)
Vicks 44D Cough & Head Congestion
  Relief Liquid
Vicks DayQuil Multi-Symptom
  Cold/Flu Relief LiquiCaps
Vicks DayQuil Multi-Symptom
  Cold/Flu Relief Liquid
▲ Vicoprofen Tablets (3% to 9%)
Vivaglobin (0.1%)
▲ Vivitrol (8% to 12%)
Voltaren Tablets (Occasionally)
Voltaren-XR Tablets (Occasionally)
▲ VoSpire ER Tablets (0.085)
▲ Wellbutrin SR Sustained-Release
  Tablets (3% to 5%)
Wellbutrin Tablets
▲ Wellbutrin XL Extended-Release
  Tablets (3% to 5%)
▲ Xopenex HFA Inhalation Aerosol
  (2.8% to 9.6%)
▲ Xopenex Inhalation Solution
  (2.8% to 9.6%)
▲ Xopenex Inhalation Solution
  Concentrate (2.8% to 9.6%)
Xyrem Oral Solution (Frequent)
Yasmin 28 Tablets (Greater than 1%)
YAZ Tablets
Zegerid Capsules (Less than 1%)
Zegerid Powder for Oral Solution
  (Less than 1%)
Zelapar Tablets
Zmax for Oral Suspension
▲ Zoloft Oral Concentrate (6%)
▲ Zoloft Tablets (6%)
Zomig Nasal Spray (Infrequent)

Zonegran Capsules (2%)
Zovia 1/35E Tablets
Zovia 1/50E Tablets
▲ Zyban Sustained-Release Tablets (4%)
Zyflo Tablets (Greater than 1%)
▲ Zyprexa Tablets (16%)
▲ Zyprexa ZYDIS Orally Disintegrating
  Tablets (16%)
Zyrtec Chewable Tablets
  (Less than 2%)
Zyrtec Syrup (Less than 2%)
Zyrtec Tablets (Less than 2%)
Zyrtec-D 12 Hour Extended Release
  Tablets (Less than 2%)

Neuropsychometrics performance, decrease

Corzide 40/5 Tablets
Cosopt Sterile Ophthalmic Solution
Inderal LA Long-Acting Capsules
InnoPran XL Capsules
Lopressor HCT 100/25 Tablets
Lopressor HCT 100/50 Tablets
Lopressor HCT 50/25 Tablets
Lopressor Injection
Lopressor Tablets
Nadolol Tablets
Timoptic in Ocudose
Timoptic Sterile Ophthalmic Solution
Timoptic-XE Sterile Ophthalmic Gel
  Forming Solution
Toprol-XL Tablets

Neurosis, unspecified

Ambien CR Tablets (Rare)
Ambien Tablets (Rare)
Atripla Tablets
Azilect Tablets (Infrequent)
Campral Tablets (Infrequent)
Evoxac Capsules
Exelon Capsules (Infrequent)
Exelon Oral Solution (Infrequent)
Gabitril Tablets (Infrequent)
▲ Intron A for Injection (Less than 5%)
Keppra Oral Solution
Keppra Tablets
Lamictal Chewable Dispersible
  Tablets (Rare)
Lamictal Tablets (Rare)
Lunesta Tablets (Infrequent)
Namenda Oral Solution (Infrequent)
Namenda Tablets (Infrequent)
Neurontin Capsules (Rare)
Neurontin Oral Solution (Rare)
Neurontin Tablets (Rare)

Nipent for Injection (Less than 3%)
Paxil CR Controlled-Release Tablets
(Infrequent)
Paxil Oral Suspension (Infrequent)
Paxil Tablets (Infrequent)
Permax Tablets (Infrequent)
Pexeva Tablets (Infrequent)
Prevacid Delayed-Release Capsules
(Less than 1%)
Prevacid for Delayed-Release Oral
Suspension (Less than 1%)
Prevacid NapraPAC 375
(Less than 1%)
Prevacid NapraPAC 500
(Less than 1%)
Prevacid SoluTab Delayed-Release
Orally Disintegrating Tablets (Less
than 1%)
PREVPAC (Less than 1%)
Prozac Pulvules and Liquid
(Infrequent)
Relpax Tablets (Rare)
Requip Tablets (Infrequent)
Rythmol SR Capsules
Sustiva Capsules
Sustiva Tablets
Symbyax Capsules (Infrequent)
Topamax Sprinkle Capsules (1%)
Topamax Tablets (1%)
Uniretic Tablets (Less than 1%)

Nightmares
Aldoril Tablets
Axert Tablets (Rare)
Biaxin Filmtab Tablets
Biaxin Granules
Biaxin XL Filmtab Tablets
Catapres Tablets
Catapres-TTS (0.5% or less)
Chantix Tablets (1% to 2%)
Cipro I.V. (1% or less)
Cipro Oral Suspension (Less than 1%)
Cipro Tablets (Less than 1%)
Cipro XR Tablets
Clorpres Tablets
▲ Clozaril Tablets (4%)
Cosopt Sterile Ophthalmic Solution
Cymbalta Delayed-Release Capsules
(Frequent)
Depade Tablets (Less than 1%)
▲ Effexor XR Capsules (4% to 7%)
Eldepryl Capsules
▲ FazaClo Orally Disintegrating Tablets
(4%)
Klonopin Tablets (Infrequent)

Klonopin Wafers (Infrequent)
Levaquin in 5% Dextrose Injection
Levaquin Injection
Levaquin Oral Solution
Levaquin Tablets
Lexapro Oral Suspension
Lexapro Tablets
▲ Lopressor HCT 100/25 Tablets (10%)
▲ Lopressor HCT 100/50 Tablets (10%)
▲ Lopressor HCT 50/25 Tablets (10%)
Lopressor Injection
Lopressor Tablets
Marinol Capsules (Less than 1%)
Matulane Capsules
Meridia Capsules
Mirapex Tablets
Nembutal Sodium Solution, USP
(Less than 1%)
Parcopa Orally Disintegrating Tablets
Phenergan Tablets and Suppositories
PREVPAC
Prezista Tablets (Less than 2%)
Proquin XR Tablets
Restoril Capsules (1.2%)
Risperdal M-Tab Orally Disintegrating
Tablets (Rare)
Risperdal Oral Solution (Rare)
Risperdal Tablets (Rare)
Rythmol SR Capsules
Stalevo Tablets
Timolide Tablets
Timoptic in Ocudose
Timoptic Sterile Ophthalmic Solution
Timoptic-XE Sterile Ophthalmic Gel
Forming Solution
Toprol-XL Tablets
Vantin Tablets and Oral Suspension
(Less than 1%)
▲ Xyrem Oral Solution (2.9% to 6.1%)

Obsessive compulsive symptoms
Mirapex Tablets
▲ Vivitrol (8% to 12%)
Zyprexa Tablets (Infrequent)
Zyprexa ZYDIS Orally Disintegrating
Tablets (Infrequent)

Orgasmic dysfunction, female
▲ Effexor XR Capsules (2% to 8%)
▲ Pexeva Tablets (2% to 9%)

Overstimulation
Adderall Tablets
Adderall XR Capsules
Adipex-P Capsules

Adipex-P Tablets
Desoxyn Tablets, USP
Dexedrine Spansule Capsules
Dexedrine Tablets
DextroStat Tablets
Eldepryl Capsules
Parnate Tablets
Restoril Capsules (Less than 0.5%)
Twinject 0.15
Twinject 0.3
Vyvanse Capsules

Panic attack
Abilify Discmelt Orally Disintegrating
  Tablets (Infrequent)
Abilify Oral Solution (Infrequent)
Abilify Tablets (Infrequent)
Ambien CR Tablets (Rare)
Ambien Tablets (Rare)
Amerge Tablets (Rare)
Celexa Oral Solution (Infrequent)
Celexa Tablets (Infrequent)
Cesamet Capsules
Cozaar Tablets (Less than 1%)
Effexor Tablets
Effexor XR Capsules
Hyzaar 100-12.5 Tablets
Hyzaar 100-25 Tablets
Hyzaar 50-12.5 Tablets
Imitrex Injection
Imitrex Nasal Spray
Imitrex Tablets
Lamictal Chewable Dispersible
  Tablets (Infrequent)
Lamictal Tablets (Infrequent)
Lariam Tablets (Occasional)
Lexapro Oral Suspension (Infrequent)
Lexapro Tablets (Infrequent)
Parnate Tablets
Paxil CR Controlled-Release Tablets
Paxil Tablets
Prozac Pulvules and Liquid
Romazicon Injection
Seroquel Tablets
Symbyax Capsules
Tasmar Tablets (1%)
Trileptal Oral Suspension
Trileptal Tablets
▲ Vivitrol (8% to 12%)
Wellbutrin SR Sustained-Release
  Tablets
Wellbutrin Tablets
Wellbutrin XL Extended-Release
  Tablets

Zoloft Oral Concentrate
Zoloft Tablets
Zyban Sustained-Release Tablets

Paranoia
Adalat CC Tablets (Rare)
Allegra-D 12 Hour Extended-Release
  Tablets (Less than 1%)
Allegra-D 24 Hour Extended-Release
  Tablets (Less than 1%)
Aricept ODT Tablets (Infrequent)
Aricept Tablets (Infrequent)
Arthrotec Tablets (Rare)
Atripla Tablets
Avelox I.V.
Avelox Tablets
Celexa Oral Solution (Infrequent)
Celexa Tablets (Infrequent)
Cesamet Capsules
Cipro I.V. (1% or less)
Cipro Oral Suspension
Cipro Tablets
Cipro XR Tablets
Clozaril Tablets (Less than 1%)
Copaxone for Injection (Infrequent)
Depade Tablets (Less than 1%)
Duragesic Transdermal System
  (1% or greater)
Effexor Tablets (Infrequent)
Effexor XR Capsules (Infrequent)
Evoxac Capsules
Exelon Capsules (2% or more)
Exelon Oral Solution (2% or more)
FazaClo Orally Disintegrating Tablets
  (Less than 1%)
Gabitril Tablets (Frequent)
Lamictal Chewable Dispersible
  Tablets (Infrequent)
Lamictal Tablets (Infrequent)
Lariam Tablets (Occasional)
Levaquin in 5% Dextrose Injection
  (0.1% to 0.9%)
Levaquin Injection (0.1% to 0.9%)
Levaquin Oral Solution (0.1% to
  0.9%)
Levaquin Tablets (0.1% to 0.9%)
Lexapro Oral Suspension
Lexapro Tablets
▲ Marinol Capsules (3% to 10%)
Neurontin Capsules (Infrequent)
Neurontin Oral Solution (Infrequent)
Neurontin Tablets (Infrequent)
Orthoclone OKT3 Sterile Solution
  (Less than 1%)

Paxil CR Controlled-Release Tablets
(Infrequent)
Paxil Oral Suspension (Infrequent)
Paxil Tablets (Infrequent)
Permax Tablets (Frequent)
Proquin XR Tablets
Prozac Pulvules and Liquid
(Infrequent)
Razadyne ER Extended-Release
Capsules (Infrequent)
Razadyne Oral Solution (Infrequent)
Razadyne Tablets (Infrequent)
Requip Tablets (Infrequent)
Rescriptor Tablets
Rilutek Tablets (Infrequent)
▲ Romazicon Injection (1% to 3%)
Sandostatin Injection (Less than 1%)
Sandostatin LAR Depot (Rare)
Seroquel Tablets (Infrequent)
Stalevo Tablets
Sustiva Capsules (0.4%)
Sustiva Tablets (0.4%)
Symmetrel Tablets
Tasmar Tablets (Infrequent)
Topamax Sprinkle Capsules
(Infrequent)
Topamax Tablets (Infrequent)
Trileptal Oral Suspension
Trileptal Tablets
Wellbutrin SR Sustained-Release
Tablets
Wellbutrin Tablets (Infrequent)
Wellbutrin XL Extended-Release
Tablets
Xyrem Oral Solution (Infrequent)
Zelapar Tablets
Zoloft Oral Concentrate (Infrequent)
Zoloft Tablets (Infrequent)
Zyban Sustained-Release Tablets
Zyprexa Tablets
Zyprexa ZYDIS Orally Disintegrating
Tablets

Personality changes

Ambien Tablets (Rare)
Cardizem LA Extended Release
Tablets (Less than 2%)
Decadron Tablets
▲ Depacon Injection (1% to 5%)
▲ Depakene Capsules (1% to 5%)
▲ Depakene Oral Solution (1% to 5%)
▲ Depakote ER Tablets (1% to 5%)
▲ Depakote Sprinkle Capsules (1% to 5%)
▲ Depakote Tablets (1% to 5%)
Eldepryl Capsules

Enbrel for Injection
Evoxac Capsules
Exelon Capsules (Infrequent)
Exelon Oral Solution (Infrequent)
Frova Tablets (Rare)
Gabitril Tablets (Frequent)
Geodon for Injection (Up to 2%)
Hydrocortone Tablets
Imitrex Tablets (Rare)
▲ Intron A for Injection (Less than 5%)
▲ Keppra Oral Solution (8%)
▲ Keppra Tablets (8%)
Lamictal Chewable Dispersible
Tablets (Infrequent)
Lamictal Tablets (Infrequent)
▲ Lupron Depot 3.75 mg (Among most
frequent)
▲ Lupron Depot-3 Month 11.25 mg
(Less than 5%)
Lupron Depot-PED 7.5 mg, 11.25 mg
and 15 mg (Less than 2%)
Lupron Injection Pediatric
(Less than 2%)
Nalfon Capsules (Less than 1%)
Namenda Oral Solution (Infrequent)
Namenda Tablets (Infrequent)
Neurontin Capsules (Rare)
Neurontin Oral Solution (2.8%)
Neurontin Tablets (Rare)
Norvir Oral Solution (Less than 2%)
Norvir Soft Gelatin Capsules (Less
than 2%)
Permax Tablets (2.1%)
▲ Prometrium Capsules (100 mg,
200 mg) (Less than 5%)
Prozac Pulvules and Liquid
(At least 2%)
Requip Tablets (Infrequent)
Rilutek Tablets (Infrequent)
Tiazac Capsules (Less than 2%)
Topamax Sprinkle Capsules
(Frequent)
Topamax Tablets (Frequent)
Trileptal Oral Suspension
Trileptal Tablets
▲ Zyprexa Tablets (8%)
▲ Zyprexa ZYDIS Orally Disintegrating
Tablets (8%)

Phobia, unspecified

Cipro XR Tablets
Imitrex Injection
Proquin XR Tablets

Phobic disorder

Cipro I.V. (1% or less)

Cipro Oral Suspension (Less than 1%)
Cipro Tablets (Less than 1%)
Imitrex Tablets (Rare)
Zyprexa Tablets (Infrequent)
Zyprexa ZYDIS Orally Disintegrating
Tablets (Infrequent)

Phonophobia

Imitrex Tablets (Frequent)
Abilify Discmelt Orally Disintegrating
Tablets (Rare)
Abilify Oral Solution (Rare)
Abilify Tablets (Rare)
Accutane Capsules
▲ Alphagan P Ophthalmic Solution (1%
to 4%)
Amerge Tablets (Frequent)
▲ Betimol Ophthalmic Solution (More
than 5%)
Betoptic S Ophthalmic Suspension
(Small number of patients)
BOTOX Purified Neurotoxin
Complex
Calcijex Injection
Campral Tablets (Rare)
Celexa Oral Solution (Infrequent)
Celexa Tablets (Infrequent)
Cesamet Capsules
Chantix Tablets (Rare)
Ciloxan Ophthalmic Ointment (Less
than 1%)
Copaxone for Injection (Infrequent)
Cosopt Sterile Ophthalmic Solution
(Less than 1%)
CytoGam Intravenous (Infrequent)
Depakote ER Tablets (Greater than
1%)
Effexor Tablets (Infrequent)
Effexor XR Capsules (Infrequent)
Flulaval Injection
Gabitril Tablets (Infrequent)
Geodon Capsules (Infrequent)
Havrix Vaccine (Less than 1%)
Hectorol Capsules
Hectorol Injection
▲ Imdur Tablets (Less than or equal to
5%)
Imitrex Injection (Infrequent)
Imitrex Tablets (Frequent)
▲ Intron A for Injection (Less than 5%)
Lacrisert Sterile Ophthalmic Insert
Lamictal Chewable Dispersible
Tablets (Infrequent)
Lamictal Tablets (Infrequent)
Levitra Tablets (Less than 2%)

Lotronex Tablets (Rare)
▲ Lumigan Ophthalmic Solution
(1% to 3%)
Lunesta Tablets (Rare)
Lyrica Capsules (0.1% to 1%)
Matulane Capsules
Maxalt Tablets (Rare)
Maxalt-MLT Orally Disintegrating
Tablets (Rare)
Migranal Nasal Spray (Infrequent)
Mirapex Tablets
Neurontin Capsules (Infrequent)
Neurontin Oral Solution (Infrequent)
Neurontin Tablets (Infrequent)
Nipent for Injection (Less than 3%)
Norvir Oral Solution (Less than 2%)
Norvir Soft Gelatin Capsules (Less
than 2%)
▲ Orthoclone OKT3 Sterile Solution
(10%)
Paxil CR Controlled-Release Tablets
(Rare)
Paxil Oral Suspension (Rare)
Paxil Tablets (Rare)
Permax Tablets (Infrequent)
Pexeva Tablets (Rare)
Photofrin for Injection
Prevacid Delayed-Release Capsules
(Less than 1%)
Prevacid for Delayed-Release Oral
Suspension (Less than 1%)
Prevacid NapraPAC 375 (Less than 1%)
Prevacid NapraPAC 500 (Less than 1%)
Prevacid SoluTab Delayed-Release
Orally Disintegrating Tablets (Less
than 1%)
PREVPAC (Less than 1%)
Prinivil Tablets (0.3% to 1.0%)
Prinzide Tablets
Prograf Capsules and Injection
ProSom Tablets (Infrequent)
Prozac Pulvules and Liquid
(Infrequent)
▲ Quixin Ophthalmic Solution
(1% to 3%)
Relpax Tablets (Infrequent)
Requip Tablets (Infrequent)
Rescriptor Tablets
Retrovir Capsules
Retrovir IV Infusion
Retrovir Syrup
Retrovir Tablets
Rilutek Tablets (Rare)
Risperdal M-Tab Orally Disintegrating
Tablets (Rare)

Risperdal Oral Solution (Rare)
Risperdal Tablets (Rare)
Rocaltrol Capsules
Rocaltrol Oral Solution
Sonata Capsules (Infrequent)
▲ Soriatane Capsules (1% to 10%)
Tambocor Tablets (Less than 1%)
Topamax Sprinkle Capsules (Infrequent)
Topamax Tablets (Infrequent)
▲ Travatan Ophthalmic Solution
(1% to 4%)
▲ Travatan Z Ophthalmic Solution (1%
to 4%)
Trileptal Oral Suspension
Trileptal Tablets
▲ Trusopt Sterile Ophthalmic Solution
(Approximately 1% to 5%)
Twinrix Vaccine (Less than 1%)
▲ VFEND I.V. (1.7% to 21%)
▲ VFEND Oral Suspension (1.7% to
21%)
▲ VFEND Tablets (1.7% to 21%)
Viagra Tablets (Less than 2%)
▲ Xalatan Sterile Ophthalmic Solution
(1% to 4%)
Zoloft Oral Concentrate (Rare)
Zoloft Tablets (Rare)
Zomig Nasal Spray (Rare)
Zonegran Capsules (Rare)
Zosyn (1.0% or less)

Psychiatric disturbances

Accutane Capsules
Advicor Tablets
Aldoril Tablets
Altoprev Extended-Release Tablets
Arthrotec Tablets (Rare)
Clinoril Tablets (Less than 1 in 100)
Cosopt Sterile Ophthalmic Solution
Cuprimine Capsules
Decadron Tablets
Didronel Tablets
▲ Focalin XR Capsules (26% to 46%)
▲ Gengraf Capsules (5%)
Hydrocortone Tablets
Indocin Capsules (Less than 1%)
Indocin Oral Suspension
(Less than 1%)
Indocin Suppositories (Less than 1%)
Infergen
Invirase Capsules (Less than 2%)
Invirase Tablets (Less than 2%)
Lariam Tablets (Occasional)
Lescol Capsules

Lescol XL Tablets
▲ Leukine (15%)
Mintezol Chewable Tablets
Mintezol Suspension
Nembutal Sodium Solution, USP
(Less than 1%)
Neoral Oral Solution
Neoral Soft Gelatin Capsules
Noroxin Tablets
Pepcid for Oral Suspension
(Infrequent)
Pepcid Injection (Infrequent)
Pepcid Injection Premixed
(Infrequent)
Pepcid Tablets (Infrequent)
Primaxin I.M.
Primaxin I.V. (Less than 0.2%)
Pulmicort Respules (Less than 1%)
Pulmicort Turbuhaler Inhalation
Powder (Rare)
Sandimmune I.V. Ampuls for Infusion
Sandimmune Oral Solution
Sandimmune Soft Gelatin Capsules
Thioridazine Hydrochloride Tablets
(Extremely rare)
Timoptic in Ocudose (Less frequent)
Timoptic Sterile Ophthalmic Solution
(Less frequent)
Timoptic-XE Sterile Ophthalmic Gel
Forming Solution
Vytorin 10/10 Tablets
Vytorin 10/20 Tablets
Vytorin 10/40 Tablets
Vytorin 10/80 Tablets
Zegerid Capsules (Less than 1%)
Zegerid Powder for Oral Solution
(Less than 1%)
Zocor Tablets

Psychoses

Abilify Discmelt Orally Disintegrating
Tablets
Abilify Oral Solution
Abilify Tablets
Accutane Capsules
Adderall Tablets (Rare)
Adderall XR Capsules
Adipex-P Capsules
Adipex-P Tablets
Aldoril Tablets
▲ Aredia for Injection (Up to 4%)
Avelox I.V.
Avelox Tablets
Azilect Tablets (Infrequent)

Biaxin Filmtab Tablets
Biaxin Granules
Biaxin XL Filmtab Tablets
BiDil Tablets
Buprenex Injectable (Less than 1%)
Campral Tablets (Rare)
Celexa Oral Solution (Infrequent)
Celexa Tablets (Infrequent)
▲ CellCept Capsules (3% to less than 20%)
▲ CellCept Intravenous (3% to less than 20%)
▲ CellCept Oral Suspension (3% to less than 20%)
▲ CellCept Tablets (3% to less than 20%)
Cesamet Capsules
Chantix Tablets (Rare)
Clinoril Tablets (Less than 1 in 100)
Concerta Extended-Release Tablets
Copegus Tablets (Less than 1%)
Covera-HS Tablets (Less than 2%)
Dapsone Tablets USP
Decadron Tablets
Depacon Injection
Depakene Capsules
Depakene Oral Solution
Depakote ER Tablets (Greater than 1%)
Depakote Sprinkle Capsules
Depakote Tablets
Desoxyn Tablets, USP (Rare)
Dexedrine Spansule Capsules (Rare at recommended doses)
Dexedrine Tablets (Rare at recommended doses)
DextroStat Tablets (Rare)
Effexor Tablets (Rare)
Effexor XR Capsules (Infrequent)
Exelon Capsules (Infrequent)
Exelon Oral Solution (Infrequent)
Gabitril Tablets (Infrequent)
Geodon for Injection (Up to 1%)
Guanidine Hydrochloride Tablets
Hydrocortone Tablets
Indocin Capsules (Less than 1%)
Indocin Oral Suspension (Less than 1%)
Indocin Suppositories (Less than 1%)
Invirase Capsules (Less than 2%)
Invirase Tablets (Less than 2%)
Klonopin Tablets
Klonopin Wafers
Lamictal Chewable Dispersible Tablets (Infrequent)

Lamictal Tablets (Infrequent)
Lanoxicaps Capsules
Lanoxin Injection
Lanoxin Injection Pediatric
Lariam Tablets (Occasional)
Levaquin in 5% Dextrose Injection
Levaquin Injection
Levaquin Oral Solution
Levaquin Tablets
Levbid Extended-Release Tablets
Levsin Drops
Levsin Elixir
Levsin Injection
Levsin Tablets
Levsin/SL Tablets
Levsinex Timecaps
Mirapex Tablets (Less than 1%)
Namenda Oral Solution (Infrequent)
Namenda Tablets (Infrequent)
Neurontin Capsules (Infrequent)
Neurontin Oral Solution (Infrequent)
Neurontin Tablets (Infrequent)
Noroxin Tablets
Orthoclone OKT3 Sterile Solution
Paxil CR Controlled-Release Tablets (Rare)
Paxil Oral Suspension (Rare)
Paxil Tablets (Rare)
PegIntron Powder for Injection (1%)
Permax Tablets (2.1%; Frequent)
Pexeva Tablets (Rare)
PREVPAC
▲ Prograf Capsules and Injection (3% to 15%)
Provigil Tablets
Prozac Pulvules and Liquid (Infrequent)
Pulmicort Respules (Less than 1%)
Pulmicort Turbuhaler Inhalation Powder (Rare)
Reyataz Capsules (Less than 3%)
Rilutek Tablets (Rare)
Ritalin Hydrochloride Tablets
Ritalin LA Capsules
Ritalin-SR Tablets
Rocaltrol Capsules (Rare)
Rocaltrol Oral Solution (Rare)
Seromycin Capsules
Stalevo Tablets
Sustiva Capsules (Less than 2%)
Sustiva Tablets (Less than 2%)
Symmetrel Tablets (0.1% to 1%)
Tarka Tablets

Tasmar Tablets (Infrequent)
Thalomid Capsules
Topamax Sprinkle Capsules
  (Frequent)
Topamax Tablets (Frequent)
Trecator Tablets
▲ Valcyte Tablets (Less than 5%)
Valtrex Caplets
▲ Velcade for Injection (35%)
Verelan PM Extended-Release
  Capsules, Controlled-Onset
  (2% or less)
Verelan Sustained-Release Capsules
  (1% or less)
VFEND I.V. (Less than 2%)
VFEND Oral Suspension
  (Less than 2%)
VFEND Tablets (Less than 2%)
Vyvanse Capsules
Wellbutrin SR Sustained-Release
  Tablets
Wellbutrin Tablets (Infrequent)
Wellbutrin XL Extended-Release
  Tablets
Zoloft Oral Concentrate
Zoloft Tablets
Zomig Nasal Spray (Rare)
Zovirax Capsules
Zovirax Suspension
Zovirax Tablets
Zyban Sustained-Release Tablets

Psychoses, aggravation
Clozaril Tablets
Decadron Tablets
FazaClo Orally Disintegrating Tablets
Hydrocortone Tablets
Seroquel Tablets (Infrequent)
Thioridazine Hydrochloride Tablets

Psychoses, toxic
Cesamet Capsules
Cipro I.V. (1% or less)
Cipro Oral Suspension
Cipro Tablets
Cipro XR Tablets
Concerta Extended-Release Tablets
Daytrana Transdermal Patch
Focalin Tablets (Rare)
Focalin XR Capsules
Levaquin in 5% Dextrose Injection
Levaquin Injection
Levaquin Oral Solution
Levaquin Tablets
Metadate CD Capsules

Proquin XR Tablets
Ritalin Hydrochloride Tablets
Ritalin LA Capsules
Ritalin-SR Tablets

Psychosis, activation
Carbatrol Capsules
FazaClo Orally Disintegrating Tablets
Pegasys (Less than 1%)
Risperdal Consta Long-Acting
  Injection (Frequent)
Tegretol Chewable Tablets
Tegretol Suspension
Tegretol Tablets
Tegretol-XR Tablets
Wellbutrin SR Sustained-Release
  Tablets
Wellbutrin XL Extended-Release
  Tablets
Zyban Sustained-Release Tablets

Psychotic symptoms, paradoxical exacerbation
DextroStat Tablets
Thiothixene Capsules

Rage
Niravam Orally Disintegrating Tablets
  (Rare)
Valium Tablets

Sedation
Aldoril Tablets
Amerge Tablets (Rare)
▲ Buprenex Injectable (Most frequent)
▲ Catapres Tablets (About 10 in 100
  patients)
Catapres-TTS (3 of 101 patients)
▲ Cesamet Capsules (3%)
▲ Clorpres Tablets (About 10%)
▲ Clozaril Tablets (More than 5% to 39%)
Corzide 40/5 Tablets (6 of 1000
  patients)
Dalmane Capsules
▲ Demser Capsules (Almost all patients)
Depacon Injection
Depakene Capsules
Depakene Oral Solution
Depakote ER Tablets
Depakote Tablets
Dilaudid Ampules
Dilaudid Multiple Dose Vials
Dilaudid Non-Sterile Powder
Dilaudid Oral Liquid
Dilaudid Rectal Suppositories
Dilaudid Tablets

Dilaudid Tablets - 8 mg
▲ Dilaudid-HP Injection (Among most frequent)
▲ Dilaudid-HP Lyophilized Powder 250 mg (Among most frequent)
▲ FazaClo Orally Disintegrating Tablets (Greater than 5% to 39%)
Hycodan Syrup
Hycodan Tablets
Hycotuss Expectorant Syrup
▲ Imitrex Injection (3%)
Imitrex Nasal Spray (Infrequent)
Imitrex Tablets
Invega Extended-Release Tablets
Kadian Capsules (Less than 3%)
Lotronex Tablets (Rare)
▲ Maxidone Tablets C-III (Among most frequent)
Mirapex Tablets
▲ MS Contin Tablets (Among most frequent)
Nadolol Tablets (6 of 1000 patients)
Niravam Orally Disintegrating Tablets
▲ Norco Tablets C-III (Among most frequent)
▲ Opana ER Tablets (5.9% to greater than or equal to 10%)
▲ Opana Tablets (1% to less than 10%)
Oramorph SR Tablets (Most frequent)
▲ OxyFast Oral Concentrate Solution (Among most frequent)
▲ OxyIR Capsules (Among most frequent)
▲ Percocet Tablets (Among most frequent)
▲ Percodan Tablets (Among most frequent)
Phenergan Tablets and Suppositories
▲ Seroquel Tablets (30%)
Sonata Capsules
▲ Strattera Capsules (2% to 4%)
Tessalon Capsules
Tessalon Perles
Thiothixene Capsules
Tussionex Pennkinetic Extended-Release Suspension
▲ Tylenol with Codeine Elixir (Among most frequent)
▲ Tylenol with Codeine Tablets (Among most frequent)
Ultram ER Tablets (0.5% to less than 1%)
Valcyte Tablets
▲ Vicodin ES Tablets (Among most frequent)
▲ Vicodin HP Tablets (Among most frequent)

▲ Vicodin Tablets (Among most frequent)
▲ Vivitrol (4% to 12%)
▲ Wellbutrin Tablets (19.8%)
▲ Xeloda Tablets (Less than 5%)
Xyrem Oral Solution (Infrequent)
▲ Zofran Injection (8%)
▲ Zofran Injection Premixed (8%)
▲ Zofran ODT Orally Disintegrating Tablets (20%)
▲ Zofran Oral Solution (20%)
▲ Zofran Tablets (20%)
▲ Zydone Tablets (Among most frequent)

Sensorium, clouded
Corzide 40/5 Tablets
Cosopt Sterile Ophthalmic Solution
Inderal LA Long-Acting Capsules
InnoPran XL Capsules
Lopressor HCT 100/25 Tablets
Lopressor HCT 100/50 Tablets
Lopressor HCT 50/25 Tablets
Lopressor Injection
Lopressor Tablets
Nadolol Tablets
Timolide Tablets
Timoptic in Ocudose
Timoptic Sterile Ophthalmic Solution
Timoptic-XE Sterile Ophthalmic Gel Forming Solution
Toprol-XL Tablets

Sensory disturbances
Arranon Injection (1%)
▲ Chantix Tablets (Greater than 5%)
Depo-Medrol Single-Dose Vial
▲ Eloxatin for Injection (8%)
Emend Capsules (Less than or equal to 0.5%)
▲ Foscavir Injection (Between 1% and 5%)
Hectorol Capsules
Hectorol Injection
▲ Leukine (6%)
Mirapex Tablets
Paxil CR Controlled-Release Tablets
Paxil Oral Suspension
Paxil Tablets
▲ Prograf Capsules and Injection (Approximately 55%)
▲ Proleukin for Injection (10%)
Rocaltrol Capsules
Rocaltrol Oral Solution
Topamax Sprinkle Capsules (Greater than 1%)

Topamax Tablets (Greater than 1%)
▲ Wellbutrin Tablets (4%)
▲ Wellbutrin XL Extended-Release
   Tablets (4%)

Serotonin syndrome
Celexa Oral Solution
Celexa Tablets
Effexor Tablets
Effexor XR Capsules
Geodon Capsules (Rare)
Geodon for Injection (Rare)
Imitrex Injection
Imitrex Tablets
Lexapro Oral Suspension
Lexapro Tablets
Maxalt Tablets
Maxalt-MLT Orally Disintegrating
   Tablets
Meridia Capsules
Paxil CR Controlled-Release Tablets
Paxil Oral Suspension
Paxil Tablets
Prozac Pulvules and Liquid
Zoloft Oral Concentrate
Zoloft Tablets
Zomig Nasal Spray
Zomig Tablets
Zomig-ZMT Tablets
Zyvox for Oral Suspension
Zyvox Injection
Zyvox Tablets

Sexual activity, decrease
▲ Catapres Tablets (About 3 in
   100 patients)
Catapres-TTS (0.5% or less)
▲ Clorpres Tablets (About 3%)
Depade Tablets (Less than 1%)
Risperdal M-Tab Orally Disintegrating
   Tablets (Frequent)
Risperdal Oral Solution (Frequent)
Risperdal Tablets (Frequent)

Sexual dysfunction
Aceon Tablets (2 mg, 4 mg, 8 mg)
   (0.3% to 1.4%)
Avalide Tablets
Avapro Tablets (Less than 1%)
Bentyl Capsules
Bentyl Injection
Bentyl Syrup
Bentyl Tablets
Caduet Tablets (Greater that 0.1%
   to 2%)

Campral Tablets (Infrequent)
Cardizem LA Extended Release
   Tablets (Less than 2%)
Catapres-TTS (2 of 101 patients)
Celexa Oral Solution
Celexa Tablets
Chantix Tablets (Rare)
Copaxone for Injection (Infrequent)
Effexor Tablets (2%)
Effexor XR Capsules
Eldepryl Capsules
Evoxac Capsules (Less than 1%)
Geodon Capsules (Infrequent)
Gleevec Tablets (Infrequent)
Lexapro Oral Suspension
Lexapro Tablets
Lithobid Tablets
Lotronex Tablets (Rare)
Micardis HCT Tablets
Mirapex Tablets
Neurontin Capsules (Infrequent)
Neurontin Oral Solution (Infrequent)
Neurontin Tablets (Infrequent)
▲ Nexavar Tablets (Common)
▲ Niravam Orally Disintegrating Tablets
   (7.4%)
Norvasc Tablets (Less than 1% to 2%)
▲ Paxil CR Controlled-Release Tablets
   (3.7% to 10.0%)
▲ Paxil Oral Suspension (3.7% to 10.0%)
▲ Paxil Tablets (3.7% to 10.0%)
Risperdal M-Tab Orally Disintegrating
   Tablets (Frequent)
Risperdal Oral Solution (Frequent)
Risperdal Tablets (Frequent)
▲ Strattera Capsules (3% or greater)
Tiazac Capsules (Less than 2%)
Vantas (Less than 2%)
Viracept Oral Powder (Less than 2%)
Viracept Tablets (Less than 2%)
Wellbutrin Tablets (Frequent)
Zoloft Oral Concentrate (Frequent)
Zoloft Tablets (Frequent)

Sleep disturbances
Aceon Tablets (2 mg, 4 mg, 8 mg)
   (2.5%)
Adalat CC Tablets (Rare)
▲ Advair Diskus 100/50 (1% to 3%)
▲ Advair Diskus 250/50 (1% to 3%)
▲ Advair Diskus 500/50 (1% to 3%)
▲ Advair HFA Inhalation Aerosol
   (1% to 3%)
Allegra-D 12 Hour Extended-Release
   Tablets (Less than 1%)

Allegra-D 24 Hour Extended-Release
Tablets (Less than 1%)
Ambien CR Tablets (Infrequent)
Ambien Tablets (Infrequent)
Amerge Tablets (Infrequent)
Anzemet Injection (Infrequently)
Anzemet Tablets (Infrequently)
Aptivus Capsules (Less than 2%)
Astelin Nasal Spray (Infrequent)
Avalide Tablets
Avapro Tablets (Less than 1%)
Avelox I.V. (Less than 0.1%)
Avelox Tablets (Less than 0.1%)
Celexa Oral Solution (At least 2%)
Celexa Tablets (At least 2%)
▲ Cesamet Capsules (11%)
▲ Chantix Tablets (2% to greater
than 5%)
▲ Clozaril Tablets (4%)
▲ Combivir Tablets (11%)
Copaxone for Injection (At least 2%)
Coreg CR Extended-Release Capsules
(0.1% to less than or equal to 1%)
Coreg Tablets (Greater than 0.1%
to 1%)
Corzide 40/5 Tablets
Cozaar Tablets (Less than 1%)
Cymbalta Delayed-Release Capsules
(Frequent)
▲ Depade Tablets (More than 10%)
Depakote ER Tablets (Greater than
1%)
Effexor Tablets (Infrequent)
Eldepryl Capsules
▲ Entocort EC Capsules (Less than 5%)
▲ Epivir Oral Solution (11%)
▲ Epivir Tablets (11%)
▲ FazaClo Orally Disintegrating Tablets
(4%)
▲ Flovent Diskus 100 mcg (1% to 3%)
▲ Flovent Diskus 250 mcg (1% to 3%)
▲ Flovent Diskus 50 mcg (1% to 3%)
▲ Hectorol Capsules (3.3%)
▲ Hectorol Injection (3.3%)
HibTITER
Hyzaar 100-12.5 Tablets
Hyzaar 100-25 Tablets
Hyzaar 50-12.5 Tablets
Imitrex Injection (Rare)
Imitrex Nasal Spray (Infrequent)
Imitrex Tablets (Rare to infrequent)
Klonopin Tablets (Infrequent)
Klonopin Wafers (Infrequent)
Lamictal Chewable Dispersible
Tablets (1.4%)

Lamictal Tablets (1.4%)
▲ Lariam Tablets (Among most frequent)
Levaquin in 5% Dextrose Injection
(0.1% to 0.9%)
Levaquin Injection (0.1% to 0.9%)
Levaquin Oral Solution (0.1% to 0.9%)
Levaquin Tablets (0.1% to 0.9%)
Lopressor Injection
Lopressor Tablets
▲ Lotronex Tablets (3%)
▲ Lupron Depot 3.75 mg (16%)
▲ Lupron Depot 7.5 mg (Less than 5%)
▲ Lupron Depot-3 Month 11.25 mg
(16%)
Lupron Injection Pediatric
Mirapex Tablets (Less than or
equal to 1%)
▲ MoviPrep Oral Solution (39.1%)
Nadolol Tablets
Namenda Oral Solution (Infrequent)
Namenda Tablets (Infrequent)
Nexium Delayed-Release Capsules
(Less than 1%)
Nexium Delayed-Release Oral
Suspension (Less than 1%)
Nexium I.V. (Less than 1%)
Noroxin Tablets (Less frequent)
Numorphan Injection
Ortho Evra Transdermal System
▲ Pediarix Vaccine (0.4% to 46.7%)
Prevacid Delayed-Release Capsules
(Less than 1%)
Prevacid for Delayed-Release Oral
Suspension (Less than 1%)
Prevacid NapraPAC 375 (Less than 1%)
Prevacid NapraPAC 500 (Less than 1%)
Prevacid SoluTab Delayed-Release
Orally Disintegrating Tablets (Less
than 1%)
▲ Prevnar for Injection (15.3% to 25.2%)
PREVPAC (Less than 1%)
Prochieve 4% Gel
Prochieve 8% Gel
ProQuad (Greater than or equal to
0.2% to less than 1%)
ProSom Tablets (Infrequent)
Protonix I.V. (Less than 1%)
Protonix Tablets (Less than 1%)
Provigil Tablets (At least 1%)
Prozac Pulvules and Liquid (Frequent)
Recombivax HB (Less than 1%)
Relpax Tablets (Rare)
Rescriptor Tablets
Reyataz Capsules (Less than 3%)

Risperdal M-Tab Orally Disintegrating Tablets (Frequent)
Risperdal Oral Solution (Frequent)
Risperdal Tablets (Frequent)
Rythmol SR Capsules
▲ Serevent Diskus (1% to 3%)
Sonata Capsules (Rare)
▲ Strattera Capsules (4%)
Symbyax Capsules (1% to 2%)
▲ Tasmar Tablets (24% to 25%)
Tricor Tablets
▲ Trizivir Tablets (7% to 11%)
Ultram ER Tablets (0.5% to less than 1%)
Univasc Tablets (Less than 1%)
Valium Tablets
Varivax (Greater than or equal to 1%)
Verelan Sustained-Release Capsules (1.4%)
Viracept Oral Powder (Less than 2%)
Viracept Tablets (Less than 2%)
▲ Visudyne for Injection (1% to 10%)
▲ Wellbutrin Tablets (4%)
▲ Wellbutrin XL Extended-Release Tablets (4%)
▲ Xenical Capsules (3.9%)
▲ Xyrem Oral Solution (2.9% to 6.1%)
Zelapar Tablets
▲ Ziagen Oral Solution (10%)
▲ Ziagen Tablets (10%)
Zyrtec Chewable Tablets (Less than 2%)
Zyrtec Syrup (Less than 2%)
Zyrtec Tablets (Less than 2%)
Zyrtec-D 12 Hour Extended Release Tablets (Less than 2%)

Sleep talking
Mirapex Tablets
Sonata Capsules (Rare)
Xyrem Oral Solution (Infrequent)

Sleep walking
Mirapex Tablets
Neurontin Capsules
Neurontin Oral Solution
Neurontin Tablets
Sonata Capsules (Rare)
▲ Xyrem Oral Solution (5.7%)

Sluggishness
Cymbalta Delayed-Release Capsules (Infrequent)
Lexapro Oral Suspension (Infrequent)
Lexapro Tablets (Infrequent)
Thyrolar Tablets
▲ Vivitrol (12% to 23%)
Xyrem Oral Solution (Infrequent)

Smell disturbances
Amerge Tablets (Infrequent)
Astelin Nasal Spray (Infrequently)
Beconase AQ Nasal Spray (Rare)
Biaxin Filmtab Tablets
Biaxin Granules
Biaxin XL Filmtab Tablets
Eligard 7.5 mg (Less than 2%)
Flonase Nasal Spray
Imitrex Injection (Rare)
Imitrex Nasal Spray (Infrequent)
Imitrex Tablets (Infrequent)
Lotronex Tablets (Rare)
Maxair Autohaler (0.60%)
Maxalt Tablets (Rare)
Maxalt-MLT Orally Disintegrating Tablets (Rare)
Migranal Nasal Spray (Infrequent)
Nasonex Nasal Spray (Very rare)
PREVPAC
Testim 1% Gel (1% or less)
Timentin ADD-Vantage
Timentin Injection Galaxy Container
Timentin IV Infusion
Timentin Pharmacy Bulk Package

Sociopathy
DextroStat Tablets
Neurontin Capsules (Rare)
Neurontin Oral Solution (Rare)
Neurontin Tablets (Rare)
Paxil CR Controlled-Release Tablets (Rare)
Paxil Oral Suspension (Rare)
Paxil Tablets (Rare)
Zyprexa Tablets (Infrequent)
Zyprexa ZYDIS Orally Disintegrating Tablets (Infrequent)

Speech difficulties
Clozaril Tablets (Less than 1%)
▲ Demser Capsules (10%)
FazaClo Orally Disintegrating Tablets (Less than 1%)
Geodon for Injection (Up to 2%)
Marinol Capsules (Less than 1%)
▲ Zyprexa Tablets (2% to 7%)
▲ Zyprexa ZYDIS Orally Disintegrating Tablets (2% to 7%)

Speech disturbances
Actiq (Less than 1%)
Adderall XR Capsules (2% to 4%)
Ambien Tablets (Infrequent)

Arranon Injection (1%)
Avelox I.V. (Less than 0.1%)
Avelox Tablets (Less than 0.1%)
Bentyl Capsules
Bentyl Injection
Bentyl Syrup
Bentyl Tablets
Brevibloc Concentrate (Less than 1%)
Brevibloc Double Strength Injection
  (Less than 1%)
Brevibloc Double Strength Premixed
  Injection (Less than 1%)
Brevibloc Injection (Less than 1%)
Brevibloc Premixed Injection (Less
  than 1%)
Carbatrol Capsules
Copaxone for Injection (2%)
Dantrium Capsules (Less frequent)
▲ Depakote ER Tablets (1% to 5%)
▲ Depakote Tablets (1% to 5%)
Diastat Rectal Delivery System
  (Greater than or equal to 1%)
Duragesic Transdermal System (1% or
  greater)
Effexor Tablets (Infrequent)
Effexor XR Capsules (Infrequent)
Eldepryl Capsules
▲ Equetro Extended-Release Capsules (6%)
Estrace Tablets
Estrace Vaginal Cream
Evoxac Capsules (Less than 1%)
Frova Tablets (Infrequent)
▲ Gabitril Tablets (4%)
Geodon Capsules (2%)
Imitrex Injection
▲ Intron A for Injection (Less than 5%)
Invirase Capsules (Less than 2%)
Invirase Tablets (Less than 2%)
▲ Lamictal Chewable Dispersible Tablets
  (3%)
▲ Lamictal Tablets (3%)
Levaquin in 5% Dextrose Injection
  (0.1% to 0.9%)
Levaquin Injection (0.1% to 0.9%)
Levaquin Oral Solution (0.1% to 0.9%)
Levaquin Tablets (0.1% to 0.9%)
Levbid Extended-Release Tablets
Levsin Drops
Levsin Elixir
Levsin Injection
Levsin Tablets
Levsin/SL Tablets
Levsinex Timecaps
Meridia Capsules

Migranal Nasal Spray (Rare)
Neurontin Capsules (Infrequent)
Neurontin Oral Solution (Infrequent)
Neurontin Tablets (Infrequent)
NuLev Orally Disintegrating Tablets
Ortho Evra Transdermal System
Ortho Tri-Cyclen Lo Tablets
Ortho Tri-Cyclen Tablets
Ortho-Cyclen Tablets
OxyContin Tablets (Less than 1%)
Permax Tablets (1.1%)
Prevacid Delayed-Release Capsules
  (Less than 1%)
Prevacid for Delayed-Release Oral
  Suspension (Less than 1%)
Prevacid NapraPAC 375
Prevacid NapraPAC 500
Prevacid SoluTab Delayed-Release
  Orally Disintegrating Tablets (Less
  than 1%)
PREVPAC
▲ Proleukin for Injection (7%)
▲ Prometrium Capsules (100 mg,
  200 mg) (Less than 5%)
Protonix I.V.
Protonix Tablets
Relpax Tablets (Infrequent)
Romazicon Injection (Less than 1%)
Rythmol SR Capsules
Symbyax Capsules (Up to 2%)
Tambocor Tablets (Less than 1%)
Tasmar Tablets (Frequent)
Tegretol Chewable Tablets
Tegretol Suspension
Tegretol Tablets
Tegretol-XR Tablets
▲ Topamax Sprinkle Capsules (Less
  than 1% to 13%)
▲ Topamax Tablets (Less than 1% to 13%)
▲ Trileptal Oral Suspension (1% to 3%)
▲ Trileptal Tablets (1% to 3%)
▲ Vesanoid Capsules (3%)
Zomig Nasal Spray (Infrequent)
▲ Zonegran Capsules (5%)
▲ Zyprexa Tablets (2% to 7%)
▲ Zyprexa ZYDIS Orally Disintegrating
  Tablets (2% to 7%)

Speech, incoherent
Clozaril Tablets (Less than 1%)

Speech, slurring
Clozaril Tablets (1%)
Corzide 40/5 Tablets (1 to 5 of
  1000 patients)

Dalmane Capsules (Rare)
Diastat Rectal Delivery System (Infrequent)
FazaClo Orally Disintegrating Tablets (1%)
Kadian Capsules (Less than 3%)
Klonopin Tablets
Klonopin Wafers
Lithobid Tablets
Matulane Capsules
Nadolol Tablets (1 to 5 of 1000 patients)
Niravam Orally Disintegrating Tablets
▲ Phenytek Capsules (Among most common)
Sonata Capsules (Rare)
Symmetrel Tablets (0.1% to 1%)
Tranxene T-TAB Tablets
Tranxene-SD Half Strength Tablets
Tranxene-SD Tablets
Valium Tablets (Infrequent)
Vicoprofen Tablets (Less than 1%)

Stimulation

Dalmane Capsules (Rare)
Parcopa Orally Disintegrating Tablets
Sonata Capsules (Rare)
Stalevo Tablets
Valium Tablets

Stupor

Abilify Discmelt Orally Disintegrating Tablets (Infrequent)
Abilify Oral Solution (Infrequent)
Abilify Tablets (Infrequent)
Ambien CR Tablets (Infrequent)
Ambien Tablets (Infrequent)
Azilect Tablets
Celexa Oral Solution (Rare)
Celexa Tablets (Rare)
Cesamet Capsules
Copaxone for Injection (Frequent)
Duragesic Transdermal System (Less than 1%)
Effexor Tablets (Infrequent)
Effexor XR Capsules (Infrequent)
▲ Foscavir Injection (Between 1% and 5%)
Gabitril Tablets (Frequent)
▲ Invanz for Injection (3.3% to 5.1%)
Lamictal Chewable Dispersible Tablets (Infrequent)
Lamictal Tablets (Infrequent)
Levaquin in 5% Dextrose Injection (0.1% to 0.9%)

Levaquin Injection (0.1% to 0.9%)
Levaquin Oral Solution (0.1% to 0.9%)
Levaquin Tablets (0.1% to 0.9%)
Lithobid Tablets
Lunesta Tablets (Rare)
Lyrica Capsules (Greater than or equal to 1%)
Maxipime for Injection
Migranal Nasal Spray (Rare)
Mirapex Tablets
Moduretic Tablets (Less than or equal to 1%)
Namenda Oral Solution (Infrequent)
Namenda Tablets (Infrequent)
Neurontin Capsules (Infrequent)
Neurontin Oral Solution (Infrequent)
Neurontin Tablets (Infrequent)
Orthoclone OKT3 Sterile Solution
OxyContin Tablets (Less than 1%)
Paxil CR Controlled-Release Tablets (Rare)
Paxil Oral Suspension (Rare)
Paxil Tablets (Rare)
Percodan Tablets
Permax Tablets (Rare)
PhosLo GelCaps
ProSom Tablets (Infrequent)
Prozac Pulvules and Liquid (Rare)
Relpax Tablets (Infrequent)
Requip Tablets (Infrequent)
Rilutek Tablets (Infrequent)
Risperdal M-Tab Orally Disintegrating Tablets (Infrequent)
Risperdal Oral Solution (Infrequent)
Risperdal Tablets (Infrequent)
Romazicon Injection (Less than 1%)
Seroquel Tablets (Infrequent)
Sonata Capsules (Rare)
Stromectol Tablets
Symmetrel Tablets
Tambocor Tablets (Less than 1%)
Topamax Sprinkle Capsules (1% to 2%)
Topamax Tablets (1% to 2%)
Trileptal Oral Suspension
Trileptal Tablets
Zyprexa Tablets (Infrequent)
Zyprexa ZYDIS Orally Disintegrating Tablets (Infrequent)

Stuttering

FazaClo Orally Disintegrating Tablets (Less than 1%)
Seroquel Tablets (Rare)

Zyprexa Tablets (Infrequent)
Zyprexa ZYDIS Orally Disintegrating
  Tablets (Infrequent)

Suicidal ideation

Abilify Discmelt Orally Disintegrating
  Tablets (Frequent)
Abilify Oral Solution (Frequent)
Abilify Tablets (Frequent)
Accutane Capsules
Ambien Tablets
Avelox I.V.
Avelox Tablets
Betaseron for SC Injection
Campral Tablets (Infrequent)
Chantix Tablets (Rare)
Cipro XR Tablets (Rare)
Copegus Tablets (Less than 1%)
Depade Tablets
Depakote Tablets
Effexor Tablets (Rare)
Effexor XR Capsules (Rare)
Exelon Capsules (Infrequent)
Exelon Oral Solution (Infrequent)
Infergen
Intron A for Injection (Rare)
Keppra Oral Solution (Rare)
Keppra Tablets (Rare)
Klonopin Tablets (Infrequent)
Klonopin Wafers (Infrequent)
Lamictal Chewable Dispersible
  Tablets (Rare)
Lamictal Tablets (Rare)
Lariam Tablets (Rare)
Levaquin in 5% Dextrose Injection
  (Rare)
Levaquin Injection (Rare)
Levaquin Oral Solution (Rare)
Levaquin Tablets (Rare)
Lexapro Oral Suspension (Infrequent)
Lexapro Tablets (Infrequent)
Lupron Depot 3.75 mg (Very rare)
Lupron Depot-3 Month 11.25 mg
  (Very rare)
Meridia Capsules
Namenda Oral Solution
Namenda Tablets
Neurontin Capsules (Infrequent)
Neurontin Oral Solution (Infrequent)
Neurontin Tablets (Infrequent)
Parcopa Orally Disintegrating Tablets
▲ Parnate Tablets (4%)
Paxil CR Controlled-Release Tablets
Paxil Oral Suspension

Paxil Tablets
Pegasys (Less than 1%)
PegIntron Powder for Injection (1%)
Proquin XR Tablets
Prozac Pulvules and Liquid
Razadyne Oral Solution (Rare)
Razadyne Tablets (Rare)
Rebetol Capsules
Rebetol Oral Solution
Rebetron Combination Therapy (Less
  than 1%)
Rebif Prefilled Syringe for Injection
Seromycin Capsules
Seroquel Tablets
Soriatane Capsules
Stalevo Tablets
Sustiva Capsules (0.7%)
Sustiva Tablets (0.7%)
Symbyax Capsules
Symmetrel Tablets (Less than 0.1%)
Topamax Sprinkle Capsules
  (Very rare)
Topamax Tablets (Very rare)
VFEND I.V. (Less than 2%)
VFEND Oral Suspension
  (Less than 2%)
VFEND Tablets (Less than 2%)
Viracept Oral Powder (Less than 2%)
Viracept Tablets (Less than 2%)
Wellbutrin SR Sustained-Release
  Tablets (Infrequent)
Wellbutrin Tablets (Rare)
Wellbutrin XL Extended-Release
  Tablets (Infrequent)
Zoloft Oral Concentrate (Rare)
Zoloft Tablets (Rare)
Zyban Sustained-Release Tablets
  (Infrequent)
Zyrtec Chewable Tablets (Rare)
Zyrtec Syrup (Rare)
Zyrtec Tablets (Rare)
Zyrtec-D 12 Hour Extended Release
  Tablets (Rare)

Suicide, attempt of

Abilify Discmelt Orally Disintegrating
  Tablets (Infrequent)
Abilify Oral Solution (Infrequent)
Abilify Tablets (Infrequent)
Accutane Capsules
Ambien CR Tablets (Rare)
Ambien Tablets (Rare)
Campral Tablets (Frequent)
Celexa Oral Solution (Frequent)

Celexa Tablets (Frequent)
Copaxone for Injection (Infrequent)
Cymbalta Delayed-Release Capsules
  (Infrequent)
Depade Tablets
Effexor Tablets (Infrequent)
Effexor XR Capsules (Infrequent)
▲ Equetro Extended-Release Capsules
  (Less than 5%)
Exelon Capsules (Infrequent)
Exelon Oral Solution (Infrequent)
Fuzeon Injection
Gabitril Tablets (Infrequent)
Imitrex Tablets (Rare)
Infergen
▲ Intron A for Injection (Rare; less than
  5%)
Invirase Capsules (Rare)
Invirase Tablets (Rare)
Keppra Injection
Klonopin Tablets (Infrequent)
Klonopin Wafers (Infrequent)
Lamictal Chewable Dispersible
  Tablets (Rare)
Lamictal Tablets (Rare)
Lariam Tablets (Rare)
Levaquin in 5% Dextrose Injection
  (Rare)
Levaquin Injection (Rare)
Levaquin Oral Solution (Rare)
Levaquin Tablets (Rare)
Lexapro Oral Suspension (Infrequent)
Lexapro Tablets (Infrequent)
Lupron Depot 3.75 mg (Very rare)
Lupron Depot-3 Month 11.25 mg
  (Very rare)
Lyrica Capsules (0.1% to 1%)
Mirapex Tablets (Less than 1%)
Namenda Oral Solution (Infrequent)
Namenda Tablets (Infrequent)
Neurontin Capsules (Infrequent)
Neurontin Oral Solution (Infrequent)
Neurontin Tablets (Infrequent)
▲ Parnate Tablets (4%)
Paxil CR Controlled-Release Tablets
Paxil Oral Suspension
Paxil Tablets
PegIntron Powder for Injection (1%)
Proleukin for Injection
Prozac Pulvules and Liquid
  (Infrequent)
Rebetron Combination Therapy (Less
  than 1%)
Rebif Prefilled Syringe for Injection

Remicade for IV Injection (Greater
  than or equal to 0.2%)
Requip Tablets (Rare)
Reyataz Capsules (Less than 3%)
Rilutek Tablets (Infrequent)
▲ Risperdal Consta Long-Acting
  Injection (1% to 4%)
Risperdal M-Tab Orally Disintegrating
  Tablets (1.2%)
Risperdal Oral Solution (1.2%)
Risperdal Tablets (1.2%)
Sandostatin LAR Depot (Rare)
Seroquel Tablets (Infrequent)
Sustiva Capsules (0.5%)
Sustiva Tablets (0.5%)
Symbyax Capsules (Infrequent)
Symmetrel Tablets (Less than 0.1%)
Thalomid Capsules
Topamax Sprinkle Capsules (Frequent)
Topamax Tablets (Frequent)
Zoloft Oral Concentrate
Zoloft Tablets
Zyprexa Tablets (Infrequent)
Zyprexa ZYDIS Orally Disintegrating
  Tablets (Infrequent)

Talkativeness
Carbatrol Capsules
Dalmane Capsules
Equetro Extended-Release Capsules
▲ Niravam Orally Disintegrating Tablets
  (2.2%)
Tegretol Chewable Tablets
Tegretol Suspension
Tegretol Tablets
Tegretol-XR Tablets

Tenseness
Allegra-D 12 Hour Extended-Release
  Tablets
Allegra-D 24 Hour Extended-Release
  Tablets
▲ Indapamide Tablets (Greater than or
  equal to 5%)
Zyrtec-D 12 Hour Extended Release
  Tablets

Thinking abnormality
Actiq (1% to 2%)
Ambien CR Tablets (Rare)
Ambien Tablets (Rare)
AmBisome for Injection (Less common)
Astelin Nasal Spray (Infrequent)
Avelox I.V. (Less than 0.1%)

Avelox Tablets (Less than 0.1%)
▲ Avinza Capsules (Less than 5%)
Brevibloc Concentrate (Less than 1%)
Brevibloc Double Strength Injection (Less than 1%)
Brevibloc Double Strength Premixed Injection (Less than 1%)
Brevibloc Injection (Less than 1%)
Brevibloc Premixed Injection (Less than 1%)
Campath Ampules
Campral Tablets (Frequent)
▲ CellCept Capsules (3% to less than 20%)
▲ CellCept Intravenous (3% to less than 20%)
▲ CellCept Oral Suspension (3% to less than 20%)
▲ CellCept Tablets (3% to less than 20%)
Cesamet Capsules
Chantix Tablets (Infrequent)
Coreg CR Extended-Release Capsules (0.1% to less than or equal to 1%)
Coreg Tablets (Greater than 0.1% to 1%)
▲ Depacon Injection (6%)
Depade Tablets
▲ Depakene Capsules (6%)
▲ Depakene Oral Solution (6%)
▲ Depakote ER Tablets (6%)
▲ Depakote Sprinkle Capsules (6%)
▲ Depakote Tablets (1% to 6%)
Diastat Rectal Delivery System (Greater than or equal to 1%)
Dilacor XR Capsules
Doxil Injection (Less than 1%)
Duragesic Transdermal System (1% or greater)
Effexor Tablets (2%)
Effexor XR Capsules (Frequent)
Evoxac Capsules (Less than 1%)
Frova Tablets (Infrequent)
▲ Gabitril Tablets (6%)
▲ Infergen (8% to 10%)
▲ Intron A for Injection (Less than 5%)
Kadian Capsules (Less than 3%)
Kaletra Oral Solution (Less than 2%)
Kaletra Tablets (Less than 2%)
Keppra Injection
Keppra Oral Solution (1% to 2%)
Keppra Tablets (1% to 2%)
▲ Lamictal Chewable Dispersible Tablets (3%)
▲ Lamictal Tablets (3%)
Lunesta Tablets

▲ Lyrica Capsules (1% to 9%)
▲ Marinol Capsules (3% to 10%)
▲ Megace ES Oral Suspension (1% to 3%)
Meridia Capsules (Greater than or equal to 1%)
▲ Mirapex Tablets (2% to 3%)
Namenda Oral Solution (Infrequent)
Namenda Tablets (Infrequent)
Nembutal Sodium Solution, USP (Less than 1%)
Neurontin Capsules (1.7% to 2.7%)
Neurontin Oral Solution (1.7% to 2.7%)
Neurontin Tablets (1.7% to 2.7%)
Nipent for Injection (Less than 3%)
Norvir Oral Solution (0% to 0.9%)
Norvir Soft Gelatin Capsules (0% to 0.9%)
▲ OxyContin Tablets (Between 1% and 5%)
Paxil CR Controlled-Release Tablets (Infrequent)
Paxil Oral Suspension (Infrequent)
Paxil Tablets (Infrequent)
Permax Tablets (Frequent)
Prevacid Delayed-Release Capsules (Less than 1%)
Prevacid for Delayed-Release Oral Suspension (Less than 1%)
Prevacid NapraPAC 375 (Less than 1%)
Prevacid NapraPAC 500 (Less than 1%)
Prevacid SoluTab Delayed-Release Orally Disintegrating Tablets (Less than 1%)
PREVPAC (Less than 1%)
ProAmatine Tablets (Less frequent)
▲ Prograf Capsules and Injection (3% to 15%)

Propofol Injectable Emulsion 1% (Less than 1%)
ProSom Tablets (2%)
Protonix I.V. (Less than 1%)
Protonix Tablets (Less than 1%)
Protopic Ointment (0.2% to less than 1%)
Provigil Tablets (At least 1%)
Prozac Pulvules and Liquid (25)
Relpax Tablets (Infrequent)
ReoPro Vials (2.1%)
Rilutek Tablets (Infrequent)
▲ Risperdal Consta Long-Acting Injection (Up to 3%)

Seroquel Tablets (Infrequent)
Sonata Capsules (Frequent)
Sular Tablets (Less than or
    equal to 1%)
▲ Symbyax Capsules (Greater than or
    equal to 5% to 6%)
Symmetrel Tablets (0.1% to 1%)
Tasmar Tablets (Infrequent)
Thalomid Capsules
Trileptal Oral Suspension (2%)
Trileptal Tablets (2%)
Vicoprofen Tablets (Less than 3%)
Wellbutrin Tablets (Infrequent)

Zelapar Tablets
Zomig Nasal Spray (Infrequent)
Zyban Sustained-Release Tablets (1%)
Zyprexa Tablets
Zyprexa ZYDIS Orally Disintegrating
    Tablets
Zyrtec Chewable Tablets
    (Less than 2%)
Zyrtec Syrup (Less than 2%)
Zyrtec Tablets (Less than 2%)
Zyrtec-D 12 Hour Extended Release
    Tablets (Less than 2%)

Part 2.
Side Effects by Brand

Abelcet Injection
Diplopia

Abilify Discmelt Orally Disintegrating Tablets
▲ Agitation (25%)
▲ Anxiety (20%)
  Apathy (Infrequent)
  Confusion (Frequent)
  Delirium (Infrequent)
  Delusions (Frequent)
  Depersonalization (Infrequent)
  Depression (Frequent)
  Diplopia (Rare)
  Dreaming abnormalities (Frequent)
  Emotional lability (Infrequent)
  Euphoria (Rare)
  Hallucinations (Infrequent to frequent)
  Hostility (Frequent)
  Hyperactivity (Infrequent)
  Libido, decreased (Infrequent)
  Libido, increased (Infrequent)
  Manic behavior (Frequent)
  Memory impairment (Infrequent)
  Nervousness (Frequent)
  Panic attack (Infrequent)
  Photophobia (Rare)
  Psychoses
  Stupor (Infrequent)
  Suicidal ideation (Frequent)
  Suicide, attempt of (Infrequent)

Abilify Oral Solution
▲ Agitation (25%)
▲ Anxiety (20%)
  Apathy (Infrequent)
  Confusion (Frequent)
  Delirium (Infrequent)
  Delusions (Frequent)
  Depersonalization (Infrequent)
  Depression (Frequent)
  Diplopia (Rare)
  Dreaming abnormalities (Frequent)
  Emotional lability (Infrequent)
  Euphoria (Rare)
  Hallucinations (Infrequent to frequent)
  Hostility (Frequent)
  Hyperactivity (Infrequent)
  Libido, decreased (Infrequent)
  Libido, increased (Infrequent)

Manic behavior (Frequent)
  Memory impairment (Infrequent)
  Nervousness (Frequent)
  Panic attack (Infrequent)
  Photophobia (Rare)
  Psychoses
  Stupor (Infrequent)
  Suicidal ideation (Frequent)
  Suicide, attempt of (Infrequent)

Abilify Tablets
▲ Agitation (25%)
▲ Anxiety (20%)
  Apathy (Infrequent)
  Confusion (Frequent)
  Delirium (Infrequent)
  Delusions (Frequent)
  Depersonalization (Infrequent)
  Depression (Frequent)
  Diplopia (Rare)
  Dreaming abnormalities (Frequent)
  Emotional lability (Infrequent)
  Euphoria (Rare)
  Hallucinations (Infrequent to frequent)
  Hostility (Frequent)
  Hyperactivity (Infrequent)
▲ Insomnia (20%)
  Libido, decreased (Infrequent)
  Libido, increased (Infrequent)
  Manic behavior (Frequent)
  Memory impairment (Infrequent)
  Nervousness (Frequent)
  Panic attack (Infrequent)
  Photophobia (Rare)
  Psychoses
  Stupor (Infrequent)
  Suicidal ideation (Frequent)
  Suicide, attempt of (Infrequent)

Accolate Tablets
Insomnia

Accutane Capsules
  Aggression
  Depression
  Emotional disturbances
  Emotional lability
  Insomnia
  Nervousness
  Photophobia
  Psychiatric disturbances

Psychoses
Suicidal ideation
Suicide, attempt of

Aceon Tablets (2 mg, 4 mg, 8 mg)
Anxiety (0.3% to 1%)
Depression (2%)
Nervousness (1.1%)
Sexual dysfunction (0.3% to 1.4%)
Sleep disturbances (2.5%)

AcipHex Tablets
Agitation (Rare)
Anxiety
Confusion (Rare)
Delirium
Depression
Diplopia
Disorientation
Dreaming abnormalities
Hangover (Rare)
Insomnia
Libido, decreased
Nervousness

Actigall Capsules
Insomnia (1.9%)

Actimmune
Confusion (Rare)
▲ Depression (3%)
Disorientation (Rare)
Hallucinations (Rare)

Actiq
Agitation (Less than 1%)
▲ Confusion (1% to 6%)
Dreaming abnormalities (Less than 1%)
Emotional lability (Less than 1%)
Euphoria (Less than 1%)
Hallucinations (1% to 2%)
Insomnia (1% to 2%)
Libido, decreased (Less than 1%)
Nervousness (1% to 2%)
Speech disturbances (Less than 1%)
Thinking abnormality (1% to 2%)

Actonel Tablets
▲ Anxiety (0.6% to 4.3%)
▲ Depression (2.3% to 6.8%)
▲ Insomnia (4.7%)

Actonel with Calcium Tablets
▲ Anxiety (0.6% to 4.7%)
▲ Depression (2.3% to 6.8%)
▲ Insomnia (4.3%)

Adalat CC Tablets
Anxiety (Less than 1%)
Confusion (Less than 1%)
Depression (Less than 1%)
Diplopia (Less than 1%)
Insomnia (Less than 1%)
Libido, decreased (Less than 1%)
Mood changes (Rare)
Nervousness (Rare)
Paranoia (Rare)
Sleep disturbances (Rare)

Adderall Tablets
Delusions
Depression
Euphoria
Hallucinations
Insomnia
Libido, changes
Overstimulation
Psychoses (Rare)

Adderall XR Capsules
Aggression
▲ Agitation (8%)
▲ Anxiety (8%)
Depression (0.70%)
▲ Emotional lability (1% to 9%)
Euphoria
Hostility
▲ Insomnia (1.5% to 27%)
Libido, changes
▲ Libido, decreased (2% to 4%)
▲ Nervousness (6%)
Overstimulation
Psychoses
▲ Speech disturbances (2% to 4%)

Adenoscan
Emotional lability (Less than 1%)
Nervousness (2%)

Adipex-P Capsules
CNS stimulation
Euphoria
Insomnia
Libido, changes
Overstimulation
Psychoses

Adipex-P Tablets
CNS stimulation
Euphoria
Insomnia
Libido, changes
Overstimulation
Psychoses

Advair Diskus 100/50
Aggression
Agitation
Depression
▲ Sleep disturbances (1% to 3%)

Advair Diskus 250/50
Aggression
Agitation
Depression
▲ Sleep disturbances (1% to 3%)

Advair Diskus 500/50
Aggression
Agitation
Depression
▲ Sleep disturbances (1% to 3%)

Advair HFA Inhalation Aerosol
Aggression
Agitation
Anxiety
Behavioral changes (Very Rare)
Depression
▲ Hangover (0% to 3%)
Hyperactivity (Very Rare)
Irritability (Very Rare)
▲ Sleep disturbances (1% to 3%)

Advicor Tablets
Anxiety
Insomnia
Libido, loss of
Psychiatric disturbances

Aerobid Inhaler System
▲ Anxiety (1% to 3%)
▲ Depression (1% to 3%)
▲ Hyperactivity (1% to 3%)
▲ Insomnia (1% to 3%)
▲ Irritability (3% to 9%)
▲ Mood changes (1% to 3%)
▲ Nervousness (3% to 9%)

Aerobid-M Inhaler System
▲ Anxiety (1% to 3%)
▲ Depression (1% to 3%)
▲ Hyperactivity (1% to 3%)
▲ Insomnia (1% to 3%)
▲ Irritability (3% to 9%)
▲ Mood changes (1% to 3%)
▲ Nervousness (3% to 9%)

Agenerase Capsules
▲ Depression (4% to 16%)

Agenerase Oral Solution
▲ Depression (4% to 16%)
▲ Mood changes (4% to 16%)

Aggrenox Capsules
Agitation (Less than 1%)
Confusion (1.1%)

Agrylin Capsules
▲ Confusion (1% to 5%)
▲ Depression (1% to 5%)
▲ Diplopia (1% to 5%)
▲ Insomnia (1% to 5%)
▲ Nervousness (1% to 5%)

Aldara Cream, 5%
Agitation
Depression
Insomnia

Aldoril Tablets
Confusion
Depression
Libido, decreased
Mental performance, impairment
Nightmares
Psychiatric disturbances
Psychoses
Sedation

Alferon N Injection
▲ Confusion (One patient to 3%)
▲ Depression (One patient to 3%)
Disorientation (1%)
Insomnia (2%)
Mental performance, impairment (1%)
Nervousness (1%)

Alimta for Injection
▲ Depression (Up to 14%)
▲ Mood changes (Up to 14%)

Alinia for Oral Suspension
Insomnia (Less than 1%)

Alinia Tablets
Insomnia (Less than 1%)

Allegra Capsules
Insomnia (Less than 1%)
Nervousness (Less than 1%)

Allegra Oral Solution
Insomnia (Less than 1%)
Nervousness (Less than 1%)

Allegra Tablets
Insomnia (Less than 1%)
Nervousness (Less than 1%)

Allegra-D 12 Hour Extended-Release Tablets
Agitation (1.9%)
Anxiety (1.4%)

Hallucinations
▲ Insomnia (12.6%)
Nervousness (1.4%)
Paranoia (Less than 1%)
Sleep disturbances (Less than 1%)
Tenseness

Allegra-D 24 Hour Extended-Release Tablets
Agitation (1.9%)
Anxiety (1.4%)
Hallucinations
▲ Insomnia (12.6%)
Nervousness (1.4%)
Paranoia (Less than 1%)
Sleep disturbances (Less than 1%)
Tenseness

Aloprim for Injection
Agitation (Less than 1%)

Alora ETS Patch
▲ Insomnia (1% to 8%)
Libido, changes

Aloxi Injection
Anxiety (1%)
Insomnia (Less than 1%)
Mood changes (Less than 1%)

Alphagan P Ophthalmic Solution
Depression
▲ Insomnia (1% to 4%)
▲ Photophobia (1% to 4%)

Altace Capsules
Anxiety (Less than 1%)
Depression (Less than 1%)
Insomnia (Less than 1%)
Nervousness (Less than 1%)

Altoprev Extended-Release Tablets
Anxiety
Depression
Insomnia
Libido, loss of
Memory loss, short-term
Psychiatric disturbances

Alupent Inhalation Aerosol
▲ Nervousness (14.1%)

Ambien CR Tablets
Agitation (Infrequent)
▲ Anxiety (2% to 3%)

Apathy (Rare)
Confusion (Frequent)
Delusions (Rare)
Dementia (Rare)
Depersonalization (Rare to 1%)
Depression (1%)
Diplopia (Frequent)
▲ Disorientation (3%)
Dreaming abnormalities (Infrequent)
Emotional lability (Infrequent)
Euphoria (1% to frequent)
Feeling, drugged (Frequent)
Feeling, intoxicated (Rare)
Feeling, strange (Rare)
▲ Hallucinations (Infrequent to 4%)
Illusion, unspecified (Infrequent)
Insomnia (Frequent)
Libido, decreased (Rare)
Mood changes (1%)
Nervousness (Infrequent)
Neurosis, unspecified (Rare)
Panic attack (Rare)
Sleep disturbances (Infrequent)
Stupor (Infrequent)
Suicide, attempt of (Rare)
Thinking abnormality (Rare)

Ambien Tablets
Aggression (Rare)
Agitation (Infrequent)
Anxiety (1%)
Apathy (Rare)
Behavioral changes
Cognitive dysfunction (Infrequent)
Confusion (Frequent)
Delusions (Rare)
Dementia (Rare)
Depersonalization (Rare)
Depression (2%)
Diplopia (Frequent)
Dreaming abnormalities (1%)
Emotional lability (Infrequent)
Euphoria (Frequent)
▲ Feeling, drugged (3%)
Feeling, intoxicated (Rare)
Feeling, strange (Rare)
Hallucinations (Infrequent)
Hysteria (Rare)
Illusion, unspecified (Infrequent)
Insomnia (Frequent)
Libido, decreased (Rare)
Manic behavior (Rare)
Mental performance, impairment
  (Infrequent)

Nervousness (1%)
Neurosis, unspecified (Rare)
Panic attack (Rare)
Personality changes (Rare)
Sleep disturbances (Infrequent)
Speech disturbances (Infrequent)
Stupor (Infrequent)
Suicidal ideation
Suicide, attempt of (Rare)
Thinking abnormality (Rare)

AmBisome for Injection
Agitation (Less common)
▲ Anxiety (7.4% to 13.7%)
Coma (Less common)
▲ Confusion (8.6% to 12.9%)
Depression (Less common)
Hallucinations (Less common)
Nervousness (Less common)
Thinking abnormality (Less common)

Amerge Tablets
Aggression (Rare)
Agitation (Rare)
Anxiety (Infrequent)
Cognitive dysfunction (Infrequent)
Confusion (Rare)
Consciousness, disorders of (Rare)
Depression (Infrequent)
Dreaming (Rare)
Feeling, strange (Infrequent)
Hallucinations (Rare)
Hostility (Rare)
Hyperactivity (Rare)
Libido, decreased (Rare)
Mental performance, impairment
 (Infrequent)
Panic attack (Rare)
Photophobia (Frequent)
Sedation (Rare)
Sleep disturbances (Infrequent)
Smell disturbances (Infrequent)

Amitiza Capsules
Anxiety (0% to 1.4%)
Depression (0% to 1.4%)
Insomnia (0% to 1.4%)
Nervousness (Less than 0.2%)

Amoxil Capsules
Agitation (Rare)
Anxiety (Rare)
Behavioral changes (Rare)
Confusion (Rare)
Hyperactivity (Rare)
Insomnia (Rare)

Amoxil Chewable Tablets
Agitation (Rare)
Anxiety (Rare)
Behavioral changes (Rare)
Confusion (Rare)
Hyperactivity (Rare)
Insomnia (Rare)

Amoxil Pediatric Drops for Oral Suspension
Agitation (Rare)
Anxiety (Rare)
Behavioral changes (Rare)
Confusion (Rare)
Hyperactivity (Rare)
Insomnia (Rare)

Amoxil Powder for Oral Suspension
Agitation (Rare)
Anxiety (Rare)
Behavioral changes (Rare)
Confusion (Rare)
Hyperactivity (Rare)
Insomnia (Rare)

Amoxil Tablets
Agitation (Rare)
Anxiety (Rare)
Behavioral changes (Rare)
Confusion (Rare)
Hyperactivity (Rare)
Insomnia (Rare)

Anaprox DS Tablets
Anxiety (Less than 1%)
CNS depression (Less than 1%)
Cognitive dysfunction (Rare)
Coma (Less than 1%)
Confusion (Less than 1%)
Dreaming abnormalities (Less than
 1%)
Hallucinations (Less than 1%)
Insomnia (Less than 1%)
Mental performance, impairment
 (Less than 1%)
Nervousness (Less than 1%)

Anaprox Tablets
Anxiety (Less than 1%)
CNS depression (Less than 1%)
Cognitive dysfunction (Rare)
Coma (Less than 1%)
Confusion (Less than 1%)
Dreaming abnormalities (Less than
 1%)

Hallucinations (Less than 1%)
Insomnia (Less than 1%)
Mental performance, impairment
(Less than 1%)
Nervousness (Less than 1%)

AndroGel
Anxiety (Fewer than 1%)
Depression (Up to 1%)
▲ Emotional lability (Up to 3%)
▲ Libido, decreased (Up to 3%)
Libido, increased (One patient)
Nervousness (Up to 3%)

Androxy Tablets
Anxiety
Depression
Libido, decreased
Libido, increased

Angeliq Tablets
Dementia
Depression
Irritability
Mood changes
Nervousness

Anzemet Injection
Agitation (Infrequently)
Anxiety (Infrequently)
Confusion (Infrequently)
Depersonalization (Infrequently)
Dreaming abnormalities (Infrequently)
Sleep disturbances (Infrequently)
Agitation (Infrequently)
Anxiety (Infrequently)
Confusion (Infrequently)
Depersonalization (Infrequently)
Dreaming abnormalities (Infrequently)
Sleep disturbances (Infrequently)

Aptivus Capsules
Depression (2%)
Insomnia (1.2% to less than 2%)
Sleep disturbances (Less than 2%)

Aredia for Injection
▲ Anxiety (14.3%)
▲ Insomnia (22.2%)
▲ Psychoses (Up to 4%)

Aricept ODT Tablets
Aggression (Frequent)
Agitation (Frequent)
Anxiety (Frequent)
Apathy (Infrequent)
Confusion (2%)

Delusions (Infrequent)
Dementia (Infrequent)
Depression (2%)
Dreaming abnormalities (Infrequent)
Emotional lability (2%)
Euphoria (Infrequent)
▲ Hallucinations (3%)
▲ Hostility (3%)
▲ Insomnia (5%)
Irritability (Frequent)
Libido, decreased (Infrequent)
Libido, increased (Frequent)
Listlessness (Infrequent)
▲ Nervousness (3%)
Paranoia (Infrequent)

Aricept Tablets
Aggression (Frequent)
Agitation (Frequent)
Anxiety (Frequent)
Apathy (Infrequent)
Confusion (2%)
Delusions (Infrequent)
Dementia (Infrequent)
Depression (2%)
Dreaming abnormalities (Infrequent)
Emotional lability (2%)
Euphoria (Infrequent)
▲ Hallucinations (3%)
▲ Hostility (3%)
▲ Insomnia (5%)
Irritability (Frequent)
Libido, decreased (Infrequent)
Libido, increased (Frequent)
Listlessness (Infrequent)
▲ Nervousness (3%)
Paranoia (Infrequent)

Arimidex Tablets
▲ Anxiety (2% to 6%)
▲ Confusion (2% to 5%)
▲ Depression (2% to 13%)
▲ Insomnia (2% to 10%)
▲ Mood changes (17% to 19%)
▲ Nervousness (2% to 5%)

Arixtra Injection
Anxiety (0.8%)
▲ Confusion (1.2% to 3.1%)
▲ Insomnia (0.9% to 5%)

Aromasin Tablets
▲ Anxiety (4.1% to 10%)
▲ Confusion (2% to 5%)
▲ Depression (6.2% to 13%)
▲ Insomnia (11% to 13.7%)

Arranon Injection

Coma (1%)
▲ Confusion (0% to 8%)
▲ Depression (0% to 6%)
▲ Insomnia (0% to 7%)
Mental performance, impairment (1%)
Sensory disturbances (1%)
Speech disturbances (1%)

Arthrotec Tablets

Anxiety (Rare)
Coma (Rare)
Confusion (Rare)
Depression (Rare)
Diplopia (Rare)
Disorientation (Rare)
Dreaming abnormalities (Rare)
Hallucinations (Rare)
Insomnia (Rare)
Irritability (Rare)
Mental performance, impairment
  (Rare)
Nervousness (Rare)
Paranoia (Rare)
Psychiatric disturbances (Rare)

Asacol Delayed-Release Tablets

Anxiety (2% or greater)
Confusion
Depression
Disorientation
Emotional lability
Insomnia (2%)
Libido, decreased
Nervousness (2% or greater)

Asmanex Twisthaler

▲ Depression (11%)
Insomnia (1% to less than 3%)

Astelin Nasal Spray

Anxiety (Infrequent)
Confusion
Depersonalization (Infrequent)
Depression (Infrequent)
Nervousness (Infrequent)
Sleep disturbances (Infrequent)
Smell disturbances (Infrequently)
Thinking abnormality (Infrequent)

Atacand HCT 16-12.5 Tablets

Anxiety (0.5% or greater)
Depression (0.5% or greater)
Insomnia (0.5% or greater)

Atacand HCT 32-12.5 Tablets

Anxiety (0.5% or greater)
Depression (0.5% or greater)
Insomnia (0.5% or greater)

Atacand Tablets

Anxiety (0.5% or greater)
Depression (0.5% or greater)

Atripla Tablets

Agitation
Anxiety (Greater than or equal to 2%)
Delusions
▲ Depression (4%)
▲ Dreaming abnormalities (4%)
Emotional lability
▲ Insomnia (4%)
Nervousness (Greater than or
  equal to 2%)
Neurosis, unspecified
Paranoia

Atrovent Inhalation Solution

Insomnia (0.9%)
Nervousness (0.5%)

Attenuvax

CNS reactions
Irritability

Augmentin Chewable Tablets

Agitation (Rare)
Anxiety (Rare)
Behavioral changes (Rare)
Confusion (Rare)
Hyperactivity (Rare)
Insomnia (Rare)

Augmentin ES-600 Powder for Oral Suspension

Agitation (Rare)
Anxiety (Rare)
Behavioral changes (Rare)
Confusion (Rare)
Hyperactivity (Rare)
Insomnia (Rare)

Augmentin Powder for Oral Suspension

Agitation (Rare)
Anxiety (Rare)
Behavioral changes (Rare)
Confusion (Rare)
Hyperactivity (Rare)
Insomnia (Rare)

Augmentin Tablets
Agitation (Rare)
Anxiety (Rare)
Behavioral changes (Rare)
Confusion (Rare)
Hyperactivity (Rare)
Insomnia (Rare)

Augmentin XR Extended-Release Tablets
Agitation (Rare)
Anxiety (Rare)
Behavioral changes (Rare)
Confusion (Rare)
Hyperactivity (Rare)
Insomnia (Rare)

Avalide Tablets
Anxiety (1% or greater)
Confusion
Depression
Emotional disturbances
Libido, changes
Nervousness (1% or greater)
Sexual dysfunction
Sleep disturbances

Avapro Tablets
Anxiety (Less than 1%)
Depression (Less than 1%)
Emotional disturbances
  (Less than 1%)
Libido, changes (Less than 1%)
Nervousness (1% or greater)
Sexual dysfunction (Less than 1%)
Sleep disturbances (Less than 1%)

Avastin IV
▲ Confusion (1% to 6%)

Avelox I.V.
Agitation (Less than 0.1%)
Anxiety (0.1% to less than 2%)
CNS stimulation
Confusion (Less than 0.1%)
Depersonalization (Less than 0.1%)
Depression
Dreaming abnormalities
  (Less than 0.1%)
Emotional lability (Less than 0.1%)
Hallucinations (Less than 0.1%)
Insomnia (0.1% to less than 2%)
Nervousness (0.1% to less than 2%)
Paranoia
Psychoses
Sleep disturbances (Less than 0.1%)
Speech disturbances (Less than 0.1%)
Suicidal ideation
Thinking abnormality (Less than 0.1%)

Avelox Tablets
Agitation (Less than 0.1%)
Anxiety (0.1% to less than 2%)
CNS stimulation
Confusion (Less than 0.1%)
Depersonalization (Less than 0.1%)
Depression
Dreaming abnormalities
  (Less than 0.1%)
Emotional lability (Less than 0.1%)
Hallucinations (Less than 0.1%)
Insomnia (0.1% to less than 2%)
Nervousness (0.1% to less than 2%)
Paranoia
Psychoses
Sleep disturbances (Less than 0.1%)
Speech disturbances (Less than 0.1%)
Suicidal ideation
Thinking abnormality (Less than 0.1%)

Avinza Capsules
▲ Agitation (Less than 5%)
▲ Anxiety (Less than 5%)
▲ Coma (Less than 5%)
▲ Confusion (Less than 5%)
▲ Delirium (Less than 5%)
▲ Dreaming abnormalities
  (Less than 5%)
▲ Euphoria (Less than 5%)
▲ Hallucinations (Less than 5%)
▲ Insomnia (5% to 10%)
▲ Libido, decreased (Less than 5%)
▲ Nervousness (Less than 5%)
▲ Thinking abnormality (Less than 5%)

Avodart Soft Gelatin Capsules
▲ Libido, decreased (0.3% to 3%)

Axert Tablets
Anxiety (Infrequent)
CNS stimulation (Infrequent)
Depression (Rare)
Diplopia (Rare)
Dreaming abnormalities (Rare)
Euphoria (Rare)
Insomnia (Infrequent)
Nervousness (Rare)
Nightmares (Rare)

Axid Oral Solution
Anxiety (1.8%)
Confusion (Rare)
Dreaming abnormalities (1.9%)

Insomnia (2.7%)
Libido, decreased
Nervousness (1.1%)

Azilect Tablets
Agitation (Infrequent)
Anxiety (Frequent)
Apathy (Rare)
Delirium (Rare)
Delusions (Infrequent)
Dementia (Infrequent)
▲ Depression (5%)
Depression, psychotic (Rare)
▲ Dreaming abnormalities (4%)
Emotional lability (Infrequent)
▲ Hallucinations (4%)
Hostility (Rare)
Libido, decreased (Greater than 1%)
Neurosis, unspecified (Infrequent)
Psychoses (Infrequent)
Stupor

Azmacort Inhalation Aerosol
Depression

Azopt Ophthalmic Suspension
Diplopia (Less than 1%)

Baraclude Oral Solution
Insomnia (Less than 1%)

Baraclude Tablets
Insomnia (Less than 1%)

Bayer Aspirin
Agitation
Coma
Confusion

Beconase AQ Nasal Spray
Depression
Smell disturbances (Rare)

Benicar Tablets
Insomnia (Greater than 0.5%)

Bentyl Capsules
Confusion
Diplopia
Excitability
Insomnia
▲ Nervousness (6%)
Sexual dysfunction
Speech disturbances

Bentyl Injection
Confusion
Diplopia

Excitability
Insomnia
▲ Nervousness (6%)
Sexual dysfunction
Speech disturbances

Bentyl Syrup
Confusion
Diplopia
Excitability
Insomnia
▲ Nervousness (6%)
Sexual dysfunction
Speech disturbances

Bentyl Tablets
Confusion
Diplopia
Excitability
Insomnia
▲ Nervousness (6%)
Sexual dysfunction
Speech disturbances

Betaseron for SC Injection
▲ Anxiety (10%)
Confusion
Depersonalization
▲ Depression (34%)
Emotional lability
▲ Insomnia (24%)
▲ Nervousness (7%)
Suicidal ideation

Betimol Ophthalmic Solution
Depression
Diplopia
▲ Photophobia (More than 5%)

Betoptic S Ophthalmic Suspension
Depression (Rare)
Insomnia (Rare)
Photophobia (Small number of patients)

Biaxin Filmtab Tablets
Anxiety
Behavioral changes
Confusion
Depersonalization
Disorientation
Hallucinations
Insomnia
Nightmares
Psychoses
Smell disturbances

Biaxin Granules
Anxiety
Behavioral changes
Confusion
Depersonalization
Disorientation
Hallucinations
Insomnia
Nightmares
Psychoses
Smell disturbances

Biaxin XL Filmtab Tablets
Anxiety
Behavioral changes
Confusion
Depersonalization
Disorientation
Hallucinations
Insomnia
Nightmares
Psychoses
Smell disturbances

Bicillin C-R Injectable Suspension
Agitation
Anxiety
Coma
Confusion
Euphoria
Hallucinations, auditory
Hallucinations, visual
Nervousness

BiDil Tablets
Disorientation
Psychoses

Boniva Injection
Insomnia (0.8% to 2%)

Boniva Tablets
Insomnia (0.8% to 2%)

BOTOX Purified Neurotoxin Complex
▲ Anxiety (3% to 10%)
Diplopia (Rare)
Disorientation
Photophobia

Bravelle for Intramuscular or Subcutaneous Injection
Depression (2.7%)
Emotional lability (2% to 2.7%)

Brevibloc Concentrate
Speech disturbances (Less than 1%)
Thinking abnormality (Less than 1%)

Brevibloc Double Strength Injection
Speech disturbances (Less than 1%)
Thinking abnormality (Less than 1%)

Brevibloc Double Strength Premixed Injection
Speech disturbances (Less than 1%)
Thinking abnormality (Less than 1%)

Brevibloc Injection
Speech disturbances (Less than 1%)
Thinking abnormality (Less than 1%)

Brevibloc Premixed Injection
Speech disturbances (Less than 1%)
Thinking abnormality (Less than 1%)

Brevicon Tablets
Libido, changes
Nervousness

Brovana Inhalation Solution
Agitation (Less than 2%)
Insomnia
Nervousness

Buprenex Injectable
Agitation (Rare)
Coma (Infrequent)
Depersonalization (Infrequent)
Diplopia (Less than 1%)
Dreaming abnormalities (Less than 1%)
Hallucinations (Infrequent)
Psychoses (Less than 1%)
▲ Sedation (Most frequent)

Byetta Injection
▲ Jitteriness (9%)

Caduet Tablets
Agitation (Less than or equal to 0.1%)
Anxiety (Greater than 0.1% to less than or equal to 1%)
Apathy (Less than or equal to 0.1%)
Depersonalization (Greater than 0.1% to less than or equal to 1%)
Depression (Greater than 0.1% to less than 2%)
Diplopia (Greater than 0.1% to less than or equal to 1%)
Dreaming abnormalities (Greater than 0.1% to less than 2%)

Emotional lability (Less than 2%)
Insomnia (Greater than 0.1%)
Libido, decreased (Less than 2%)
Nervousness (Greater than 0.1% to
  less than or equal to 1%)
Sexual dysfunction (Greater than
  0.1% to 2%)

Cafcit Injection
CNS stimulation
Irritability
Jitteriness

Cafcit Oral Solution
CNS stimulation
Irritability
Jitteriness

Calcijex Injection
Libido, decreased
Photophobia

Campath Ampules
Apathy
Coma
Confusion
▲ Depression (1% to 7%)
Hallucinations
▲ Insomnia (10%)
Nervousness
Thinking abnormality

Campral Tablets
Agitation (Infrequent)
▲ Anxiety (5% to 8%)
Apathy (Infrequent)
Confusion (Infrequent)
Depersonalization (Rare)
▲ Depression (4% to 8%)
Diplopia (Rare)
Dreaming abnormalities (Infrequent)
Hallucinations (Infrequent)
Hostility (Infrequent)
▲ Insomnia (6% to 9%)
Libido, decreased (Frequent)
Libido, increased (Infrequent)
Manic behavior (Rare)
Neurosis, unspecified (Infrequent)
Photophobia (Rare)
Psychoses (Rare)
Sexual dysfunction (Infrequent)
Suicidal ideation (Infrequent)
Suicide, attempt of (Frequent)
Thinking abnormality (Frequent)

Camptosar Injection
Confusion (0% to 2.7%)
▲ Insomnia (0% to 19%)

Cancidas for Injection
Insomnia (0% to 1.2%)

Captopril Tablets
Confusion
Depression
Insomnia (About 0.5 to 2%)
Nervousness

Carafate Suspension
Insomnia (Less than 0.5%)

Carafate Tablets
Insomnia (Less than 0.5%)

Carbatrol Capsules
Agitation
Confusion
Depression
Diplopia
Hallucinations, visual
Psychosis, activation
Speech disturbances
Talkativeness

Cardene I.V.
Confusion (Rare)

Cardene SR Capsules
Anxiety (Rare)
Confusion (Rare)
Depression (Rare)

Cardizem LA Extended
Release Tablets
Depression (Less than 2%)
Dreaming abnormalities
  (Less than 2%)
Hallucinations (Less than 2%)
Insomnia (Less than 2%)
Nervousness (Less than 2%)
Personality changes
  (Less than 2%)
Sexual dysfunction (Less than 2%)

Cardura XL Tablets
Agitation
Libido, decreased (Less than 1%)
Nervousness

Carimune NF
Coma

Carnitor Injection
Anxiety (1% to 2%)
▲ Depression (5% to 6%)
▲ Insomnia (1% to 3%)

Catapres Tablets

Agitation (About 3 in 100 patients)
Anxiety
Behavioral changes
Delirium
Depression (About 1 in 100 patients)
Dreaming abnormalities
Hallucinations
Hallucinations, auditory (Rare)
Hallucinations, visual (Rare)
Insomnia (About 5 in 1,000 patients)
Libido, loss of (About 3 in 100 patients)
▲ Nervousness (About 3 in 100 patients)
Nightmares
▲ Sedation (About 10 in 100 patients)
▲ Sexual activity, decrease (About 3 in 100 patients)

Catapres-TTS

Agitation (0.5% or less)
Anxiety (0.5% or less)
Behavioral changes (0.5% or less)
Delirium (0.5% or less)
Depression (0.5% or less)
Dreaming abnormalities (0.5% or less)
Hallucinations, auditory (0.5% or less)
Hallucinations, visual (0.5% or less)
Insomnia (2 of 101 patients)
Irritability (0.5% or less)
Libido, loss of (0.5% or less)
Nervousness (1 of 101 patients)
Nightmares (0.5% or less)
Sedation (3 of 101 patients)
Sexual activity, decrease (0.5% or less)
Sexual dysfunction (2 of 101 patients)

Ceftin for Oral Suspension

Hyperactivity (0.1% to 1%)
Irritability (0.1% to 1%)

Celebrex Capsules

Anxiety (0.1% to 1.9%)
Depression (0.1% to 1.9%)
Insomnia (2.3%)
Nervousness (0.1% to 1.9%)

Celexa Oral Solution

Aggression (Infrequent)
▲ Agitation (3%)
▲ Anxiety (4%)
Apathy (Infrequent)
Behavioral changes
Catatonia (Rare)
Coma
Confusion (Frequent)
Delirium
Delusions (Rare)
Depersonalization (Infrequent)
Depression (Frequent)
Depression, aggravation of (Frequent)
Depression, psychotic (Infrequent)
Diplopia (Rare)
Emotional lability (Infrequent)
Euphoria (Infrequent)
Hallucinations (Infrequent)
▲ Insomnia (15%)
Libido, decreased (2%)
Libido, increased (Infrequent)
Manic behavior
Mental performance, impairment (Frequent)
Mental status, altered
Panic attack (Infrequent)
Paranoia (Infrequent)
Photophobia (Infrequent)
Psychoses (Infrequent)
Serotonin syndrome
Sexual dysfunction
Sleep disturbances (At least 2%)
Stupor (Rare)
Suicide, attempt of (Frequent)

Celexa Tablets

Aggression (Infrequent)
▲ Agitation (3%)
▲ Anxiety (4%)
Apathy (Infrequent)
Behavioral changes
Catatonia (Rare)
Coma
Confusion (Frequent)
Delirium
Delusions (Rare)
Depersonalization (Infrequent)
Depression (Frequent)
Depression, aggravation of (Frequent)
Depression, psychotic (Infrequent)
Diplopia (Rare)
Emotional lability (Infrequent)
Euphoria (Infrequent)
Hallucinations (Infrequent)
▲ Insomnia (15%)
Libido, decreased (2%)
Libido, increased (Infrequent)
Manic behavior
Mental performance, impairment (Frequent)
Mental status, altered

Panic attack (Infrequent)
Paranoia (Infrequent)
Photophobia (Infrequent)
Psychoses (Infrequent)
Serotonin syndrome
Sexual dysfunction
Sleep disturbances (At least 2%)
Stupor (Rare)
Suicide, attempt of (Frequent)

CellCept Capsules

▲ Agitation (3% to less than 20%)
▲ Anxiety (3% to 28.4%)
▲ Confusion (3% to less than 20%)
▲ Delirium (3% to less than 20%)
▲ Depression (3% to less than 20%)
▲ Emotional lability (3% to less than 20%)
▲ Hallucinations (3% to less than 20%)
▲ Insomnia (40.8%)
▲ Nervousness (3% to less than 20%)
▲ Psychoses (3% to less than 20%)
▲ Thinking abnormality (3% to less than 20%)

CellCept Intravenous

▲ Agitation (3% to less than 20%)
▲ Anxiety (3% to 28.4%)
   Confusion (3% to less than 20%)
▲ Delirium (3% to less than 20%)
▲ Depression (3% to less than 20%)
▲ Emotional lability (3% to less than 20%)
▲ Hallucinations (3% to less than 20%)
▲ Insomnia (40.8%)
▲ Nervousness (3% to less than 20%)
▲ Psychoses (3% to less than 20%)
▲ Thinking abnormality (3% to less than 20%)

CellCept Oral Suspension

▲ Agitation (3% to less than 20%)
▲ Anxiety (3% to 28.4%)
▲ Confusion (3% to less than 20%)
▲ Delirium (3% to less than 20%)
▲ Depression (3% to less than 20%)
▲ Emotional lability (3% to less than 20%)
▲ Hallucinations (3% to less than 20%)
▲ Insomnia (40.8%)
▲ Nervousness (3% to less than 20%)
▲ Psychoses (3% to less than 20%)
▲ Thinking abnormality (3% to less than 20%)

CellCept Tablets

▲ Agitation (3% to less than 20%)
▲ Anxiety (3% to 28.4%)

▲ Confusion (3% to less than 20%)
▲ Delirium (3% to less than 20%)
▲ Depression (3% to less than 20%)
▲ Emotional lability (3% to less than 20%)
▲ Hallucinations (3% to less than 20%)
▲ Insomnia (40.8%)
▲ Nervousness (3% to less than 20%)
▲ Psychoses (3% to less than 20%)
▲ Thinking abnormality (3% to less than 20%)

Cesamet Capsules

   Anxiety
   Apathy
   CNS depression
   CNS stimulation
   Confusion
   Depersonalization (2%)
▲ Depression (14%)
   Disorientation (2%)
   Dreaming abnormalities
   Emotional disturbances
   Emotional lability
▲ Euphoria (11% to 38%)
   Hallucinations
   Hyperactivity
   Inebriated feeling
   Insomnia
   Irritability
   Mood changes
   Nervousness
   Panic attack
   Paranoia
   Photophobia
   Psychoses
   Psychoses, toxic
▲ Sedation (3%)
▲ Sleep disturbances (11%)
   Stupor
   Thinking abnormality

Chantix Tablets

   Aggression (Infrequent)
   Agitation (Infrequent)
   Anxiety (Frequent)
   Depression (Frequent)
   Disorientation (Infrequent)
▲ Dreaming abnormalities (9% to 13%)
   Emotional disturbances (Frequent)
   Euphoria (Rare)
   Hallucinations (Rare)
▲ Insomnia (18% to 19%)
   Irritability (Frequent)
   Libido, decreased (Infrequent)
   Mental performance, impairment (Rare)

Mood changes (Infrequent)
Nightmares (1% to 2%)
Photophobia (Rare)
Psychoses (Rare)
▲ Sensory disturbances (Greater than 5%)
Sexual dysfunction (Rare)
▲ Sleep disturbances (2% to greater than 5%)
Suicidal ideation (Rare)
Thinking abnormality (Infrequent)

Children's Tylenol Plus Cold & Allergy Suspension Liquid
Excitability

Children's Tylenol Plus Cold Suspension Liquid
Excitability
Insomnia
Nervousness

Children's Tylenol Plus Cough & Runny Nose Suspension Liquid
Excitability

Children's Tylenol Plus Flu Suspension Liquid
Excitability
Insomnia
Nervousness

Children's Tylenol Plus Multi-Symptom Cold Suspension Liquid
Excitability
Insomnia
Nervousness

Children's Vicks NyQuil Cold/Cough Relief Liquid
Excitability
Insomnia
Nervousness

Cialis Tablets
Insomnia (Less than 2%)

Ciloxan Ophthalmic Ointment
Photophobia (Less than 1%)

Cipro I.V.
Agitation
Anxiety (1% or less)
CNS stimulation
Confusion (1% or less)

Delirium
Depersonalization (1% or less)
Depression (1% or less)
Diplopia (1% or less)
Hallucinations (1% or less)
Insomnia (1% or less)
Irritability (1% or less)
Manic behavior (1% or less)
Nervousness
Nightmares (1% or less)
Paranoia (1% or less)
Phobic disorder (1% or less)
Psychoses, toxic (1% or less)

Cipro Oral Suspension
Agitation
Anxiety
CNS stimulation
Confusion
Delirium
Depersonalization (Less than 1%)
Depression (Less than 1%)
Diplopia (Less than 1%)
Hallucinations (Less than 1%)
Insomnia (Less than 1%)
Irritability (Less than 1%)
Manic behavior (Less than 1%)
Nervousness
Nightmares (Less than 1%)
Paranoia
Phobic disorder (Less than 1%)
Psychoses, toxic

Cipro Tablets
Agitation
Anxiety
CNS stimulation
Confusion
Delirium
Depersonalization (Less than 1%)
Depression (Less than 1%)
Diplopia (Less than 1%)
Hallucinations (Less than 1%)
Insomnia (Less than 1%)
Irritability (Less than 1%)
Manic behavior (Less than 1%)
Nervousness
Nightmares (Less than 1%)
Paranoia
Phobic disorder (Less than 1%)
Psychoses, toxic

Cipro XR Tablets
Agitation
Anxiety

CNS stimulation
Confusion
Delirium
Depersonalization (Less than 1%)
Depression (Less than 1%)
Diplopia (Less than 1%)
Dreaming abnormalities (Less than 1%)
Hallucinations
Insomnia (Less than 1%)
Irritability
Manic behavior
Nervousness
Nightmares
Paranoia
Phobia, unspecified
Psychoses, toxic
Suicidal ideation (Rare)

Ciprodex Otic Suspension
Irritability (0.5%)

Clarinex Syrup
▲ Emotional lability (3.1%)
▲ Insomnia (4.5%)
▲ Irritability (12.1%)

Clarinex-D 12-Hour Extended-Release Tablets
▲ Insomnia (10%)

Clarinex-D 24-Hour Extended-Release Tablets
CNS stimulation
Hyperactivity (2%)
▲ Insomnia (5%)
Nervousness (2%)

Climara Pro Transdermal System
▲ Depression (5.7%)
Irritability
Libido, changes
Mood changes
Nervousness

Climara Transdermal System
▲ Depression (1% to 8%)
Irritability
Libido, changes
Mood changes
Nervousness

Clinoril Tablets
Depression (Less than 1%)
Insomnia (Less than 1%)
Nervousness (Greater than 1%)

Psychiatric disturbances (Less than 1 in 100)
Psychoses (Less than 1 in 100)

Clolar for Intravenous Infusion
▲ Anxiety (22%)
▲ Depression (11%)
▲ Irritability (11%)

Clorpres Tablets
▲ Agitation (About 3%)
Anxiety
Behavioral changes
Delirium
Depression (About 1%)
Dreaming abnormalities
Hallucinations, auditory
Hallucinations, visual
Insomnia (About 5 in 1,000)
▲ Libido, loss of (About 3%)
▲ Nervousness (About 3%)
Nightmares
▲ Sedation (About 10%)
▲ Sexual activity, decrease (About 3%)

Clozaril Tablets
▲ Agitation (4%)
Anxiety (1%)
CNS reactions
▲ Confusion (3%)
Delirium
Delusions (Less than 1%)
Depression (1%)
Hallucinations (Less than 1%)
▲ Insomnia (2% to 20%)
Irritability (Less than 1%)
Libido, decreased (Less than 1%)
Libido, increased (Less than 1%)
Memory loss, short-term (Less than 1%)
Mental performance, impairment
Mental status, altered
▲ Nightmares (4%)
Paranoia (Less than 1%)
Psychoses, aggravation
▲ Sedation (More than 5% to 39%)
▲ Sleep disturbances (4%)
Speech difficulties (Less than 1%)
Speech, incoherent (Less than 1%)
Speech, slurring (1%)

Colazal Capsules
Anxiety
Depression
Insomnia (2%)
Nervousness

Combivent Inhalation Aerosol
CNS stimulation
Insomnia (Less than 2%)
Nervousness (Less than 2%)

Combivir Tablets
▲ Depressive reactions (9%)
▲ Insomnia (11%)
▲ Sleep disturbances (11%)

Comtan Tablets
Agitation (1%)
Anxiety (2%)
Consciousness, disorders of
Hallucinations

Comvax
Agitation
▲ Irritability (32.2% to 57.0%)

Concentrated Tylenol Infants' Drops Plus Cold
Insomnia
Nervousness

Concentrated Tylenol Infants' Drops Plus Cold and Cough
Insomnia
Nervousness

Concerta Extended-Release Tablets
Aggression
Depression
Emotional lability (0.7%)
▲ Insomnia (1.5% to 5%)
Manic behavior
▲ Nervousness (Greater than 0.7%)
Psychoses
Psychoses, toxic

Condylox Topical Solution
▲ Insomnia (Less than 5%)

Copaxone for Injection
▲ Agitation (4%)
▲ Anxiety (23%)
Coma (Infrequent)
Confusion (2%)
Depersonalization (Infrequent)
Depression (At least 2%)
Depression, psychotic (Infrequent)
Diplopia (At least 2%)
Dreaming abnormalities (Frequent)
Emotional lability (At least 2%)
Euphoria (At least 2%)
Hallucinations (Infrequent)

Hostility (Infrequent)
Insomnia (At least 2%)
Libido, decreased (Infrequent)
Manic behavior (Infrequent)
Memory impairment (Infrequent)
Mental performance, impairment (Infrequent)
Nervousness (2%)
Paranoia (Infrequent)
Photophobia (Infrequent)
Sexual dysfunction (Infrequent)
Sleep disturbances (At least 2%)
Speech disturbances (2%)
Stupor (Frequent)
Suicide, attempt of (Infrequent)

Copegus Tablets
Aggression (Less than 1%)
▲ Anxiety (33%)
Coma (Less than 1%)
▲ Depression (20%)
▲ Insomnia (30%)
▲ Irritability (33%)
▲ Memory impairment (6%)
▲ Mood changes (5% to 9%)
▲ Nervousness (33%)
Psychoses (Less than 1%)
Suicidal ideation (Less than 1%)

Coreg CR Extended-Release Capsules
Depression (Greater than 1% to less than or equal to 3%)
Depression, aggravation of (0.1% to less than or equal to 1%)
Emotional lability (0.1% to less than or equal to 1%)
Insomnia (1% to 2%)
Libido, decreased (0.1% to less than or equal to 1%)
Nervousness (0.1% to less than or equal to 1%)
Sleep disturbances (0.1% to less than or equal to 1%)
Thinking abnormality (0.1% to less than or equal to 1%)

Coreg Tablets
▲ Depression (Greater than 1% to 3%)
Depression, aggravation of (Greater than 0.1% to 1%)
Emotional lability (Greater than 0.1% to 1%)
Insomnia (2%)

Libido, decreased (Greater than 0.1% to 1%)

Nervousness (Greater than 0.1% to 1%)

Sleep disturbances (Greater than 0.1% to 1%)

Thinking abnormality (Greater than 0.1% to 1%)

Cortifoam Rectal Foam
Insomnia

Corzide 40/5 Tablets
Libido, decreased (1 to 5 of 1000 patients)

Memory loss, short-term

Neuropsychometrics performance, decrease

Sedation (6 of 1000 patients)

Sensorium, clouded

Sleep disturbances

Speech, slurring (1 to 5 of 1000 patients)

Cosopt Sterile Ophthalmic Solution
Anxiety

Behavioral changes

Catatonia

Confusion

Depression (Less than 1%)

Diplopia

Disorientation

Disorientation, place

Disorientation, time

Emotional lability

Hallucinations

Insomnia

Libido, decreased

Memory loss, short-term

Mental performance, impairment

Nervousness

Neuropsychometrics performance, decrease

Nightmares

Photophobia (Less than 1%)

Psychiatric disturbances

Sensorium, clouded

Covera-HS Tablets
Confusion (Less than 2%)

Insomnia (Less than 2%)

Psychoses (Less than 2%)

Cozaar Tablets
Anxiety (Less than 1%)

Confusion (Less than 1%)

Depression (Less than 1%)

Dreaming abnormalities (Less than 1%)

Insomnia (1% or greater)

Libido, decreased (Less than 1%)

Memory impairment (Less than 1%)

▲ Nervousness (Less than 1% to 4%)

Panic attack (Less than 1%)

Sleep disturbances (Less than 1%)

Crestor Tablets
Anxiety (Greater than or equal to 1%)

Depression (Greater than or equal to 2%)

Insomnia (Greater than or equal to 2%)

Crixivan Capsules
Anxiety (Less than 2%)

Depression

Cubicin for Injection
▲ Anxiety (1% to 5%)

Confusion (1% to 2%)

Hallucinations (Less than 1%)

▲ Insomnia (4.5% to 11.2%)

Jitteriness (Less than 1%)

Mental status, altered (Less than 1%)

Cuprimine Capsules
Agitation

Anxiety

Mental status, altered

Psychiatric disturbances

Cyanokit
Memory impairment

Cymbalta Delayed-Release Capsules
▲ Anxiety (3%)

Diplopia (Infrequent)

Hallucinations

▲ Insomnia (8% to 13%)

Irritability (Frequent)

Jitteriness (Infrequent)

▲ Libido, decreased (1% to 6%)

Mood changes (Infrequent)

Nervousness (Frequent)

Nightmares (Frequent)

Sleep disturbances (Frequent)

Sluggishness (Infrequent)

Suicide, attempt of (Infrequent)

CytoGam Intravenous
Photophobia (Infrequent)

Dacogen Injection
▲ Anxiety (11%)
▲ Confusion (12%)
  Depression (Greater than or equal to 1%)
▲ Insomnia (28%)
  Mental status, altered

Dalmane Capsules
  Coma
  Confusion (Rare)
  Depression (Rare)
  Disorientation
  Euphoria (Rare)
  Hallucinations (Rare)
  Hyperactivity (Rare)
  Irritability
  Nervousness
  Sedation
  Speech, slurring (Rare)
  Stimulation (Rare)
  Talkativeness

Dantrium Capsules
  Confusion (Less frequent)
  Depression (Less frequent)
  Diplopia (Less frequent)
  Insomnia (Less frequent)
  Nervousness (Less frequent)
  Speech disturbances (Less frequent)

Dapsone Tablets USP
  Insomnia
  Psychoses

DAPTACEL Vaccine
▲ Anxiety (23.6% to 39.6%)
▲ Irritability (36.9% to 41.4%)

Daytrana Transdermal Patch
  Confusion
  Depression
▲ Insomnia (4% to 30%)
  Irritability
  Nervousness
  Psychoses, toxic

Decadron Tablets
  Depression
  Emotional disturbances
  Euphoria
  Insomnia
  Mood changes
  Personality changes
  Psychiatric disturbances
  Psychoses
  Psychoses, aggravation

Demadex Injection
  Insomnia (1.2%)
  Nervousness (1.1%)

Demadex Tablets
  Insomnia (1.2%)
  Nervousness (1.1%)

Demser Capsules
  Anxiety
  Awareness, heightened
  Confusion
  Depression
  Disorientation
  Hallucinations
  Insomnia
▲ Sedation (Almost all patients)
▲ Speech difficulties (10%)

Depacon Injection
  Aggression
  Agitation (1% or more)
▲ Anxiety (1% to 5%)
  Catatonia (1% or more)
  CNS depression
  Coma (Rare)
▲ Confusion (1% to 5%)
  Dementia (Several reports)
▲ Depression (4% to 5%)
▲ Diplopia (16%)
▲ Dreaming abnormalities (1% to 5%)
  Emotional disturbances
▲ Emotional lability (6%)
  Euphoria (0.9%)
  Hallucinations
  Hostility
  Hyperactivity
▲ Insomnia (9% to 15%)
▲ Nervousness (0.9% to 11%)
▲ Personality changes (1% to 5%)
  Psychoses
  Sedation
▲ Thinking abnormality (6%)

Depade Tablets
▲ Insomnia (3%)
▲ Irritability (Less than 10%)
▲ Nervousness (More than 10%)
  Nightmares (Less than 1%)
  Paranoia (Less than 1%)
  Sexual activity, decrease (Less than 1%)
▲ Sleep disturbances (More than 10%)
  Suicidal ideation
  Suicide, attempt of
  Thinking abnormality

Depakene Capsules

Aggression
Agitation (1% or more)
▲ Anxiety (1% to 5%)
Catatonia (1% or more)
CNS depression
▲ Coma (Rare)
▲ Confusion (1% to 5%)
Dementia (Several reports)
▲ Depression (5%)
▲ Diplopia (16%)
▲ Dreaming abnormalities (1% to 5%)
Emotional disturbances
▲ Emotional lability (6%)
Hallucinations
Hostility
Hyperactivity
▲ Insomnia (15%)
▲ Nervousness (11%)
▲ Personality changes (1% to 5%)
Psychoses
Sedation
▲ Thinking abnormality (6%)

Depakene Oral Solution

Aggression
Agitation (1% or more)
▲ Anxiety (1% to 5%)
Catatonia (1% or more)
CNS depression
Coma (Rare)
▲ Confusion (1% to 5%)
Dementia (Several reports)
▲ Depression (5%)
▲ Diplopia (16%)
▲ Dreaming abnormalities (1% to 5%)
Emotional disturbances
▲ Emotional lability (6%)
Hallucinations
Hostility
Hyperactivity
▲ Insomnia (15%)
▲ Nervousness (11%)
▲ Personality changes (1% to 5%)
Psychoses
Sedation
▲ Thinking abnormality (6%)

Depakote ER Tablets

Aggression
Agitation (Greater than 1%)
▲ Anxiety (1% to 5%)
Catatonia (Greater than 1%)
CNS depression
Coma (Rare)
▲ Confusion (1% to 5%)

Dementia (Several reports)
▲ Depression (4% to 5%)
▲ Diplopia (16%)
▲ Dreaming abnormalities (1% to 5%)
Emotional disturbances
▲ Emotional lability (6%)
Hallucinations (Greater than 1%)
Hostility
Hyperactivity
▲ Insomnia (Greater than 1% to 15%)
▲ Nervousness (Greater than 1% to 11%)
▲ Personality changes (1% to 5%)
Photophobia (Greater than 1%)
Psychoses (Greater than 1%)
Sedation
Sleep disturbances (Greater than 1%)
▲ Speech disturbances (1% to 5%)
▲ Thinking abnormality (6%)

Depakote Sprinkle Capsules

Aggression
Agitation
▲ Anxiety (1% to 5%)
Catatonia
Coma (Rare)
▲ Confusion (1% to 5%)
Dementia (Several reports)
▲ Depression (4% to 5%)
▲ Diplopia (16%)
▲ Dreaming abnormalities (1% to 5%)
Emotional disturbances
▲ Emotional lability (6%)
Hallucinations
Hostility
Hyperactivity
▲ Insomnia (9% to 15%)
▲ Nervousness (7% to 11%)
▲ Personality changes (1% to 5%)
Psychoses
▲ Thinking abnormality (6%)

Depakote Tablets

Aggression
▲ Agitation (1% to 5%)
▲ Anxiety (1% to 5%)
▲ Catatonia (1% to 5%)
CNS depression
Coma (Rare)
▲ Confusion (1% to 5%)
Dementia (Several reports)
▲ Depression (1% to 5%)
▲ Diplopia (1% to 16%)
▲ Dreaming abnormalities (1% to 5%)
Emotional disturbances

▲ Emotional lability (1% to 6%)
▲ Hallucinations (1% to 5%)
  Hostility
  Hyperactivity
▲ Insomnia (1% to 15%)
▲ Nervousness (1% to 11%)
▲ Personality changes (1% to 5%)
  Psychoses
  Sedation
▲ Speech disturbances (1% to 5%)
  Suicidal ideation
▲ Thinking abnormality (1% to 6%)

DepoCyt Injection
▲ Confusion (4% to 14%)

DepoDur Extended-Release Injection
▲ Anxiety (2% to 5%)
▲ Insomnia (5% to 10%)

Depo-Medrol Single-Dose Vial
  Sensory disturbances

Depo-Provera Contraceptive Injection
▲ Depression (1% to 5%)
▲ Insomnia (1% to 5%)
▲ Libido, decreased (1% to 5%)
  Libido, increased (Less than 1%)
▲ Nervousness (Greater than 5%)

depo-subQ provera 104 Injectable Suspension
▲ Anxiety (1% to less than 5%)
▲ Depression (1% to less than 5%)
▲ Insomnia (1% to less than 5%)
▲ Irritability (1% to less than 5%)
▲ Libido, decreased (1% to less than 5%)
  Libido, increased
  Nervousness

Desoxyn Tablets, USP
  Euphoria
  Insomnia
  Libido, changes
  Overstimulation
  Psychoses (Rare)

Detrol LA Capsules
  Anxiety (1%)
  Confusion
  Delusions
  Disorientation
  Hallucinations
  Memory impairment

Detrol Tablets
  Hallucinations
  Nervousness (1.1%)

Dexedrine Spansule Capsules
  Agitation
  Euphoria
  Insomnia
  Libido, changes
  Overstimulation
  Psychoses (Rare at recommended doses)

Dexedrine Tablets
  Agitation
  Euphoria
  Insomnia
  Libido, changes
  Overstimulation
  Psychoses (Rare at recommended doses)

DextroStat Tablets
  Aggression
  Euphoria
  Insomnia
  Libido, changes
  Overstimulation
  Psychoses (Rare)
  Psychotic symptoms, paradoxical exacerbation
  Sociopathy

Diastat Rectal Delivery System
  Agitation (Greater than or equal to 1%)
  Anxiety, paradoxical
  CNS depression
  CNS stimulation, paradoxical
  Confusion (Greater than or equal to 1%)
  Depression (Infrequent)
  Emotional lability (Greater than or equal to 1%)
▲ Euphoria (3%)
  Libido, changes (Infrequent)
  Nervousness (Greater than or equal to 1%)
  Speech disturbances (Greater than or equal to 1%)
  Speech, slurring (Infrequent)
  Thinking abnormality (Greater than or equal to 1%)

Didronel Tablets
  Confusion
  Depression

Hallucinations
Psychiatric disturbances

Dilacor XR Capsules
Insomnia (1%)
Thinking abnormality

Dilaudid Ampules
Agitation
Anxiety
Diplopia
Disorientation
Euphoria
Fear
Hallucinations
Insomnia
Mental clouding
Mental performance, impairment
Mood changes
Sedation

Dilaudid Multiple Dose Vials
Agitation
Anxiety
Diplopia
Disorientation
Euphoria
Fear
Hallucinations
Insomnia
Mental performance, impairment
Mood changes
Sedation

Dilaudid Non-Sterile Powder
Agitation
Anxiety
Diplopia
Disorientation
Euphoria
Fear
Hallucinations
Insomnia
Mental clouding
Mental performance, impairment
Mood changes
Sedation

Dilaudid Oral Liquid
Agitation (Less frequent)
Depression (Less frequent)
Diplopia (Less frequent)
Disorientation (Less frequent)
Dreaming (Less frequent)
Euphoria
Floating feeling (Less frequent)

Hallucinations (Less frequent)
Insomnia (Less frequent)
Mood changes (Less frequent)
Nervousness (Less frequent)
Sedation

Dilaudid Rectal Suppositories
Agitation
Anxiety
Diplopia
Disorientation
Euphoria
Fear
Hallucinations
Insomnia
Mental clouding
Mental performance, impairment
Mood changes
Sedation

Dilaudid Tablets
Agitation
Anxiety
Diplopia
Disorientation
Euphoria
Fear
Hallucinations
Insomnia
Mental clouding
Mental performance, impairment
Mood changes
Sedation

Dilaudid Tablets - 8 mg
Agitation (Less frequent)
Depression (Less frequent)
Diplopia (Less frequent)
Disorientation (Less frequent)
Dreaming (Less frequent)
Euphoria
Floating feeling (Less frequent)
Hallucinations (Less frequent)
Insomnia (Less frequent)
Mood changes (Less frequent)
Nervousness (Less frequent)
Sedation

Dilaudid-HP Injection
Agitation (Less frequent)
Depression (Less frequent)
Diplopia (Less frequent)
Disorientation (Less frequent)
Dreaming abnormalities
  (Less frequent)

Euphoria (Less frequent)
Floating feeling (Less frequent)
Hallucinations (Less frequent)
Insomnia (Less frequent)
Mood changes (Less frequent)
Nervousness
▲ Sedation (Among most frequent)

Dilaudid-HP Lyophilized Powder 250 mg
Agitation (Less frequent)
Depression (Less frequent)
Diplopia (Less frequent)
Disorientation (Less frequent)
Dreaming abnormalities
  (Less frequent)
Euphoria (Less frequent)
Floating feeling (Less frequent)
Hallucinations (Less frequent)
Insomnia (Less frequent)
Mood changes (Less frequent)
Nervousness
▲ Sedation (Among most frequent)

Diovan HCT Tablets
Anxiety (Greater than 0.2%)
Confusion
Depression (Less frequent)
Insomnia (Greater than 0.2%)
Libido, decreased
  (Less frequent)

Diovan Tablets
Anxiety
Insomnia

Ditropan XL Extended-Release Tablets
▲ Confusion (2% to less than 5%)
Hallucinations (Rare)
▲ Insomnia (2% to less than 5%)
▲ Nervousness (2% to less than 5%)

Diuril Oral Suspension
Confusion

Diuril Sodium Intravenous
Confusion

Dolobid Tablets
Confusion (Less than 1 in 100)
Depression (Less than 1 in 100)
Disorientation (Less than 1 in 100)
Hallucinations (Less than 1 in 100)
Insomnia (Greater than 1 in 100)
Nervousness (Less than 1 in 100)

Donnatal Extentabs
Agitation
Excitability
Insomnia
Nervousness

Doxil Injection
▲ Agitation (1% to 10%)
▲ Anxiety (Less than 1% to 10%)
▲ Confusion (1% to 10%)
▲ Depression (Less than 1% to 10%)
▲ Emotional lability (1% to 5%)
▲ Insomnia (Less than 1% to 10%)
Nervousness (Less than 1%)
Thinking abnormality (Less than 1%)

Duragesic Transdermal System
Agitation (1% or greater)
▲ Anxiety (3% to 10%)
▲ Confusion (10% or more)
Depersonalization (Less than 1%)
▲ Depression (3% to 10%)
Dreaming abnormalities (1% or
  greater)
▲ Euphoria (3% to 10%)
▲ Hallucinations (3% to 10%)
Hostility (Less than 1%)
▲ Insomnia (3% to 10%)
Libido, decreased (Less than 1%)
▲ Nervousness (3% to 10%)
Paranoia (1% or greater)
Speech disturbances (1% or greater)
Stupor (Less than 1%)
Thinking abnormality (1% or greater)

Dyazide Capsules
Confusion

DynaCirc CR Tablets
Depression (0.5% to 1%)
Insomnia (0.5% to 1%)
Libido, decreased (0.5% to 1%)
Nervousness (0.5% to 1%)

EC-Naprosyn Delayed-Release Tablets
Anxiety (Less than 1%)
CNS depression (Less than 1%)
Cognitive dysfunction (Rare)
Coma (Less than 1%)
Confusion (Less than 1%)
Dreaming abnormalities (Less
  than 1%)
Hallucinations (Less than 1%)
Insomnia (Less than 1%)

Mental performance, impairment
(Less than 1%)
Nervousness (Less than 1%)

Edecrin Sodium Intravenous
Confusion

Edecrin Tablets
Confusion

Effexor Tablets
Aggression
▲ Agitation (2% to 4.5%)
Alcohol abuse (Rare)
▲ Anxiety (2% to 11.2%)
Apathy (Infrequent)
Behavioral changes
Catatonia
CNS stimulation (Infrequent)
Confusion (2%)
Delirium
Delusions (Rare)
Dementia (Rare)
Depersonalization (1%)
Depression (1%)
Depression, psychotic (Rare)
Diplopia (Infrequent)
▲ Dreaming abnormalities (4%)
Emotional lability (Infrequent)
Euphoria (Infrequent)
Hallucinations (Infrequent)
Hangover (Infrequent)
Hostility (Infrequent)
▲ Insomnia (3% to 22.5%)
Irritability
▲ Libido, decreased (2% to 5.7%)
Libido, increased (Infrequent)
Manic behavior (0.5%)
▲ Nervousness (2% to 21.3%)
Panic attack
Paranoia (Infrequent)
Photophobia (Infrequent)
Psychoses (Rare)
Serotonin syndrome
Sexual dysfunction (2%)
Sleep disturbances (Infrequent)
Speech disturbances (Infrequent)
Stupor (Infrequent)
Suicidal ideation (Rare)
Suicide, attempt of (Infrequent)
Thinking abnormality (2%)

Effexor XR Capsules
Aggression
▲ Agitation (4%)
Alcohol abuse (Rare)

Anxiety (1%)
Apathy (Infrequent)
Behavioral changes
Catatonia
CNS stimulation (Infrequent)
Confusion (Frequent)
Delirium
Delusions (Rare)
Dementia (Rare)
Depersonalization (Frequent)
▲ Depression (3%)
Depression, psychotic (Infrequent)
Diplopia (Infrequent)
▲ Dreaming abnormalities (3% to 7%)
Emotional lability (Infrequent)
Euphoria (Infrequent)
Feeling, intoxicated (Rare)
Hallucinations (Infrequent)
Hangover (Infrequent)
Hostility (Infrequent)
▲ Insomnia (3% to 23%)
Irritability
▲ Libido, decreased (3% to 9%)
Libido, increased (Infrequent)
Manic behavior (0.5%)
▲ Nervousness (5% to 11%)
▲ Nightmares (4% to 7%)
▲ Orgasmic dysfunction, female
(2% to 8%)
Panic attack
Paranoia (Infrequent)
Photophobia (Infrequent)
Psychoses (Infrequent)
Serotonin syndrome
Sexual dysfunction
Speech disturbances (Infrequent)
Stupor (Infrequent)
Suicidal ideation (Rare)
Suicide, attempt of (Infrequent)
Thinking abnormality (Frequent)

Efudex Topical Cream
Emotional disturbances (Infrequent)
Insomnia
Irritability

Efudex Topical Solutions
Emotional disturbances (Infrequent)
Insomnia
Irritability

Eldepryl Capsules
Agitation
Anxiety (1 of 49 patients)
Apathy
Behavioral changes

▲ Confusion (3 of 49 patients)
Delusions
Depression
Diplopia
Disorientation
▲ Dreaming abnormalities (2 of 49 patients)
Euphoria
▲ Hallucinations (3 of 49 patients)
Insomnia (1 of 49 patients)
Irritability
Memory impairment
Mental status, altered
Mood changes
Nervousness
Nightmares
Overstimulation
Personality changes
Sexual dysfunction
Sleep disturbances
Speech disturbances

Eligard 30 mg
Depression (1.1%)
Insomnia (1.1%)
▲ Libido, decreased (3.3%)

Eligard 45 mg
Libido, decreased (1%)

Eligard 7.5 mg
Depression (Less than 2%)
Insomnia (Less than 2%)
Libido, decreased (Less than 2%)
Smell disturbances (Less than 2%)

Elmiron Capsules
Depression
Emotional lability
Insomnia

Eloxatin for Injection
▲ Anxiety (2% to 5%)
▲ Depression (2% to 5%)
▲ Insomnia (9% to 11%)
▲ Nervousness (2% to 5%)
▲ Sensory disturbances (8%)

Elspar for Injection
Agitation
Coma
Confusion
Depression
Hallucinations
Irritability

Emcyt Capsules
Anxiety (1%)
Emotional lability (2%)
▲ Insomnia (3%)

Emend Capsules
Anxiety (Greater than 0.5%)
Confusion (Greater than 0.5%)
Depression (Greater than 0.5%)
Disorientation (Isolated cases)
▲ Insomnia (2.1% to 4.1 %)
Sensory disturbances (Less than or equal to 0.5%)

Emsam Transdermal System
Anxiety
▲ Insomnia (12%)
Libido, decreased (0.7%)
Nervousness

Emtriva Capsules
▲ Depression (6% to 9%)
▲ Dreaming abnormalities (2% to 11%)
▲ Insomnia (7% to 16%)

Emtriva Oral Solution
▲ Depression (6% to 9%)
▲ Dreaming abnormalities (2% to 11%)
▲ Insomnia (7% to 16%)

Enbrel for Injection
Depression (Infrequent)
Mood changes
Personality changes

Engerix-B Vaccine
Agitation (Less than 1%)
Insomnia (Less than 1%)
Irritability (Less than 1%)

Enjuvia Tablets
Dementia
Depression
Irritability
Libido, changes
Mood changes
Nervousness

Entocort EC Capsules
▲ Agitation (Less than 5%)
▲ Confusion (Less than 5%)
▲ Insomnia (Less than 5%)
▲ Nervousness (Less than 5%)
▲ Sleep disturbances (Less than 5%)

EpiPen Auto-Injector
Anxiety

EpiPen Jr. Auto-Injector
Anxiety
Nervousness

Epivir Oral Solution
▲ Depressive reactions (9%)
▲ Insomnia (11%)
▲ Sleep disturbances (11%)

Epivir Tablets
▲ Depressive reactions (9%)
▲ Insomnia (11%)
▲ Sleep disturbances (11%)

Epogen for Injection
▲ Anxiety (2% to 7%)
▲ Insomnia (13% to 21%)

Epzicom Tablets
▲ Anxiety (3% to 5%)
▲ Depression (7%)
▲ Dreaming abnormalities (4% to 5%)
▲ Insomnia (7% to 9%)

Equetro Extended-Release Capsules
Agitation
▲ Anxiety (7%)
Confusion
▲ Depersonalization (Less than 5%)
▲ Depression (7%)
▲ Diplopia (Less than 5%)
Hallucinations
▲ Insomnia (Less than 5%)
▲ Nervousness (Less than 5%)
▲ Speech disturbances (6%)
▲ Suicide, attempt of (Less than 5%)
Talkativeness

Erbitux
Confusion (2%)
▲ Depression (7% to 10%)
▲ Insomnia (Less than 1% to 12%)

Ery-Tab Tablets
Confusion (Isolated reports)
Hallucinations (Isolated reports)

Erythrocin Stearate Filmtab Tablets
Confusion (Isolated reports)
Hallucinations (Isolated reports)

Erythromycin Base Filmtab Tablets
Confusion (Isolated reports)
Hallucinations (Isolated reports)

Erythromycin Delayed-Release Capsules, USP
Confusion (Isolated reports)
Hallucinations (Isolated reports)

Estrace Tablets
Libido, changes
Speech disturbances

Estrace Vaginal Cream
Libido, changes
Speech disturbances

Estrasorb Topical Emulsion
Dementia
Depression
Irritability
Libido, changes
Mood changes
Nervousness

Estratest H.S. Tablets
Anxiety
Dementia (1.8%)
Depression
Irritability
Libido, changes
Mood changes
Nervousness

Estratest Tablets
Anxiety
Dementia (1.8%)
Depression
Irritability
Libido, changes
Mood changes
Nervousness

Estring Vaginal Ring
▲ Anxiety (1% to 3%)
Depression
▲ Insomnia (4%)
Libido, decreased
Nervousness

Eulexin Capsules
Anxiety (1%)
Confusion (1%)
Depression (1%)
▲ Libido, loss of (36%)
Nervousness (1%)

Evista Tablets
▲ Depression (6.4%)
▲ Insomnia (5.5%)

Evoxac Capsules
Aggression
Agitation (Less than 1%)

Anxiety (1.3%)
Apathy
Coma (Less than 1%)
Confusion (Less than 1%)
Delirium
Delusions
Dementia
Depersonalization (Less than 1%)
▲ Depression (1% to 3%)
Depression, aggravation of (Less than 1%)
Diplopia (Less than 1%)
Dreaming abnormalities (Less than 1%)
Emotional lability (Less than 1%)
Hallucinations (Less than 1%)
Illusion, unspecified
Insomnia (2.4%)
Manic behavior (Less than 1%)
Neurosis, unspecified
Paranoia
Personality changes
Sexual dysfunction (Less than 1%)
Speech disturbances (Less than 1%)
Thinking abnormality (Less than 1%)

Exelon Capsules
▲ Aggression (3%)
Agitation (2% or more)
▲ Anxiety (4% to 5%)
Apathy (Infrequent)
▲ Confusion (8%)
Delirium (Infrequent)
Delusions (2% or more)
Dementia (Infrequent)
Depersonalization (Infrequent)
▲ Depression (6%)
Diplopia (Infrequent)
Dreaming abnormalities (Infrequent)
Emotional lability (Infrequent)
▲ Hallucinations (4%)
▲ Insomnia (3% to 9%)
Libido, decreased (Infrequent)
Libido, increased (Infrequent)
Mental performance, impairment (Infrequent)
Nervousness (2% or more)
Neurosis, unspecified (Infrequent)
Paranoia (2% or more)
Personality changes (Infrequent)
Psychoses (Infrequent)
Suicidal ideation (Infrequent)
Suicide, attempt of (Infrequent)

Exelon Oral Solution
▲ Aggression (3%)
Agitation (2% or more)
▲ Anxiety (4% to 5%)
Apathy (Infrequent)
▲ Confusion (8%)
Delirium (Infrequent)
Delusions (2% or more)
Dementia (Infrequent)
Depersonalization (Infrequent)
▲ Depression (6%)
Diplopia (Infrequent)
Dreaming abnormalities (Infrequent)
Emotional lability (Infrequent)
▲ Hallucinations (4%)
▲ Insomnia (3% to 9%)
Libido, decreased (Infrequent)
Libido, increased (Infrequent)
Mental performance, impairment (Infrequent)
Nervousness (2% or more)
Neurosis, unspecified (Infrequent)
Paranoia (2% or more)
Personality changes (Infrequent)
Psychoses (Infrequent)
Suicidal ideation (Infrequent)
Suicide, attempt of (Infrequent)

Extra Strength Tylenol PM Caplets, Vanilla Caplets, Geltabs, Gelcaps and Liquid
Insomnia

Fabrazyme for Intravenous Infusion
▲ Anxiety (8%)
▲ Depression (3%)

Famvir Tablets
Confusion (Infrequent)
Delirium (Infrequent)
Disorientation (Infrequent)
Hallucinations (Infrequent)
Insomnia (1.5% to 2.5%)

Fansidar Tablets
Apathy
Depression
Hallucinations
Insomnia
Nervousness

Faslodex Injection
▲ Anxiety (5%)
▲ Depression (5.7%)
▲ Insomnia (6.9%)

FazaClo Orally Disintegrating Tablets
▲ Agitation (4%)
  Anxiety (1%)
▲ Confusion (3%)
  Delirium
  Delusions (Less than 1%)
  Depression (1%)
  Hallucinations (Less than 1%)
▲ Insomnia (2% to 20%)
  Irritability (Less than 1%)
  Libido, decreased (Less than 1%)
  Libido, increased (Less than 1%)
▲ Nightmares (4%)
  Paranoia (Less than 1%)
  Psychoses, aggravation
  Psychosis, activation
▲ Sedation (Greater than 5% to 39%)
▲ Sleep disturbances (4%)
  Speech difficulties (Less than 1%)
  Speech, slurring (1%)
  Stuttering (Less than 1%)

Femara Tablets
  Anxiety (Less frequent)
  Depression (Less frequent)
▲ Insomnia (Less than 0.1% to 7%)
  Insomnia
  Libido, changes
▲ Nervousness (5.4%)

Femring Vaginal Ring
  Irritability
  Libido, changes
  Mood changes
  Nervousness

Femtrace Tablets
  Irritability
  Libido, changes
  Mood changes
  Nervousness

Fentora Tablets
▲ Confusion (1% to 16%)
▲ Depression (3% to 11%)
  Disorientation (Greater than 1%)
  Hallucinations (Greater than 1%)
▲ Insomnia (1% to 11%)
  Nervousness (Greater than 1%)

Ferrlecit Injection
  Agitation
  Nervousness (Two or more patients)

Flebogamma 5%, Immune Globulin Intravenous (Human)
  Anxiety
  Coma

Flomax Capsules
  Insomnia (1.4% to 2.4%)
  Libido, decreased (1.0% to 2.0%)

Flonase Nasal Spray
  Smell disturbances

Flovent Diskus 100 mcg
  Aggression
  Agitation
  Depression
▲ Sleep disturbances (1% to 3%)

Flovent Diskus 250 mcg
  Aggression
  Agitation
  Depression
▲ Sleep disturbances (1% to 3%)

Flovent Diskus 50 mcg
  Aggression
  Agitation
  Depression
▲ Sleep disturbances (1% to 3%)

Flovent HFA 110 mcg Inhalation Aerosol
  Aggression
  Agitation
  Confusion
  Depression

Flovent HFA 220 mcg Inhalation Aerosol
  Aggression
  Agitation
  Confusion
  Depression

Flovent HFA 44 mcg Inhalation Aerosol
  Aggression
  Agitation
  Confusion
  Depression

Floxin Otic Solution
  Insomnia (Single report)

Flulaval Injection
  Insomnia
  Photophobia

Flumadine Syrup
  Agitation (0.3% to 1%)
  Confusion (Less than 0.3%)
  Depression (0.3% to 1%)
  Euphoria (Less than 0.3%)

Hallucinations (Less than 0.3%)
Insomnia (2.1% to 3.4%)
Mental performance, impairment
  (0.3% to 2.1%)
Nervousness (1.3% to 2.1%)

Flumadine Tablets
Agitation (0.3% to 1%)
Confusion (Less than 0.3%)
Depression (0.3% to 1%)
Euphoria (Less than 0.3%)
Hallucinations (Less than 0.3%)
Insomnia (2.1% to 3.4%)
Mental performance, impairment
  (0.3% to 2.1%)
Nervousness (1.3% to 2.1%)

Flumist Vaccine
▲ Irritability (9.9% to 17.8%)

Focalin Tablets
Depression
Hallucinations
▲ Insomnia (Among most common)
▲ Nervousness (Among most common)
Psychoses, toxic (Rare)

Focalin XR Capsules
▲ Anxiety (5% to 11%)
Depression
Insomnia
▲ Jitteriness (12%)
Nervousness
▲ Psychiatric disturbances (26% to 46%)
Psychoses, toxic

Foradil Aerolizer
Anxiety (1.5%)
Insomnia (1.5%)
Nervousness

Fortaz for Injection
Coma

Fortaz Injection
Coma

Forteo for Injection
▲ Depression (4.1%)
▲ Insomnia (4.3%)

Fortical Nasal Spray
Insomnia (Less than 1%)

Foscavir Injection
▲ Insomnia (Between 1% and 5%)
▲ Nervousness (Between 1% and 5%)

▲ Sensory disturbances (Between 1%
  and 5%)
▲ Stupor (Between 1% and 5%)

Frova Tablets
Agitation (Infrequent)
Anxiety (Frequent)
Confusion (Infrequent)
Depersonalization (Infrequent)
Depression (Infrequent)
Depression, aggravation of (Rare)
Dreaming abnormalities (Rare)
Emotional lability (Infrequent)
Euphoria (Infrequent)
Insomnia (Frequent)
Mental performance, impairment
  (Infrequent)
Nervousness (Infrequent)
Personality changes (Rare)
Speech disturbances (Infrequent)
Thinking abnormality (Infrequent)

Fuzeon Injection
Anxiety
Depression
Insomnia
Suicide, attempt of

Gabitril Tablets
Agitation (1%)
Anxiety (1% or more)
Apathy (Infrequent)
Coma (Infrequent)
▲ Confusion (5%)
Delusions (Infrequent)
Depersonalization (Frequent)
▲ Depression (3%)
Diplopia (1% or more)
Dreaming abnormalities (Infrequent)
▲ Emotional lability (3%)
Euphoria (Frequent)
Hallucinations (Frequent)
Hostility (2%)
▲ Insomnia (6%)
▲ Irritability (10%)
Libido, decreased (Infrequent)
Libido, increased (Infrequent)
▲ Mental performance, impairment (6%)
▲ Nervousness (10%)
Neurosis, unspecified (Infrequent)
Paranoia (Frequent)
Personality changes (Frequent)
Photophobia (Infrequent)
Psychoses (Infrequent)
▲ Speech disturbances (4%)
Stupor (Frequent)

Suicide, attempt of (Infrequent)
▲ Thinking abnormality (6%)

Gammagard Liquid
Coma

Gammagard S/D
Coma (Rare)

Gamunex Immune Globulin I.V., 10%
Coma (Rare)

Gantrisin Pediatric Suspension
Anxiety
Apathy
Depression
Disorientation
Hallucinations
Insomnia

Garamycin Injectable
Confusion
Depression

Gardasil Injection
Insomnia (1.2%)

Gemzar for Injection
Insomnia (Infrequent)

Gengraf Capsules
Anxiety (1% to less than 3%)
Confusion (1% to less than 3%)
Depression (Rare)
Emotional lability (1% to less than 3%)
Insomnia (1% to less than 3%)
Libido, decreased (1% to less than 3%)
Libido, increased (1% to less than 3%)
Mental performance, impairment (1% to less than 3%)
Nervousness (1% to less than 3%)
▲ Psychiatric disturbances (5%)

Genotropin Lyophilized Powder
Aggression

Geodon Capsules
Agitation (Frequent)
▲ Anxiety (5%)
Confusion (Frequent)
Delirium (Frequent)
Depression

Diplopia (Frequent)
Hostility (Frequent)
Insomnia (Rare)
Photophobia (Infrequent)
Serotonin syndrome (Rare)
Sexual dysfunction (Infrequent)
Speech disturbances (2%)

Geodon for Injection
Anxiety (Up to 2%)
Insomnia (Rare)
Personality changes (Up to 2%)
Psychoses (Up to 1%)
Serotonin syndrome (Rare)
Speech difficulties (Up to 2%)

Gleevec Tablets
▲ Anxiety (0% to 12%)
Confusion (Rare)
▲ Depression (0.5% to 12.7%)
▲ Insomnia (0% to 19%)
Memory impairment (Infrequent)
Sexual dysfunction (Infrequent)

Gris-PEG Tablets
Confusion (Occasional)
Insomnia (Occasional)

Guanidine Hydrochloride Tablets
Confusion
Emotional lability
Hallucinations
Irritability
Jitteriness
Mood changes
Psychoses

Havrix Vaccine
Insomnia (Less than 1%)
▲ Irritability (24% to 36%)
Photophobia (Less than 1%)

Hectorol Capsules
Apathy
▲ Depression (Greater than or equal to 5%)
▲ Insomnia (Greater than or equal to 5%)
Libido, decreased
Photophobia
Sensory disturbances
▲ Sleep disturbances (3.3%)

Hectorol Injection
Apathy
Libido, decreased

Photophobia
Sensory disturbances
▲ Sleep disturbances (3.3%)

Herceptin I.V.
Confusion (At least one of the 958 patients)
▲ Depression (6%)
▲ Insomnia (14%)
Manic behavior (At least one of the 958 patients)

HibTITER
Irritability (133 of 1,118 vaccinations)
Sleep disturbances

Humira Injection
▲ Confusion (Less than 5%)

Hycodan Syrup
Anxiety
Fear
Mental clouding
Mental performance, impairment
Mood changes
Sedation

Hycodan Tablets
Anxiety
Fear
Mental clouding
Mental performance, impairment
Mood changes
Sedation

Hycotuss Expectorant Syrup
Anxiety
Fear
Mental clouding
Mental performance, impairment
Mood changes
Sedation

Hydrocortone Tablets
Depression
Euphoria
Insomnia
Mood changes
Personality changes
Psychiatric disturbances
Psychoses
Psychoses, aggravation

Hyperstat I.V.
Anxiety
Confusion
Euphoria
Libido, decreased

Hytrin Capsules
Anxiety (At least 1%)
Depression (0.3%)
Insomnia (At least 1%)
Libido, decreased (0.6%)
Nervousness (2.3%)

Hyzaar 100-12.5 Tablets
Anxiety
Confusion
Depression
Dreaming abnormalities
Insomnia
Libido, decreased
Memory impairment
Nervousness
Panic attack
Sleep disturbances

Hyzaar 100-25 Tablets
Anxiety
Confusion
Depression
Dreaming abnormalities
Insomnia
Libido, decreased
Memory impairment
Nervousness
Panic attack
Sleep disturbances

Hyzaar 50-12.5 Tablets
Anxiety
Confusion
Depression
Dreaming abnormalities
Insomnia
Libido, decreased
Memory impairment
Nervousness
Panic attack
Sleep disturbances

I.V. Busulfex
Agitation (2%)
▲ Anxiety (72% to 75%)
Coma (One patient)
▲ Confusion (11%)
Delirium (2%)
▲ Depression (23%)
▲ Hallucinations (5%)
▲ Insomnia (84%)

Imdur Tablets
▲ Anxiety (Less than or equal to 5%)
▲ Confusion (Less than or equal to 5%)

▲ Depression (Less than or equal to 5%)
▲ Insomnia (Less than or equal to 5%)
▲ Libido, decreased (Less than or equal to 5%)
▲ Nervousness (Less than or equal to 5%)
▲ Photophobia (Less than or equal to 5%)

Imitrex Injection

Aggression
Agitation (Infrequent)
Anxiety (Frequent)
Apathy
Confusion (Infrequent)
Depression (Rare)
Euphoria (Infrequent)
Feeling, intoxicated (Rare)
Feeling, strange (2%)
Hallucinations
Hysteria (Rare)
Mental performance, impairment (Rare)
Panic attack
Phobia, unspecified
Photophobia (Infrequent)
▲ Sedation (3%)
Serotonin syndrome
Sleep disturbances (Rare)
Smell disturbances (Rare)
Speech disturbances

Imitrex Nasal Spray

Agitation (Infrequent)
Anxiety (Infrequent)
Apathy (Rare)
Confusion (Infrequent)
Depression (Infrequent)
Emotional disturbances (Rare)
Euphoria (Infrequent)
Feeling, strange (Infrequent)
Memory impairment (Rare)
Mental performance, impairment (Rare)
Panic attack
Sedation (Infrequent)
Sleep disturbances (Infrequent)
Smell disturbances (Infrequent)

Imitrex Tablets

Aggression (Rare)
Agitation (Up to 2%)
Anxiety
Apathy (Rare)
Awareness, heightened (Rare)
Confusion (Infrequent)

Depression (Infrequent)
Euphoria (Infrequent)
Feeling, strange
Hallucinations (Rare)
Hysteria (Rare)
Memory impairment (Rare)
Mental performance, impairment (Infrequent)
Panic attack
Personality changes (Rare)
Phobic disorder (Rare)
Phonophobia (Frequent)
Photophobia (Frequent)
Sedation
Serotonin syndrome
Sleep disturbances (Rare to infrequent)
Smell disturbances (Infrequent)
Suicide, attempt of (Rare)

Indapamide Tablets

▲ Agitation (Greater than or equal to 5%)
▲ Anxiety (Greater than or equal to 5%)
▲ Depression (Less than 5%)
▲ Insomnia (Less than 5%)
▲ Irritability (Greater than or equal to 5%)
▲ Libido, decreased (Less than 5%)
▲ Nervousness (Less than 5%)
▲ Tenseness (Greater than or equal to 5%)

Inderal LA Long-Acting Capsules

Catatonia
Depression
Disorientation, place
Disorientation, time
Dreaming abnormalities
Emotional lability
Hallucinations
Insomnia
Memory loss, short-term
Neuropsychometrics performance, decrease
Sensorium, clouded

Indocin Capsules

Anxiety (Less than 1%)
Coma (Less than 1%)
Confusion (Less than 1%)
Depersonalization (Less than 1%)
Depression (Greater than 1%)
Diplopia (Less than 1%)
Insomnia (Less than 1%)

Listlessness (Greater than 1%)
Nervousness (Less than 1%)
Psychiatric disturbances (Less than 1%)
Psychoses (Less than 1%)

Indocin I.V.
Coma (Less than 1%)

Indocin Oral Suspension
Anxiety (Less than 1%)
Coma (Less than 1%)
Confusion (Less than 1%)
Depersonalization (Less than 1%)
Depression (Greater than 1%)
Diplopia (Less than 1%)
Insomnia (Less than 1%)
Listlessness (Greater than 1%)
Nervousness (Less than 1%)
Psychiatric disturbances (Less than 1%)
Psychoses (Less than 1%)

Indocin Suppositories
Anxiety (Less than 1%)
Coma (Less than 1%)
Confusion (Less than 1%)
Depersonalization (Less than 1%)
Depression (Greater than 1%)
Diplopia (Less than 1%)
Insomnia (Less than 1%)
Listlessness (Greater than 1%)
Nervousness (Less than 1%)
Psychiatric disturbances (Less than 1%)
Psychoses (Less than 1%)

Infanrix Vaccine
▲ Anxiety (3.3% to 9.2%)
▲ Irritability (28.8% to 61.5%)

Infed Injection
Disorientation

Infergen
▲ Agitation (4% to 6%)
▲ Anxiety (10% to 19%)
▲ Confusion (4%)
▲ Depression (18% to 26%)
▲ Emotional lability (6% to 12%)
▲ Insomnia (24% to 39%)
▲ Libido, decreased (5%)
▲ Nervousness (16% to 31%)
Psychiatric disturbances
Suicidal ideation
Suicide, attempt of
▲ Thinking abnormality (8% to 10%)

InnoPran XL Capsules
Catatonia
Depression
Disorientation, place
Disorientation, time
Emotional lability
Hallucinations
Insomnia
Memory loss, short-term
Neuropsychometrics performance, decrease
Sensorium, clouded

Intron A for Injection
▲ Aggression (Less than 5%)
▲ Agitation (Less than 5%)
▲ Anxiety (Up to 5%)
▲ Apathy (Less than 5%)
▲ CNS reactions (Less than 5%)
▲ Coma (Less than 5%)
▲ Confusion (Up to 12%)
▲ Consciousness, disorders of (Less than 5%)
▲ Depression (2% to 40%)
▲ Depression, aggravation of (Less than 5%)
▲ Diplopia (Less than 5%)
▲ Dreaming abnormalities (Less than 5%)
▲ Emotional lability (Less than 5%)
▲ Insomnia (Up to 12%)
▲ Irritability (Up to 16%)
▲ Libido, decreased (Up to 5%)
▲ Manic behavior (Less than 5%)
▲ Mental performance, impairment (Up to 14%)
▲ Nervousness (Up to 3%)
▲ Neurosis, unspecified (Less than 5%)
▲ Personality changes (Less than 5%)
▲ Photophobia (Less than 5%)
▲ Speech disturbances (Less than 5%)
Suicidal ideation (Rare)
▲ Suicide, attempt of (Rare; less than 5%)
▲ Thinking abnormality (Less than 5%)

Invanz for Injection
▲ Agitation (3.3% to 5.1%)
Anxiety (0.8% to 1.1%)
▲ Confusion (3.3% to 5.1%)
Depression (Greater than 0.1%)
▲ Disorientation (3.3% to 5.1%)
Hallucinations (Very rare)
▲ Insomnia (3% to 3.2%)
▲ Mental status, altered (3.3% to 5.1%)
Nervousness (Greater than 0.1%)
▲ Stupor (3.3% to 5.1%)

Invega Extended-Release Tablets

Agitation
▲ Anxiety (5% to 9%)
Confusion (Infrequent)
Insomnia
Sedation

Invirase Capsules

Agitation (Less than 2%)
Anxiety (Greater than or equal to 2%)
Confusion (Less than 2%)
Depression (Greater than or equal to 2%)
Dreaming abnormalities (Less than 2%)
Euphoria (Less than 2%)
Hallucinations (Less than 2%)
Insomnia (Greater than or equal to 2%)
Irritability (Less than 2%)
Libido, changes (Greater than or equal to 2%)
Mental performance, impairment (Less than 2%)
Psychiatric disturbances (Less than 2%)
Psychoses (Less than 2%)
Speech disturbances (Less than 2%)
Suicide, attempt of (Rare)

Invirase Tablets

Agitation (Less than 2%)
Anxiety (Greater than or equal to 2%)
Confusion (Less than 2%)
Depression (Greater than or equal to 2%)
Dreaming abnormalities (Less than 2%)
Euphoria (Less than 2%)
Hallucinations (Less than 2%)
Insomnia (Greater than or equal to 2%)
Irritability (Less than 2%)
Libido, changes (Greater than or equal to 2%)
Mental performance, impairment (Less than 2%)
Psychiatric disturbances (Less than 2%)
Psychoses (Less than 2%)
Speech disturbances (Less than 2%)
Suicide, attempt of (Rare)

Ionsys Transdermal System

Agitation (.1% to less than 1%)

▲ Anxiety (1% to less than 10%)
Confusion (.1% to less than 1%)
Dreaming abnormalities (.1% to less than 1%)
▲ Insomnia (3%)
Nervousness (.1% to less than 1%)

Kadian Capsules

Agitation (Less than 3%)
▲ Anxiety (Less than 3% to 6%)
Apathy (Less than 3%)
Confusion (Less than 3%)
Depression (Less than 3%)
Diplopia (Less than 3%)
Dreaming abnormalities (Less than 3%)
Euphoria (Less than 3%)
Hallucinations (Less than 3%)
Insomnia (Less than 3%)
Libido, decreased (Less than 3%)
Mental performance, impairment (Less than 3%)
Sedation (Less than 3%)
Speech, slurring (Less than 3%)
Thinking abnormality (Less than 3%)

Kaletra Oral Solution

Agitation (Less than 2%)
Anxiety (Less than 2%)
Confusion (Less than 2%)
Depression (Up to 2%)
Dreaming abnormalities (Less than 2%)
Emotional lability (Less than 2%)
Insomnia (Up to 2%)
Libido, decreased (Up to 2%)
Nervousness (Less than 2%)
Thinking abnormality (Less than 2%)

Kaletra Tablets

Agitation (Less than 2%)
Anxiety (Less than 2%)
Confusion (Less than 2%)
Depression (0% to 2%)
Dreaming abnormalities (Less than 2%)
Emotional lability (Less than 2%)
Insomnia (0% to 2%)
Libido, decreased (0% to 2%)
Nervousness (Less than 2%)
Thinking abnormality (Less than 2%)

Keflex Capsules

Agitation
Confusion
Hallucinations

Keppra Injection
Anxiety (2%)
Confusion
▲ Depression (4%)
Diplopia (2%)
Emotional lability (2%)
Hostility (2%)
Insomnia
▲ Nervousness (4%)
Suicide, attempt of
Thinking abnormality

Keppra Oral Solution
Aggression
▲ Agitation (6%)
Anxiety (2%)
Apathy
▲ Behavioral changes (38%)
Confusion (1% to 2%)
Depersonalization
▲ Depression (3% to 5%)
Diplopia (2%)
▲ Emotional lability (2% to 6%)
▲ Hostility (2% to 12%)
Insomnia (1% to 2%)
▲ Irritability (6%)
▲ Mood changes (5%)
▲ Nervousness (4% to 10%)
Neurosis, unspecified
▲ Personality changes (8%)
Suicidal ideation (Rare)
Thinking abnormality (1% to 2%)

Keppra Tablets
Aggression
▲ Agitation (6%)
Anxiety (2%)
Apathy
▲ Behavioral changes (38%)
Confusion (1% to 2%)
Depersonalization
▲ Depression (3% to 5%)
Diplopia (2%)
▲ Emotional lability (2% to 6%)
▲ Hostility (2% to 12%)
Insomnia (1% to 2%)
▲ Irritability (6%)
▲ Mood changes (5%)
▲ Nervousness (4% to 10%)
Neurosis, unspecified
▲ Personality changes (8%)
Suicidal ideation (Rare)
Thinking abnormality (1% to 2%)

Ketek Tablets
Anxiety (Less than 0.2%)
Diplopia (Greater than or equal to
0.2% to less than 2%)

Insomnia (Greater than or equal to
0.2% to less than 2%)

Klonopin Tablets
Aggression (Infrequent)
Agitation
Anxiety (Infrequent)
Apathy (Infrequent)
▲ Behavioral changes (5% to 25%)
▲ CNS depression (Most frequent)
Coma
Confusion (1%)
Depersonalization (Infrequent)
▲ Depression (4% to 7%)
Diplopia (Infrequent)
Dreaming abnormalities (Infrequent)
Emotional lability (1%)
Excitability (Infrequent)
Hallucinations
Hostility
Hyperactivity (Infrequent)
Hysteria
Illusion, unspecified (Infrequent)
Inebriated feeling (Infrequent)
Insomnia (Infrequent)
Libido, decreased (1%)
Libido, increased (Infrequent)
Libido, loss of (Infrequent)
▲ Memory impairment (4%)
Mental performance, impairment (1%
to 2%)
Nervousness (1% to 3%)
Nightmares (Infrequent)
Psychoses
Sleep disturbances (Infrequent)
Speech, slurring
Suicidal ideation (Infrequent)
Suicide, attempt of (Infrequent)

Klonopin Wafers
Aggression (Infrequent)
Agitation
Anxiety (Infrequent)
Apathy (Infrequent)
▲ Behavioral changes (5% to 25%)
▲ CNS depression (Most frequent)
Coma
Confusion (1%)
Depersonalization (Infrequent)
▲ Depression (4% to 7%)
Diplopia (Infrequent)
Dreaming abnormalities (Infrequent)
Emotional lability (1%)
Excitability (Infrequent)
Hallucinations

Hostility
Hyperactivity (Infrequent)
Hysteria
Illusion, unspecified (Infrequent)
Inebriated feeling (Infrequent)
Insomnia (Infrequent)
Libido, decreased (1%)
Libido, increased (Infrequent)
Libido, loss of (Infrequent)
▲ Memory impairment (4%)
Mental performance, impairment (1% to 2%)
Nervousness (1% to 3%)
Nightmares (Infrequent)
Psychoses
Sleep disturbances (Infrequent)
Speech, slurring
Suicidal ideation (Infrequent)
Suicide, attempt of (Infrequent)

Kogenate FS
Depersonalization

Kogenate FS with Bio-Set
Depersonalization (1 case)

K-Phos Neutral Tablets
Confusion

K-Phos Original (Sodium Free) Tablets
Confusion (Less frequent)

Kytril Injection
Agitation (Less than 2%)
▲ Anxiety (Less than 2% to 3.4%)
CNS stimulation (Less than 2%)
▲ Insomnia (Less than 2% to 4.9%)

Kytril Oral Solution
Anxiety (2%)
▲ Insomnia (3% to 5%)

Kytril Tablets
Anxiety (2%)
▲ Insomnia (3% to 5%)

Lacrisert Sterile Ophthalmic Insert
Photophobia

Lamictal Chewable Dispersible Tablets
▲ Agitation (Greater than 1% to less than 5%)
▲ Anxiety (4% to 5%)
Apathy (Infrequent)
CNS depression (Infrequent)

CNS stimulation (Rare)
Confusion (Frequent)
Delirium (Rare)
Delusions (Rare)
Depersonalization (Infrequent)
▲ Depression (Greater than 1% to less than 5%)
▲ Diplopia (5% to 49%)
Dreaming abnormalities (Infrequent)
▲ Emotional lability (Greater than 1% to 5%)
Euphoria (Infrequent)
Hallucinations (Infrequent)
Hostility (Infrequent)
▲ Insomnia (5% to 10%)
▲ Irritability (3%)
Libido, decreased (Infrequent)
Libido, increased (Rare)
▲ Manic behavior (5%)
Memory impairment (2.4%)
Mental performance, impairment (1.7%)
Nervousness (2%)
Neurosis, unspecified (Rare)
Panic attack (Infrequent)
Paranoia (Infrequent)
Personality changes (Infrequent)
Photophobia (Infrequent)
Psychoses (Infrequent)
Sleep disturbances (1.4%)
▲ Speech disturbances (3%)
Stupor (Infrequent)
Suicidal ideation (Rare)
Suicide, attempt of (Rare)
▲ Thinking abnormality (3%)

Lamictal Tablets
▲ Agitation (Greater than 1% to less than 5%)
▲ Anxiety (4% to 5%)
Apathy (Infrequent)
CNS depression (Infrequent)
CNS stimulation (Rare)
Confusion (Frequent)
Delirium (Rare)
Delusions (Rare)
Depersonalization (Infrequent)
▲ Depression (Greater than 1% to less than 5%)
▲ Diplopia (5% to 49%)
Dreaming abnormalities (Infrequent)
▲ Emotional lability (Greater than 1% to 5%)
Euphoria (Infrequent)
Hallucinations (Infrequent)

Hostility (Infrequent)
▲ Insomnia (5% to 10%)
▲ Irritability (3%)
Libido, decreased (Infrequent)
Libido, increased (Rare)
▲ Manic behavior (5%)
Memory impairment (2.4%)
Mental performance, impairment (1.7%)
Nervousness (2%)
Neurosis, unspecified (Rare)
Panic attack (Infrequent)
Paranoia (Infrequent)
Personality changes (Infrequent)
Photophobia (Infrequent)
Psychoses (Infrequent)
Sleep disturbances (1.4%)
▲ Speech disturbances (3%)
Stupor (Infrequent)
Suicidal ideation (Rare)
Suicide, attempt of (Rare)
▲ Thinking abnormality (3%)

Lanoxicaps Capsules
Anxiety
Apathy
CNS reactions (Rare)
Confusion
Delirium
Depression
Hallucinations
Mental status, altered
Psychoses

Lanoxin Injection
Anxiety
Apathy
CNS reactions
Confusion
Delirium
Depression
Hallucinations
Mental status, altered
Psychoses

Lanoxin Injection Pediatric
Anxiety
Apathy
CNS reactions
Confusion
Delirium
Depression
Hallucinations
Mental status, altered
Psychoses

Lanoxin Tablets
Anxiety
Apathy
CNS reactions
Confusion
Delirium
Depression
Hallucinations
Mental status, altered

Lariam Tablets
Agitation (Occasional)
Anxiety (Occasional)
CNS reactions
Confusion (Occasional)
Depression (Occasional)
▲ Dreaming abnormalities (Among most frequent)
Emotional disturbances (Less than 1%)
Hallucinations (Occasional)
▲ Insomnia (Among most frequent)
Mood changes (Occasional)
Panic attack (Occasional)
Paranoia (Occasional)
Psychiatric disturbances (Occasional)
Psychoses (Occasional)
▲ Sleep disturbances (Among most frequent)
Suicidal ideation (Rare)
Suicide, attempt of (Rare)

Lescol Capsules
Anxiety
Depression
Insomnia (2.7%)
Libido, loss of
Memory loss, short-term
Psychiatric disturbances

Lescol XL Tablets
Anxiety
Depression
Insomnia (0.8%)
Libido, loss of
Memory loss, short-term
Psychiatric disturbances

Leukeran Tablets
Agitation (Rare)
Confusion (Rare)
Hallucinations (Rare)

Leukine
▲ Anxiety (11%)
▲ CNS reactions (11%)
▲ Insomnia (0.11)

▲ Psychiatric disturbances (15%)
▲ Sensory disturbances (6%)

Leustatin Injection
▲ Insomnia (7%)

Levaquin in 5% Dextrose Injection
Aggression (0.1% to 0.9%)
Agitation (0.1% to 0.9%)
Anxiety (1.2%)
Coma (0.1% to 0.9%)
Confusion (0.1% to 0.9%)
Delirium (0.1% to 0.9%)
Depression (0.1% to 0.9%)
Diplopia
Dreaming abnormalities (0.1% to 0.9%)
Emotional lability (0.1% to 0.9%)
Hallucinations (0.1% to 0.9%)
▲ Insomnia (0.4% to 4.6%)
Manic behavior (0.1% to 0.9%)
Mental performance, impairment (0.1% to 0.9%)
Nervousness (0.1% to 0.9%)
Nightmares
Paranoia (0.1% to 0.9%)
Psychoses
Psychoses, toxic
Sleep disturbances (0.1% to 0.9%)
Speech disturbances (0.1% to 0.9%)
Stupor (0.1% to 0.9%)
Suicidal ideation (Rare)
Suicide, attempt of (Rare)

Levaquin Injection
Aggression (0.1% to 0.9%)
Agitation (0.1% to 0.9%)
Anxiety (1.2%)
Coma (0.1% to 0.9%)
Confusion (0.1% to 0.9%)
Delirium (0.1% to 0.9%)
Depression (0.1% to 0.9%)
Diplopia
Dreaming abnormalities (0.1% to 0.9%)
Emotional lability (0.1% to 0.9%)
Hallucinations (0.1% to 0.9%)
▲ Insomnia (0.4% to 4.6%)
Manic behavior (0.1% to 0.9%)
Mental performance, impairment (0.1% to 0.9%)
Nervousness (0.1% to 0.9%)
Nightmares
Paranoia (0.1% to 0.9%)
Psychoses
Psychoses, toxic

Sleep disturbances (0.1% to 0.9%)
Speech disturbances (0.1% to 0.9%)
Stupor (0.1% to 0.9%)
Suicidal ideation (Rare)
Suicide, attempt of (Rare)

Levaquin Oral Solution
Aggression (0.1% to 0.9%)
Agitation (0.1% to 0.9%)
Anxiety (1.2%)
Coma (0.1% to 0.9%)
Confusion (0.1% to 0.9%)
Delirium (0.1% to 0.9%)
Depression (0.1% to 0.9%)
Diplopia
Dreaming abnormalities (0.1% to 0.9%)
Emotional lability (0.1% to 0.9%)
Hallucinations (0.1% to 0.9%)
▲ Insomnia (0.4% to 4.6%)
Manic behavior (0.1% to 0.9%)
Mental performance, impairment (0.1% to 0.9%)
Nervousness (0.1% to 0.9%)
Nightmares
Paranoia (0.1% to 0.9%)
Psychoses
Psychoses, toxic
Sleep disturbances (0.1% to 0.9%)
Speech disturbances (0.1% to 0.9%)
Stupor (0.1% to 0.9%)
Suicidal ideation (Rare)
Suicide, attempt of (Rare)

Levaquin Tablets
Aggression (0.1% to 0.9%)
Agitation (0.1% to 0.9%)
Anxiety (0.012)
Coma (0.1% to 0.9%)
Confusion (0.1% to 0.9%)
Delirium (0.1% to 0.9%)
Depression (0.1% to 0.9%)
Diplopia
Dreaming abnormalities (0.1% to 0.9%)
Emotional lability (0.1% to 0.9%)
Hallucinations (0.1% to 0.9%)
▲ Insomnia (0.4% to 4.6%)
Manic behavior (0.1% to 0.9%)
Mental performance, impairment (0.1% to 0.9%)
Nervousness (0.1% to 0.9%)
Nightmares
Paranoia (0.1% to 0.9%)
Psychoses
Psychoses, toxic

Sleep disturbances (0.1% to 0.9%)
Speech disturbances (0.1% to 0.9%)
Stupor (0.1% to 0.9%)
Suicidal ideation (Rare)
Suicide, attempt of (Rare)

Levbid Extended-Release Tablets
Insomnia
Manic behavior
Memory loss, short-term
Mental performance, impairment
Nervousness
Psychoses
Speech disturbances

Levitra Tablets
Insomnia (Less than 2%)
Photophobia (Less than 2%)
Libido, changes
Nervousness

Levothroid Tablets
Anxiety
Emotional lability
Hyperactivity
Insomnia
Irritability
Nervousness

Levoxyl Tablets
Anxiety
Emotional lability
Hyperactivity
Insomnia
Irritability
Nervousness

Levsin Drops
Insomnia
Manic behavior
Memory loss, short-term
Mental performance, impairment
Nervousness
Psychoses
Speech disturbances

Levsin Elixir
Insomnia
Manic behavior
Memory loss, short-term
Mental performance, impairment
Nervousness
Psychoses
Speech disturbances

Levsin Injection
Insomnia
Manic behavior
Memory loss, short-term
Mental performance, impairment
Nervousness
Psychoses
Speech disturbances

Levsin Tablets
Insomnia
Manic behavior
Memory loss, short-term
Mental performance, impairment
Nervousness
Psychoses
Speech disturbances

Levsin/SL Tablets
Insomnia
Manic behavior
Memory loss, short-term
Mental performance, impairment
Nervousness
Psychoses
Speech disturbances

Levsinex Timecaps
Insomnia
Manic behavior
Memory loss, short-term
Mental performance, impairment
Nervousness
Psychoses
Speech disturbances

Lexapro Oral Suspension
Aggression (Infrequent)
Agitation (Infrequent)
Anxiety (At least 2%)
Apathy (Infrequent)
Behavioral changes
Coma
Confusion (Infrequent)
Delirium
Delusions
Depersonalization (Infrequent)
Depression (Infrequent)
Depression, aggravation of (Infrequent)
Diplopia
Disorientation (Infrequent)
▲ Dreaming abnormalities (3%)
Emotional lability (Infrequent)
Excitability (Infrequent)

Feeling, strange (Infrequent)
Hallucinations, auditory (Infrequent)
Hallucinations, visual
▲ Insomnia (5% to 14%)
Irritability (Frequent)
Jitteriness (Infrequent)
▲ Libido, decreased (3% to 7%)
Mental performance, impairment
  (Frequent)
Nervousness (Infrequent)
Nightmares
Panic attack (Infrequent)
Paranoia
Serotonin syndrome
Sexual dysfunction
Sluggishness (Infrequent)
Suicidal ideation (Infrequent)
Suicide, attempt of (Infrequent)

Lexapro Tablets
Aggression (Infrequent)
Agitation (Infrequent)
Anxiety (At least 2%)
Apathy (Infrequent)
Behavioral changes
Coma
Confusion (Infrequent)
Delirium
Delusions
Depersonalization (Infrequent)
Depression (Infrequent)
Depression, aggravation of
  (Infrequent)
Diplopia
Disorientation (Infrequent)
▲ Dreaming abnormalities (3%)
Emotional lability (Infrequent)
Excitability (Infrequent)
Feeling, strange (Infrequent)
Hallucinations, auditory
  (Infrequent)
Hallucinations, visual
▲ Insomnia (5% to 14%)
Irritability (Frequent)
Jitteriness (Infrequent)
▲ Libido, decreased (3% to 7%)
Mental performance, impairment
  (Frequent)
Nervousness (Infrequent)
Nightmares
Panic attack (Infrequent)
Paranoia
Serotonin syndrome
Sexual dysfunction
Sluggishness (Infrequent)

Suicidal ideation (Infrequent)
Suicide, attempt of (Infrequent)

Lexiva Tablets
▲ Depression (Less than 1% to 11%)
▲ Mood changes (Less than 1% to 11%)

Librium Capsules
Confusion
Libido, decreased
Libido, increased

Lidoderm Patch
CNS depression
CNS stimulation
Confusion
Diplopia
Disorientation
Euphoria
Nervousness

Lipitor Tablets
Depression (Less than 2%)
Dreaming abnormalities (Less than 2%)
Emotional lability (Less than 2%)
Insomnia (Greater than or
  equal to 2%)
Libido, decreased (Less than 2%)

Liquid PedvaxHIB
Irritability

Lithobid Tablets
Coma
Confusion
Hallucinations
Memory impairment
Sexual dysfunction
Speech, slurring
Stupor

Lithostat Tablets
▲ Anxiety (20%)
▲ Depression (20%)
▲ Nervousness (20%)

Lopressor HCT 100/25 Tablets
Catatonia
Confusion
▲ Depression (5%)
Disorientation
Emotional lability
Hallucinations
Insomnia
Memory loss, short-term
Neuropsychometrics performance,
  decrease

▲ Nightmares (10%)
Sensorium, clouded

Lopressor HCT 100/50 Tablets
Catatonia
Confusion
▲ Depression (5%)
Disorientation
Emotional lability
Hallucinations
Insomnia
Memory loss, short-term
Neuropsychometrics performance,
  decrease
▲ Nightmares (10%)
Sensorium, clouded

Lopressor HCT 50/25 Tablets
Catatonia
Confusion
▲ Depression (5%)
Disorientation
Emotional lability
Hallucinations
Insomnia
Memory loss, short-term
Neuropsychometrics performance,
  decrease
▲ Nightmares (10%)
Sensorium, clouded

Lopressor Injection
Catatonia
Confusion
▲ Depression (5%)
Disorientation
Emotional lability
Hallucinations
Insomnia
Libido, decreased
Memory loss, short-term
Neuropsychometrics performance,
  decrease
Nightmares
Sensorium, clouded
Sleep disturbances

Lopressor Tablets
Catatonia
Confusion
▲ Depression (5%)
Disorientation
Emotional lability
Hallucinations
Insomnia
Libido, decreased

Memory loss, short-term
Neuropsychometrics performance,
  decrease
Nightmares
Sensorium, clouded
Sleep disturbances

Lotensin HCT Tablets
Dreaming abnormalities
  (0.3% or more)
Insomnia (0.3% to 1%)
Libido, decreased (0.3% to 1%)
Nervousness (0.3% to 1%)

Lotensin Tablets
Anxiety (Less than 1%)
Insomnia (Less than 1%)
Libido, increased (Less than 1%)
Nervousness (Less than 1%)

Lotrel Capsules
Anxiety
Insomnia
Libido, decreased
Nervousness

Lotronex Tablets
Anxiety (Infrequent)
Confusion (Rare)
Depression (2%)
Dreaming abnormalities (Rare)
Photophobia (Rare)
Sedation (Rare)
Sexual dysfunction (Rare)
▲ Sleep disturbances (3%)
Smell disturbances (Rare)

Lovenox Injection
Confusion (2.2%)

Low-Ogestrel Tablets
Libido, changes
Nervousness

Lumigan Ophthalmic Solution
▲ Photophobia (1% to 3%)

Lunesta Tablets
Agitation (Infrequent)
Anxiety (Infrequent)
Apathy
▲ Confusion (0% to 3%)
▲ Depression (1% to 4%)
▲ Dreaming abnormalities (1% to 3%)
Emotional lability (Infrequent)
Euphoria (Rare)
▲ Hallucinations (1% to 3%)

Hostility (Infrequent)
Insomnia (Infrequent)
▲ Libido, decreased (0% to 3%)
Memory impairment (Infrequent)
▲ Nervousness (0% to 5%)
Neurosis, unspecified (Infrequent)
Photophobia (Rare)
Stupor (Rare)
Thinking abnormality

Lupron Depot 3.75 mg
▲ Anxiety (3%)
Confusion
▲ Delusions (Among most frequent)
▲ Depression (16%)
Depression, aggravation of
▲ Emotional lability (16%)
▲ Insomnia (16%)
▲ Libido, changes (16%)
▲ Libido, decreased (Less than 5%)
▲ Memory impairment (Among most frequent)
Mood changes
▲ Nervousness (4%)
▲ Personality changes (Among most frequent)
▲ Sleep disturbances (16%)
Suicidal ideation (Very rare)
Suicide, attempt of (Very rare)

Lupron Depot 7.5 mg
▲ Agitation (Less than 5%)
▲ Insomnia (Less than 5%)
▲ Libido, decreased (5.4%)
▲ Sleep disturbances (Less than 5%)

Lupron Depot-3 Month 11.25 mg
Agitation
▲ Anxiety (Less than 5%)
▲ Delusions (Less than 5%)
▲ Depression (16%)
Depression, aggravation of (Possible)
▲ Emotional lability (16%)
▲ Insomnia (16%)
▲ Libido, changes (16%)
▲ Libido, decreased (1.8% to 11%)
▲ Memory impairment (Less than 5%)
▲ Nervousness (4%)
▲ Personality changes (Less than 5%)
▲ Sleep disturbances (16%)
Suicidal ideation (Very rare)
Suicide, attempt of (Very rare)

Lupron Depot-PED 7.5 mg, 11.25 mg and 15 mg
Emotional lability (Less than 2%)
Nervousness (Less than 2%)
Personality changes (Less than 2%)

Lupron Injection Pediatric
Emotional lability (Less than 2%)
Nervousness (Less than 2%)
Personality changes (Less than 2%)
Sleep disturbances

Lyrica Capsules
Agitation (0.1% to 1%)
Anxiety (Greater than or equal to 1%)
Apathy (0.1% to 1%)
Coma (Rare)
▲ Confusion (1% to 7%)
Delirium (Rare)
Delusions (Rare)
Depersonalization (Greather than or equal to 1%)
Depression, psychotic (Rare)
▲ Diplopia (2% to 12%)
Dreaming abnormalities (0.1% to 1%)
▲ Euphoria (2% to 3%)
Hallucinations (0.1% to 1%)
Hangover (Rare)
Hostility (0.1% to 1%)
Libido, decreased (Greater than or equal to 1%)
Libido, increased (0.1% to 1%)
Nervousness (1% to greater than or equal to 2%)
Photophobia (0.1% to 1%)
Stupor (Greater than or equal to 1%)
Suicide, attempt of (0.1% to 1%)
▲ Thinking abnormality (1% to 9%)

Malarone Pediatric Tablets
Anxiety (Less than 1%)
Depression (Less than 1%)
▲ Dreaming (2% to 7%)
▲ Insomnia (2% to 3%)

Malarone Tablets
Anxiety (Less than 1%)
Depression (Less than 1%)
▲ Dreaming (2% to 7%)
▲ Insomnia (2% to 3%)

Marinol Capsules
Anxiety (Greater than 1%)
▲ Awareness, heightened (8% to 24%)
Confusion (Greater than 1%)
Depersonalization (Greater than 1%)
Depression (Less than 1%)
▲ Euphoria (3% to 10%)
Hallucinations (Greater than 1%)
Mood changes
Nervousness (Greater than 1%)
Nightmares (Less than 1%)

▲ Paranoia (3% to 10%)
  Speech difficulties (Less than 1%)
▲ Thinking abnormality (3% to 10%)

Matulane Capsules
  Coma
  Confusion
  Depression
  Diplopia
  Hallucinations
  Insomnia
  Nervousness
  Nightmares
  Photophobia
  Speech, slurring

Mavik Tablets
  Anxiety (0.3% to 1.0%)
  Insomnia (0.3% to 1.0%)
  Libido, decreased (0.3% to 1.0%)

Maxair Autohaler
  Anxiety
  Confusion
  Depression
  Insomnia
▲ Nervousness (4.5% to 6.9%)
  Smell disturbances (0.6%)

Maxalt Tablets
  Agitation (Infrequent)
  Anxiety (Infrequent)
  Confusion (Infrequent)
  Depersonalization (Rare)
  Depression (Infrequent)
  Disorientation (Infrequent)
  Dreaming abnormalities
    (Infrequent)
  Euphoria (Frequent)
  Hangover (Infrequent)
  Insomnia (Infrequent)
  Irritability (Infrequent)
  Memory impairment (Infrequent)
  Mental performance, impairment
    (Frequent)
  Nervousness (Infrequent)
  Photophobia (Rare)
  Serotonin syndrome
  Smell disturbances (Rare)

Maxalt-MLT Orally
Disintegrating Tablets
  Agitation (Infrequent)
  Anxiety (Infrequent)
  Confusion (Infrequent)
  Depersonalization (Rare)
  Depression (Infrequent)
  Disorientation (Infrequent)
  Dreaming abnormalities
    (Infrequent)
  Euphoria (Frequent)
  Hangover (Infrequent)
  Insomnia (Infrequent)
  Irritability (Infrequent)
  Memory impairment (Infrequent)
  Mental performance, impairment
    (Infrequent)
  Nervousness (Infrequent)
  Photophobia (Rare)
  Serotonin syndrome
  Smell disturbances (Rare)

Maxidone Tablets C-III
  Mental clouding
  Mental performance, impairment
  Mood changes
▲ Sedation (Among most frequent)

Maxipime for Injection
  Coma
  Confusion
  Hallucinations
  Stupor

Megace ES Oral Suspension
▲ Confusion (1% to 3%)
▲ Depression (1% to 3%)
▲ Insomnia (0% to 6%)
▲ Libido, decreased (0% to 5%)
▲ Thinking abnormality (1% to 3%)

Menostar Transdermal System
  Dementia
  Depression
  Irritability
  Libido, changes
  Nervousness

Mepron Suspension
▲ Anxiety (7%)
▲ Insomnia (10% to 19%)

Meridia Capsules
  Agitation (Greater than or
    equal to 1%)
▲ Anxiety (4.5%)
  CNS stimulation (1.5%)
  Confusion
▲ Depression (4.3%)
  Depression, aggravation of
  Dreaming abnormalities
  Emotional lability (1.3%)

▲ Insomnia (10.7%)
Libido, decreased
Libido, increased
Memory loss, short-term
Mental performance, impairment
Mood changes
▲ Nervousness (5.2%)
Nightmares
Serotonin syndrome
Speech disturbances
Suicidal ideation
Thinking abnormality (Greater than or
equal to 1%)

Merrem I.V.
Agitation (Greater than 0.1% to 1%)
Anxiety (Greater than 0.1% to 1%)
Confusion (Greater than 0.1% to 1%)
Delirium (Greater than 0.1% to 1%)
Depression (Greater than 0.1%
to 1%)
Hallucinations (Greater than
0.1% to 1%)
Insomnia (Greater than 0.1% to 1%)
Nervousness (Greater than 0.1% to 1%)

Meruvax II
Irritability

Metadate CD Capsules
Depression
▲ Insomnia (5%)
▲ Nervousness (Among most common)
Psychoses, toxic

MetroGel-Vaginal Gel
Depression (Less than 1%)

Mevacor Tablets
Anxiety (0.5% to 1.0%)
Depression (0.5% to 1.0%)
Insomnia (0.5% to 1.0%)
Libido, loss of (0.5% to 1.0%)
Memory loss, short-term (0.5%
to 1.0%)

Miacalcin Nasal Spray
Agitation (Less than 1%)
Anxiety (Less than 1%)
▲ Depression (1% to 3%)
Insomnia (Less than 1%)

Micardis HCT Tablets
Anxiety
Depression
Insomnia

Nervousness
Sexual dysfunction

Micardis Tablets
Anxiety (More than 0.3%)
Depression (More than 0.3%)
Insomnia (More than 0.3%)

Microgestin 1.5/30 Tablets
Libido, changes
Nervousness

Microgestin 1/20 Tablets
Libido, changes
Nervousness

Microgestin Fe 1.5/30 Tablets
Libido, changes
Nervousness

Microgestin Fe 1/20 Tablets
Libido, changes
Nervousness

Midamor Tablets
Confusion (Less than or equal to 1%)
Depression (Less than or equal to 1%)
Insomnia (Less than or equal to 1%)
Libido, decreased (Less than or equal
to 1%)
Nervousness (Less than or equal to 1%)

Migranal Nasal Spray
Anxiety (Rare)
Confusion (Infrequent)
Depression (Rare)
Euphoria (Infrequent)
Insomnia (Infrequent)
Mental performance, impairment
(Infrequent)
Nervousness (Infrequent)
Photophobia (Infrequent)
Smell disturbances (Infrequent)
Speech disturbances (Rare)
Stupor (Rare)

Mintezol Chewable Tablets
Confusion
Depression
Floating feeling
Psychiatric disturbances

Mintezol Suspension
Confusion
Depression
Floating feeling
Psychiatric disturbances

Mirapex Tablets

Aggression
Agitation (Less than 1%)
Anxiety (1% or more)
Apathy (1% or more)
Cognitive dysfunction
Coma
▲ Confusion (4% to 10%)
Delirium
Delusions (1%)
Dementia
Depression (1% or more)
Diplopia (1% or more)
Disorientation
▲ Dreaming abnormalities (11%)
▲ Hallucinations (9% to 17%)
Hallucinations, auditory
Hallucinations, visual
▲ Insomnia (13% to 27%)
Libido, decreased (1%)
Libido, increased
Memory impairment
Mood changes
Nervousness (1% or more)
Nightmares
Obsessive compulsive symptoms
Photophobia
Psychoses (Less than 1%)
Sedation
Sensory disturbances
Sexual dysfunction
Sleep disturbances (Less than or equal to 1%)
Sleep talking
Sleep walking
Stupor
Suicide, attempt of (Less than 1%)
▲ Thinking abnormality (2% to 3%)

Mircette Tablets

Depression
Libido, changes
Nervousness

Mirena Intrauterine System

▲ Depression (5% or more)
▲ Libido, decreased (5% or more)
▲ Nervousness (5% or more)

M-M-R II

Irritability

Moban Tablets

Depression (Less frequent)
Euphoria (Less frequent)
Hyperactivity (Less frequent)
Libido, increased
Mental status, altered

Mobic Oral Suspension

Anxiety (Less than 2%)
Confusion (Less than 2%)
Depression (Less than 2%)
Dreaming abnormalities (Less than 2%)
▲ Insomnia (0% to 3.6%)
Nervousness (Less than 2%)

Mobic Tablets

Anxiety (Less than 2%)
Confusion (Less than 2%)
Depression (Less than 2%)
Dreaming abnormalities (Less than 2%)
▲ Insomnia (0% to 3.6%)
Nervousness (Less than 2%)

Moduretic Tablets

Confusion (Less than or equal to 1%)
Depression (Less than or equal to 1%)
Insomnia (Less than or equal to 1%)
Libido, decreased
Nervousness (Less than or equal to 1%)
Stupor (Less than or equal to 1%)

MoviPrep Oral Solution

▲ Sleep disturbances (39.1%)

MS Contin Tablets

Agitation (Less frequent)
Depression (Less frequent)
Diplopia (Less frequent)
Disorientation (Less frequent)
Dreaming (Less frequent)
▲ Euphoria (Among most frequent)
Feeling, strange (Less frequent)
Floating feeling (Less frequent)
Hallucinations (Less frequent)
Insomnia (Less frequent)
Libido, decreased (Less frequent)
Mental performance, impairment
Mood changes (Less frequent)
Nervousness (Less frequent)
▲ Sedation (Among most frequent)

Mumpsvax

Irritability

Mycamine for Injection

Delirium (0.8%)

Myfortic Tablets

▲ Anxiety (3% to less than 20%)
▲ Depression (3% to less than 20%)
▲ Insomnia (23.5%)

Mylotarg for Injection
▲ Anxiety (7% to 10%)
▲ Depression (8% to 10%)
▲ Insomnia (11% to 13%)

Myobloc Injection
Anxiety (Greater than 2%)
Confusion (Greater than 2%)

Myozyme for Intravenous Infusion
Agitation
Irritability

Nadolol Tablets
Behavioral changes (6 of 1000 patients)
Catatonia
Depression
Disorientation, place
Disorientation, time
Emotional lability
Hallucinations
Libido, decreased (1 to 5 of 1000 patients)
Memory loss, short-term
Neuropsychometrics performance, decrease
Sedation (6 of 1000 patients)
Sensorium, clouded
Sleep disturbances
Speech, slurring (1 to 5 of 1000 patients)

Nalfon Capsules
Confusion (1.4%)
Depression (Less than 1%)
Diplopia (Less than 1%)
Disorientation (Less than 1%)
Insomnia (Less than 1%)
▲ Nervousness (5.7%)
Personality changes (Less than 1%)

Namenda Oral Solution
Agitation (Greater than or equal to 2%)
Anxiety (Greater than or equal to 2%)
Apathy (Infrequent)
Coma
▲ Confusion (6%)
Delirium (Infrequent)
Delusions (Infrequent)
Depersonalization (Infrequent)
Depression (Greater than or equal to 2%)
Diplopia (Infrequent)
Emotional lability (Infrequent)
Hallucinations
Hallucinations, auditory
Hallucinations, visual
Insomnia (Greater than or equal to 2%)
Libido, increased (Infrequent)
Nervousness (Infrequent)
Neurosis, unspecified (Infrequent)
Personality changes (Infrequent)
Psychoses (Infrequent)
Sleep disturbances (Infrequent)
Stupor (Infrequent)
Suicidal ideation
Suicide, attempt of (Infrequent)
Thinking abnormality (Infrequent)

Namenda Tablets
Agitation (Greater than or equal to 2%)
Anxiety (Greater than or equal to 2%)
Apathy (Infrequent)
Coma
▲ Confusion (6%)
Delirium (Infrequent)
Delusions (Infrequent)
Depersonalization (Infrequent)
Depression (Greater than or equal to 2%)
Diplopia (Infrequent)
Emotional lability (Infrequent)
Hallucinations
Hallucinations, auditory
Hallucinations, visual
Insomnia (Greater than or equal to 2%)
Libido, increased (Infrequent)
Nervousness (Infrequent)
Neurosis, unspecified (Infrequent)
Personality changes (Infrequent)
Psychoses (Infrequent)
Sleep disturbances (Infrequent)
Stupor (Infrequent)
Suicidal ideation
Suicide, attempt of (Infrequent)
Thinking abnormality (Infrequent)

Naprosyn Suspension
Anxiety (Less than 1%)
CNS depression (Less than 1%)
Cognitive dysfunction (Rare)
Coma (Less than 1%)
Confusion (Less than 1%)
Dreaming abnormalities (Less than 1%)

Hallucinations (Less than 1%)
Insomnia (Less than 1%)
Mental performance, impairment
  (Less than 1%)
Nervousness (Less than 1%)

Naprosyn Tablets
Anxiety (Less than 1%)
CNS depression (Less than 1%)
Cognitive dysfunction (Rare)
Coma (Less than 1%)
Confusion (Less than 1%)
Dreaming abnormalities (Less than 1%)
Hallucinations (Less than 1%)
Insomnia (Less than 1%)
Mental performance, impairment
  (Less than 1%)
Nervousness (Less than 1%)

Nasonex Nasal Spray
Smell disturbances (Very rare)

Natrecor for Injection
▲ Anxiety (2% to 3%)
Confusion (Greater than or
  equal to 1%)
▲ Insomnia (2% to 6%)

Necon 0.5/35 Tablets
Libido, changes
Nervousness

Necon 1/35 Tablets
Libido, changes
Nervousness

Necon 1/50 Tablets
Libido, changes
Nervousness

Necon 10/11 Tablets
Libido, changes
Nervousness

Nembutal Sodium Solution, USP
Agitation (Less than 1%)
Anxiety (Less than 1%)
CNS depression (Less than 1%)
Confusion (Less than 1%)
Hallucinations (Less than 1%)
Insomnia (Less than 1%)
Nervousness (Less than 1%)
Nightmares (Less than 1%)
Psychiatric disturbances (Less than 1%)
Thinking abnormality (Less than 1%)

Neoral Oral Solution
Anxiety (1% to less than 3%)
Confusion (1% to less than 3%)
Consciousness, disorders of
Depression (1%)
Emotional lability (1% to less
  than 3%)
Insomnia (1% to 3%)
Libido, decreased (1% to less
  than 3%)
Libido, increased (1% to less
  than 3%)
Mental performance, impairment (1%
  to less than 3%)
Nervousness (1% to less than 3%)
Psychiatric disturbances

Neoral Soft Gelatin Capsules
Anxiety (1% to less than 3%)
Confusion (1% to less than 3%)
Consciousness, disorders of
Depression (1%)
Emotional lability (1% to less
  than 3%)
▲ Insomnia (1% to 3%)
Libido, decreased (1% to less
  than 3%)
Libido, increased (1% to less
  than 3%)
Mental performance, impairment
  (1% to less than 3%)
Nervousness (1% to less than 3%)
Psychiatric disturbances

Neulasta Injection
▲ Insomnia (15% to 72%)

Neumega for Injection
Confusion
▲ Insomnia (33%)
Mental status, altered
Nervousness (Greater than or
  equal to 10%)

Neurontin Capsules
Aggression
Agitation (Infrequent)
Anxiety (Frequent)
Apathy (Infrequent)
Behavioral changes
CNS depression
Confusion
Depersonalization (Infrequent)
Depression (1.8%)
▲ Diplopia (1.2% to 5.9%)
Dreaming abnormalities (Infrequent)

▲ Emotional lability (4.2% to 6%)
Euphoria (Infrequent)
Feeling, drugged (Infrequent)
Feeling, high (Rare)
Feeling, strange (Rare)
Hallucinations (Infrequent)
Hangover (Rare)
▲ Hostility (5.2% to 7.6%)
Hyperactivity
Hysteria (Rare)
Insomnia
Libido, changes (Infrequent)
Libido, decreased (Infrequent)
Libido, increased (Rare)
Manic behavior (Rare)
Nervousness (2.4%)
Neurosis, unspecified (Rare)
Paranoia (Infrequent)
Personality changes (Rare)
Photophobia (Infrequent)
Psychoses (Infrequent)
Sexual dysfunction (Infrequent)
Sleep walking
Sociopathy (Rare)
Speech disturbances (Infrequent)
Stupor (Infrequent)
Suicidal ideation (Infrequent)
Suicide, attempt of (Infrequent)
Thinking abnormality (1.7% to 2.7%)

Neurontin Oral Solution

Aggression
Agitation (Infrequent)
Anxiety (Frequent)
Apathy (Infrequent)
Behavioral changes
CNS depression
Confusion
Depersonalization (Infrequent)
Depression (1.8%)
▲ Diplopia (1.2 to 5.9%)
Dreaming abnormalities (Infrequent)
▲ Emotional lability (4.2% to 6%)
Euphoria (Infrequent)
Feeling, drugged (Infrequent)
Feeling, high (Rare)
Feeling, strange (Rare)
Hallucinations (Infrequent)
Hangover (Rare)
▲ Hostility (5.2% to 7.6%)
Hyperactivity
Hysteria (Rare)
Insomnia
Libido, changes (Infrequent)
Libido, decreased (Infrequent)

Libido, increased (Rare)
Manic behavior (Rare)
Nervousness (2.4%)
Neurosis, unspecified (Rare)
Paranoia (Infrequent)
Personality changes (2.8%)
Photophobia (Infrequent)
Psychoses (Infrequent)
Sexual dysfunction (Infrequent)
Sleep walking
Sociopathy (Rare)
Speech disturbances (Infrequent)
Stupor (Infrequent)
Suicidal ideation (Infrequent)
Suicide, attempt of (Infrequent)
Thinking abnormality (1.7% to 2.7%)

Neurontin Tablets

Aggression
Agitation (Infrequent)
Anxiety (Frequent)
Apathy (Infrequent)
Behavioral changes
CNS depression
Confusion
Depersonalization (Infrequent)
Depression (1.8%)
▲ Diplopia (1.2% to 5.9%)
Dreaming abnormalities (Infrequent)
▲ Emotional lability (4.2% to 6%)
Euphoria (Infrequent)
Feeling, drugged (Infrequent)
Feeling, high (Rare)
Feeling, strange (Rare)
Hallucinations (Infrequent)
Hangover (Rare)
▲ Hostility (5.2% to 7.6%)
Hyperactivity
Hysteria (Rare)
Insomnia
Libido, changes (Infrequent)
Libido, decreased (Infrequent)
Libido, increased (Rare)
Manic behavior (Rare)
Nervousness (2.4%)
Neurosis, unspecified (Rare)
Paranoia (Infrequent)
Personality changes (Rare)
Photophobia (Infrequent)
Psychoses (Infrequent)
Sexual dysfunction (Infrequent)
Sleep walking
Sociopathy (Rare)
Speech disturbances (Infrequent)

Stupor (Infrequent)
Suicidal ideation (Infrequent)
Suicide, attempt of (Infrequent)
Thinking abnormality (1.7% to 2.7%)

Nexavar Tablets
▲ Depression (Common)
▲ Sexual dysfunction (Common)

Nexium Delayed-Release Capsules
Aggression
Agitation
Apathy (Less than 1%)
Confusion (Less than 1%)
Depression
Depression, aggravation of (Less than 1%)
Hallucinations
Insomnia (Less than 1%)
Nervousness (Less than 1%)
Sleep disturbances (Less than 1%)

Nexium Delayed-Release Oral Suspension
Aggression
Agitation
Apathy (Less than 1%)
Confusion (Less than 1%)
Depression
Depression, aggravation of (Less than 1%)
Hallucinations
Insomnia (Less than 1%)
Nervousness (Less than 1%)
Sleep disturbances (Less than 1%)

Nexium I.V.
Aggression
Agitation
Apathy (Less than 1%)
Confusion (Less than 1%)
Depression (Rare)
Depression, aggravation of (Less than 1%)
Hallucinations
Insomnia (Less than 1%)
Nervousness (Less than 1%)
Sleep disturbances (Less than 1%)

Niaspan Extended-Release Tablets
Insomnia
Nervousness

Nimotop Capsules
Depression (Up to 1.4%)

Nipent for Injection
▲ Anxiety (3% to 10%)
▲ CNS reactions (1% to 11%)
▲ Depression (3% to 10%)
Dreaming abnormalities (Less than 3%)
Emotional lability (Less than 3%)
Hallucinations (Less than 3%)
Hangover (Less than 3%)
Hostility (Less than 3%)
▲ Insomnia (3% to 10%)
Libido, changes (Less than 3%)
▲ Nervousness (3% to 10%)
Neurosis, unspecified (Less than 3%)
Photophobia (Less than 3%)
Thinking abnormality (Less than 3%)

Niravam Orally Disintegrating Tablets
Aggression (Rare)
Agitation (2.9%)
▲ Anxiety (16.6% to 19.2%)
CNS stimulation, paradoxical (Rare)
▲ Cognitive dysfunction (10.3% to 28.8%)
▲ Confusion (5% to 10.4%)
Depersonalization
▲ Depression (5.1% to 13.9%)
Diplopia
Dreaming abnormalities (1.8%)
Fear (1.4%)
Hallucinations
▲ Insomnia (8.9% to 29.5%)
▲ Irritability (10.5% to 33.1%)
▲ Libido, changes (7.1%)
▲ Libido, decreased (14.4%)
▲ Libido, increased (7.7%)
▲ Memory impairment (5.5% to 33.1%)
▲ Nervousness (4.1%)
Rage (Rare)
Sedation
▲ Sexual dysfunction (7.4%)
Speech, slurring
▲ Talkativeness (2.2%)

Norco Tablets C-III
Mental clouding
Mental performance, impairment
Mood changes
▲ Sedation (Among most frequent)

Norflex Injection
Agitation
Confusion (Infrequent)
Hallucinations

Norinyl 1 + 35 Tablets
Libido, changes
Nervousness

Norinyl 1 + 50 Tablets
Libido, changes
Nervousness

Noroxin Tablets
Anxiety (Less frequent)
CNS reactions
CNS stimulation
Confusion
Depression (Less frequent)
Diplopia
Hallucinations
Insomnia (Less frequent)
Psychiatric disturbances
Psychoses
Sleep disturbances (Less frequent)

Norvasc Tablets
Agitation (Less than 0.1%)
Anxiety (More than 0.1% to 1%)
Apathy (Less than 0.1%)
Depersonalization (More than 0.1% to 1%)
Depression (More than 0.1% to 1%)
Diplopia (More than 0.1% to 1%)
Dreaming abnormalities (More than 0.1% to 1%)
Insomnia (More than 0.1% to 1%)
Nervousness (More than 0.1% to 1%)
Sexual dysfunction (Less than 1% to 2%)

Norvir Oral Solution
Agitation (Less than 2%)
Anxiety (0% to 1.7%)
Confusion (0.6% to 0.9%)
Depression (1.7%)
Diplopia (Less than 2%)
Dreaming abnormalities (Less than 2%)
Emotional lability (Less than 2%)
Euphoria (Less than 2%)
Hallucinations (Less than 2%)
Insomnia (2% to 2.6%)
Libido, decreased (Less than 2%)
Nervousness (Less than 2%)
Personality changes (Less than 2%)
Photophobia (Less than 2%)
Thinking abnormality (0% to 0.9%)

Norvir Soft Gelatin Capsules
Agitation (Less than 2%)
Anxiety (0 to 1.7%)
Confusion (0.6% to 0.9%)
Depression (1.7%)
Diplopia (Less than 2%)
Dreaming abnormalities (Less than 2%)
Emotional lability (Less than 2%)
Euphoria (Less than 2%)
Hallucinations (Less than 2%)
Insomnia (2% to 2.6%)
Libido, decreased (Less than 2%)
Nervousness (Less than 2%)
Personality changes (Less than 2%)
Photophobia (Less than 2%)
Thinking abnormality (0% to 0.9%)

Noxafil Oral Suspension
▲ Anxiety (9%)
▲ Insomnia (1% to 17%)

NuLev Orally Disintegrating Tablets
Insomnia
Nervousness
Speech disturbances

Numorphan Injection
CNS stimulation, paradoxical
Confusion
Depression
Diplopia
Euphoria
Hallucinations
Mental clouding
Nervousness
Sleep disturbances

NuvaRing
Depression
Nervousness

Omacor Capsules
Depression
Emotional lability
Insomnia
Insomnia (0.2%)

Omnicef for Oral Suspension
Insomnia (0.2%)

Ontak Vials
▲ Confusion (8%)
▲ Insomnia (9%)
▲ Nervousness (11%)

Opana ER Tablets

Agitation (Less than 1%)
▲ Anxiety (1% to less than 10%)
CNS depression (Less than 1%)
Depression (Less than 1%)
Disorientation (Less than 1%)
Euphoria (Less than 1%)
Hallucinations (Less than 1%)
▲ Insomnia (4%)
Jitteriness (Less than 1%)
Mental performance, impairment
(Less than 1%)
Mental status, altered (Less than 1%)
Nervousness (Less than 1%)
▲ Sedation (5.9% to greater than or
equal to 10%)

Opana Tablets

Agitation (Less than 1%)
▲ Anxiety (1% to less than 10%)
CNS depression (Less than 1%)
Confusion (2.7%)
Depression (Less than 1%)
Disorientation (Less than 1%)
Euphoria (Less than 1%)
Hallucinations (Less than 1%)
Insomnia (Less than 1%)
Jitteriness (Less than 1%)
Mental performance, impairment
(Less than 1%)
Mental status, altered (Less than 1%)
Nervousness (Less than 1%)
▲ Sedation (1% to less than 10%)

Oracea Capsules

Anxiety (1.5%)

Oramorph SR Tablets

Agitation (Less frequent)
Depression (Less frequent)
Diplopia (Less frequent)
Disorientation (Less frequent)
Dreaming (Less frequent)
Euphoria (Most frequent)
Floating feeling (Less frequent)
Insomnia (Less frequent)
Libido, decreased (Less frequent)
Mood changes (Less frequent)
Nervousness (Less frequent)
Sedation (Most frequent)

Ortho Evra Transdermal System

Depression
Emotional lability (1% to 2.4%)
Libido, changes

Mood changes
Nervousness
Sleep disturbances
Speech disturbances

Ortho Tri-Cyclen Lo Tablets

Depression
Diplopia
Insomnia
Libido, changes
Mood changes
Nervousness
Speech disturbances

Ortho Tri-Cyclen Tablets

Depression
Diplopia (Rare)
Insomnia
Libido, changes
Mood changes
Nervousness
Speech disturbances

Orthoclone OKT3 Sterile Solution

Agitation
CNS reactions
Cognitive dysfunction
Coma
Combativeness
Confusion
Delirium (Less than 1%)
Diplopia
Disorientation
Hallucinations, auditory
Hallucinations, visual
Manic behavior (Less than 1%)
Mental status, altered (Less than 1%)
Mood changes
Paranoia (Less than 1%)
▲ Photophobia (10%)
Psychoses
Stupor

Ortho-Cyclen Tablets

Depression
Diplopia (Rare)
Insomnia
Libido, changes
Mood changes
Nervousness
Speech disturbances

Ovcon 50 Tablets

Libido, changes
Nervousness

Ovidrel Prefilled Syringe for Injection

Insomnia (Less than 2%)

Oxandrin Tablets

Depression
Excitability
Insomnia
Libido, changes

Oxsoralen-Ultra Capsules

Depression
Insomnia
Nervousness

OxyContin Tablets

Agitation (Less than 1%)
▲ Anxiety (Between 1% and 5%)
▲ Confusion (Between 1% and 5%)
Depersonalization (Less than 1%)
Depression (Less than 1%)
▲ Dreaming abnormalities (Between 1% and 5%)
Emotional lability (Less than 1%)
▲ Euphoria (Between 1% and 5%)
Hallucinations (Less than 1%)
▲ Insomnia (Between 1% and 5%)
Libido, decreased
▲ Nervousness (Between 1% and 5%)
Speech disturbances (Less than 1%)
Stupor (Less than 1%)
▲ Thinking abnormality (Between 1% and 5%)

OxyFast Oral Concentrate Solution

Euphoria
▲ Sedation (Among most frequent)

OxyIR Capsules

Euphoria
▲ Sedation (Among most frequent)

Parcopa Orally Disintegrating Tablets

Agitation
Anxiety
Confusion
Delusions
Dementia
Depression
Diplopia
Disorientation
Dreaming abnormalities
Euphoria
Hallucinations

Insomnia
Libido, increased
Memory impairment
Nervousness
Nightmares
Stimulation
Suicidal ideation

Parnate Tablets

Aggression
Agitation
Anxiety
Confusion
Disorientation
Insomnia
Manic behavior
Memory loss, short-term
Overstimulation
Panic attack
▲ Suicidal ideation (4%)
▲ Suicide, attempt of (4%)

Paxil CR Controlled-Release Tablets

Aggression
▲ Agitation (1.1% to 5%)
Alcohol abuse (Infrequent)
▲ Anxiety (1% to 5.9%)
Behavioral changes
Bulimia (Rare)
CNS stimulation (Frequent)
Confusion (1%)
Delirium (Rare)
Delusions (Rare)
Depersonalization (Infrequent)
Depression (Frequent)
Depression, psychotic (Rare)
Diplopia (Rare)
▲ Dreaming abnormalities (3% to 4%)
Emotional disturbances (Infrequent)
Emotional lability (Frequent)
Euphoria (Rare)
Feeling, drugged (2%)
Hallucinations (Infrequent)
Hostility (Infrequent)
Hysteria (Rare)
▲ Insomnia (1.3% to 24%)
Irritability
▲ Libido, decreased (3% to 9%)
Libido, increased (Rare)
Manic behavior (Infrequent)
Mental performance, impairment (Frequent)
Mood changes
▲ Nervousness (4% to 9%)

Neurosis, unspecified (Infrequent)
Panic attack
Paranoia (Infrequent)
Photophobia (Rare)
Psychoses (Rare)
Sensory disturbances
Serotonin syndrome
▲ Sexual dysfunction (3.7% to 10.0%)
Sociopathy (Rare)
Stupor (Rare)
Suicidal ideation
Suicide, attempt of
Thinking abnormality (Infrequent)

Paxil Oral Suspension
Aggression
▲ Agitation (1.1% to 5%)
Alcohol abuse (Infrequent)
▲ Anxiety (1% to 5.9%)
Behavioral changes
Bulimia (Rare)
CNS stimulation (Frequent)
Confusion (1%)
Delirium (Rare)
Delusions (Rare)
Depersonalization (Infrequent)
Depression (Frequent)
Depression, psychotic (Rare)
Diplopia (Rare)
▲ Dreaming abnormalities (3% to 4%)
Emotional disturbances (Infrequent)
Emotional lability (Frequent)
Euphoria (Rare)
Feeling, drugged (2%)
Hallucinations (Infrequent)
Hostility (Infrequent)
Hysteria (Rare)
▲ Insomnia (1.3% to 24%)
▲ Libido, decreased (3% to 9%)
Libido, increased (Rare)
Manic behavior (Infrequent)
Mental performance, impairment
   (Frequent)
Mood changes
▲ Nervousness (4% to 9%)
Neurosis, unspecified (Infrequent)
Paranoia (Infrequent)
Photophobia (Rare)
Psychoses (Rare)
Sensory disturbances
Serotonin syndrome
▲ Sexual dysfunction (3.7% to 10.0%)
Sociopathy (Rare)
Stupor (Rare)
Suicidal ideation

Suicide, attempt of
Thinking abnormality (Infrequent)

Paxil Tablets
Aggression
▲ Agitation (1.1% to 5%)
Alcohol abuse (Infrequent)
▲ Anxiety (1% to 5.9%)
Behavioral changes
Bulimia (Rare)
CNS stimulation (Frequent)
Confusion (1%)
Delirium (Rare)
Delusions (Rare)
Depersonalization (Infrequent)
Depression (Frequent)
Depression, psychotic (Rare)
Diplopia (Rare)
▲ Dreaming abnormalities (3% to 4%)
Emotional disturbances (Infrequent)
Emotional lability (Frequent)
Euphoria (Rare)
Feeling, drugged (2%)
Hallucinations (Infrequent)
Hostility (Infrequent)
Hysteria (Rare)
▲ Insomnia (1.3% to 24%)
Irritability
▲ Libido, decreased (3% to 9%)
Libido, increased (Rare)
Manic behavior (Infrequent)
Mental performance, impairment
   (Frequent)
Mood changes
▲ Nervousness (4% to 9%)
Neurosis, unspecified (Infrequent)
Panic attack
Paranoia (Infrequent)
Photophobia (Rare)
Psychoses (Rare)
Sensory disturbances
Serotonin syndrome
▲ Sexual dysfunction (3.7% to 10.0%)
Sociopathy (Rare)
Stupor (Rare)
Suicidal ideation
Suicide, attempt of
Thinking abnormality (Infrequent)

Pediarix Vaccine
▲ Irritability (1.7% to 63.8%)
▲ Sleep disturbances (0.4% to 46.7%)

Pediatric Vicks Formula 44m Cough & Cold Relief Liquid
Excitability

Pegasys

Aggression (Less than 1%)
▲ Anxiety (19%)
Coma (Less than 1%)
▲ Depression (18%)
▲ Insomnia (19%)
▲ Irritability (0.19)
▲ Memory impairment (5%)
▲ Mood changes (3%)
▲ Nervousness (19%)
Psychosis, activation (Less than 1%)
Suicidal ideation (Less than 1%)

PegIntron Powder for Injection

Aggression (1%)
Agitation (2%)
▲ Anxiety (28%)
▲ Depression (1% to 29%)
▲ Emotional lability (0.28)
▲ Insomnia (23%)
▲ Irritability (28%)
Memory loss, short-term
▲ Nervousness (4%)
Psychoses (1%)
Suicidal ideation (1%)
Suicide, attempt of (1%)

Pentasa Capsules

Depression (Less than 1%)
Insomnia (Less than 1%)

Pepcid for Oral Suspension

Agitation (Infrequent)
Anxiety (Infrequent)
Confusion (Infrequent)
Depression (Infrequent)
Hallucinations (Infrequent)
Insomnia (Infrequent)
Libido, decreased (Infrequent)
Psychiatric disturbances (Infrequent)

Pepcid Injection

Agitation (Infrequent)
Anxiety (Infrequent)
Confusion (Infrequent)
Depression (Infrequent)
Hallucinations (Infrequent)
Insomnia (Infrequent)
Libido, decreased (Infrequent)
Psychiatric disturbances (Infrequent)

Pepcid Injection Premixed

Agitation (Infrequent)
Anxiety (Infrequent)
Confusion (Infrequent)
Depression (Infrequent)
Hallucinations (Infrequent)
Insomnia (Infrequent)
Libido, decreased (Infrequent)
Psychiatric disturbances (Infrequent)

Pepcid Tablets

Agitation (Infrequent)
Anxiety (Infrequent)
Confusion (Infrequent)
Depression (Infrequent)
Hallucinations (Infrequent)
Insomnia (Infrequent)
Libido, decreased (Infrequent)
Psychiatric disturbances (Infrequent)

Percocet Tablets

Euphoria
Mental performance, impairment
▲ Sedation (Among most frequent)

Percodan Tablets

Agitation
Anxiety
Coma
Confusion
Depression
Euphoria
Hallucinations
Mental performance, impairment
Nervousness
▲ Sedation (Among most frequent)
Stupor

Permax Tablets

Agitation (Infrequent)
▲ Anxiety (6.4%)
Apathy (Infrequent)
Coma (Infrequent)
▲ Confusion (11.1%)
Consciousness, disorders of
Delusions (Infrequent)
▲ Depression (3.2%)
Diplopia (2.1%)
Dreaming abnormalities (2.7%)
Emotional lability (Infrequent)
Euphoria (Infrequent)
▲ Hallucinations (13.8%)
Hostility (Infrequent)
▲ Insomnia (7.9%)
Libido, decreased (Infrequent)
Libido, increased (Infrequent)
Manic behavior (Infrequent)
Nervousness (Frequent)
Neurosis, unspecified (Infrequent)
Paranoia (Frequent)

Personality changes (2.1%)
Photophobia (Infrequent)
Psychoses (2.1%; Frequent)
Speech disturbances (1.1%)
Stupor (Rare)
Thinking abnormality (Frequent)

Pexeva Tablets
▲ Agitation (1.1% to 5%)
Alcohol abuse (Infrequent)
Antisocial reaction (Rare)
▲ Anxiety (2% to 5.9%)
Bulimia (Rare)
Confusion (1%)
Delirium (Rare)
Delusions (Rare)
▲ Depersonalization (3%)
Depression, psychotic (Rare)
Diplopia (Rare)
▲ Dreaming abnormalities (4%)
Emotional disturbances (Infrequent)
Emotional lability (Frequent)
Euphoria (Infrequent)
Feeling, drugged (2%)
Hallucinations (Infrequent)
Hostility (Infrequent)
Hysteria (Rare)
▲ Insomnia (1.3% to 24%)
▲ Libido, decreased (1% to 14%)
Libido, increased (Infrequent)
▲ Nervousness (2.9% to 9%)
Neurosis, unspecified (Infrequent)
▲ Orgasmic dysfunction, female
   (2% to 9%)
Photophobia (Rare)
Psychoses (Rare)

Phenergan Tablets and Suppositories
Agitation
Catatonia
Confusion
Delirium
Diplopia
Disorientation
Euphoria
Excitability
Hallucinations
Hysteria
Insomnia
Mental performance, impairment
Nervousness
Nightmares
Sedation

Phenytek Capsules
▲ Confusion (Among most common)
Insomnia
Nervousness
▲ Speech, slurring (Among most
   common)

PhosLo GelCaps
Coma
Confusion
Delirium
Stupor

Photofrin for Injection
▲ Anxiety (3% to 7%)
▲ Confusion (8%)
Diplopia
▲ Insomnia (4% to 14%)
Photophobia

Plavix Tablets
Anxiety (1% to 2.5%)
Confusion
▲ Depression (3.6%)
Hallucinations
Insomnia (1% to 2.5%)
Anxiety (Less than 2%)
Diplopia (Less than 2%)
Insomnia (Less than 2%)

Podocon-25 Liquid
Coma

Premarin Intravenous
Dementia
Depression
Libido, changes
Nervousness

Premarin Tablets
Dementia
▲ Depression (5% to 8%)
▲ Insomnia (6% to 7%)
Irritability
Libido, changes
Mood changes
▲ Nervousness (2% to 5%)

Premarin Vaginal Cream
Dementia
Depression
Irritability
Libido, changes
Mood changes
Nervousness

Premphase Tablets

▲ Anxiety (2% to 5%)
   Dementia
▲ Depression (6% to 11%)
   Diplopia
▲ Insomnia (6% to 7%)
   Irritability
   Libido, changes
   Mood changes
▲ Nervousness (2% to 3%)

Prempro Tablets

▲ Anxiety (2% to 5%)
   Dementia
▲ Depression (6% to 11%)
   Diplopia
▲ Insomnia (6% to 7%)
   Irritability
   Libido, changes
   Mood changes
▲ Nervousness (2% to 3%)

Prevacid Delayed-Release Capsules

   Agitation (Less than 1%)
   Anxiety (Less than 1%)
   Apathy (Less than 1%)
   Confusion (Less than 1%)
   Depersonalization (Less than 1%)
   Depression (Less than 1%)
   Diplopia (Less than 1%)
   Dreaming abnormalities
    (Less than 1%)
   Emotional lability (Less than 1%)
   Hallucinations (Less than 1%)
   Hostility (Less than 1%)
   Libido, decreased (Less than 1%)
   Libido, increased (Less than 1%)
   Nervousness (Less than 1%)
   Neurosis, unspecified (Less than 1%)
   Photophobia (Less than 1%)
   Sleep disturbances (Less than 1%)
   Speech disturbances (Less than 1%)
   Thinking abnormality (Less than 1%)

Prevacid for Delayed-Release Oral Suspension

   Agitation (Less than 1%)
   Anxiety (Less than 1%)
   Apathy (Less than 1%)
   Confusion (Less than 1%)
   Depersonalization (Less than 1%)
   Depression (Less than 1%)
   Diplopia (Less than 1%)
   Dreaming abnormalities (Less than 1%)

   Emotional lability (Less than 1%)
   Hallucinations (Less than 1%)
   Hostility (Less than 1%)
   Libido, decreased (Less than 1%)
   Libido, increased (Less than 1%)
   Nervousness (Less than 1%)
   Neurosis, unspecified (Less than 1%)
   Photophobia (Less than 1%)
   Sleep disturbances (Less than 1%)
   Speech disturbances (Less than 1%)
   Thinking abnormality (Less than 1%)

Prevacid NapraPAC 375

   Agitation (Less than 1%)
   Anxiety (Less than 1%)
   Apathy (Less than 1%)
   Cognitive dysfunction (Less than 1%)
   Confusion (Less than 1%)
   Depersonalization (Less than 1%)
   Depression (Less than 1%)
   Diplopia (Less than 1%)
   Dreaming abnormalities
    (Less than 1%)
   Emotional lability (Less than 1%)
   Hallucinations (Less than 1%)
   Hostility (Less than 1%)
   Insomnia (Less than 1%)
   Libido, decreased (Less than 1%)
   Libido, increased (Less than 1%)
   Nervousness (Less than 1%)
   Neurosis, unspecified (Less than 1%)
   Photophobia (Less than 1%)
   Sleep disturbances (Less than 1%)
   Speech disturbances
   Thinking abnormality (Less than 1%)

Prevacid NapraPAC 500

   Agitation (Less than 1%)
   Anxiety (Less than 1%)
   Apathy (Less than 1%)
   Cognitive dysfunction (Less than 1%)
   Confusion (Less than 1%)
   Depersonalization (Less than 1%)
   Depression (Less than 1%)
   Diplopia (Less than 1%)
   Dreaming abnormalities
    (Less than 1%)
   Emotional lability (Less than 1%)
   Hallucinations (Less than 1%)
   Hostility (Less than 1%)
   Insomnia (Less than 1%)
   Libido, decreased (Less than 1%)
   Libido, increased (Less than 1%)
   Nervousness (Less than 1%)
   Neurosis, unspecified (Less than 1%)

Photophobia (Less than 1%)
Sleep disturbances (Less than 1%)
Speech disturbances
Thinking abnormality (Less than 1%)

Prevacid SoluTab Delayed-Release Orally Disintegrating Tablets

Agitation (Less than 1%)
Anxiety (Less than 1%)
Apathy (Less than 1%)
Confusion (Less than 1%)
Depersonalization (Less than 1%)
Depression (Less than 1%)
Diplopia (Less than 1%)
Dreaming abnormalities
  (Less than 1%)
Emotional lability (Less than 1%)
Hallucinations (Less than 1%)
Hostility (Less than 1%)
Libido, decreased (Less than 1%)
Libido, increased (Less than 1%)
Nervousness (Less than 1%)
Neurosis, unspecified (Less than 1%)
Photophobia (Less than 1%)
Sleep disturbances (Less than 1%)
Speech disturbances (Less than 1%)
Thinking abnormality (Less than 1%)

Prevnar for Injection

▲ Irritability (44.2% to 58.7%)
▲ Sleep disturbances (15.3% to 25.2%)

PREVPAC

Agitation (Less than 1%)
Anxiety (Less than 1%)
Apathy (Less than 1%)
Behavioral changes
▲ Confusion (Less than 1% to 3%)
Depersonalization
Depression (Less than 1%)
Diplopia (Less than 1%)
Disorientation
Dreaming abnormalities
  (Less than 1%)
Emotional lability (Less than 1%)
Hallucinations (Less than 1%)
Hostility (Less than 1%)
Hyperactivity
Insomnia
Libido, decreased (Less than 1%)
Libido, increased (Less than 1%)
Nervousness (Less than 1%)
Neurosis, unspecified (Less than 1%)
Nightmares

Photophobia (Less than 1%)
Psychoses
Sleep disturbances (Less than 1%)
Smell disturbances
Speech disturbances
Thinking abnormality (Less than 1%)

Prezista Tablets

Anxiety (Less than 2%)
Confusion (Less than 2%)
Disorientation (Less than 2%)
Irritability (Less than 2%)
Memory impairment (Less than 2%)
Mood changes (Less than 2%)
Nightmares (Less than 2%)

Primaxin I.M.

Confusion
Hallucinations
Psychiatric disturbances

Primaxin I.V.

Confusion (Less than 0.2%)
Hallucinations
Psychiatric disturbances
  (Less than 0.2%)

Prinivil Tablets

Confusion (0.3% to 1.0%)
Depression (Greater than 1%)
Diplopia (0.3% to 1.0%)
Insomnia (0.3% to 1.0%)
Irritability (0.3% to 1.0%)
Libido, decreased (0.4%)
Memory impairment (0.3% to 1.0%)
Nervousness (0.3% to 1.0%)
Photophobia (0.3% to 1.0%)

Prinzide Tablets

Confusion
Depression (0.3% to 1%)
Diplopia
Insomnia
Irritability
Libido, decreased (0.3% to 1%)
Memory impairment
Nervousness
Photophobia

ProAir HFA Inhalation Aerosol

Anxiety (Less than 3%)
Nervousness (Frequent)

ProAmatine Tablets

Anxiety (Less frequent)
Confusion (Less frequent)
Insomnia (Rare)

Nervousness (Less frequent)
Thinking abnormality (Less frequent)

Prochieve 4% Gel
Aggression
▲ Depression (8% to 11%)
Emotional lability
Insomnia
▲ Libido, decreased (10%)
▲ Nervousness (16%)
Sleep disturbances

Prochieve 8% Gel
Aggression
▲ Depression (8% to 11%)
Emotional lability
Insomnia
▲ Libido, decreased (10%)
▲ Nervousness (16%)
Sleep disturbances

Procrit for Injection
▲ Anxiety (2% to 11%)
▲ Insomnia (13% to 21%)

Prograf Capsules and Injection
▲ Agitation (3% to 15%)
▲ Anxiety (3% to 15%)
Coma
▲ Confusion (3% to 15%)
Delirium
▲ Depression (3% to 15%)
▲ Dreaming abnormalities (3% to 15%)
▲ Emotional lability (3% to 15%)
▲ Hallucinations (3% to 15%)
▲ Insomnia (32% to 64%)
Jitteriness
▲ Mental status, altered (Approximately 55%)
▲ Nervousness (3%)
Photophobia
▲ Psychoses (3% to 15%)
▲ Sensory disturbances (Approximately 55%)
▲ Thinking abnormality (3% to 15%)

Proleukin for Injection
Agitation
▲ Anxiety (12%)
Coma (1%)
▲ Confusion (34%)
Depression (Less than 1%)
Insomnia
Irritability
▲ Mental status, altered (73%)
▲ Sensory disturbances (10%)

▲ Speech disturbances (7%)
Suicide, attempt of

Prometrium Capsules (100 mg, 200 mg)
▲ Anxiety (Less than 5%)
▲ Confusion (Less than 5%)
▲ Depression (5% to 19%)
▲ Emotional lability (6%)
▲ Insomnia (Less than 5%)
▲ Irritability (5% to 8%)
▲ Mental performance, impairment (Less than 5%)
Nervousness
▲ Personality changes (Less than 5%)
▲ Speech disturbances (Less than 5%)

Propecia Tablets
▲ Libido, decreased (1.8% - 6.4%)

Propofol Injectable Emulsion 1%
Hysteria (Less than 1%)
Insomnia (Less than 1%)
Thinking abnormality (Less than 1%)

ProQuad
Agitation
Apathy
Dreaming abnormalities
Insomnia (0.2% to less than 1%)
▲ Irritability (6.7%)
Nervousness
Sleep disturbances (0.2% to less than 1%)

Proquin XR Tablets
Agitation
Anxiety
Confusion
Delirium
Depression
Diplopia
Hallucinations
Insomnia
Nightmares
Paranoia
Phobia, unspecified
Psychoses, toxic
Suicidal ideation

Proscar Tablets
▲ Libido, decreased (2.6% to 6.4%)
Agitation (Infrequent)
Anxiety (Frequent)
Apathy (Infrequent)
Confusion (2%)

Depression (2%)
Diplopia (Rare)
Dreaming abnormalities (2%)
Emotional lability (Infrequent)
Euphoria (Infrequent)
Excitement, paradoxical
Hallucinations (Rare)
▲ Hangover (3%)
Hostility (Infrequent)
Libido, decreased (Rare)
Mental performance, impairment
▲ Nervousness (8%)
Photophobia (Infrequent)
Sleep disturbances (Infrequent)
Stupor (Infrequent)
Thinking abnormality (2%)

Protonix I.V.
Anxiety (Greater than or equal to 1%)
Confusion (Less than 1%)
Depression (Less than 1%)
Diplopia (Less than 1%)
Dreaming abnormalities
  (Less than 1%)
Emotional lability (Less than 1%)
Hallucinations (Less than 1%)
Insomnia (Greater than
  or equal to 1%)
Libido, decreased (Less than 1%)
Nervousness (Less than 1%)
Sleep disturbances (Less than 1%)
Speech disturbances
Thinking abnormality (Less than 1%)

Protonix Tablets
Anxiety (Greater than or equal to 1%)
Confusion (Less than 1%)
Depression (Less than 1%)
Diplopia (Less than 1%)
Dreaming abnormalities
  (Less than 1%)
Emotional lability (Less than 1%)
Hallucinations (Less than 1%)
Insomnia (Less than or equal to 1%)
Libido, decreased (Less than 1%)
Nervousness (Less than 1%)
Sleep disturbances (Less than 1%)
Speech disturbances
Thinking abnormality (Less than 1%)

**Protopam Chloride for
Injection, USP**
Manic behavior (Several cases)

Protopic Ointment
Depression (1% to 2%)
▲ Insomnia (Up to 4%)
Thinking abnormality (0.2% to less
  than 1%)

**Proventil HFA Inhalation
Aerosol**
Anxiety (Less than 3%)
CNS stimulation
Depression (Less than 3%)
Insomnia
▲ Nervousness (7%)

Proventil Inhalation Aerosol
CNS stimulation
Insomnia
▲ Nervousness (Less than 10%)

**Proventil Inhalation
Solution 0.083%**
▲ Insomnia (1% to 3.1%)
▲ Nervousness (4%)

Provigil Tablets
Agitation (1%)
▲ Anxiety (5%)
Confusion (1%)
Depression (2%)
Emotional lability (1%)
Hallucinations (At least 1%)
▲ Insomnia (0.05)
Libido, decreased (At least 1%)
Manic behavior
▲ Nervousness (7%)
Psychoses
Sleep disturbances (At least 1%)
Thinking abnormality (At least 1%)

Prozac Pulvules and Liquid
Aggression
Agitation (At least 2%)
Antisocial reaction (Rare)
▲ Anxiety (4% to 17%)
Apathy (Infrequent)
CNS depression (Infrequent)
CNS stimulation (Infrequent)
Coma (Rare)
Confusion (Frequent)
Delusions (Rare)
Depersonalization (Infrequent)
Depression
Diplopia (Rare)
▲ Dreaming abnormalities (1% to 5%)
Emotional lability (Frequent)
Euphoria (Infrequent)
Hallucinations (Infrequent)

Hostility (Infrequent)
▲ Insomnia (10% to 33%)
Irritability
▲ Libido, decreased (1% to 11%)
Libido, increased (Infrequent)
▲ Nervousness (8% to 16%)
Neurosis, unspecified (Infrequent)
Panic attack
Paranoia (Infrequent)
Personality changes (At least 2%)
Photophobia (Infrequent)
Psychoses (Infrequent)
Serotonin syndrome
Sleep disturbances (Frequent)
Stupor (Rare)
Suicidal ideation
Suicide, attempt of (Infrequent)
Thinking abnormality (2%)

Pulmicort Respules

Aggression (Less than 1%)
Anxiety (Less than 1%)
Depression (Less than 1%)
▲ Emotional lability (1% to 3%)
Irritability (Less than 1%)
Psychiatric disturbances (Less than 1%)
Psychoses (Less than 1%)

Pulmicort Turbuhaler Inhalation Powder

▲ Insomnia (1% to 3%)
Irritability (Rare)
Psychiatric disturbances (Rare)
Psychoses (Rare)

Quixin Ophthalmic Solution

▲ Photophobia (1% to 3%)

Raniclor Tablets, Chewable

Agitation (Rare)
Confusion (Rare)
Hallucinations (Rare)
Hyperactivity (Rare)
Insomnia (Rare)
Nervousness (Rare)

Rapamune Oral Solution and Tablets

▲ Anxiety (3% to 20%)
▲ Confusion (3% to 20%)
▲ Depression (3% to 20%)
▲ Emotional lability (3% to 20%)
▲ Insomnia (13% to 22%)

Razadyne ER Extended-Release Capsules

Aggression
Agitation (Greater than or equal to 2%)

Anxiety (Greater than or equal to 2%)
Apathy (Infrequent)
Confusion (Greater than or equal to 2%)
Delirium (Infrequent)
▲ Depression (7%)
Hallucinations (Greater than or equal to 2%)
▲ Insomnia (5%)
Libido, increased (Infrequent)
Paranoia (Infrequent)

Razadyne Oral Solution

Aggression
Agitation (Greater than or equal to 2%)
Anxiety (Greater than or equal to 2%)
Apathy (Infrequent)
Confusion (Greater than or equal to 2%)
Delirium (Infrequent)
▲ Depression (7%)
Hallucinations (Greater than or equal to 2%)
▲ Insomnia (5%)
Libido, increased (Infrequent)
Paranoia (Infrequent)
Suicidal ideation (Rare)

Razadyne Tablets

Aggression
Agitation (Greater than or equal to 2%)
Anxiety (Greater than or equal to 2%)
Apathy (Infrequent)
Confusion (Greater than or equal to 2%)
Delirium (Infrequent)
▲ Depression (7%)
Hallucinations (Greater than or equal to 2%)
▲ Insomnia (5%)
Libido, increased (Infrequent)
Paranoia (Infrequent)
Suicidal ideation (Rare)

Rebetol Capsules

▲ Agitation (5% to 8%)
▲ Anxiety (47%)
▲ Depression (13% to 36%)
▲ Emotional lability (7% to 47%)
▲ Insomnia (14% to 41%)
▲ Irritability (10% to 47%)

▲ Nervousness (3% to 6%)
Suicidal ideation

Rebetol Oral Solution
▲ Agitation (5% to 8%)
▲ Anxiety (47%)
▲ Depression (13% to 36%)
▲ Emotional lability (7% to 47%)
▲ Insomnia (14% to 41%)
▲ Irritability (10% to 47%)
▲ Nervousness (3% to 6%)
Suicidal ideation

Rebetron Combination Therapy
▲ Depression (23% to 36%)
▲ Emotional lability (7% to 12%)
▲ Insomnia (26% to 39%)
▲ Irritability (23% to 32%)
Mental performance, impairment
▲ Nervousness (4% to 5%)
Suicidal ideation (Less than 1%)
Suicide, attempt of (Less than 1%)

Rebif Prefilled Syringe for Injection
▲ Depression (25%)
Suicidal ideation
Suicide, attempt of

Recombivax HB
Agitation
Insomnia (Less to greater than 1%)
Irritability (Greater than 1%)
Sleep disturbances (Less than 1%)

ReFacto Vials
Insomnia

Relpax Tablets
Agitation (Infrequent)
Anxiety (Infrequent)
Apathy (Infrequent)
Catatonia (Rare)
Confusion (Infrequent)
Dementia (Rare)
Depersonalization (Infrequent)
Depression (Infrequent)
Depression, psychotic (Rare)
Diplopia (Rare)
Dreaming abnormalities (Infrequent)
Emotional lability (Infrequent)
Euphoria (Infrequent)
Hallucinations (Rare)
Hysteria (Rare)
Insomnia (Infrequent)
Manic behavior (Rare)

Nervousness (Infrequent)
Neurosis, unspecified (Rare)
Photophobia (Infrequent)
Sleep disturbances (Rare)
Speech disturbances (Infrequent)
Stupor (Infrequent)
Thinking abnormality (Infrequent)

Remicade for IV Injection
Confusion (Greater than or equal to 0.2%)
Suicide, attempt of (Greater than or equal to 0.2%)

ReoPro Vials
Agitation (0.70%)
Anxiety (1.7%)
Coma (0.4%)
Confusion (0.6%)
Diplopia (0.1%)
Insomnia (0.3%)
Thinking abnormality (2.1%)

Requip Tablets
Aggression (Infrequent)
Agitation (Infrequent)
Anxiety (1% or more)
Apathy (Infrequent)
Coma (Infrequent)
▲ Confusion (5%)
Delirium (Infrequent)
Delusions (Infrequent)
Dementia (Infrequent)
Depersonalization (Infrequent)
Depression (1% or more)
Diplopia (2%)
▲ Dreaming abnormalities (11%)
Emotional lability (Infrequent)
Euphoria (Infrequent)
▲ Hallucinations (5% to 10%)
Insomnia (1% or more)
Libido, decreased (Infrequent)
Libido, increased (Infrequent)
Manic behavior (Infrequent)
Mental performance, impairment (Infrequent)
Nervousness (1% or more)
Neurosis, unspecified (Infrequent)
Paranoia (Infrequent)
Personality changes (Infrequent)
Photophobia (Infrequent)
Stupor (Infrequent)
Suicide, attempt of (Rare)

Rescriptor Tablets
Agitation
▲ Anxiety (2.4% to 6.7%)
Cognitive dysfunction
Confusion
▲ Depressive reactions (4.9% to 12.6%)
Diplopia
Disorientation
Dreaming abnormalities
Emotional lability
Euphoria
Hallucinations
▲ Insomnia (1.2% to 5%)
Libido, decreased
Manic behavior
Nervousness
Paranoia
Photophobia
Sleep disturbances

Restoril Capsules
Agitation (Less than 0.5%)
Anxiety (2%)
Confusion (1.3%)
Depression (1.7%)
Euphoria (1.5%)
Hallucinations (Less than 0.5%)
Hangover (2.5%)
▲ Nervousness (4.6%)
Nightmares (1.2%)
Overstimulation (Less than 0.5%)

Retrovir Capsules
Anxiety
Confusion
Depression
Emotional lability
▲ Insomnia (2.4% to 5%)
Irritability (1.6%)
Nervousness (1.6%)
Photophobia

Retrovir IV Infusion
Anxiety
Confusion
Depression
Emotional lability
▲ Insomnia (3% to 5%)
Irritability (2%)
Manic behavior
Mental acuity, loss of
Nervousness (2%)
Photophobia

Retrovir Syrup
Anxiety
Confusion
Depression
Emotional lability
▲ Insomnia (2.4% to 5%)
Irritability (1.6%)
Mental acuity, loss of
Nervousness (1.6%)
Photophobia

Retrovir Tablets
Anxiety
Confusion
Depression
Emotional lability
▲ Insomnia (2.4% to 5%)
Irritability (1.6%)
Mental acuity, loss of
Nervousness (1.6%)
Photophobia

Revatio Tablets
▲ Insomnia (7%)

Revlimid Capsules
Confusion (1.7% to 2.3%)
Delirium
Delusions
▲ Depression (0.3% to 5.4%)
▲ Insomnia (10.1% to 32.1%)
Memory impairment
Mental status, altered

Reyataz Capsules
Agitation (Less than 3%)
Anxiety (Less than 3%)
Confusion (Less than 3%)
▲ Depression (3% to 8%)
Dreaming abnormalities
  (Less than 3%)
Emotional lability (Less than 3%)
Hallucinations (Less than 3%)
Hostility (Less than 3%)
▲ Insomnia (Less than 1% to 5%)
Libido, decreased (Less than 3%)
Nervousness (Less than 3%)
Psychoses (Less than 3%)
Sleep disturbances (Less than 3%)
Suicide, attempt of (Less than 3%)

Ribavirin, USP Capsules
▲ Agitation (5% to 8%)
▲ Anxiety (47%)
▲ Depression (13% to 36%)
▲ Emotional lability (7% to 47%)

▲ Insomnia (14% to 41%)
▲ Irritability (10% to 47%)
▲ Nervousness (3% to 6%)

Rilutek Tablets

Agitation (Frequent)
Apathy (Infrequent)
CNS depression (Rare)
Coma (Infrequent)
Confusion (Infrequent)
Delirium (Infrequent)
Delusions (Infrequent)
Dementia (Rare)
Depersonalization (Infrequent)
▲ Depression (4.2% to 6.1%)
Depression, psychotic (Rare)
Diplopia (Rare)
Dreaming abnormalities (Rare)
Emotional lability (Infrequent)
Euphoria (Rare)
Hallucinations (Infrequent)
Hostility (Frequent)
Insomnia (2.1% to 2.9%)
Libido, decreased (Infrequent)
Libido, increased (Infrequent)
Manic behavior (Infrequent)
Paranoia (Infrequent)
Personality changes (Infrequent)
Photophobia (Rare)
Psychoses (Rare)
Stupor (Infrequent)
Suicide, attempt of (Infrequent)
Thinking abnormality (Infrequent)

Risperdal Consta Long-Acting Injection

Agitation (Frequent)
Anxiety (Frequent)
Apathy (Frequent)
Confusion (Infrequent)
Delirium (Infrequent)
Delusions (Frequent)
Dementia (Infrequent)
Depersonalization (Infrequent)
Depression (Frequent)
Depression, psychotic (Infrequent)
Dreaming abnormalities (Up to 2%)
Emotional lability (Infrequent)
Euphoria (Infrequent)
▲ Hallucinations (6% to 7%)
▲ Insomnia (13% to 16%)
Libido, decreased (Infrequent)
Manic behavior (Infrequent)
Nervousness (Frequent)
Psychosis, activation (Frequent)

▲ Suicide, attempt of (1% to 4%)
▲ Thinking abnormality (Up to 3%)

Risperdal M-Tab Orally Disintegrating Tablets

▲ Aggression (1% to 3%)
▲ Agitation (8% to 26%)
▲ Anxiety (4% to 20%)
Apathy (Infrequent)
Catatonia (Infrequent)
Cognitive dysfunction
Coma (Rare)
Confusion (Infrequent)
Delirium (Rare)
Depression (Infrequent)
Diplopia (Rare)
Dreaming abnormalities (Frequent)
Emotional lability (Rare)
Euphoria (Infrequent)
▲ Insomnia (23% to 26%)
Libido, increased (Infrequent)
▲ Manic behavior (8%)
Mental performance, impairment (Infrequent)
Mental status, altered
Nervousness (Frequent)
Nightmares (Rare)
Photophobia (Rare)
Sexual activity, decrease (Frequent)
Sexual dysfunction (Frequent)
Sleep disturbances (Frequent)
Stupor (Infrequent)
Suicide, attempt of (1.2%)

Risperdal Oral Solution

▲ Aggression (1% to 3%)
▲ Agitation (8% to 26%)
▲ Anxiety (4% to 20%)
Apathy (Infrequent)
Catatonia (Infrequent)
Cognitive dysfunction
Coma (Rare)
Confusion (Infrequent)
Delirium (Rare)
Depression (Infrequent)
Diplopia (Rare)
Dreaming abnormalities (Frequent)
Emotional lability (Rare)
Euphoria (Infrequent)
▲ Insomnia (23% to 26%)
Libido, increased (Infrequent)
▲ Manic behavior (8%)
Mental performance, impairment (Infrequent)
Mental status, altered

Nervousness (Frequent)
Nightmares (Rare)
Photophobia (Rare)
Sexual activity, decrease (Frequent)
Sexual dysfunction (Frequent)
Sleep disturbances (Frequent)
Stupor (Infrequent)
Suicide, attempt of (1.2%)

Risperdal Tablets
▲ Aggression (1% to 3%)
▲ Agitation (8% to 26%)
▲ Anxiety (4% to 20%)
  Apathy (Infrequent)
  Catatonia (Infrequent)
  Cognitive dysfunction
  Coma (Rare)
  Confusion (Infrequent)
  Delirium (Rare)
  Depression (Infrequent)
  Diplopia (Rare)
  Dreaming abnormalities (Frequent)
  Emotional lability (Rare)
  Euphoria (Infrequent)
▲ Insomnia (23% to 26%)
  Libido, increased (Infrequent)
▲ Manic behavior (8%)
  Mental performance, impairment
    (Infrequent)
  Mental status, altered
  Nervousness (Frequent)
  Nightmares (Rare)
  Photophobia (Rare)
  Sexual activity, decrease (Frequent)
  Sexual dysfunction (Frequent)
  Sleep disturbances (Frequent)
  Stupor (Infrequent)
  Suicide, attempt of (1.2%)

Ritalin Hydrochloride Tablets
  Aggression
  Depression
  Hallucinations
▲ Insomnia (One of the two most
    common)
▲ Nervousness (One of the two most
    common)
  Psychoses
  Psychoses, toxic

Ritalin LA Capsules
  Aggression
  Depression
  Hallucinations
  Hostility
▲ Insomnia (3.1%)
▲ Nervousness (Among most common)

  Psychoses
  Psychoses, toxic

Ritalin-SR Tablets
  Aggression
  Depression
  Hallucinations
▲ Insomnia (One of the two most
    common)
▲ Nervousness (One of the two most
    common)
  Psychoses
  Psychoses, toxic

Rituxan I.V.
▲ Anxiety (1% to 5%)

Rocaltrol Capsules
  Apathy
  Libido, decreased
  Photophobia
  Psychoses (Rare)
  Sensory disturbances

Rocaltrol Oral Solution
  Apathy
  Libido, decreased
  Photophobia
  Psychoses (Rare)
  Sensory disturbances

Romazicon Injection
▲ Agitation (3% to 9%)
▲ Anxiety (3% to 9%)
  Confusion (Less than 1%)
  Delirium (Less than 1%)
▲ Depersonalization (1% to 3%)
▲ Depression (1% to 3%)
▲ Diplopia (1% to 3%)
  Emotional lability (1% to 3%)
▲ Euphoria (1% to 3%)
  Fear
▲ Insomnia (3% to 9%)
▲ Nervousness (3% to 9%)
  Panic attack
▲ Paranoia (1% to 3%)
  Speech disturbances (Less than 1%)
  Stupor (Less than 1%)

RotaTeq
▲ Irritability (2.9% to 8.1%)

Rozerem Tablets
  Depression (2%)
▲ Insomnia (3%)

Rythmol SR Capsules
▲ Anxiety (10% to 13%)
  Dementia

▲ Depression (1% to 3%)
Emotional disturbances
Insomnia
Libido, decreased
Neurosis, unspecified
Nightmares
Sleep disturbances
Speech disturbances

Sanctura Tablets
Delirium
Hallucinations

Sandimmune I.V. Ampuls for Infusion
Anxiety (Rare)
Confusion (2% or less)
Consciousness, disorders of
Depression (Rare)
Psychiatric disturbances

Sandimmune Oral Solution
Anxiety (Rare)
Confusion (2% or less)
Consciousness, disorders of
Depression (Rare)
Psychiatric disturbances

Sandimmune Soft Gelatin Capsules
Anxiety (Rare)
Confusion (2% or less)
Consciousness, disorders of
Depression (Rare)
Psychiatric disturbances

Sandostatin Injection
Anxiety (Less than 1%)
▲ Depression (1% to 4%)
Libido, decreased (Less than 1%)
Paranoia (Less than 1%)

Sandostatin LAR Depot
▲ Anxiety (5% to 15%)
▲ Confusion (5% to 15%)
▲ Depression (5% to 15%)
▲ Hallucinations (1% to 4%)
▲ Insomnia (5% to 15%)
Libido, decreased (Rare)
▲ Nervousness (1% to 4%)
Paranoia (Rare)
Suicide, attempt of (Rare)

Seasonique Tablets
Depression
Libido, changes
Mood changes
Nervousness

Septra Tablets
Insomnia
Nervousness

Serevent Diskus
Anxiety (1% to less than 3%)
▲ Sleep disturbances (1% to 3%)

Seromycin Capsules
Aggression
Coma
Confusion
Disorientation
Memory impairment
Psychoses
Suicidal ideation

Seroquel Tablets
Aggression
▲ Agitation (6% to 20%)
▲ Anxiety (4%)
Apathy (Infrequent)
Behavioral changes
Catatonia (Infrequent)
Confusion (Infrequent)
Delirium (Rare)
Delusions (Infrequent)
Depersonalization (Infrequent)
Dreaming abnormalities (Infrequent)
Emotional lability (Rare)
Euphoria (Rare)
Hallucinations (Infrequent)
Hostility
Insomnia
Irritability
Libido, decreased (Rare)
Libido, increased (Infrequent)
Manic behavior (Infrequent)
Mental performance, impairment
Mental status, altered
Panic attack
Paranoia (Infrequent)
Psychoses, aggravation (Infrequent)
▲ Sedation (30%)
Stupor (Infrequent)
Stuttering (Rare)
Suicidal ideation
Suicide, attempt of (Infrequent)
Thinking abnormality (Infrequent)

Serostim for Injection
▲ Insomnia (3.9% to 5.9%)

Simulect for Injection
▲ Agitation (3% to 10%)
▲ Anxiety (3% to 10%)

▲ Depression (3% to 10%)
▲ Insomnia (Greater than or
  equal to 10%)

Singulair Chewable Tablets
Aggression
Agitation
Depression
Dreaming abnormalities (Very rare)
Hallucinations
Insomnia
Irritability (Very rare)

Singulair Oral Granules
Aggression
Agitation
Depression
Dreaming abnormalities (Very rare)
Hallucinations
Insomnia
Irritability (Very rare)

Singulair Tablets
Aggression
Agitation
Depression
Dreaming abnormalities (Very rare)
Hallucinations
Insomnia
Irritability (Very rare)

Skelaxin Tablets
CNS depression
▲ Irritability (Most frequent)
▲ Nervousness (Most frequent)

Solodyn Extended Release Tablets
▲ Mood changes (3%)

Soltamox Oral Solution
Depression (2%)
Libido, loss of
▲ Mood changes (11.6%)

Sonata Capsules
Agitation (Infrequent)
Anxiety (Frequent)
Apathy (Frequent)
Confusion (1% or less)
Delusions (Rare)
Depersonalization (Less than 1%
  to 2%)
Depression (Frequent)
Diplopia (Infrequent)
Emotional lability (Frequent)
Euphoria (Frequent)

Hallucinations (Less than 1%)
Hangover (Infrequent)
Hostility (Rare)
Insomnia (Infrequent)
Libido, decreased (Infrequent)
Nervousness (Frequent)
Photophobia (Infrequent)
Sedation
Sleep disturbances (Rare)
Sleep talking (Rare)
Sleep walking (Rare)
Speech, slurring (Rare)
Stimulation (Rare)
Stupor (Rare)
Thinking abnormality (Frequent)

Soriatane Capsules
Aggression
Anxiety (Less than 1%)
▲ Depression (1% to 10%)
▲ Diplopia (1% to 5%)
▲ Insomnia (1% to 10%)
  Libido, decreased (Less than 1%)
▲ Photophobia (1% to 10%)
  Suicidal ideation

Spiriva HandiHaler
▲ Depression (1% to 3%)

St. Joseph 81 mg Aspirin Chewable and Enteric Coated Tablets
Agitation
Coma
Confusion

Stalevo Tablets
Agitation (1%)
Anxiety (2%)
CNS reactions
Confusion
Delusions
Dementia
Depression
Diplopia
Disorientation
Dreaming abnormalities
Euphoria
▲ Hallucinations (4%)
Insomnia
Libido, increased
Memory impairment
Mental acuity, loss of
Mental status, altered
Nervousness
Nightmares

Paranoia
Psychoses
Stimulation
Suicidal ideation

Strattera Capsules
Aggression (0.5%)
▲ Depression (2% to 6%)
▲ Dreaming abnormalities (4%)
Hostility
▲ Insomnia (5% to 16%)
▲ Irritability (0.5% to 8%)
▲ Libido, decreased (5% or greater)
▲ Mood changes (Greater than 5%)
▲ Sedation (2% to 4%)
▲ Sexual dysfunction (3% or greater)
▲ Sleep disturbances (4%)

Striant Mucoadhesive
Anxiety
Depression
Emotional lability

Stromectol Tablets
Coma
Confusion
Mental status, altered
Stupor

Suboxone Tablets
▲ Anxiety (12%)
▲ Depression (11%)
▲ Insomnia (14% to 25%)
▲ Nervousness (6%)

Subutex Tablets
▲ Anxiety (12%)
▲ Depression (11%)
▲ Insomnia (21.4% to 25%)
▲ Nervousness (6%)

Sular Tablets
Anxiety (Less than or equal to 1%)
Confusion (Less than or equal to 1%)
Depression (Less than or equal to 1%)
Dreaming abnormalities (Less than or equal to 1%)
Insomnia (Less than or equal to 1%)
Libido, decreased (Less than or equal to 1%)
Nervousness (Less than or equal to 1%)
Thinking abnormality (Less than or equal to 1%)

Supprelin LA Implant
Mood changes

Sustiva Capsules
Aggression (0.4%)
Agitation (Less than 2%)
▲ Anxiety (2% to 13%)
Apathy (Less than 2%)
Confusion (Less than 2%)
Delusions
▲ Depression (2% to 19%)
Depression, aggravation of (Less than 2%)
Diplopia (Less than 2%)
▲ Dreaming abnormalities (1% to 4%)
Emotional lability (Less than 2%)
Euphoria (Less than 2%)
Hallucinations (Less than 2%)
▲ Insomnia (1% to 7%)
Manic behavior (0.2%)
▲ Mental performance, impairment (1% to 9%)
▲ Nervousness (1% to 7%)
Neurosis, unspecified
Paranoia (0.4%)
Psychoses (Less than 2%)
Suicidal ideation (0.7%)
Suicide, attempt of (0.5%)

Sustiva Tablets
Aggression (0.4%)
Agitation (Less than 2%)
▲ Anxiety (2% to 13%)
Apathy (Less than 2%)
Confusion (Less than 2%)
Delusions
▲ Depression (2% to 19%)
Depression, aggravation of (Less than 2%)
Diplopia (Less than 2%)
▲ Dreaming abnormalities (1% to 4%)
Emotional lability (Less than 2%)
Euphoria (Less than 2%)
Hallucinations (Less than 2%)
▲ Insomnia (1% to 7%)
Manic behavior (0.2%)
▲ Mental performance, impairment (1% to 9%)
▲ Nervousness (1% to 7%)
Neurosis, unspecified
Paranoia (0.4%)
Psychoses (Less than 2%)
Suicidal ideation (0.7%)
Suicide, attempt of (0.5%)

Sutent Capsules
Mental performance, impairment

Symbyax Capsules
Aggression
Agitation
Anxiety
Coma (Infrequent)
Confusion (Infrequent)
Depersonalization (Infrequent)
Diplopia (Infrequent)
Emotional lability (Infrequent)
Euphoria (Infrequent)
Hostility (Infrequent)
Insomnia
Irritability
▲ Libido, decreased (2% to 4%)
Libido, increased (Rare)
Neurosis, unspecified (Infrequent)
Panic attack
Sleep disturbances (1% to 2%)
Speech disturbances (Up to 2%)
Suicidal ideation
Suicide, attempt of (Infrequent)
▲ Thinking abnormality (5% to 6%)

Symmetrel Tablets
Aggression
▲ Agitation (1% to 5%)
▲ Anxiety (1% to 5%)
Coma
▲ Confusion (0.1% to 5%)
Consciousness, disorders of
  (Uncommon)
Delirium
Delusions
▲ Depression (1% to 5%)
▲ Dreaming abnormalities (1% to 5%)
Euphoria (0.1% to 1%)
▲ Hallucinations (1% to 5%)
▲ Insomnia (5% to 10%)
▲ Irritability (1% to 5%)
Libido, decreased (0.1% to 1%)
Manic behavior
▲ Nervousness (1% to 5%)
Paranoia
Psychoses (0.1% to 1%)
Speech, slurring (0.1% to 1%)
Stupor
Suicidal ideation (Less than 0.1%)
Suicide, attempt of (Less than 0.1%)
Thinking abnormality (0.1% to 1%)

Synagis Intramuscular Powder
Nervousness (More than 1%)
Nervousness (More than 1%)

Synera Topical Patch
CNS depression
CNS stimulation
Confusion
Diplopia
Euphoria
Nervousness

Tambocor Tablets
▲ Anxiety (1% to 3%)
Apathy (Less than 1%)
Confusion (Less than 1%)
Depersonalization (Less than 1%)
▲ Depression (1% to 3%)
▲ Diplopia (1% to 3%)
Dreaming abnormalities
  (Less than 1%)
Euphoria (Less than 1%)
▲ Insomnia (1% to 3%)
Libido, decreased (Less than 1%)
Photophobia (Less than 1%)
Speech disturbances (Less than 1%)
Stupor (Less than 1%)

Tamiflu Capsules
Confusion
Delirium
Insomnia (1%)

Tamiflu Oral Suspension
Confusion
Delirium
Insomnia (1.1% to 1.2%)

Tarceva Tablets
▲ Anxiety (0% to 13%)
▲ Depression (0% to 19%)
▲ Insomnia (0% to 15%)

Targretin Capsules
Agitation
Confusion
Depression
▲ Insomnia (4.8% to 11.3%)

Targretin Gel
▲ Insomnia (4.8% to 11.3%)

Tarka Tablets
Anxiety (0.3% or more)
Confusion
Insomnia (Less frequent)
Libido, decreased
Mental performance, impairment
  (Less frequent)
Psychoses

Tasmar Tablets
Agitation (1%)
Anxiety (1% or more)
Apathy (Infrequent)
▲ Confusion (10% to 11%)
Consciousness, disorders of (Four cases)
Delirium (Rare)
Delusions (Infrequent)
Depression (Frequent)
Diplopia (Infrequent)
▲ Dreaming abnormalities (16% to 21%)
Emotional lability (Frequent)
Euphoria (1%)
▲ Hallucinations (8% to 10%)
Hostility (Infrequent)
Hyperactivity (1%)
Irritability (1%)
Libido, decreased (Infrequent)
Libido, increased (Infrequent)
Manic behavior (Infrequent)
Mental acuity, loss of (1%)
Nervousness (Infrequent)
Panic attack (1%)
Paranoia (Infrequent)
Psychoses (Infrequent)
▲ Sleep disturbances (24% to 25%)
Speech disturbances (Frequent)
Thinking abnormality (Infrequent)

Taxotere Injection Concentrate
Confusion

Tegretol Chewable Tablets
Agitation
Confusion
Depression
Diplopia
Hallucinations, visual
Psychosis, activation
Speech disturbances
Talkativeness

Tegretol Suspension
Agitation
Confusion
Depression
Diplopia
Hallucinations, visual
Psychosis, activation
Speech disturbances
Talkativeness

Tegretol Tablets
Agitation
Confusion

Depression
Diplopia
Hallucinations, visual
Psychosis, activation
Speech disturbances
Talkativeness

Tegretol-XR Tablets
Agitation
Confusion
Depression, aggravation of
Diplopia
Hallucinations, visual
Psychosis, activation
Speech disturbances
Talkativeness

Temodar Capsules
▲ Anxiety (7%)
▲ Confusion (1% to 5%)
▲ Depression (6%)
▲ Diplopia (5%)
▲ Insomnia (10%)
▲ Memory impairment (7%)

Tessalon Capsules
Confusion
Hallucinations, visual
Sedation
Confusion
Hallucinations, visual
Sedation

Testim 1% Gel
Depression
Insomnia (1% or less)
Mood changes (1% or less)
Smell disturbances (1% or less)

Teveten HCT Tablets
Anxiety (Less than 1%)
Depression (Less than 1%)
Insomnia (Less than 1%)
Nervousness (Less than 1%)

Teveten Tablets
Anxiety (Less than 1%)
Depression (1%)
Insomnia (Less than 1%)
Nervousness (Less than 1%)

Thalomid Capsules
Agitation
Anxiety
Confusion
Depression
Diplopia

Emotional lability
Euphoria
Hangover
Hostility
Insomnia
Libido, decreased
▲ Nervousness (2.8% to 9.4%)
Psychoses
Suicide, attempt of
Thinking abnormality

Thioridazine Hydrochloride Tablets
Agitation
Behavioral changes
Confusion, nocturnal
  (Extremely rare)
Dreaming abnormalities
Hyperactivity (Extremely rare)
Libido, changes
Psychiatric disturbances
  (Extremely rare)
Psychoses, aggravation

Thiothixene Capsules
Agitation
Insomnia
Psychotic symptoms, paradoxical
  exacerbation
Sedation

Thyrolar Tablets
Anxiety
Depression
Insomnia
Sluggishness

Tiazac Capsules
Depression (Less than 2%)
Dreaming abnormalities
  (Less than 2%)
Hallucinations (Less than 2%)
Insomnia (Less than 2%)
Nervousness (Less than 2%)
Personality changes (Less than 2%)
Sexual dysfunction (Less than 2%)

Timentin ADD-Vantage
Smell disturbances

Timentin Injection Galaxy Container
Smell disturbances

Timentin IV Infusion
Smell disturbances

Timentin Pharmacy Bulk Package
Smell disturbances

Timolide Tablets
Catatonia
Confusion (Less than 1%)
Depression
Diplopia
Disorientation, place
Disorientation, time
Emotional lability
Hallucinations
Insomnia (Less than 1%)
Libido, decreased (Less than 1%)
Memory impairment
Mental performance, impairment
Nervousness (Less than 1%)
Nightmares
Sensorium, clouded

Timoptic in Ocudose
Anxiety (Less frequent)
Behavioral changes (Less frequent)
Catatonia
Confusion (Less frequent)
Depression (Less frequent)
Diplopia (Less frequent)
Disorientation (Less frequent)
Disorientation, place
Disorientation, time
Emotional lability
Hallucinations (Less frequent)
Insomnia (Less frequent)
Libido, decreased
Memory loss, short-term
Mental performance, impairment
Nervousness (Less frequent)
Neuropsychometrics performance,
  decrease
Nightmares
Psychiatric disturbances
  (Less frequent)
Sensorium, clouded

Timoptic Sterile Ophthalmic Solution
Anxiety (Less frequent)
Behavioral changes (Less frequent)
Catatonia
Confusion (Less frequent)
Depression (Less frequent)
Diplopia (Less frequent)
Disorientation (Less frequent)
Disorientation, place

Disorientation, time
Emotional lability
Hallucinations (Less frequent)
Insomnia
Libido, decreased
Memory loss, short-term
Mental performance, impairment
Nervousness (Less frequent)
Neuropsychometrics performance, decrease
Nightmares
Psychiatric disturbances (Less frequent)
Sensorium, clouded

Timoptic-XE Sterile Ophthalmic Gel Forming Solution

Anxiety
Behavioral changes
Catatonia
Confusion
Depression
Diplopia
Disorientation
Disorientation, place
Disorientation, time
Emotional lability
Hallucinations
Insomnia
Libido, decreased
Memory loss, short-term
Mental performance, impairment
Nervousness
Neuropsychometrics performance, decrease
Nightmares
Psychiatric disturbances
Sensorium, clouded

Tindamax Tablets

Coma (Rare)
Confusion (Rare)
Depression (Rare)
Insomnia

Topamax Sprinkle Capsules

▲ Aggression (2% to 9%)
▲ Agitation (1% to 3%)
▲ Anxiety (4% to 24%)
▲ Apathy (1% to 3%)
▲ Cognitive dysfunction (0% to 7%)
▲ Confusion (2% to 14%)
Delirium (Infrequent)
Delusions (Infrequent)

Depersonalization (1% to 2%)
▲ Depression (1% to 13%)
▲ Diplopia (1% to 10%)
Dreaming abnormalities (Infrequent)
▲ Emotional lability (3%)
Euphoria (Infrequent)
Hallucinations (Frequent)
▲ Insomnia (6% to 9%)
▲ Libido, decreased (0% to 3%)
Libido, increased (Rare)
Manic behavior (Rare)
▲ Memory impairment (2% to 14%)
▲ Mental performance, impairment (5% to 14%)
▲ Mental slowness (8% to 15.4%)
▲ Mood changes (2% to 11%)
▲ Nervousness (4% to 19%)
Neurosis, unspecified (1%)
Paranoia (Infrequent)
Personality changes (Frequent)
Photophobia (Infrequent)
Psychoses (Frequent)
Sensory disturbances (Greater than 1%)
▲ Speech disturbances (Less than 1% to 13%)
Stupor (1% to 2%)
Suicidal ideation (Very rare)
Suicide, attempt of (Frequent)

Topamax Tablets

▲ Aggression (2% to 9%)
▲ Agitation (1% to 3%)
▲ Anxiety (4% to 24%)
▲ Apathy (1% to 3%)
▲ Cognitive dysfunction (0% to 7%)
▲ Confusion (2% to 14%)
Delirium (Infrequent)
Delusions (Infrequent)
Depersonalization (1% to 2%)
▲ Depression (1% to 13%)
▲ Diplopia (1% to 10%)
Dreaming abnormalities (Infrequent)
▲ Emotional lability (3%)
Euphoria (Infrequent)
Hallucinations (Frequent)
▲ Insomnia (6% to 9%)
▲ Libido, decreased (0% to 3%)
Libido, increased (Rare)
Manic behavior (Rare)
▲ Memory impairment (2% to 14%)
▲ Mental performance, impairment (5% to 14%)
▲ Mental slowness (8% to 15.4%)
▲ Mood changes (2% to 11%)
▲ Nervousness (4% to 19%)

Neurosis, unspecified (1%)
Paranoia (Infrequent)
Personality changes (Frequent)
Photophobia (Infrequent)
Psychoses (Frequent)
Sensory disturbances
  (Greater than 1%)
▲ Speech disturbances (Less than 1%
  to 13%)
Stupor (1% to 2%)
Suicidal ideation (Very rare)
Suicide, attempt of (Frequent)
Anxiety
Catatonia
Confusion
▲ Depression (About 5 of 100 patients)
Disorientation, place
Disorientation, time
Emotional lability
Hallucinations
Insomnia
Libido, decreased
Memory loss, short-term
Nervousness
Neuropsychometrics performance,
  decrease
Nightmares
Sensorium, clouded

Transderm Scop Transdermal Therapeutic System

Confusion (Infrequent)
Disorientation (Infrequent)
Hallucinations (Infrequent)
Memory impairment (Infrequent)

Tranxene T-TAB Tablets

Confusion (Less common)
Depression
Diplopia
Insomnia
Irritability
Nervousness (Less common)
Speech, slurring

Tranxene-SD Half Strength Tablets

Confusion (Less common)
Depression
Diplopia
Insomnia
Irritability
Nervousness (Less common)
Speech, slurring

Tranxene-SD Tablets

Confusion (Less common)
Depression
Diplopia
Insomnia
Irritability
Nervousness (Less common)
Speech, slurring

Trasylol Injection

Agitation (1% to 2%)
Anxiety (1% to 2%)
▲ Confusion (4%)
▲ Insomnia (3%)

Travatan Ophthalmic Solution

▲ Anxiety (1% to 5%)
▲ Depression (1% to 5%)
▲ Photophobia (1% to 4%)

Travatan Z Ophthalmic Solution

▲ Anxiety (1% to 5%)
▲ Depression (1% to 5%)
▲ Photophobia (1% to 4%)

Trecator Tablets

Depression
Diplopia
Psychoses

Trelstar Depot

Emotional lability (1.4%)
Insomnia (2.1%)

Trelstar LA Suspension

Insomnia (1.7%)
Libido, decreased (2.3%)

Tricor Tablets

Anxiety
Confusion
Depression
Insomnia
Libido, decreased
Nervousness
Sleep disturbances

Trileptal Oral Suspension

Aggression
Agitation (1% to 2%)
▲ Anxiety (5% to 7%)
Apathy
Confusion (1% to 2%)
Delirium
Delusions
▲ Diplopia (5% to 40%)

▲ Emotional lability (2% to 3%)
Euphoria
Feeling, intoxicated
Feeling, strange (1% to 2%)
Hysteria
▲ Insomnia (2% to 4%)
Libido, decreased
Libido, increased
Manic behavior
▲ Nervousness (2% to 4%)
Panic attack
Paranoia
Personality changes
Photophobia
▲ Speech disturbances (1% to 3%)
Stupor
Thinking abnormality (2%)

Trileptal Tablets
Aggression
Agitation (1% to 2%)
▲ Anxiety (5% to 7%)
Apathy
Confusion (1% to 2%)
Delirium
Delusions
▲ Diplopia (5% to 40%)
▲ Emotional lability (2% to 3%)
Euphoria
Feeling, intoxicated
Feeling, strange (1% to 2%)
Hysteria
▲ Insomnia (2% to 4%)
Libido, decreased
Libido, increased
Manic behavior
▲ Nervousness (2% to 4%)
Panic attack
Paranoia
Personality changes
Photophobia
▲ Speech disturbances (1% to 3%)
Stupor
Thinking abnormality (2%)

Tri-Norinyl Tablets
Libido, changes
Nervousness

Trisenox Injection
▲ Agitation (5%)
▲ Anxiety (30%)
▲ Coma (5%)
▲ Confusion (5%)
▲ Depression (20%)
▲ Insomnia (43%)

Trivora-28 Tablets
Libido, changes
Nervousness

Trizivir Tablets
▲ Depression (9%)
▲ Insomnia (7% to 13%)
▲ Nervousness (Greater than or
equal to 5%)
▲ Sleep disturbances (7% to 11%)

**Trusopt Sterile Ophthalmic
Solution**
▲ Photophobia (Approximately 1% to 5%)

Truvada Tablets
Anxiety
▲ Depression (4%)
Depressive reactions
▲ Dreaming abnormalities (4%)
▲ Insomnia (4%)

**Tussionex Pennkinetic
Extended-Release Suspension**
Anxiety
Euphoria
Fear
Mental clouding
Mental performance, impairment
Mood changes
Sedation

Twinject 0.15
Anxiety
Overstimulation

Twinject 0.3
Anxiety
Overstimulation

Twinrix Vaccine
Agitation (Less than 1%)
Insomnia (Less than 1%)
Irritability (Less than 1%)
Photophobia (Less than 1%)

Tygacil for Injection
Insomnia (2.3%)

Tykerb Tablets
▲ Insomnia (0% to 10%)

**Tylenol Allergy Multi-Symptom
Caplets with Cool Burst and
Gelcaps**
Excitability
Insomnia
Nervousness

Tylenol Allergy Multi-Symptom Nighttime Caplets with Cool Burst
Excitability
Insomnia
Nervousness

Tylenol Cold Head Congestion Daytime Caplets with Cool Burst
Insomnia
Nervousness

Tylenol Cold Head Congestion Nighttime Caplets with Cool Burst
Excitability
Insomnia
Nervousness

Tylenol Cold Head Congestion Severe Caplets with Cool Burst
Insomnia
Nervousness

Tylenol Cold Multi-Symptom Daytime Caplets with Cool Burst and Gelcaps
Insomnia
Nervousness

Tylenol Cold Multi-Symptom Daytime Liquid with Citrus Burst
Insomnia
Nervousness

Tylenol Cold Multi-Symptom Nighttime Caplets with Cool Burst
Excitability
Insomnia
Nervousness

Tylenol Cold Multi-Symptom Nighttime Liquid with Cool Burst
Excitability
Insomnia
Nervousness

Tylenol Cold Multi-Symptom Severe Caplets with Cool Burst
Insomnia
Nervousness

Tylenol Cold Multi-Symptom Severe Daytime Liquid with Citrus Burst
Insomnia
Nervousness

Tylenol Cold Severe Congestion Non-Drowsy Caplets with Cool Burst
Insomnia
Nervousness

Tylenol Cough & Sore Throat Nighttime Liquid with Cool Burst
Excitability

Tylenol Severe Allergy Caplets
Excitability

Tylenol Sinus Congestion & Pain Daytime Caplets with Cool Burst and Gelcaps
Insomnia
Nervousness

Tylenol Sinus Congestion & Pain Nighttime Caplets with Cool Burst
Excitability
Insomnia
Nervousness

Tylenol Sinus Congestion & Pain Severe Caplets with Cool Burst
Insomnia
Nervousness

Tylenol Sinus Severe Congestion Caplets with Cool Burst
Insomnia
Nervousness

Tylenol Sore Throat Nighttime Liquid with Cool Burst
Excitability

Tylenol with Codeine Elixir
Mental performance, impairment
▲ Sedation (Among most frequent)

Tylenol with Codeine Tablets
Euphoria
Mental performance, impairment
▲ Sedation (Among most frequent)

Tyzeka Tablets
▲ Insomnia (3%)

Ultane Liquid for Inhalation
▲ Agitation (7% to 15%)
 Confusion (Less than 1%)
 Insomnia (Less than 1%)
 Nervousness (Less than 1%)

Ultram ER Tablets
 Agitation (0.5% to less than 1%)
▲ Anxiety (1% to less than 5%)
▲ Confusion (1% to greater than 5%)
▲ Depression (1% to less than 5%)
▲ Disorientation (0.5% to less than 1%)
 Dreaming abnormalities (0.5% to less than 1%)
 Euphoria (0.5% to less than 1%)
▲ Insomnia (6.5% to 10.9%)
 Irritability (0.5% to less than 1%)
 Jitteriness (0.5% to less than 1%)
 Libido, decreased (0.5% to less than 1%)
▲ Nervousness (1% to less than 5%)
 Sedation (0.5% to less than 1%)
 Sleep disturbances (0.5% to less than 1%)

Uniphyl Tablets
 Behavioral changes
 Insomnia
 Irritability

Uniretic Tablets
 Anxiety (Less than 1%)
 Depression (Less than 1%)
 Emotional lability (Less than 1%)
 Insomnia (Less than 1%)
 Libido, decreased (Less than 1%)
 Nervousness (Less than 1%)
 Neurosis, unspecified (Less than 1%)

Univasc Tablets
 Anxiety (Less than 1%)
 Mood changes (Less than 1%)
 Nervousness (Less than 1%)
 Sleep disturbances (Less than 1%)

Uroqid-Acid No. 2 Tablets
 Confusion

Vagifem Tablets
▲ Insomnia (3% to 5%)

Valcyte Tablets
▲ Agitation (Less than 5%)
▲ Confusion (Less than 5%)
▲ Depression (Less than 5%)

▲ Hallucinations (Less than 5%)
▲ Insomnia (16%)
▲ Psychoses (Less than 5%)
 Sedation

Valium Tablets
 Anxiety, paradoxical
 Confusion (Infrequent)
 Depression (Infrequent)
 Diplopia (Infrequent)
 Excitement, paradoxical
 Hallucinations
 Insomnia
 Libido, changes (Infrequent)
 Rage
 Sleep disturbances
 Speech, slurring (Infrequent)
 Stimulation

Valtrex Caplets
 Agitation
 Behavioral changes
 Coma
 Confusion
 Consciousness, disorders of
▲ Depression (Less than 1% to 7%)
 Hallucinations, auditory
 Hallucinations, visual
 Manic behavior
 Psychoses

Vandazole Vaginal Gel
 Insomnia (Less than 1%)

Vantas
 Depression (Less than 2%)
 Insomnia (2.9%)
 Irritability (Less than 2%)
 Libido, decreased (2.3%)
 Sexual dysfunction (Less than 2%)

Vantin Tablets and Oral Suspension
 Anxiety (Less than 1%)
 Confusion (Less than 1%)
 Dreaming abnormalities (Less than 1%)
 Hallucinations (Less than 1%)
 Insomnia (Less than 1%)
 Nervousness (Less than 1%)
 Nightmares (Less than 1%)

Vaprisol
▲ Confusion (3.8%)
▲ Insomnia (3.3%)

Vaqta
▲ Irritability (10.8%)

Varivax
Irritability (Greater than or
equal to 1%)
Nervousness (Greater than or
equal to 1%)
Sleep disturbances (Greater than or
equal to 1%)

Velcade for Injection
▲ Anxiety (14%)
▲ Insomnia (18%)
▲ Psychoses (35%)

Ventavis Inhalation Solution
▲ Insomnia (8%)

**Ventolin HFA Inhalation
Aerosol**
CNS stimulation
Insomnia

Veramyst Nasal Spray
Depression

Verdeso Foam
Irritability (0% to 1%)

**Verelan PM Extended-Release
Capsules, Controlled-Onset**
Confusion (2% or less)
Insomnia (2% or less)
Psychoses (2% or less)

**Verelan Sustained-Release
Capsules**
Insomnia (1% or less)
Psychoses (1% or less)
Sleep disturbances (1.4%)

Vesanoid Capsules
▲ Agitation (9%)
▲ Anxiety (17%)
▲ CNS depression (3%)
▲ Coma (3%)
▲ Confusion (14%)
▲ Dementia (3%)
▲ Depression (14%)
▲ Hallucinations (6%)
▲ Insomnia (14%)
▲ Memory impairment (3%)
▲ Speech disturbances (3%)

VESIcare Tablets
Depression (0.8% to 1.2%)

VFEND I.V.
Agitation (Less than 2%)
Anxiety (Less than 2%)

Coma (Less than 2%)
Confusion (Less than 2%)
Delirium (Less than 2%)
Dementia (Less than 2%)
Depersonalization (Less than 2%)
Depression (Less than 2%)
Diplopia (Less than 2%)
Dreaming abnormalities (Less than
2%)
Euphoria (Less than 2%)
Hallucinations (0% to 2.8%)
Insomnia (Less than 2%)
Libido, decreased (Less than 2%)
▲ Photophobia (1.7% to 21%)
Psychoses (Less than 2%)
Suicidal ideation (Less than 2%)

VFEND Oral Suspension
Agitation (Less than 2%)
Anxiety (Less than 2%)
Coma (Less than 2%)
Confusion (Less than 2%)
Delirium (Less than 2%)
Dementia (Less than 2%)
Depersonalization (Less than 2%)
Depression (Less than 2%)
Diplopia (Less than 2%)
Dreaming abnormalities
(Less than 2%)
Euphoria (Less than 2%)
Hallucinations (0% to 2.8%)
Insomnia (Less than 2%)
Libido, decreased (Less than 2%)
▲ Photophobia (1.7% to 21%)
Psychoses (Less than 2%)
Suicidal ideation (Less than 2%)

VFEND Tablets
Agitation (Less than 2%)
Anxiety (Less than 2%)
Coma (Less than 2%)
Confusion (Less than 2%)
Delirium (Less than 2%)
Dementia (Less than 2%)
Depersonalization (Less than 2%)
Depression (Less than 2%)
Diplopia (Less than 2%)
Dreaming abnormalities
(Less than 2%)
Euphoria (Less than 2%)
Hallucinations (0% to 2.8%)
Insomnia (Less than 2%)
Libido, decreased (Less than 2%)
▲ Photophobia (1.7% to 21%)
Psychoses (Less than 2%)
Suicidal ideation (Less than 2%)

Viadur Implant
Anxiety (Less than 2%)
▲ Depression (5.3%)

Viagra Tablets
Anxiety
Depression (Less than 2%)
Diplopia
Dreaming abnormalities
  (Less than 2%)
Insomnia (Less than 2%)
Photophobia (Less than 2%)

Vicks 44D Cough & Head Congestion Relief Liquid
Insomnia
Nervousness

Vicks DayQuil Multi-Symptom Cold/Flu Relief LiquiCaps
Insomnia
Nervousness

Vicks DayQuil Multi-Symptom Cold/Flu Relief Liquid
Insomnia
Nervousness

Vicks NyQuil Multi-Symptom Cold/Flu Relief LiquiCaps
Excitability

Vicks NyQuil Multi-Symptom Cold/Flu Relief Liquid
Excitability

Vicodin ES Tablets
Anxiety
Fear
Mental clouding
Mental performance, impairment
Mood changes
▲ Sedation (Among most frequent)

Vicodin HP Tablets
Anxiety
Fear
Mental clouding
Mental performance, impairment
Mood changes
▲ Sedation (Among most frequent)

Vicodin Tablets
Anxiety
Fear
Mental clouding
Mental performance, impairment
Mood changes
▲ Sedation (Among most frequent)

Vicoprofen Tablets
Agitation (Less than 1%)
▲ Anxiety (3% to 9%)
Confusion (Less than 3%)
Depression (Less than 1%)
Dreaming abnormalities (Less than 1%)
Euphoria (Less than 1%)
▲ Insomnia (3% to 9%)
Libido, decreased (Less than 1%)
Mood changes (Less than 1%)
▲ Nervousness (3% to 9%)
Speech, slurring (Less than 1%)
Thinking abnormality (Less than 3%)

Viracept Oral Powder
Anxiety (Less than 2%)
Depression (Less than 2%)
Emotional lability (Less than 2%)
Insomnia (Less than 2%)
Sexual dysfunction (Less than 2%)
Sleep disturbances (Less than 2%)
Suicidal ideation (Less than 2%)

Viracept Tablets
Anxiety (Less than 2%)
Depression (Less than 2%)
Emotional lability (Less than 2%)
Insomnia (Less than 2%)
Sexual dysfunction (Less than 2%)
Sleep disturbances (Less than 2%)
Suicidal ideation (Less than 2%)

Viread Tablets
▲ Anxiety (6%)
▲ Depression (4% to 11%)
▲ Insomnia (3% to 4%)

Visudyne for Injection
▲ Diplopia (1% to 10%)
▲ Sleep disturbances (1% to 10%)

Vivaglobin
Nervousness (0.1%)

Vivitrol
▲ Agitation (8% to 12%)
▲ Anxiety (8% to 12%)
Delirium
▲ Depression (3% to 8%)
Dreaming abnormalities
Euphoria
▲ Insomnia (8% to 14%)
Irritability

Libido, decreased
Mental performance, impairment
▲ Nervousness (8% to 12%)
▲ Obsessive compulsive symptoms (8% to 12%)
▲ Panic attack (8% to 12%)
▲ Sedation (4% to 12%)
▲ Sluggishness (12% to 23%)

Voltaren Ophthalmic Solution
▲ Insomnia (Less than or equal to 3%)

Voltaren Tablets
Anxiety (Occasionally)
Coma (Rarely)
Confusion (Occasionally)
Depression (Occasionally)
Dreaming abnormalities (Occasionally)
Hallucinations (Rarely)
Insomnia (Occasionally)
Nervousness (Occasionally)

Voltaren-XR Tablets
Anxiety (Occasionally)
Coma (Rarely)
Confusion (Occasionally)
Depression (Occasionally)
Dreaming abnormalities (Occasionally)
Hallucinations (Rarely)
Insomnia (Occasionally)
Nervousness (Occasionally)

VoSpire ER Tablets
CNS stimulation
Insomnia (2.4%)
Irritability (Less frequent)
▲ Nervousness (8.5%)

Vytorin 10/10 Tablets
Anxiety
Depression
Insomnia
Libido, loss of
Psychiatric disturbances

Vytorin 10/20 Tablets
Anxiety
Depression
Insomnia
Libido, loss of
Psychiatric disturbances

Vytorin 10/40 Tablets
Anxiety
Depression

Insomnia
Libido, loss of
Psychiatric disturbances

Vytorin 10/80 Tablets
Anxiety
Depression
Insomnia
Libido, loss of
Psychiatric disturbances

Vyvanse Capsules
Delusions
Depression
Euphoria
Hallucinations
▲ Insomnia (10% to 19%)
▲ Irritability (10%)
Libido, changes
Overstimulation
Psychoses

Wellbutrin SR Sustained-Release Tablets
Aggression
▲ Agitation (3% to 9%)
▲ Anxiety (5% to 6%)
Behavioral changes
CNS stimulation (1% to 2%)
Coma
Confusion
Delirium
Delusions
Depersonalization (Infrequent)
Depression
Depression, aggravation of
▲ Diplopia (2% to 3%)
Dreaming abnormalities (At least 1%)
Emotional lability (Infrequent)
Euphoria
Hallucinations
Hostility (Infrequent)
▲ Insomnia (5% to 16%)
▲ Irritability (2% to 3%)
Libido, decreased (Infrequent)
Libido, increased
Manic behavior
▲ Memory impairment (Up to 3%)
▲ Nervousness (3% to 5%)
Panic attack
Paranoia
Psychoses
Psychosis, activation
Suicidal ideation (Infrequent)

Wellbutrin Tablets
Aggression
▲ Agitation (31.9%)
▲ Anxiety (3.1%)
Behavioral changes
Coma
▲ Confusion (8.4%)
Delirium
Delusions (1.2%)
Depersonalization (Infrequent)
Depression (Frequent)
Depression, aggravation of
Diplopia (Rare)
Dreaming abnormalities
Euphoria (1.2%)
Hallucinations (Frequent)
▲ Hostility (5.6%)
▲ Insomnia (18.6%)
▲ Libido, decreased (3.1%)
Libido, increased (Frequent)
Manic behavior (Frequent)
Memory impairment (Infrequent)
Mood changes (Infrequent)
Nervousness
Panic attack
Paranoia (Infrequent)
Psychoses (Infrequent)
▲ Sedation (19.8%)
▲ Sensory disturbances (4%)
Sexual dysfunction (Frequent)
▲ Sleep disturbances (4%)
Suicidal ideation (Rare)
Thinking abnormality (Infrequent)

Wellbutrin XL Extended-Release Tablets
Aggression
▲ Agitation (2% to 9%)
▲ Anxiety (5% to 7%)
Behavioral changes
CNS stimulation (1% to 2%)
Coma
▲ Confusion (8%)
Delirium
Delusions
Depersonalization (Infrequent)
Depression
Depression, aggravation of
▲ Diplopia (2% to 3%)
▲ Dreaming abnormalities (At least 1% to 3%)
Emotional lability (Infrequent)
Euphoria
Hallucinations
Hostility (Infrequent)

▲ Insomnia (11% to 20%)
▲ Irritability (2% to 3%)
▲ Jitteriness (3%)
▲ Libido, decreased (3%)
Libido, increased
Manic behavior
▲ Memory impairment (3%)
▲ Nervousness (3% to 5%)
Panic attack
Paranoia
Psychoses
Psychosis, activation
▲ Sensory disturbances (4%)
▲ Sleep disturbances (4%)
Suicidal ideation (Infrequent)

Xalatan Sterile Ophthalmic Solution
Diplopia (Less than 1%)
▲ Photophobia (1% to 4%)

Xeloda Tablets
▲ Confusion (Less than 5%)
▲ Depression (Less than 5%)
▲ Insomnia (Less than 5%)
▲ Irritability (Less than 5%)
▲ Mood changes (5%)
▲ Sedation (Less than 5%)

Xenical Capsules
▲ Anxiety (2.8% to 4.4%)
▲ Depression (3.4%)
▲ Sleep disturbances (3.9%)

Xifaxan Tablets
Dreaming abnormalities (Less than 2%)
Insomnia (Less than 2%)

Xopenex HFA Inhalation Aerosol
Anxiety (2.7%)
Insomnia
▲ Nervousness (2.8% to 9.6%)

Xopenex Inhalation Solution
Anxiety (2.7%)
Insomnia
▲ Nervousness (2.8% to 9.6%)

Xopenex Inhalation Solution Concentrate
Anxiety (2.7%)
Insomnia
▲ Nervousness (2.8% to 9.6%)

Xyrem Oral Solution
▲ Confusion (Less than 1% to 5.9%)
▲ Depression (5.9%)

▲ Disorientation (2.9% to 8.6%)
  Dreaming abnormalities (Frequent)
  Emotional disturbances (Infrequent)
  Euphoria (Infrequent)
  Fear (Infrequent)
  Hallucinations, auditory (Infrequent)
  Hangover (Infrequent)
▲ Inebriated feeling (8.6%)
  Insomnia (Frequent)
  Jitteriness (Infrequent)
  Libido, increased (Infrequent)
  Memory impairment (Frequent)
  Mental performance, impairment
    (Infrequent)
  Mood changes (Infrequent)
  Nervousness (Frequent)
▲ Nightmares (2.9% to 6.1%)
  Paranoia (Infrequent)
  Sedation (Infrequent)
▲ Sleep disturbances (2.9% to 6.1%)
  Sleep talking (Infrequent)
▲ Sleep walking (5.7%)
  Sluggishness (Infrequent)

Yasmin 28 Tablets
  Depression (Greater than 1%)
  Emotional lability
  Libido, changes
  Nervousness (Greater than 1%)

YAZ Tablets
  Depression (Greater than 1%)
  Emotional lability (Greater than 1%)
  Libido, changes
  Libido, decreased (Greater than 1%)
  Nervousness

Zantac 150 EFFERdose Tablets
  Agitation (Rare)
  Confusion (Rare)
  Depression (Rare)
  Hallucinations (Rare)
  Insomnia (Rare)
  Libido, loss of (Occasional)

Zantac 150 Tablets
  Agitation (Rare)
  Confusion (Rare)
  Depression (Rare)
  Hallucinations (Rare)
  Insomnia (Rare)
  Libido, loss of (Occasional)

Zantac 25 EFFERdose Tablets
  Agitation (Rare)
  Confusion (Rare)

  Depression (Rare)
  Hallucinations (Rare)
  Insomnia (Rare)
  Libido, loss of (Occasional)

Zantac 300 Tablets
  Agitation (Rare)
  Confusion (Rare)
  Depression (Rare)
  Hallucinations (Rare)
  Insomnia (Rare)
  Libido, loss of (Occasional)

Zantac Injection
  Agitation
  Confusion (Rare)
  Depression (Rare)
  Hallucinations
  Insomnia
  Libido, decreased

Zantac Injection Pharmacy Bulk Package
  Agitation (Rare)
  Confusion (Rare)
  Depression (Rare)
  Hallucinations (Rare)
  Insomnia (Rare)
  Libido, decreased (Infrequent)

Zantac Injection Premixed
  Agitation
  Confusion (Rare)
  Depression (Rare)
  Hallucinations
  Insomnia
  Libido, decreased

Zantac Syrup
  Agitation (Rare)
  Confusion (Rare)
  Depression (Rare)
  Hallucinations (Rare)
  Insomnia (Rare)
  Libido, loss of (Occasional)

Zegerid Capsules
  Aggression (Less than 1%)
  Anxiety (Less than 1%)
  Apathy (Less than 1%)
  Confusion (Less than 1%)
  Depression (Less than 1%)
  Diplopia (Less than 1%)
  Dreaming abnormalities
    (Less than 1%)
  Hallucinations (Less than 1%)

Insomnia (Less than 1%)
Nervousness (Less than 1%)
Psychiatric disturbances
  (Less than 1%)

Zegerid Powder for Oral Solution

Aggression (Less than 1%)
Anxiety (Less than 1%)
Apathy (Less than 1%)
Confusion (Less than 1%)
Depression (Less than 1%)
Diplopia (Less than 1%)
Dreaming abnormalities
  (Less than 1%)
Hallucinations (Less than 1%)
Insomnia (Less than 1%)
Nervousness (Less than 1%)
Psychiatric disturbances
  (Less than 1%)

Zelapar Tablets

Agitation
Dementia
Depression (2%)
Diplopia
Emotional lability
▲ Hallucinations (4%)
▲ Insomnia (7%)
Nervousness
Paranoia
Sleep disturbances
Thinking abnormality

Ziagen Oral Solution

▲ Anxiety (5%)
Depression, aggravation of
  (5 patients)
▲ Depressive reactions (6%)
▲ Sleep disturbances (10%)

Ziagen Tablets

▲ Anxiety (5%)
Depression, aggravation of
  (5 patients)
▲ Depressive reactions (6%)
▲ Sleep disturbances (10%)

Zmax for Oral Suspension

Agitation
Anxiety
Hyperactivity
Nervousness

Zocor Tablets

Anxiety
Depression

Insomnia
Libido, loss of
Memory loss, short-term
Psychiatric disturbances

Zofran Injection

▲ Agitation (2% to 6%)
▲ Anxiety (2% to 6%)
▲ Sedation (8%)

Zofran Injection Premixed

▲ Agitation (2% to 6%)
▲ Anxiety (2% to 6%)
▲ Sedation (8%)

Zofran ODT Orally Disintegrating Tablets

▲ Agitation (6%)
▲ Anxiety (6%)
▲ Sedation (20%)

Zofran Oral Solution

▲ Agitation (6%)
▲ Anxiety (6%)
▲ Sedation (20%)

Zofran Tablets

▲ Agitation (6%)
▲ Anxiety (6%)
▲ Sedation (20%)

Zoloft Oral Concentrate

Aggression (Infrequent to 2%)
▲ Agitation (1% to 6%)
▲ Anxiety (4%)
Apathy (Infrequent)
Behavioral changes
Coma (Rare)
Confusion (Infrequent)
Delusions (Infrequent)
Depersonalization (Infrequent)
Depression (Infrequent)
Depression, aggravation of
  (Infrequent)
Diplopia (Rare)
Dreaming abnormalities (Infrequent)
Emotional lability (Infrequent)
Euphoria (Infrequent)
Hallucinations (Infrequent)
Hostility
Illusion, unspecified (Rare)
▲ Insomnia (12% to 28%)
Irritability
▲ Libido, decreased (1% to 11%)
Libido, increased (Rare)
Mental performance, impairment
  (1.3% to 2%)

▲ Nervousness (6%)
Panic attack
Paranoia (Infrequent)
Photophobia (Rare)
Psychoses
Serotonin syndrome
Sexual dysfunction (Frequent)
Suicidal ideation (Rare)
Suicide, attempt of

Zoloft Tablets
Aggression (Infrequent to 2%)
▲ Agitation (1% to 6%)
▲ Anxiety (4%)
Apathy (Infrequent)
Behavioral changes
Coma (Rare)
Confusion (Infrequent)
Delusions (Infrequent)
Depersonalization (Infrequent)
Depression (Infrequent)
Depression, aggravation of
  (Infrequent)
Diplopia (Rare)
Dreaming abnormalities (Infrequent)
Emotional lability (Infrequent)
Euphoria (Infrequent)
Hallucinations (Infrequent)
Hostility
Illusion, unspecified (Rare)
▲ Insomnia (12% to 28%)
Irritability
▲ Libido, decreased (1% to 11%)
Libido, increased (Rare)
Mental performance, impairment
  (1.3% to 2%)
▲ Nervousness (6%)
Panic attack
Paranoia (Infrequent)
Photophobia (Rare)
Psychoses
Serotonin syndrome
Sexual dysfunction (Frequent)
Suicidal ideation (Rare)
Suicide, attempt of

Zometa for Intravenous Infusion
▲ Agitation (12.8%)
▲ Anxiety (11% to 14%)
▲ Confusion (7% to 12.8%)
▲ Depression (14%)
▲ Insomnia (15.1% to 16%)

Zomig Nasal Spray
Agitation (Infrequent to less than 2%)

Anxiety (Infrequent)
Apathy (Rare)
Coma
Confusion (Infrequent)
Depersonalization (Infrequent)
Depression (Infrequent)
Dreaming abnormalities (Rare)
Euphoria (Rare)
Hallucinations
Insomnia (Infrequent to less than 2%)
Irritability (Rare)
Manic behavior (Rare)
Nervousness (Infrequent)
Photophobia (Rare)
Psychoses (Rare)
Serotonin syndrome
Speech disturbances (Infrequent)
Thinking abnormality (Infrequent)

Zomig Tablets
Agitation (Infrequent)
Anxiety (Infrequent)
Apathy (Rare)
Depression (Infrequent)
Diplopia (Rare)
Emotional lability (Infrequent)
Euphoria (Rare)
Hallucinations (Rare)
Insomnia (Infrequent)
Irritability (Rare)
Serotonin syndrome

Zomig-ZMT Tablets
Agitation (Infrequent)
Anxiety (Infrequent)
Apathy (Rare)
Depression (Infrequent)
Diplopia (Rare)
Emotional lability (Infrequent)
Euphoria (Rare)
Hallucinations (Rare)
Insomnia (Infrequent)
Irritability (Rare)
Serotonin syndrome

Zonegran Capsules
▲ Agitation (9%)
▲ Anxiety (3%)
▲ Confusion (6%)
▲ Depression (6%)
▲ Diplopia (6%)
Dreaming abnormalities (Infrequent)
Euphoria (Infrequent)
▲ Insomnia (6%)
▲ Irritability (9%)

Libido, decreased (Infrequent)
▲ Memory impairment (6%)
▲ Mental performance, impairment (6%)
▲ Mental slowness (4%)
Nervousness (2%)
Photophobia (Rare)
▲ Speech disturbances (5%)

Zostavax Injection
Depression (9%)

Zosyn
▲ Agitation (2.1% to 7.1%)
▲ Anxiety (1.2% to 3.2%)
Confusion (1.0% or less)
Depression (1.0% or less)
Hallucinations (1.0% or less)
▲ Insomnia (4.5% to 6.6%)
Photophobia (1.0% or less)

Zovia 1/35E Tablets
Libido, changes
Nervousness

Zovia 1/50E Tablets
Libido, changes
Nervousness

Zovirax Capsules
Agitation
Coma
Confusion
Consciousness, disorders of
Delirium
Hallucinations
Psychoses

Zovirax Suspension
Agitation
Coma
Confusion
Consciousness, disorders of
Delirium
Hallucinations
Psychoses

Zovirax Tablets
Agitation
Coma
Confusion
Consciousness, disorders of
Delirium
Hallucinations
Psychoses

Zyban Sustained-Release Tablets
Aggression
Agitation (Frequent)

▲ Anxiety (8%)
Behavioral changes
CNS stimulation (Infrequent)
Coma
Confusion (Infrequent)
Delirium
Delusions
Depersonalization (Infrequent)
Depression (Frequent)
Diplopia (Frequent)
▲ Dreaming abnormalities (5%)
Emotional lability (Infrequent)
Euphoria
Hallucinations
Hostility (Infrequent)
▲ Insomnia (31% to 40%)
Irritability (Frequent)
Libido, decreased (Infrequent)
Libido, increased
Manic behavior
Memory impairment (Infrequent)
▲ Mental performance, impairment (9%)
▲ Nervousness (4%)
Panic attack
Paranoia
Psychoses
Psychosis, activation
Suicidal ideation (Infrequent)
Thinking abnormality (1%)

Zydone Tablets
Anxiety
Fear
Mental clouding
Mental performance, impairment
Mood changes
▲ Sedation (Among most frequent)

Zyflo Tablets
Insomnia (Greater than 1%)
Nervousness (Greater than 1%)

Zyprexa IntraMuscular
Confusion (Infrequent)
Emotional lability (Infrequent)

Zyprexa Tablets
▲ Agitation (23%)
Alcohol abuse (Infrequent)
Antisocial reaction (Infrequent)
▲ Anxiety (9%)
▲ Apathy (4%)
Behavioral changes
CNS stimulation (Infrequent)
Coma (Rare)
▲ Confusion (4%)

Delirium (Infrequent)
Delusions (Frequent)
Dementia (Infrequent)
Depersonalization (Infrequent)
▲ Depression (18%)
Diplopia (Infrequent)
Dreaming abnormalities
Emotional lability
▲ Euphoria (2% to 3%)
Hallucinations
Hangover (Infrequent)
▲ Hostility (15%)
▲ Insomnia (12% to 20%)
Libido, decreased (Infrequent)
Libido, increased
Manic behavior (Frequent)
▲ Nervousness (16%)
Obsessive compulsive symptoms (Infrequent)
Paranoia
▲ Personality changes (8%)
Phobic disorder (Infrequent)
Sociopathy (Infrequent)
▲ Speech difficulties (2% to 7%)
▲ Speech disturbances (2% to 7%)
Stupor (Infrequent)
Stuttering (Infrequent)
Suicide, attempt of (Infrequent)
Thinking abnormality

Zyprexa ZYDIS Orally Disintegrating Tablets
▲ Agitation (23%)
Alcohol abuse (Infrequent)
Antisocial reaction (Infrequent)
▲ Anxiety (9%)
▲ Apathy (4%)
Behavioral changes
CNS stimulation (Infrequent)
Coma (Rare)
▲ Confusion (4%)
Delirium (Infrequent)
Dementia (Infrequent)
Depersonalization (Infrequent)
▲ Depression (18%)
Diplopia (Infrequent)
Dreaming abnormalities
Emotional lability
▲ Euphoria (2% to 3%)
Hallucinations
Hangover (Infrequent)
▲ Hostility (15%)
▲ Insomnia (12% to 20%)
Libido, decreased (Infrequent)
Libido, increased

Manic behavior (Frequent)
▲ Nervousness (16%)
Obsessive compulsive symptoms (Infrequent)
Paranoia
▲ Personality changes (8%)
Phobic disorder (Infrequent)
Sociopathy (Infrequent)
▲ Speech difficulties (2% to 7%)
▲ Speech disturbances (2% to 7%)
Stupor (Infrequent)
Stuttering (Infrequent)
Suicide, attempt of (Infrequent)
Thinking abnormality

Zyrtec Chewable Tablets
Agitation (Less than 2%)
Anxiety (Less than 2%)
Confusion (Less than 2%)
Depersonalization (Less than 2%)
Depression (Less than 2%)
Emotional lability (Less than 2%)
Euphoria (Less than 2%)
Hallucinations (Rare)
▲ Insomnia (Less than 2% to 9%)
Irritability
Libido, decreased (Less than 2%)
Mental performance, impairment (Less than 2%)
Nervousness (Less than 2%)
Sleep disturbances (Less than 2%)
Suicidal ideation (Rare)
Thinking abnormality (Less than 2%)

Zyrtec Syrup
Agitation (Less than 2%)
Anxiety (Less than 2%)
Confusion (Less than 2%)
Depersonalization (Less than 2%)
Depression (Less than 2%)
Emotional lability (Less than 2%)
Euphoria (Less than 2%)
Hallucinations (Rare)
▲ Insomnia (Less than 2% to 9%)
Irritability
Libido, decreased (Less than 2%)
Mental performance, impairment (Less than 2%)
Nervousness (Less than 2%)
Sleep disturbances (Less than 2%)
Suicidal ideation (Rare)
Thinking abnormality (Less than 2%)

Zyrtec Tablets
Agitation (Less than 2%)
Anxiety (Less than 2%)

Confusion (Less than 2%)
Depersonalization (Less than 2%)
Depression (Less than 2%)
Emotional lability (Less than 2%)
Euphoria (Less than 2%)
Hallucinations (Rare)
▲ Insomnia (Less than 2% to 9%)
Irritability
Libido, decreased (Less than 2%)
Mental performance, impairment
  (Less than 2%)
Nervousness (Less than 2%)
Sleep disturbances (Less than 2%)
Suicidal ideation (Rare)
Thinking abnormality (Less than 2%)

Zyrtec-D 12 Hour Extended Release Tablets

Agitation (Less than 2%)
Anxiety (Less than 2%)
CNS stimulation
Confusion (Less than 2%)
Depersonalization (Less than 2%)
Depression (Less than 2%)
Emotional lability (Less than 2%)
Euphoria (Less than 2%)

Excitability
Fear
Hallucinations
▲ Insomnia (4%)
Libido, decreased (Less than 2%)
Mental performance, impairment
  (Less than 2%)
Nervousness (Less than 2%)
Sleep disturbances (Less than 2%)
Suicidal ideation (Rare)
Tenseness
Thinking abnormality (Less than 2%)

Zyvox for Oral Suspension

Cognitive dysfunction
Insomnia (2.5%)
Serotonin syndrome

Zyvox Injection

Cognitive dysfunction
Insomnia (2.5%)
Serotonin syndrome

Zyvox Tablets

Cognitive dysfunction
Insomnia (2.5%)
Serotonin syndrome

Section 6

Psychotropic Herbs and Supplements

Various herbs and nutritional supplements are commonly used to relieve a variety of mental and emotional problems, ranging from memory loss to nervousness and depression. The profiles in this section describe the verified effects of these products, as well as other claims made by their proponents. Also included is a brief discussion of their proposed mechanism of action and the contraindications, precautions, and potential interactions associated with their use. Information on use in pregnancy, typical dosage, and the effects of overdosage can be found as well. The profiles are organized alphabetically by the substance's most commonly used name.

The information in these profiles is drawn from in-depth monographs in two alternative medicine handbooks published by *Physicians' Desk Reference®—PDR® for Herbal Medicines* and *PDR® for Nutritional Supplements*.

5-HTP

Why people take it

5-HTP (5-hydroxytryptophan) is valued primarily for its effect on depression. In one carefully designed study, it was found to work slightly better than the serotonin-boosting drug fluvoxamine. Other trials, however, have been less encouraging.

5-HTP has also been used as a weight-loss aid. In one carefully controlled clinical trial—and again in a follow-up study—it trimmed 5 percent off the subjects' body weight in a matter of weeks.

Although more research is needed, 5-HTP also seems to act as a mild painkiller. Clinical studies have shown it to be helpful for treating insomnia, fibromyalgia, and chronic tension headache.

What it is; how it works

As the name suggests, 5-HTP is a chemical cousin of the amino acid tryptophan. In fact, the body needs tryptophan to make 5-HTP, which is then converted to serotonin in the brain. Scientists believe it is this conversion that accounts for the antidepressant effects of 5-HTP.

5-HTP is commercially derived from the seeds of an African plant. Small amounts are also found in food, including bananas, tomatoes, plums, avocados, eggplant, walnuts, and pineapples.

Avoid if...

5-HTP should be strictly avoided by anyone with carcinoid tumors (small growths usually found in the intestinal tract). It is not recommended for people with heart disease, chest pain, or high blood pressure, as well as those who have suffered heart attacks. It should not be taken by patients who show signs of an allergic reaction to any component of the supplement. It should also be avoided during treatment with, or within 2 weeks of stopping, a drug classified as an MAO inhibitor, such as the antidepressants Nardil and Parnate.

Special cautions

A severe, life-threatening condition known as eosinophilia-myalgia syndrome (EMS) has been reported in a few people taking 5-HTP. Marked by muscle pain and excessive white blood cell counts, the syndrome has been linked to contaminants in the 5-HTP preparation, rather than 5-HTP itself. Switching preparations in one group of patients resolved the problem.

Supplemental 5-HTP has been know to cause side effects such as nausea, diarrhea, loss of appetite, vomiting, difficulty breathing, and irregular heartbeat. In high doses it can also cause neurological problems such as dilated pupils, abnormally sensitive reflexes, loss of muscle coordination, and blurred vision.

Possible drug interactions

Remember that 5-HTP should never be used while taking a prescription MAO inhibitor such as Nardil or Parnate, or within 2 weeks of stopping an MAO inhibitor. At least in theory, a dangerous interaction is possible.

It's also best to avoid combining 5-HTP with serotonin-boosting drugs such as Luvox and the antidepressant medications Paxil, Prozac, Serzone, and Zoloft. The excessive levels of serotonin that may result can trigger sweating, tremors, flushing, confusion, and agitation. Likewise, 5-HTP should not be combined with tricyclic antidepressants such as Elavil and Tofranil or with the antidepressant herb St. John's wort.

Similarly, patients should not use 5-HTP while taking migraine drugs such as Amerge, Imitrex, and Zomig, since the combination could increase the risk of adverse reactions. In addition, combining 5-HTP with the migraine remedy Sansert reduces its effectiveness; and 5-HTP can also decrease the effectiveness of the antihistamine Periactin.

Patients should also be aware that certain drugs, such as the blood pressure drugs Aldomet and Dibenzyline, inhibit 5-HTP's effect, while Carbidopa enhances its delivery to the brain.

Special information about pregnancy and breastfeeding

Pregnant women and nursing mothers should not take 5-HTP.

Available preparations and dosage

Because of its potential side effects, experts advise against taking 5-HTP by itself. In Europe, doctors prescribe 5-HTP along with carbidopa, which suppresses the conversion of 5-HTP to serotonin outside the brain, reducing serotonin-induced side effects in the body. High daily doses of 100 milligrams to 2 grams of 5-HTP are needed to gain the desired effects; and only when taken with carbidopa are such doses considered reasonably safe. The lower doses of 5-HTP found in dietary supplements are not likely to have any effect.

Overdosage

No overdoses have been reported. However, the first symptoms of overdose would likely be those of excessive serotonin levels, such as sweating, tremors, flushing, confusion, agitation, and rapid heartbeat. Untreated, the patient's condition could progress to coma, seizures, and death. If an overdose is suspected, seek medical help immediately.

Acetylcysteine

Why people take it

Acetylcysteine—also known as N-acetylcysteine or NAC—is available as a supplement and as a prescription drug. Doctors use it to treat acetaminophen overdose. They also prescribe it to thin the excess mucus that occurs with certain lung disorders, such as acute and chronic bronchitis.

As a nutritional supplement, acetylcysteine shows potential as a treatment for age-related memory loss, and may be helpful for a broad range of disorders. The evidence so far shows that it is an effective treatment for chronic obstructive pulmonary disease. Preliminary studies suggest supplemental acetylcysteine may be helpful for treating, and possibly preventing, heart disease. It also shows promise in treating diabetes, certain cancers, and immune system disorders, although more studies are needed.

Because of its liver-protecting abilities, some researchers suggest that acetylcysteine could help treat infectious liver diseases such as hepatitis C, although this remains to be seen.

What it is; how it works

Acetylcysteine is derived from the amino acid L-cysteine. It is preferred over L-cysteine because it is more stable and possibly better absorbed. As a drug, acetylcysteine is well known for its ability to increase liver stores of the antioxidant glutathione, which is why it's routinely given to treat liver damage due to acetaminophen poisoning. This versatile drug is also available as an inhalant called Mucomyst, which binds to mucus proteins, making the gluey substance more watery.

When given as a supplement, acetylcysteine may protect certain cells from damage and even death by increasing levels of L-cysteine and glutathione. Researchers believe this is why it may be helpful for diabetes, heart disease, and cancer, among other things. One study, however, suggested that acetylcysteine might have actually caused DNA damage in certain cells, leading the researchers to believe that the supplement may promote some cancers while inhibiting others.

Avoid if...

There are no known reasons to avoid acetylcysteine at recommended dosages.

Special cautions

Acetylcysteine may be harmful if given early in the treatment of critically ill patients and should therefore be used cautiously, if at all. Caution is also advised for patients with a history of peptic ulcers, since the supplement's mucus-thinning properties could disrupt the stomach's protective mucosal lining. In addition, acetylcysteine metabolism is reduced in patients with chronic liver disease as well as in preterm newborns.

Potential side effects of acetylcysteine include nausea, vomiting, diarrhea, headaches, and rashes. It could also interfere with certain tests for diabetes.

There is a small possibility that acetylcysteine could cause kidney stones. Patients who tend to form kidney stones, especially those caused by excess cystine, should not take this supplement.

Possible drug interactions
Acetylcysteine can cause headaches in those taking nitrates for the treatment of chest pain. It could also decrease blood levels of certain anti-seizure drugs such as Tegretol and Carbatrol.

Special information about pregnancy and breastfeeding
Pregnant women should use acetylcysteine only if prescribed by a doctor, and nursing mothers should avoid the supplement entirely.

Available preparations and dosage
When taking a prescription form of acetylcysteine such as Mucomyst, patients should follow their doctor's instructions.

As a dietary supplement, the usual dose is 600 milligrams, taken anywhere from once daily to 3 times a day. It is available in capsule and tablet form. Common brands include NAC Fuel by TwinLab and N-A-C Sustain by Jarrow Formulas. Various generic brands are also available. Patients should follow the manufacturer's labeling whenever possible.

An important note: Patients should be sure to drink at least 6 to 8 glasses of water a day to prevent the formation of kidney stones.

Overdosage
No information on overdosage with oral supplements is available. When given intravenously for acetaminophen poisoning, high doses can produce symptoms similar to those of a severe allergic reaction, including swelling of the face and throat and heart and blood pressure irregularities.

Acetyl-L-Carnitine

Why people take it
Acetyl-L-carnitine may help slow the progression of Alzheimer's disease in some patients, especially younger ones. In one of its larger clinical trials, researchers found that acetyl-L-carnitine provided the most benefit for patients less than 62 years old. Other, smaller studies showed benefits for patients with mild to moderate symptoms. None of the studies, however, found that the supplement could reverse Alzheimer's disease.

Acetyl-L-carnitine also shows some promise in treating stroke, diabetes-related nerve disorders, and Down's syndrome. Although more research is needed, preliminary evidence suggests it may also help slow the aging process, improve depression in the elderly, treat the mental decline associated with alcoholism, and improve sperm motility.

What it is; how it works

Acetyl-L-carnitine is a close chemical relative of the amino acid compound L-carnitine. The body makes acetyl-L-carnitine in the brain, liver, and kidneys. It also occurs naturally in meat and dairy products.

Acetyl-L-carnitine helps the body's cells produce energy. It also promotes production of acetylcholine, a chemical messenger that plays a role in memory and learning. In lab studies, acetyl-L-carnitine also appears to protect cells from the damage that often occurs during aging.

Researchers aren't sure how acetyl-L-carnitine helps improve memory and nerve disorders. Some speculate it may boost brain levels of acetylcholine, which is deficient in patients with age-related dementias like Alzheimer's. Others suggest it may slow the death of nerve cells in the brain and other parts of the body.

Avoid if...

There are no known reasons to avoid acetyl-L-carnitine at recommended dosages.

Special cautions

People with seizure disorders should take acetyl-L-carnitine only under a doctor's supervision. Although the incidence is rare, a few patients have experienced an increase in the number or severity of their seizures while taking this supplement.

Caregivers of patients with Alzheimer's should be aware that acetyl-L-carnitine has caused increased agitation in some patients.

Acetyl-L-carnitine may also cause stomach upsets, including nausea, vomiting, diarrhea, and cramping.

Possible drug interactions

Certain drugs may cause a decrease in the body's acetyl-L-carnitine levels. These include the anti-HIV drugs Videx, Hivid, and Zerit, and anti-seizure drugs such as Depakote. Antibiotics that contain pivalic acid, such as Spectracef, may also decrease acetyl-L-carnitine levels, although this shouldn't pose a problem if treatment is only for a short period.

Special information about pregnancy and breastfeeding

Because the safety of acetyl-L-carnitine supplements during pregnancy hasn't been tested, women who are pregnant or breastfeeding should not take this substance.

Available preparations and dosage

Typical dosages range from 500 milligrams to 2 grams daily, given in several smaller doses. Some studies, including those for Alzheimer's, used 3 grams a day. There is no consensus on how long treatment must continue before results are observed. Patients should follow the manufacturer's labeling whenever available.

Acetyl-L-carnitine is available in tablets and capsules from various companies, including TwinLab, Now Foods, and Jarrow Formulas. It is also a common ingredient in "brain boosting" supplements.

Overdosage
There are no reports of overdosage.

Alpha-GPC

Why people take it
Alpha-GPC (L-alpha-glycerylphosphorylcholine) is promoted as a "cognitive enhancer" that helps treat age-related memory disorders, including Alzheimer's disease and the aftereffects of stroke. It is also popular among athletes and bodybuilders because of its reputed ability to boost levels of human growth hormone. Although some preliminary research does support these claims, more convincing evidence is needed before this supplement can be considered effective.

What it is; how it works
Alpha-GPC is made from a naturally occurring soybean fat known as lecithin. It is closely related to phosphatidylcholine and serves a similar purpose, acting as a source of the essential nutrient choline. (Alpha-GPC is 40 percent choline.) In theory, the body could use this to make acetylcholine, a chemical messenger that plays a role in memory and learning and also encourages the body to secrete human growth hormone.

Whether alpha-GPC does indeed get converted into acetylcholine, and how much of it actually reaches the brain, is unknown. Animal studies suggest that the conversion does occur, but researchers aren't certain whether this would have any therapeutic effect on the body. Further clinical studies, as well as safety data, are needed to confirm any potential benefits of using this supplement.

Avoid if...
Unless patients have an allergic reaction, there are no known reasons to avoid alpha-GPC supplements.

Special cautions
There are no reported precautions for alpha-GPC, although it should probably not be given to children due to the lack of safety data.

Possible drug interactions
There are no known drug interactions.

Special information about pregnancy and breastfeeding
Due to the lack of safety data, pregnant and breastfeeding women should not take alpha-GPC.

Available preparations and dosage
Typical daily dosages range from 500 milligrams to 1 gram. No information is available on how long treatment should last. Patients should follow the manufacturer's labeling whenever available.

Overdosage
No information on overdosage is available.

Arginine Pyroglutamate

Why people take it
Preliminary research suggests that arginine pyroglutamate may help improve verbal memory in the elderly. One study also found that it may be useful for treating the memory problems associated with chronic alcohol abuse. Definitive evidence for both claims, however, is still lacking.

This supplement is also used by some bodybuilders because the arginine it contains tends to promote the production of human growth hormone. Enthusiasts believe this hormone builds muscle mass and promotes endurance. Many experts, however, warn against adult use of human growth hormone—or substances that promote its release.

What it is; how it works
Arginine pyroglutamate is a water-soluble molecule made from the naturally occurring acids L-arginine and pyroglutamate. The supplement is absorbed by the small intestine, where its two acids are split and sent to various metabolic pathways in the body. Some of the pyroglutamate appears to enter the brain, although more studies are needed to confirm this.

Scientists aren't sure how arginine pyroglutamate may help memory problems, but it appears to be structurally related to the experimental drug piracetam. Piracetam has been studied in Europe as a possible "cognitive enhancer," although clinical trials give mixed results on its effectiveness. Piracetam seems to enhance membrane fluidity in the brain and also appears to interact with glutamate receptors in the brain. Some researchers speculate that arginine pyroglutamate may work in a similar fashion.

In addition to stimulating the production of human growth hormone, the arginine in this compound serves as raw material for nitric oxide, one of the factors that promotes the dilation of blood vessels.

Avoid if...
Unless patients have an allergic reaction, there are no known reasons to completely avoid arginine pyroglutamate. However, due to its impact on

the production of human growth hormone, it is not recommended for children, pregnant women, or nursing mothers.

Special cautions

Arginine pyroglutamate may cause minor stomach upsets. Because the arginine it contains affects insulin secretion, people with diabetes should take this compound with care. Arginine may also aggravate schizophrenia. Patients with this problem would be wise to avoid the substance.

Possible drug interactions

Because arginine tends to dilate blood vessels, it's best to avoid combining this supplement with Viagra, heart medicines such as nitroglycerin, and some blood pressure medicines. Patients should also check with their doctor before combining arginine pyroglutamate with any psychotropic medication.

Special information about pregnancy and breastfeeding

Due to its impact on human growth hormone, pregnant and breastfeeding women should not take arginine pyroglutamate.

Available preparations and dosage

Typical dosages range from 500 milligrams to 1,000 milligrams a day. A 500-milligram dose delivers about 150 milligrams of L-arginine and 350 milligrams of pyroglutamate. Patients should follow the manufacturer's labeling whenever available.

Overdosage

No information on overdosage is available.

Bugleweed

Latin name: Lycopus virginicus
Other names: Gypsywort, Sweet Bugle, Water Bugle, Virginia Water Horehound

Why people take it

Bugleweed is used in cases of mildly overactive thyroid, a condition which often leads to nervousness and insomnia. Bugleweed also relieves tension and pain in the breast.

What it is; how it works

Bugleweed does its work by inhibiting the action of thyroid hormones and the reproductive hormones associated with the menstrual cycle. It also reduces levels of prolactin, the hormone that triggers breast milk production.

The herb is a creeping perennial that grows to about 2 feet in height and has a mint-like smell. It was discovered on the banks of streams in

Virginia, but now grows throughout North America. A closely related plant called Gypsywort is found in Europe. Bugleweed's medicinal value lies in its fresh or dried above-ground parts collected during the flowering season.

Avoid if...

Bugleweed should not be used by people with thyroid insufficiency, those taking a thyroid medication, or anyone who will be undergoing a diagnostic test that employs radioactive isotopes.

Special cautions

Warn patients against stopping use of this herb abruptly. This could lead to excessive thyroid activity and symptoms such as breast pain.

Possible drug interactions

Do not use bugleweed if you are taking any thyroid medications.

Special information about pregnancy and breastfeeding

No harmful effects are known.

Available preparations and dosage

Bugleweed is available as a crushed dry herb, as a freshly pressed juice, and in liquid extract form. The dried herb may be used to make tea.

The best dosage of bugleweed varies according to the patient's age and weight. The daily dosage for an adult usually lies between 1 and 2 grams of bugleweed for tea. Liquid extracts should supply approximately 20 milligrams of the active ingredient.

Overdosage

Extremely high doses of bugleweed can cause enlargement of the thyroid gland. Suddenly stopping use of the herb can make the problem worse.

CDP-Choline

Why people take it

Touted as a stronger type of choline (see separate entry), CDP-choline is said to offer many of the same benefits. Like choline, it may sharpen the memory and boost learning, two traits that might help stall aging in the brain. Also like choline, it promises to alleviate some movement disorders. It has been tested in people who have trouble carrying out voluntary movements such as walking—people with Parkinson's disease, for example. And it has also been studied as a treatment for involuntary movements such as the continual chewing or writhing motions (called *tardive dyskinesia*) occasionally triggered by long-term use of antipsychotic drugs. In addition, some evidence hints that it may be useful for treating stroke, brain injury, and vision problems.

Unfortunately, results to date have been less than spectacular. A number of studies have detected small improvements when people with Alzheimer's disease, head injury, or tardive dyskinesia were treated with large doses of the substance. Minor benefits have also been observed in studies of people with multi-infarct dementia or stroke. Likewise, some people with Parkinson's disease have enjoyed small improvements in their symptoms when CDP-choline was added to their regular drug regimen. On balance, though, experts agree that bigger and better studies are needed before CDP-choline can win a passing grade.

(Note, however, that although CDP-choline may still be considered experimental in the U.S., it's sold widely under a variety of brand names in Europe and Japan for treatment of all the disorders discussed above.)

What it is; how it works

Routinely present throughout the body, CDP-choline is a necessary ingredient in the production of compounds known as phospholipids, especially the phospholipid known as phosphatidylcholine. (See separate entry for more on the use of this compound as a dietary supplement.) In turn, phosphatidylcholine and other phospholipids are used to manufacture cell membranes, the barriers protecting the intricate machinery that allows cells to function properly.

Some research suggests that CDP-choline, like other forms of choline, boosts production of acetylcholine, a chemical messenger (neurotransmitter) that's deficient in the brains of people with Alzheimer's disease. Other studies indicate that the drug promotes formation and repair of cell membranes, thereby limiting nerve damage and aiding in recovery from stroke and head injury. To some degree, CDP-choline may also increase the circulation in the brain. At this point, however, all of these possible effects need further verification.

Avoid if...

Because of its potential impact on neurotransmitters, patients who suffer from bipolar disorder or Parkinson's disease should check with their doctor before using CDP-choline. The product should not be used by patients who are allergic to choline. It is also unwise to give it to children due to the lack of safety data.

Special cautions

People in research studies have taken as much as 1,000 milligrams of CDP-choline per day with few ill effects. The most common complaints have been gastrointestinal reactions (nausea, vomiting, diarrhea, stomach pain), dizziness, rash, headache, and fatigue. A small number of people have suffered low blood pressure and changes in heart rate after taking CDP-choline.

Possible drug interactions

CDP-choline could theoretically interfere with the action of drugs that work by blocking the effect of acetylcholine (for example, the antinausea medication scopolamine). Patients who are taking such drugs should check with their doctor before using CDP-choline.

Special information about pregnancy and breastfeeding

Because the safety of CDP-choline supplements during pregnancy hasn't been evaluated, it's best for pregnant and breastfeeding women to avoid them.

Available preparations and dosage

Typically, CDP-choline is sold in capsule form in strengths of 200 to 250 milligrams. Daily dosages of 500 to 2,000 milligrams are typical. Patients should follow the manufacturer's labeling whenever available.

Overdosage

No information on overdosage is available.

Choline

Why people take it

Choline is a vitamin-like compound that has recently gained acceptance as an essential nutrient. It is so important, in fact, that the National Academy of Sciences has increased the recommended intake for pregnant and nursing women in order to ensure normal brain development in the baby. Although the body can produce a certain amount of choline on its own, we also need to get an adequate supply from food. Studies have found that a dietary deficiency can lead to liver and kidney disorders, high blood pressure, and heart disease.

Choline is one of the building blocks of acetylcholine, a key chemical messenger in the nervous system. This fact has led researchers to study it for a wide variety of neurologic disorders, including the tremors and rigidity of Parkinson's disease, the memory loss of Alzheimer's disease, and the involuntary movements of tardive dyskinesia and Huntington's disease.

Choline shows promise as a way to control mood swings and reduce memory loss. Increases in acetylcholine in the brain seem to improve mood, alertness, and mental energy, while low levels are linked to depression and lack of concentration. Many people who use choline notice an improvement in overall disposition. Athletes who take choline-based supplements report greater energy and less fatigue. And researchers have also found that choline boosts the mood of at least some Alzheimer's patients. (Choline will not, however, cure Alzheimer's, though it might play a role in staving it off.)

Choline is also reported to help prevent or treat liver disorders such as cirrhosis, fatty liver, hepatitis, and damage due to drugs or toxic substances. In addition, it may confer some benefit to those with eczema, kidney and gallbladder disorders, and manic depression. It also appears to have some positive impact on cholesterol levels, although not to the extent of two related compounds, phosphatidylcholine and lecithin.

What it is; how it works
Closely related to the B-complex family of vitamins, choline is found in all living cells, where it supports the integrity of cell membranes. In addition to its role in the production of acetylcholine, it aids in the transport of fats into the body's cells. An adequate supply of choline is essential for proper liver function. It is also needed to hold down levels of the amino acid homocysteine—which plays a role in heart disease.

Avoid if...
People suffering from ulcers should avoid choline supplements, since they can increase stomach acid. And because of its potential impact on neurotransmitters, patients who have manic depression or Parkinson's disease should check with their doctor before using choline.

Special cautions
Choline is generally safe and nontoxic even at high levels, although megadoses are usually reserved for treating manic depression and other serious psychiatric disorders. High doses (more than 3.5 grams a day) can be counterproductive, actually causing depression in some people, and can lead to a fishy body odor and other side effects such as dizziness, low blood pressure, excessive sweating, nausea, diarrhea, and abdominal cramps. Excess consumption can also overstimulate muscles, leading to tightening in the shoulders and neck and, ultimately, a tension headache.

Certain patients should be particularly cautious of high doses, including those with liver or kidney disease, depression, Parkinson's disease, and trimethylaminuria (a rare genetic disorder that interferes with choline metabolism).

Possible drug interactions
Choline could theoretically interfere with the action of drugs that work by blocking the effect of acetylcholine (for example, the antinausea medication scopolamine). It's best to check with the doctor before combining choline with such drugs.

On the other hand, the anticancer drug methotrexate could interfere with choline metabolism and possibly block its beneficial effects. Animal studies show that choline supplementation may help offset this problem.

Special information about pregnancy and breastfeeding
For healthy women who eat a balanced diet, choline supplements are usually unnecessary during pregnancy and breastfeeding.

Available preparations and dosage
The new RDI for choline ranges from 425 to 550 milligrams per day for adults. Few people suffer an outright deficiency, since Americans' average dietary intake ranges from 500 to 1,000 milligrams daily. However, since many of the foods richest in choline, such as egg yolks and liver, are also high in cholesterol, intake may be falling among people who watch their cholesterol levels.

Choline is available as tablets, capsules, softgels, powder, and liquids. The different forms of Choline (bitartrate, chloride, and dihydrogencitate) vary in potency from 36 to 75 percent choline. The optimal daily supplemental dose of choline is often pegged at 250 to 350 milligrams, although some studies have used as much as 1,200 milligrams. To lower homocysteine levels, choline requires the vitamins B_6, B_{12}, and folic acid. Aside from eggs and liver, good dietary sources of choline are wheat germ, lentils, peanuts, soybeans, iceberg lettuce, cabbage, and cauliflower. Supplements such as lecithin and phosphatidylcholine supply significant amounts of basic choline. It's also found in brewer's yeast, and is often included in B-complex and multinutrient vitamins or sold in combination with vitamin B_6 or inositol. It should be taken with meals.

Overdosage
A dose of 200 grams or more (100 times the typical dose) could prove dangerous. Sustained megadoses of 3,500 milligrams daily or more tend to cause muscle stiffness and digestive upsets.

DHA

Why people take it
DHA (docosahexaenoic acid) is an essential fatty acid that has piqued interest in the medical community due to its abundant presence in fish oil (see separate entry). Researchers suspect that DHA supplements could prove useful for treating certain brain and mood disorders. DHA deficiencies have been noted in people with attention deficit disorder, dyslexia, depression, age-related mental decline, and Alzheimer's disease. DHA levels are also inadequate in those suffering from postpartum depression or the cognitive decline associated with alcoholism. In addition, DHA has gained a reputation as a "brain booster." Japanese students, for example, take DHA supplements to improve their performance on exams.

Researchers are also studying DHA as a potential treatment for vision disorders such as age-related macular degeneration, and for certain serious congenital disorders such as cystic fibrosis. Like the fish oil in which it's found, DHA is also used to reduce triglyceride levels and protect against heart disease

What it is; how it works

One of the two omega-3 fatty acids found in fish oil, DHA is essential for proper brain and eye development in infants. DHA is abundant in breast milk, and many studies have linked breast-feeding to better vision and higher IQ in children, particularly those born prematurely. Scientists in the U.S. are still debating whether adding DHA to commercial infant formulas confers similar benefits, but the World Health Organization already recommends it. In fact, DHA-enriched formulas are widely available in Japan and countries throughout Europe, and were finally approved for use in the U.S. in 2001.

The science backing DHA supplementation for children and adults is far more questionable. While most nutritionists agree that it's important to get enough omega-3 fats from the diet, the value of supplements is unknown. In theory, DHA could be helpful for various psychiatric disorders because it's one of the main fatty acids in brain and eye tissue, and it appears to be necessary for proper brain-cell signaling. However, most of the research is preliminary, and many of the findings contradict each other. Although some studies, for example, have revealed low DHA levels in people with attention deficit disorders and Alzheimer's disease, clinical trials of DHA supplements failed to improve these conditions.

Avoid if...

Because of possible blood-thinning effects, DHA supplements should not be used by patients who have a bleeding disorder such as hemophilia or a tendency to hemorrhage.

Special cautions

There have been no reports of serious reactions, even in those taking up to 6 grams of DHA a day for 3 months. Potential minor side effects include a fishy odor or taste, belching, upset stomach, nausea, and diarrhea. Infants and children should not take DHA supplements unless monitored by a physician.

Because DHA supplements may slightly increase the risk of hemorrhage, patients should stop taking them before any type of surgery. It is also advisable to check the Special Cautions in the entry on Fish Oil. In theory, the same warnings could apply to DHA supplements.

Possible drug interactions

There have been no reported interactions to date. But patients who are taking a blood-thinning drug such as aspirin or Coumadin should still check with their doctor before taking DHA supplements, which could further thin the blood. Increased bleeding could also occur if DHA is taken with supplemental garlic or the herb ginkgo. Possible signs of an interaction could include increased bruising and nosebleeds.

Special information about pregnancy and breastfeeding
Pregnant and breastfeeding women should check with their doctor before using DHA supplements.

Available preparations and dosage
DHA supplements are made from fish or algae and are available in capsule form; a common brand is Neuromins. Typical dosages for pregnant and nursing women are 100 to 200 milligrams a day. The dosages needed to lower triglyceride levels are higher, ranging from 1 to 4 grams a day. DHA is also found in certain infant formulas and in specially raised eggs.

Patients should choose preparations that contain vitamin E to prevent oxidation of the easily damaged oil; they should also take a little extra vitamin E to prevent oxidation within the body. To prevent stomach upset, DHA supplements should be taken with meals.

Overdosage
No information on overdosage is available.

DHEA

Why people take it
Whether or not DHEA (dehydroepiandrosterone) should be taken at all as an unregulated over-the-counter supplement is a controversial issue. There is evidence that this steroid can improve feelings of well-being and increase sexual satisfaction—but only in people whose adrenal glands are functioning poorly. There are also preliminary results indicating that it may have a beneficial effect on some people with major depression.

Much of the controversy arises because DHEA is being promoted as a cure for many other ailments and has taken on the reputation of an anti-aging remedy—kind of a modern-day fountain of youth. Advocates claim that it can encourage weight loss; boost sex drive and the immune system; enhance mood, memory, and energy; and reverse the aging process. Some proponents even suggest using it as an adjunct to conventional cancer therapy. And a number of anti-aging clinics recommend taking it as early as your 40's or 50's to fight off old age and remain biologically young. Athletes take it in large doses to enhance their performance. However, much of the research behind these claims was done on laboratory animals, and experts caution that the results of such studies cannot be translated to humans. The long-term effects of DHEA supplementation are not known and since it is a powerful hormone, it should be used with great caution and only under a doctor's supervision.

What it is; how it works

DHEA is a steroid hormone produced primarily by the adrenal glands. It is the most abundant hormone in the body, with the highest concentrations found in the brain. The only known function of DHEA is as a precursor hormone, meaning that it is a source material which the body converts into other hormones, such as estrogen and testosterone. It peaks in production by the age of 25 and gradually declines until, by age 70, levels may be more than 80 percent below their earlier highs.

Low DHEA levels have been associated with certain diseases, such as Alzheimer's, cancer, diabetes, multiple sclerosis, lupus, and other immune function disorders. For this reason, researchers have been tempted to speculate that supplementation with a synthetic form of DHEA could reverse these diseases, much like hormone replacement therapy reduces some of the symptoms of menopause by returning the hormone balance to a premenopausal state. However, it has not yet been proven that either the diseases or the aging process itself are a result of lowered levels of DHEA, and it is not yet clear whether using DHEA is helpful or, in the long run, harmful.

Despite all this, there are physicians who recommend use of this hormone to treat a variety of ailments or combat the effects of aging. Anyone who decides to try DHEA should seek out a qualified physician willing to plan and monitor their treatment.

Avoid if...

DHEA should not be used by patients who have a hormone-related cancer—or a family history of one—including breast, cervical, uterine, ovarian, and prostate cancers. The hormone should also not be given to children.

Special cautions

DHEA has been known to cause acne, facial hair growth, and deepening of the voice in some women, and there are reports of breast enlargement in men taking high doses, probably because it triggers hormone production. The hormone may also lower levels of "good" HDL cholesterol and raise levels of cancer-promoting hormones. There have been a few reports of DHEA-related hepatitis and insulin resistance.

Possible drug interactions

Natural DHEA levels may be boosted by certain drugs, including Xanax, Cardizem, testosterone, and the sports supplement androstenedione. Adding even more DHEA through supplementation increases the risk of side effects.

Certain other drugs tend to lower natural DHEA levels. Drugs in this category include Danocrine (used to treat endometriosis), corticosteroids, insulin, and morphine.

Special information about pregnancy and breastfeeding
Because of its hormonal effects, DHEA should not be used during pregnancy or while breastfeeding.

Available preparations and dosage
DHEA is available in capsule, tablet, cream, and spray form in strengths ranging from 5 milligrams to 200 milligrams. The typical daily dose is 25 to 50 milligrams.

Dosage should be set by a physician following a blood test or saliva test can tell if a true deficiency exists and how much, if any, supplemental DHEA is needed. Individuals taking DHEA will also periodically need to visit their doctor to have their blood levels monitored and the dosage adjusted accordingly.

Overdosage
No information on overdosage is available.

DL-Phenylalanine

Why people take it
An "essential" amino acid that the body can't manufacture on its own, phenylalanine is one of the raw materials for three of the nervous system's most important chemical messengers: dopamine, epinephrine, and norepinephrine. The body can also convert it to phenylethylamine, a mood-boosting substance that's said to have pain-relieving effects as well.

In light of these properties, phenylalanine has been proposed as a treatment for depression, Parkinson's disease, and chronic-pain conditions such as arthritis. Trials for arthritis have yielded conflicting results, but preliminary trials for depression have proved encouraging. Phenylalanine has also been promoted as an appetite suppressant and sexual stimulant, but its effectiveness for these purposes remains unproven.

What it is; how it works
There are two types of phenylalanine: L-phenylalanine and D-phenylalanine. The "L" variety occurs primarily in animal protein and supports production of dopamine, epinephrine, norepinephrine, and the mood elevator phenylethylamine. The "D" form of the substance is typically found in plant protein and blocks an enzyme that degrades enkephalins, a group of natural substances that the body produces to deaden pain.

Because of this action, D-phenylalanine (but not L-phenylalanine) has been proposed as a treatment for chronic pain. L-phenylalanine, on the other hand, is usually taken to relieve depression. The "L" form of the substance has also been suggested as a treatment for vitiligo, a disease characterized by abnormal white blotches of skin due to loss of pigmentation.

D-phenylalanine alone is not available as a nutritional supplement, but both forms are created during the commercial manufacturing process and are typically sold as DL-phenylalanine or DLPA. Products containing only the "L" form are also available. Phenylalanine is also an ingredient of the popular artificial sweetener aspartame.

Avoid if...

Children born without the ability to process phenylalanine can build up dangerous levels of this amino acid, leading to mental retardation, seizures, extreme hyperactivity, and psychosis. Youngsters with this condition—called phenylketonuria—must follow a special diet designed to supply no more phenylalanine than necessary, and must be monitored regularly for excess phenylalanine in the blood.

Special cautions

L-phenylalanine has also been reported to exacerbate involuntary movements (tardive dyskinesia) in schizophrenic patients. Anyone with this disorder should therefore use DL-phenylalanine with extreme caution. Caution is also warranted for people with high blood pressure or an anxiety disorder; phenylalanine tends to aggravate these conditions.

DL-phenylalanine occasionally causes mild nausea, heartburn, or headache. Because it can have significant effects on mood, it's best to use this type of phenylalanine only under a doctor's supervision.

Possible drug interactions

Phenylalanine supplements should never be combined with drugs known as MAO inhibitors, including the antidepressants Nardil and Parnate; a surge in blood pressure could result. It is also best to avoid combining phenylalanine with antipsychotic drugs, since it increases the likelihood of tardive dyskinesia.

On the other hand, taking phenylalanine with the drug Eldepryl may boost the antidepressant activity of both agents.

Special information about pregnancy and breastfeeding

Phenylalanine supplements are not recommended during pregnancy and breastfeeding.

Available preparations and dosage

DL-phenylalanine is available in capsule, tablet, and powder form. Typical dosages range from 375 milligrams to 2.25 grams daily.

Overdosage
There are no reports of overdosage.

Fish Oil

Why people take it

Fish oil is one of those nutritional megastars that holds promise for a wide variety of chronic conditions. The latest buzz focuses on its potential to alleviate symptoms of several serious psychiatric illnesses, including bipolar disorder, schizophrenia, and severe depression. Preliminary research hints that it may also be helpful for warding off Alzheimer's disease and treating attention deficit disorder. Keep in mind, however, that most of this research is still in its infancy, and more definitive answers are needed before fish oil supplements can be recommended.

While the effects of fish oil on the brain are still being investigated, more is known about its benefits for the heart. Rich in omega-3 fatty acids, fish oil seems to help protect against cardiovascular disease. Studies have found that it lowers blood pressure, keeps arteries clear following angioplasty, and reduces the risk of sudden cardiac death, death from heart attack, and stroke. If all that weren't enough, there's some evidence that fish oil could be useful for treating arthritis (particularly rheumatoid arthritis), Crohn's disease, kidney disease, and ulcerative colitis.

What it is; how it works

The two omega-3 fatty acids contained in fish oil are eicosapentaenoic acid (EPA) and docosahexaenoic acid (DHA). These acids are especially prevalent in oily cold-water fish such as cod, tuna, mackerel, herring, and salmon. Because the omega-3s come from algae that are then eaten by krill that in turn are eaten by larger fish, farm-raised fish that have been fed grain alone may contain little or none of these beneficial acids.

Researchers speculate that because Western diets have changed drastically in the last century, Americans may be deficient in omega-3 fatty acids. The brain and nervous system rely on fatty acids like EPA and DHA to regulate cell membrane function. These acids may even play a role in the proper regulation of serotonin, a chemical messenger that has gained fame for its role in depression and other mental illnesses. Indeed, depression rates have soared in recent decades, and global studies show that depression is less likely to occur in countries that consume the most fish. But while the evidence so far is tantalizing, fish oil's effectiveness against psychiatric disorders has yet to be tested in major clinical trials.

In the prevention of heart disease, omega-3s are thought to work by lowering total cholesterol and triglyceride levels, raising "good" HDL cholesterol, and thinning the blood. They lower the level of fibrinogen, the blood clotting factor, and keep blood platelets from becoming too sticky, all of which helps to prevent the buildup of artery-clogging plaque. Fish oil also tends to dilate the blood vessels, which can help to lower blood pressure in those with hypertension.

Some researchers have found that the omega-3s have anti-inflammatory properties that appear to make them helpful in the treatment of arthritis, Crohn's disease, endometriosis, lupus, and ulcerative colitis. In addition, laboratory experiments suggest that these fatty acids may have an anti-cancer effect. They are also being studied for a variety of other disorders, including eczema, psoriasis, and Raynaud's phenomenon.

Avoid if...
Because of their blood-thinning effects, fish oil supplements should be used only with great caution by patients who have a bleeding disorder such as hemophilia or a tendency to hemorrhage.

Special cautions
Although fish oil tends to have beneficial effects on "good" HDL cholesterol and total cholesterol levels, high doses sometimes cause an increase in "bad" LDL cholesterol levels. A few studies have also suggested that fish oil supplements may cause an increase in the blood sugar levels of people with diabetes. Diabetics should discuss use of these supplements with their doctor and closely monitor their blood sugar for any change.

Because fish oil supplements may slightly increase the risk of hemorrhage, patients should stop taking them before any type of surgery. Patients who have had a stroke should check with their doctor before using fish oil. It could be dangerous if the stroke involved bleeding into the brain. Give fish oil supplements to children only under a doctor's supervision.

Potential side effects of fish oil capsules include a fishy odor or taste, belching, upset stomach, nausea, diarrhea, increased bleeding (including nosebleeds), and easy bruising.

To obtain the greatest heart benefits from the fatty acids found in fish and fish oils, patients should follow a low-fat diet.

Possible drug interactions
Patients who are taking a blood-thinning drug such as aspirin or Coumadin should check with their doctor before taking fish oil supplements, which could further thin the blood. Increased bleeding could also occur if fish oil is taken with supplemental garlic or the herb ginkgo. Signs to watch for include easy bruising, nosebleeds, spitting or vomiting up blood, and blood in the stool or urine. Note, however, that these reactions are rare and may be alleviated by reducing the dose of fish oil.

Special information about pregnancy and breastfeeding

Pregnant women and nursing mothers should use fish oil capsules only under a doctor's supervision.

Some types of fish can contain high amounts of mercury, which can hurt a developing baby's brain. The Food and Drug Administration advises pregnant and breastfeeding women, and those who might become pregnant, to avoid shark, swordfish, king mackerel, and tilefish.

Available preparations and dosage

Fish oil is available in liquid, softgel, or capsule form. Most fish oil supplements range in potency from 200 to 400 milligrams of omega-3 acids. Patients should check the labels carefully, since the number of milligrams in each capsule often refers to the total weight rather than its omega-3 content. Patients should choose preparations that contain vitamin E to prevent oxidation of the easily damaged oil; they should also take a little extra vitamin E to prevent oxidation within the body.

Supplements that contain 18 percent EPA and 12 percent DHA are generally considered standard. They should be taken in divided doses, with meals, to prevent stomach upset. Patients should pay attention to expiration dates and refrigerate the package after opening. Some preparations may contain pesticides.

There is no recommended dietary allowance (RDA) for omega-3 fatty acids. When taken to prevent arterial clogging after angioplasty, doses of 4 to 5 grams per day are typical. For arthritis and high blood pressure, doses of 3 grams daily are usually recommended. A dosage of 1 gram a day has been found to have a protective effect on heart attack victims. However, the American Heart Association suggests that it may be better for patients to boost their intake by eating fish 2 or 3 times a week, rather than taking large amounts of supplements. A 7-ounce serving of salmon or bluefish provides 2.4 grams of omega-3 acids. The same serving of herring contains 3.2 grams.

Overdosage

There are no reports of serious adverse effects, even with dosages as high as 15 grams a day taken for prolonged periods of time. However, it's important for patients to make sure they are using fish oil supplements rather than fish liver oils. The latter contain large amounts of vitamins A and D, which can build up in the body until they reach toxic levels. Symptoms of vitamin A toxicity include hair loss, headache, menstrual problems, stiffness, joint pain, weakness, and dry skin. Excessive intake of vitamin D can lead to irreversible kidney and cardiovascular damage.

Gamma-Tocopherol

Why people take it

Gamma-tocopherol is a member of the vitamin E family. Although *alpha*-tocopherol is the best known form of this vitamin, there is preliminary evidence that gamma-tocopherol may be more protective against cardiovascular disease and some cancers. As a form of vitamin E, gamma-tocopherol is also thought to slow the progress of Alzheimer's disease.

What it is; how it works

Gamma-tocopherol is the most common of the tocopherols. It is found in many seeds and nuts, including soybeans, corn, and walnuts, and is the principal tocopherol in the American diet.

Like other forms of vitamin E, gamma-tocopherol is an antioxidant, scavenging the free radicals that cause cellular damage. Researchers believe that it helps to prevent fat buildup in the arteries, protects cells in the artery walls, reduces the risk of blood clots, inhibits the development of certain cancers, and stimulates the immune system.

Avoid if...

Gamma-tocopherol must be avoided by anyone with a hypersensitivity to it. There are no medical conditions that completely preclude its use.

Special cautions

Those on the blood-thinning medication warfarin should be cautious in using high doses of gamma-tocopherol (doses greater than 100 milligrams daily). Also those with vitamin K deficiencies, such as people with liver failure, should be cautious about using high doses. Gamma-tocopherol must also be used cautiously by those with bleeding ulcers and similar bleeding problems, those with a history of hemorrhagic stroke, and those with hemophilia.

To reduce the risk of bleeding problems, people preparing for surgery should stop high-dose gamma-tocopherol supplementation 1 month before the procedure.

There is one study in which high blood levels of gamma-tocopherol was associated with an increased incidence of knee osteoarthritis, especially in African-Americans.

Possible drug interactions

High doses of gamma-tocopherol may boost the effects of blood-thinning drugs, such as aspirin. Some herbs, including garlic and ginkgo, also possess blood-thinning activity and high doses of gamma-tocopherol may enhance their action as well. The following drugs may reduce the impact of gamma-tocopherol:

Cholestyramine (Questran)

Colestipol (Colestid)
Isoniazid (Rifampin)
Mineral oil
Neomycin (Neosporin)
Orlistat (Xenical)
Sucralfate (Carafate)
Alpha-tocopherol
Iron

Vitamin C and selenium may increase the effectiveness of gamma-tocopherol.

Special information about pregnancy and breastfeeding
Since the effects of gamma-tocopherol during pregnancy have not been studied, the safest course is to forego supplementation.

Available preparations and dosage
Typical doses are about 200 milligrams daily.

Overdosage
There are no reports of gamma-tocopherol overdose.

Ginkgo

Latin name: Ginkgo biloba

Why people take it
Ginkgo is generally accepted as a remedy for minor deficits in brain function, such as those that occur with advancing age. It is used to improve concentration and combat short-term memory loss due to clogged arteries in the brain, and to treat dizziness, ringing in the ears, headache, and emotional hypersensitivity accompanied by anxiety. For people with intermittent circulation problems in the legs, it permits longer pain-free walks.

What it is; how it works
Although the ginkgo tree has been around for 200 million years, it's only during the last couple of decades that its true value has been recognized. Active compounds in ginkgo extract improve circulation, discourage clot formation, reinforce the walls of the capillaries, and protect nerve cells from harm when deprived of oxygen. These ingredients also appear to have an antioxidant effect, sparing brain tissue from the damage caused by free radicals. Because the active ingredients are limited to minute quantities in natural ginkgo leaves, only concentrated ginkgo extract is really effective.

The ginkgo tree grows over 100 feet high and can live for hundreds of years. The tree flowers for the first time when it is between 20 and 30 years old. Native to China, Japan, and Korea, it now grows worldwide, and is intensively cultivated in major plantations such as one in Sumter, South Carolina.

Avoid if...
Anyone who has been warned about the possibility of bleeding in the brain should avoid ginkgo. There have been reports of intracranial hemorrhage associated with this herb. It should also be avoided if it causes an allergic reaction.

Special cautions
Taken orally in customary doses, ginkgo is unlikely to have side effects. Spasms, cramps, and mild digestive problems are the most common reactions. On rare occasions, allergic skin problems may occur.

Possible drug interactions
Combining ginkgo with clot-busting drugs, blood-thinners, or aspirin may increase the risk of intracranial bleeding.

Special information about pregnancy and breastfeeding
There is no information available.

Available preparations and dosage
Ginkgo extract is produced in liquid, tablet, and capsule form, in strengths ranging from 30 to 500 milligrams. Tea made from ginkgo leaves, as in traditional Chinese medicine, is too weak to be effective.

A total daily intake of 120 milligrams is usually recommended, typically in three 40-milligram doses spaced throughout the day. Doses of up to 240 milligrams a day are taken by people with severe memory loss.

Strengths of commercial preparations may vary. Follow the manufacturer's labeling whenever available.

Overdosage
A massive overdose can reduce muscle tone, leading to severe weakness. If an overdose is suspected, seek medical attention immediately.

Glycine

Why people take it
In at least one carefully designed clinical trial, high-dose glycine has provided additional relief to schizophrenic patients taking antipsychotic drugs. Glycine has also been used successfully to help alleviate the symptoms of spasticity, primarily in patients with multiple sclerosis; and it has cured seizures caused by an inborn lack of the related amino acid L-serine.

Glycine is one of the many nutritional supplements adopted by body-builders to boost physical performance. Its popularity stems from its role in the formation of creatine, a key ingredient in the chemical reaction that powers muscles. Unfortunately, while there's some evidence that creatine may indeed be helpful during short bursts of physical activity, glycine alone does not seem to have the same effect. In fact, the American Dietetic Association notes that glycine and other supposedly ergogenic (energy-producing) substances may owe their standing more to psychological than to any physical effects.

Studies in laboratory animals suggest that glycine may combat certain types of cancer, including liver tumors and melanoma. Taken with other amino acids, it may also reduce the symptoms of benign prostatic hyperplasia (BPH), although the study suggesting this possibility has never been replicated.

What it is; how it works

Glycine is one of the "nonessential" amino acids that the body can produce for itself whenever they fall short in the diet. It's also available from high-protein foods such as meat, fish, beans, and dairy products.

Glycine combines with two other amino acids—arginine and methionine—to build energy-producing creatine. It also promotes the storage of blood sugar (glucose) in the form of glycogen. Together with the amino acids cysteine and glutamic acid, it produces the protective antioxidant glutathione. And on top of all these duties, it also serves as one of the nervous system's chemical regulators, inhibiting neurological responses in the spinal cord.

Glycine's beneficial effect on schizophrenia is believed to result from its ability to boost nerve impulses transmitted through N-methyl-D-aspartic acid (NMDA) receptors in the brain.

Avoid if...

Extra glycine and other amino acids increase the burden on the liver and kidneys, and should be avoided by anyone who has problems in these areas unless their doctor recommends otherwise.

Special cautions

Even when taken in megadoses, glycine rarely has unwanted side effects. Mild stomach problems are the most likely possibility.

Possible drug interactions

Theoretically glycine may add to the beneficial effects of antispastic drugs such as baclofen, diazepam (Valium), dantrolene (Dantrium), and tizanidine (Zanaflex). No other interactions are known.

Special information about pregnancy and breastfeeding
It's not known whether high levels of glycine are safe during pregnancy. As with any supplement not absolutely necessary for health, it's best to avoid glycine while pregnant or breastfeeding.

Available preparations and dosage
Glycine is available in tablet, capsule, and powder form in doses ranging from 100 to 600 milligrams. Those who use it as a performance-booster take up to 1 gram daily in divided doses. Doses for spasticity are 1 gram per day. Doses used for the management of schizophrenia have ranged from 40 to 90 grams daily.

Overdosage
There are no reports of glycine overdose.

Hops

Latin name: Humulus lupulus

Why people take it
This herb is an accepted remedy for edginess and insomnia. Effectiveness for its other uses—including stimulation of the appetite, increasing the flow of digestive juices, and treating ulcers, skin abrasions, and bladder inflammation—has never been scientifically verified.

What it is; how it works
Hops have long been associated with beer and ale, but the beverage originally called ale in English was made from fermented malt only, and contained no hops. The use of hops probably began in Holland in the early 14th century, and the resulting drink became known as "bier" or "beer." At first, there was much resistance to the use of hops, which was regarded as a "wicked weed that would spoil the taste… and endanger the people."

The plant's medicinal value lies in a set of light yellow scales adjoining the fruit. Compounds in these scales have a sedative effect. Hop tea induces calm, and pillows stuffed with hops assist sleep.

Avoid if...
No known medical conditions preclude the use of hops.

Special cautions
The fresh plant can occasionally cause a reaction. However, when taken at customary dosage levels, hops pose no problems.

Possible drug interactions
There are no known interactions.

Special information about pregnancy and breastfeeding
No harmful effects are known.

Available preparations and dosage
Hops are available in crushed and powdered form, and in commercial preparations for oral administration. A hop tea can be prepared by pouring boiling water over the ground herb and steeping for 10 to 15 minutes.

The usual single dose of Hops is 0.5 grams (about 1 heaping tea-spoonful). The strength of commercial preparations may vary, so follow the manufacturer's directions whenever available.

Store hops protected from light and moisture.

Overdosage
No information on overdosage is available.

Huperzine A

Why people take it
Huperzine A shows considerable promise as a treatment for Alzheimer's disease and age-related memory impairment. Numerous studies suggest that it may be as effective as Cognex and Aricept, two of the prescription drugs currently available for Alzheimer's.

What it is; how it works
Alzheimer's disease is marked by declining activity in certain nerve cells that respond to acetylcholine, one of the key chemical messengers in the brain. Huperzine A, like Cognex and Aricept, inhibits the breakdown of acetylcholine, thereby boosting the amount available to these cells.

Huperzine A is a plant alkaloid derived from the Chinese club moss plant, *Huperzia serrata*. In Chinese folk medicine, this herb has long been used as treatment for fever and inflammation, though there's no scientific evidence that it's effective for these problems.

Avoid if...
Huperzine A has a number of potential cardiac and neurological side effects. It should be avoided by those with seizure disorders, heartbeat irregularities, or asthma. People with irritable bowel disease, inflammatory bowel disease, and malabsorption syndromes should also refrain from using this medication.

Special cautions
Huperzine A has potent pharmacological effects and its long-term safety has not been verified. It should be used only under medical supervision and should never be given to children.

Side effects reported with huperzine A include nausea and diarrhea, sweating, blurred vision, twitching, and dizziness. Other possible effects include vomiting, cramping, asthma attacks, slow or irregular heartbeat, seizures, urinary incontinence, increased urination, and excessive salivation.

Possible drug interactions
Combining huperzine A with other medications that boost acetylcholine levels increases the likelihood of side effects. Drugs in this category include Aricept, Cognex, neostigmine, physostigmine, and pyridostigmine. Side effects are also more likely when huperzine A is taken with drugs that mimic the effects of acetylcholine, such as the bladder stimulant Urecholine.

Special information about pregnancy and breastfeeding
Safety of this medication during pregnancy has not been confirmed. It should be avoided by pregnant women and nursing mothers.

Available preparations and dosage
Huperzine A is available in natural and synthetic forms. The natural substance is three times as potent as its synthetic counterpart. Doses of natural huperzine A used in clinical trials have ranged from 60 to 200 micrograms daily.

Overdosage
There are no reports of huperzine A overdose.

Kava Kava

Latin name: Piper methysticum

Why people take it
In the past, kava kava has been taken for a host of ailments on which it has no appreciable effect, including asthma, arthritis, indigestion, cystitis, syphilis, and gonorrhea. For anxiety and insomnia, it is generally considered a proven remedy. The herb's safety, however, has been questioned by various governmental bodies, including the FDA (see "special cautions").

What it is; how it works
Kava kava has actually been around for centuries in the South Seas, where it's used as a ceremonial beverage. The plant's fleshy underground stem is mildly intoxicating when chewed. Prepared as a nonalcoholic drink, it is said to foster a sense of contentment and well-being, while sharpening the mind, memory, and senses.

Research shows that the active ingredients in kava kava (kava pyrones) do in fact have a calming, sedative effect. They also appear to relax the muscles, relieve spasms, and prevent convulsions. At least two scientific studies have confirmed the herb's ability to significantly reduce symptoms of anxiety. In a third study, researchers rated it as effective as prescription tranquilizers.

Avoid if...

Kava kava should not be used by women who are pregnant or nursing. It should also be avoided by anyone with a depressive disorder; it can deepen a depressed mood. In addition, this herb should not be used by anyone who has a neurological disorder.

Special cautions

Note: The FDA is advising consumers of the potential risk of severe liver injury from the use of dietary supplements containing kava kava. Recent reports from health authorities in Germany, Switzerland, France, Canada, and the United Kingdom have linked kava use to at least 25 cases of liver toxicity, including hepatitis, cirrhosis, and liver failure. Therefore, safety is a concern when taking this herb. Before using kava kava, all patients—especially those with liver disease or liver problems, or persons who are taking drugs that can affect the liver—should consult their doctor first.

Heavy long-term use can also cause an unusual scaly rash, and may lead to unwanted weight loss. This herb should not be taken for more than 3 months without a doctor's approval.

Patients may notice a slightly tired feeling in the mornings when first taking kava kava.

In rare cases, kava kava can cause an allergic reaction, a slight yellowing of the skin, gastrointestinal complaints, impaired or abnormal movement, loss of balance, pupil dilation, and difficulty focusing. Because of the possibility of visual disturbances, it's important to drive with caution while using this herb.

Possible drug interactions

Kava kava should not be combined with other substances that act on the brain, such as alcohol, barbiturates, or other mood-altering drugs. It may increase their effect. Be especially wary of taking it with the tranquilizer Xanax; the combination has caused coma.

Kava kava has an antagonistic effect on dopamine. Patients taking a levodopa-based medication for Parkinson's disease should avoid this herb.

Special information about pregnancy and breastfeeding

Remember, kava kava should be avoided during pregnancy and nursing.

Available preparations and dosage

Commercial extracts are the predominant form of kava kava. The crushed root can also be used. Daily doses delivering between 50 and 240 milligrams of the active ingredients are the customary recommendation. Commercial capsules containing between 150 and 300 milligrams of root extract may be taken twice a day. Because the potency of commercial preparations may vary, follow the manufacturer's directions whenever available. The dosage should be administered with food or liquid.

Overdosage

An overdose is usually signaled by a lack of coordination, followed by tiredness and a tendency to sleep. If an overdose is suspected, seek medical attention immediately.

Lavender

Latin name: Lavandula angustifolia

Why people take it

In Europe, lavender is considered an effective remedy for nervousness, insomnia, nervous stomach, and loss of appetite. It is also used in mineral baths to treat circulatory disorders.

Other uses remain unproven. They include migraine, cramps, asthma, and arthritis. Lavender is used in aromatherapy for sleep induction, and is added to bathwater to help treat poorly healing wounds.

What it is; how it works

Because of its wonderful fragrance, from Roman times onward lavender has always been a popular bath additive. In fact, its name derives from the Latin "lavare" meaning "to wash." Over the centuries, it has been used in a variety of forms, including oil, distilled water, and alcohol solution (tincture). One species, spike lavender, is even an effective insect repellent.

Lavender's medicinal value lies in the essential oil, customarily extracted from the flowers. Taken internally, lavender has been found to stimulate the production and flow of bile. It also has a mildly sedating effect, and gets rid of gas. Used externally, it improves circulation and brings color to the skin.

Avoid if...

No known medical conditions preclude the use of lavender.

Special cautions

Taken at customary dosage levels, lavender presents no problems, although a few people do develop a sensitivity to the oil.

Possible drug interactions
No interactions have been reported.

Special information about pregnancy and breastfeeding
No harmful effects are known.

Available preparations and dosage
Extracts, bath additives, and crushed lavender flowers are all available.

To prepare a bath additive, boil 100 grams (about one-half cup) of lavender in 2 quarts of water, then add to the tub.

The usual daily dose of lavender for internal use is:
Crushed flowers: 3 to 5 grams
Essential oil: 1 to 4 drops

Overdosage
No information on overdosage is available.

Lemon Balm

Latin name: Melissa officinalis
Other names: Balm Mint, Bee Balm, Blue Balm, Cure-all, Garden Balm, Honey Plant, Sweet Balm, Sweet Mary

Why people take it
Lemon balm is officially recognized only for its ability to calm the nerves and promote sleep. In the past it has been taken for a wide variety of problems, including bloating and gas, mood disorders, bronchial inflammation, high blood pressure, palpitations, vomiting, toothache, earache, and headache. However, its effectiveness for these purposes has never been validated by clinical trials.

Applied externally, it has also been used for arthritis, nerve pains, and stiff neck—but again without clinical validation.

What it is; how it works
Lemon balm's medicinal properties have been held in high regard for nearly two millennia. The Roman scholar Pliny believed lemon balm could prevent infection in open wounds (an action that has been clinically proven for balsamic oils in general). The noted 16th century physician Paracelsus believed lemon balm could heal even patients close to death.

Modern research on lemon balm has revealed a mild sedative effect, antibacterial and antiviral properties, and an ability to quell spasms and relieve cramps and gas. Only the plant's leaves are medicinal.

A perennial herb, lemon balm grows up to 3 feet in height. It is native to the east Mediterranean region and west Asia, but is cultivated throughout central Europe. Before flowering, it has a lemon-like taste and smell; and the fresh leaves, in addition to their medicinal applications, are commonly used in cooking.

Avoid if...
No known medical conditions preclude the use of lemon balm.

Special cautions
When taken at customary dosage levels, lemon balm poses no hazards.

Possible drug interactions
There are no known interactions.

Special information about pregnancy and breastfeeding
No harmful effects are known.

Available preparations and dosage
Lemon balm can be found in the form of dried herb, herb powder, and liquid or dry extracts, as well as various liquid and solid commercial preparations.

To make a tea, pour a cup of hot water over 1.5 to 4.5 grams (about one-quarter to 1 teaspoonful) of crushed lemon balm, steep for 10 minutes, and strain.

The usual daily dose of lemon balm is 8 to 10 grams (about 2 teaspoonfuls) Because the strength of commercial preparations may vary, follow the manufacturer's instructions whenever available.

Lemon balm can be stored in a well-sealed, non-plastic container protected from light and moisture for up to 1 year.

Overdosage
No information on overdosage is available.

L-Phenylalanine

Why people take it
An "essential" amino acid that the body can't manufacture on its own, phenylalanine is one of the raw materials for three of the nervous system's most important chemical messengers: dopamine, epinephrine, and norepinephrine. The body can also convert it to phenylethylamine, a mood-boosting substance that's said to have pain-relieving effects as well.

L-phenylalanine, the form of the substance found naturally in the diet, has shown promise as a treatment for unipolar depression. It has also proven useful in the treatment of vitiligo, a disease characterized by abnormal white blotches of skin due to loss of pigmentation. Phenylalanine has also been promoted as an appetite suppressant and sexual stimulant, but its effectiveness for these purposes remains unproven.

What it is; how it works

Researchers believe that L-phenylalanine's impact on depression stems from its role in the production of dopamine and norepinephrine, two of the chemical messengers that regulate mood. It's value in the treatment of vitiligo is thought to rest on an ability to stimulate the production of pigment-producing melanin in the affected areas of skin.

Outright deficiencies of L-phenylalanine are rare, but have been known to strike people who don't eat enough protein. (Signs of deficiency include bloodshot eyes, cataracts, and behavioral changes.) Good sources of L-phenylalanine include protein foods such as poultry, meats, fish, dairy products, soybeans, nuts, and seeds. Phenylalanine is also an ingredient of the popular artificial sweetener aspartame.

Another form of phenylalanine—D-phenylalanine—has been proposed as a treatment for chronic pain. This substance is available only in combination with L-phenylalanine, in products known as DL-phenylalanine (see separate entry).

Avoid if...

Children born without the ability to process phenylalanine can build up dangerous levels of this amino acid, leading to mental retardation, seizures, extreme hyperactivity, and psychosis. Youngsters with this condition—called phenylketonuria—must follow a special diet designed to supply no more phenylalanine than necessary, and must be monitored regularly for excess phenylalanine in the blood.

Special cautions

L-phenylalanine has also been reported to exacerbate involuntary movements (tardive dyskinesia) in schizophrenic patients. Anyone with this disorder should therefore use L-phenylalanine supplements with extreme caution. Caution is also warranted for people with high blood pressure or an anxiety disorder; phenylalanine tends to aggravate these conditions.

It's best for patients with vitiligo to use L-phenylalanine under a doctor's supervision.

Possible drug interactions

L-phenylalanine supplements should never be combined with drugs known as MAO inhibitors, including the antidepressants Nardil and Parnate; a surge in blood pressure could result. It is also best to avoid combining L-phenylalanine with antipsychotic drugs, since it increases the likelihood of tardive dyskinesia.

On the other hand, taking L-phenylalanine with the drug Eldepryl may boost the antidepressant activity of both agents.

Special information about pregnancy and breastfeeding
Phenylalanine supplements are not recommended during pregnancy and breastfeeding.

Available preparations and dosage
The estimated adult daily requirement for L-phenylalanine and the related amino acid tyrosine combined is approximately 7 milligrams per pound of body weight. Infants require almost 9 times that amount; children need 10 milligrams per pound. Most people fulfill these requirements through diet alone, but commercial L-phenylalanine supplements are available in capsule and tablet form. Typical dosages range from 500 milligrams to 1.5 grams daily. The supplements should not be taken with other amino acids or protein foods. L-phenylalanine is most effective if taken on an empty stomach prior to meals. Vitamin B_6 is said to enhance its effectiveness.

Overdosage
No overdoses have been reported

Melatonin

Why people take it
In numerous clinical studies, the hormone we call melatonin has demonstrated its value as a treatment for insomnia. For example, in one study, 14 of 18 patients taking melatonin were able to give up the sedatives they had been relying on to sleep. There is also a possibility that melatonin may relieve jet lag, though the evidence for this is mixed.

Other claims made for this hormone range from wildly exaggerated to totally baseless. Despite some hints that it may be useful for cancer and immune disorders, clinical research has yet to verify its value. Assertions that melatonin can improve the symptoms of Alzheimer's disease, lower cholesterol levels, reduce high blood pressure, prevent heart attacks, improve sexual performance, and delay the onset of aging are entirely without foundation.

What it is; how it works
Melatonin is a product of the pineal gland, where it is synthesized from the amino acid tryptophan. Under normal conditions, melatonin levels foreshadow the sleep cycle, usually increasing rapidly from the late evening until midnight, then decreasing as morning approaches. In this way, melatonin helps regulate circadian rhythm, the body's 24-hour "dark-light clock" that governs the timing of hormone production, sleep, body temperature, and more.

Not surprisingly, people with high levels of melatonin usually sleep longer and more soundly than those with a deficiency. For example, the elderly, who produce less melatonin than the young and middle-aged, are typically more susceptible to insomnia. Similarly, events that throw melatonin levels out of synch—such as a jet trip between time zones—seem to interfere with production of the hormone and thus disrupt sleep. Consumption of alcohol, tobacco, and narcotics has a similar effect.

Avoid if...
Because melatonin sometimes causes depression, those who suffer from depression should avoid it. It has been known to trigger seizures, and should not be used by anyone with epilepsy or other seizure disorders. Couples who are trying to conceive a baby should avoid this hormone. It is also not for use in children or teenagers.

Special cautions
As with other medications that cause sleepiness, melatonin should be taken only at bedtime. Patients should not drive or operate hazardous machinery after taking a dose.

Side effects are more likely with higher doses. They include stomach discomfort, morning grogginess, daytime hangover, depression, headache, lethargy, disorientation, amnesia, inhibition of fertility, increased seizures, reduced male sexual drive, low body temperature, retinal damage, and breast enlargement.

Possible drug interactions
A number of drugs can reduce melatonin levels. Among them are aspirin, other nonsteroidal anti-inflammatory drugs, and beta blockers such as Inderal, Lopressor, and Tenormin. On the other hand, Luvox can increase the effect of melatonin supplements.

Use of melatonin with benzodiazepines, sedating antihistamines, sedating antidepressants and other sedating drugs may cause additive sedation and increase the likelihood of side effects. Melatonin should never be combined with Prozac.

There is a report of melatonin enhancing the activity of the tuberculosis drug isoniazid. It may also increase the anticancer effect of interleukin-2.

Special information about pregnancy and breastfeeding
Experts advise against the use of melatonin by pregnant women and nursing mothers.

Available preparations and dosage
Melatonin is available in capsules, tablets, lozenges, and liquid. Those who use melatonin for sleep disturbance or jet lag should take no more than 0.3 to 3 milligrams at bedtime for short periods of time (no longer than 2 weeks). It's best to check with a doctor before taking higher doses or dosing for longer periods of time.

Overdosage
There are no reports of melatonin overdose.

Myo-Inositol

Why people take it
In a number of clinical trials, *myo*-inositol has proven to be an effective treatment for some patients with depression, panic disorder, and obsessive-compulsive disorder. It does not, however, have any beneficial effects on Alzheimer's disease, schizophrenia, or autism. And when tested for attention deficit disorder, it made the problem worse.

What it is; how it works
Myo-inositol is a small, but significant, component of cell membranes. The body manufactures it from glucose, and it's also obtained from dietary intake of foods such as dried beans, chickpeas, lentils, citrus fruit, nuts, oats, rice, and whole-grain products.

Researchers have noted a shortage of *myo*-inositol in the cerebrospinal fluid of many patients with depression. They believe its effects on depression and anxiety may stem from its ability to activate serotonin receptors in the brain. As one of the brain's chief chemical messengers, serotonin appears to play a key role in the modulation of moods—a fact that accounts for the success of such serotonin-boosting drugs as Luvox, Paxil, and Prozac. While *myo*-inositol has similar therapeutic effects, hopes that it might enhance the effect of these drugs have failed to be realized.

Avoid if...
There are no known reasons to avoid *myo*-inositol at recommended dosage levels.

Special cautions
Due to the theoretical possibility that this substance could exacerbate the manic symptoms of bipolar disorder, patients suffering from this problem should use *myo*-inositol supplements with caution and only under a doctor's supervision.

Possible drug interactions
Although it has not been observed in clinical trials, there is a theoretical possibility that high doses of *myo*-inositol may improve the action of serotonin-boosting drugs such as Celexa, Luvox, Paxil, Prozac, and Zoloft, and migraine medications such as Amerge, Axert, Imitrex, Maxalt, and Zomig. It might also add to the effects of St. John's wort.

Special information about pregnancy and breastfeeding
Because the safety of *myo*-inositol during pregnancy has not been confirmed, it should be avoided by pregnant women and nursing mothers. In very high doses, it can trigger uterine contractions.

Available preparations and dosage
The dosage that produced positive effects in clinical studies was 12 grams a day, divided into several smaller doses. Improvement, if any, can be expected in about 1 month.

Overdosage
There are no reports of *myo*-inositol overdose.

NADH

Why people take it
A chemical cousin of vitamin B_3, NADH (nicontinamide adenine dinucleotide) is naturally present in each of the body's cells, where it's needed to trigger conversion of nutrients into the cellular "fuel" adenosine triphosphate (ATP). Proponents of NADH have tested it for several serious diseases, including Parkinson's, Alzheimer's, depression, and chronic fatigue syndrome. Although results have been mixed, it seems to be helpful for many patients with Parkinson's disease. Trials for Alzheimer's disease and chronic fatigue syndrome have also been encouraging. Additionally, in one recent study NADH was found to significantly lower blood pressure and cholesterol levels.

What it is; how it works
Because of its role in the synthesis of ATP, NADH is a key factor in the body's production of energy. There's also some evidence that high levels of NADH in the brain may enhance production of such chemical messengers as dopamine, norepinephrine, and serotonin. The body produces NADH continuously, using vitamin B_3 as raw material. It's also readily available from such dietary sources as fish, poultry, beef, and products made with yeast. Deficiencies of NADH in the U.S. are almost unknown, except in rare cases of alcoholism.

Research on the use of NADH for treatment of chronic fatigue syndrome has produced encouraging—though not spectacular—results. The study included 26 patients with chronic fatigue, and found that 31 percent of those taking 10 milligrams of NADH daily had fewer symptoms. The researchers theorize that a shortage of ATP may contribute to the symptoms of chronic fatigue, and that NADH works by helping to replenish depleted cellular stores of the compound.

Because Parkinson's disease is caused by a shortage of dopamine at certain locations in the brain, researchers have speculated that NADH's dopamine-boosting effect might relieve the tremors and rigidity the disease produces. Preliminary studies seem to indicate that for many Parkinson's patients this may be true. In one uncontrolled trial of NADH in 885 people with Parkinson's disease, nearly 80 percent showed improvement.

Since NADH supports production of other chemical messengers in the brain, scientists are also eyeing it for use against Alzheimer's disease and depression. In one small trial, 17 patients suffering from Alzheimer's showed improvement after taking NADH for 8 to 12 weeks. Likewise, a 10-month trial of NADH in 205 depressed patients ended in improvement for 93 percent. But since these studies were small, uncontrolled, and conducted by advocates of NADH, experts say more rigorous testing is needed before any firm conclusions can be drawn.

Avoid if...
Given the lack of conclusive research, it would be unwise to use NADH as a replacement for more promising treatments. Although there are no known reasons to avoid the supplement, it's best used as part of an overall treatment plan. It is not recommended for children.

Special cautions
Little is known about the effects of long-term, high-dose use of NADH, but excessive use of the related compound nicotinic acid can lead to liver damage, so caution is in order.

NADH appears to have few significant side effects, but there have been isolated reports of such gastrointestinal side effects as nausea and loss of appetite.

Possible drug interactions
No drug interactions are known.

Special information about pregnancy and breastfeeding
Because of lack of long-term safety studies, NADH should be avoided by pregnant women and nursing mothers.

Available preparations and dosage
NADH is available in 2.5- and 5-milligram tablets. A typical dosage recommendation is 5 milligrams once or twice daily, with water, on an empty stomach. An injectable form is used by physicians to treat complications of alcoholism.

Overdosage
No information is available on overdosage.

Passion Flower

Latin name: Passiflora incarnata
Other names: Granadilla, Maypop, Passion Vine

Why people take it

Although proven effective only for edginess and insomnia, passion flower has also been used as a remedy for depression and nervous stomach. Applied externally, it has been used for hemorrhoids.

What it is; how it works

This perennial vine, which reaches 30 feet in length, grows naturally from the southeastern U.S. to Brazil and Argentina, and is cultivated in Europe as a garden plant. The blossoms are considered symbolic of Christ's Passion (their central corona, for instance, represents the Crown of Thorns), accounting for their name.

The above-ground parts of the plant hold its medicinal value. In animal tests, researchers found that the plant lowers blood pressure and slows the passage of food through the digestive tract.

Avoid if...

No known medical conditions preclude the use of passion flower.

Special cautions

At customary dosage levels, Passion Flower poses no risks.

Possible drug interactions

No interactions have been reported.

Special information about pregnancy and breastfeeding

No harmful effects are known.

Available preparations and dosage

Passion flower is available as an herb for tea. It is also an ingredient in certain sedative bath additives.

To make tea, pour 150 milliliters (about two-thirds of a cup) of hot water over 1 teaspoonful of passion flower, steep for 10 minutes, then strain.

To prepare an external rinse, particularly for hemorrhoids, put 20 grams (about 3 tablespoonfuls) of Passion Flower into 200 grams (about 1 cup) of simmering water, allow to cool, then strain.

The typical oral dosage is 2 to 3 cups of tea during the day and one-half hour before bedtime.

Overdosage

No information on overdosage is available.

Phosphatidylcholine

Why people take it

Two potential benefits have attracted interest in phosphatidylcholine: its impact on cholesterol levels and its effect on memory loss. In both roles, the substance gets mixed reviews.

Hopes that phosphatidylcholine might combat memory loss have been based on its ability to increase levels of acetylcholine in the brain. This important chemical messenger appears to play a role in maintaining memory, and has been found to be in short supply in Alzheimer's patients. Unfortunately an analysis of 11 carefully controlled clinical experiments with lecithin, a food supplement rich in phosphatidyl-choline, was unable to detect any significant benefit. The supplement may have very modest effects on patients with impaired thinking or dementia, but it doesn't seem to yield any major improvement.

Similarly, some experts once believed that phosphatidylcholine might relieve the symptoms of tardive dyskinesia, a severe neurological disorder that's brought on by long-term use of certain antipsychotic drugs. But when schizophrenic patients suffering from the signs and symptoms of the disorder—involuntary movements of the muscles of the face, mouth, and cheeks—were put on lecithin or related compounds, they experienced only slight improvement.

Phosphatidylcholine's performance against high cholesterol has been equally unexciting. Although it has produced moderate reductions in some studies, it has had no significant effect in a number of others.

It has been suggested that phosphatidylcholine might eventually have some therapeutic role in some cancers. Phosphatidylcholine is essential for normal liver function, and there is ample evidence that liver cancer is promoted in various animals by choline-deficient diets. In addition, phosphatidylcholine has demonstrated protective effects against a number of other liver disorders, including alcoholic fibrosis and viral hepatitis.

What it is; how it works

Phosphatidylcholine is a combination of choline, fatty acids, glycerol, and phosphorus. Its choline component serves as a raw material in the production of acetylcholine and has recently been classified as an essential nutrient by the National Academy of Sciences. (See entry on Choline.) As a source of extra choline, phosphatidylcholine is a better delivery form and is better tolerated than choline itself.

Phosphatidylcholine is one of several phosphorus-based compounds contained in lecithin, a naturally occurring substance derived from beef liver, eggs, soybeans, and peanuts. Lecithin products are generally composed of from 5 to 30 percent phosphatidylcholine. Choline constitutes about 13 percent of the total.

Avoid if...
Phosphatidylcholine is generally considered safe for everyone.

Special cautions
No major side effects need be expected. A few people suffer mild side effects such as nausea, diarrhea, and increased salivation.

Possible drug interactions
It's best to avoid choline-containing supplements if one is taking a prescription drug such as scopolamine (an antinausea medication) that works by blocking the effects of acetylcholine.

Special information about pregnancy and breastfeeding
For healthy women who eat a balanced diet, choline supplements are usually unnecessary during pregnancy and breastfeeding.

Available preparations and dosage
There are several ways to obtain supplemental phosphatidylcholine. Typical commercial lecithin supplements contain 20 to 30 percent phosphatidylcholine. Softgel capsules containing 55 to 90 percent phosphatidylcholine are available. There's also a liquid containing 3 grams of phosphatidylcholine per 5 milliliters. Typical dosages range from 3 to 9 grams of phosphatidylcholine daily, taken in several smaller doses.

Overdosage
The upper tolerable limit of choline is 3.5 grams a day. (It takes approximately 27 grams of phosphatidylcholine to supply this amount.) Dosages above this level may bring on dizziness, nausea, diarrhea, cramps, and a fishy body odor.

Phosphatidylserine

Why people take it
Phosphatidylserine (PS) is found in high concentrations in the brain. It may help to preserve, or even improve, some aspects of mental functioning in the elderly. In the largest study to date, 200 milligrams of phosphatidylserine daily made a small but significant improvement in patients with Alzheimer's disease. Other smaller studies also found phosphatidylserine to be mildly helpful. Keep in mind, however, that these studies lasted just a few months, and while phosphatidylserine may reduce symptoms in the short term, at best it probably slows the rate of deterioration rather than halting the progression altogether. Preliminary evidence also suggests that phosphatidylserine can boost the immune system, and it may blunt the effects of the stress hormone cortisol during exercise.

What it is; how it works

Phosphatidylserine belongs to a special category of fat-soluble substances called phospholipids, which are essential components of cell membranes. Brain tissues are especially rich in phosphatidylserine, but aging causes a decline in the phosphatidylserine content of cells throughout the body. Research has shown that in addition to improving neural function, phosphatidylserine may enhance energy metabolism in all cells. It also seems to boost levels of the brain chemical acetylcholine, which has been linked to improved memory function.

Some controversy exists about the source of phosphatidylserine supplements. Most research has been conducted with phosphatidylserine derived from cow brain tissue. Due to concerns about mad-cow disease, soy-based phosphatidylserine supplements have generally replaced cow-based ones. The two types are not structurally identical, however, and some researchers think these differences could be important.

Phosphatidylserine is found in only trace amounts in a typical diet. Very small amounts are present in egg yolks and soybeans.

Avoid if...

Aside from an allergy to them, there are no known reasons to avoid phosphatidylserine supplements.

Special cautions

Due to the lack of safety studies, phosphatidylserine supplements should not be given to children. Those who have a rare genetic condition known as antiphospholipid-antibody syndrome should talk to their doctor before taking phosphatidylserine.

Occasional side effects, such as nausea and indigestion, have been reported.

Possible drug interactions

There are no reported drug interactions with phosphatidylserine.

Special information about pregnancy and breastfeeding

Due to the lack of safety data, pregnant and breastfeeding women should not use phosphatidylserine.

Available preparations and dosage

Most phosphatidylserine supplements are made from soy. Due to concerns about mad-cow disease, it's best to avoid those made from cow, or "bovine," sources. PS capsules are available in strengths of 50, 100, and 500 milligrams. Typical doses are 100 milligrams three times a day.

Overdosage

There are no reports of overdosage.

Rauwolfia

Latin name: Rauwolfia serpentina

Why people take it

Rauwolfia is officially recognized in Europe as a treatment for nervousness, insomnia, and high blood pressure. In folk medicine, it has also been used for vomiting, gas, liver problems, and wounds. However, its effectiveness for such conditions remains unverified.

Indian medicine uses it as an antidote for poisonous snake bites, and as a remedy for fever, abdominal cramps, slow and painful urination, and wounds.

What it is; how it works

Reserpine, an extract of rauwolfia, combats high blood pressure, and is found in such prescription blood pressure medications as Diupres and Hydropres. Reserpine also combats irregular heartbeat and has a sedative effect.

Rauwolfia, a small shrub sporting white to pink flowers, is native to India, Indochina, Borneo, Sri Lanka, and Sumatra. Its medicinal properties lie in the dried root. The fresh root has a very bitter and unpleasant taste.

Avoid if...

Rauwolfia can trigger severe depression. No one suffering from depression should take this herb. The drug also tends to stimulate the lining of the digestive tract, so it should be avoided if an ulcer or ulcerative colitis exists. Rauwolfia should also be avoided during pregnancy and nursing.

Special cautions

Side effects can include nasal congestion, depression, fatigue, impotence, and slowed reaction time. Patients should use caution when handling machinery or driving.

Possible drug interactions

Rauwolfia must never be combined with drugs classified as monoamine oxidase inhibitors, such as the antidepressants Nardil and Parnate.

Rauwolfia enhances the sedative effect of alcohol and barbiturates; the combination should be avoided. Rauwolfia also increases the effects of antipsychotic drugs.

Taken with digitalis-based drugs such as Lanoxin, or quinidine products such as Quinaglute and Quinidex, rauwolfia can slow the heart and cause irregular beats.

The drug is also likely to interact with levodopa (Sinemet), causing twitching and other involuntary movements. Combining it with many common flu remedies and appetite suppressants can lead to a sharp rise in blood pressure.

Special information about pregnancy and breastfeeding

Rauwolfia may cause birth defects when taken during pregnancy; and it appears in breast milk. Women should avoid this drug while pregnant or breastfeeding.

Available preparations and dosage

Rauwolfia is available in ground form and as a powder for internal use.

The usual daily dose of rauwolfia is 600 milligrams. (Recommended dosage of the active ingredient reserpine is far smaller; 0.25 milligram is the daily maximum.)

Overdosage

Symptoms of overdosage include mental depression, heavy sedation, and a severe drop in blood pressure. If an overdose is suspected, seek medical attention immediately.

SAMe

Why people take it

In a series of small but promising clinical trials, this over-the-counter remedy for depression has proved itself the equal of traditional prescription drugs. Though some authorities dismiss it as a mild mood-lifter, others regard it as an important new medication, since it has not only performed as well as potent "tricyclic" antidepressants, but also starts working faster (within one or two weeks, versus three to four weeks or longer for standard drugs). Outside the U.S., it has been sold for years as a prescription antidepressant, mainly under the name AdoMet.

SAMe (S-adenosylmethionine) has been studied as an aid to the effectiveness of other antidepressants, with promising results. It also has been found to provide at least some relief from postpartum depression and depression associated with Parkinson's disease and epilepsy. In addition, it has been tested for a number of other neurological disorders, including schizophrenia, Alzheimer's disease, and dementia. Although these tests are far from conclusive, they've produced encouraging results.

SAMe is also used to treat osteoarthritis, the type of arthritis caused by wear and tear on the protective cartilage in the joints. Preliminary studies appear to confirm its ability to relieve stiffness, pain, and swelling. However, there's no evidence to support manufacturers' claims that it can renew damaged cartilage. SAMe also shows promise as a treatment for the painful muscle condition called fibromyalgia. And studies show that supplementation with SAMe can improve liver function, making it a candidate for treatment of cirrhosis, impaired bile flow, and liver damage from drugs or alcohol.

Claims that SAMe is useful in the treatment of heart disease and cancer are currently unsubstantiated, though preliminary clinical studies are underway. Assertions that SAMe fights the effects of aging also remain unproven.

What it is; how it works

The body manufactures a natural supply of SAMe from the essential amino acid methionine. In turn, SAMe plays an important role in the production of a wide variety of hormones, amino acids, antioxidants, and chemical messengers in the brain. Researchers have noted low levels of SAMe in people with depression, and have found that SAMe rises as depression improves. SAMe also helps maintain the strength and flexibility of cell walls, and participates in the production of DNA and RNA.

SAMe supplements are especially helpful in cases of liver disease, which depletes the body's natural supply. Extra vitamin B_6, B_{12}, and folic acid are usually recommended with SAMe supplementation. In fact, some products already have them added.

Avoid if...

People who have bipolar disorder should use SAMe only under a doctor's supervision; SAMe can cause episodes of mania. Those taking antidepressants should not discontinue their medication or start taking SAMe without consulting a physician. SAMe is not recommended for children.

Special cautions

Patients taking a prescription antidepressant may need to reduce their dosage gradually when attempting to replace their medication with SAMe or adding SAMe to their regimen.

Patients with high homocysteine levels (a condition associated with increased risk of heart disease) should consider adding the homocysteine-lowering supplement TMG to the regimen. Homocysteine is a byproduct of SAMe.

Unlike some prescription antidepressants, SAMe is said to have no serious side effects. However, some people suffer mild digestive upsets, anxiety, insomnia, mania, and hyperactive muscles.

There is no reason to believe that SAMe could cause cancer. But because people who already have cancer might react differently to this substance, they should check with their doctor before taking SAMe.

Possible drug interactions

SAMe may reduce the effectiveness of some medications, including the Parkinson's disease medication L-dopa.

Special information about pregnancy and breastfeeding

The safety of SAMe supplements during pregnancy has not been determined; it should be used only under a doctor's supervision. SAMe supplementation is not recommended for nursing mothers.

Available preparations and dosage

Synthetic SAMe is available in tablets and capsules, usually in strengths of 100 or 200 milligrams. For depression, some authorities recommend dosages of 400 to 1,600 milligrams daily. For arthritis, recommendations vary from 200 to 1,200 milligrams daily. For liver disease, daily dosages of 1,600 milligrams are common. The daily total is divided into smaller doses. They should be taken 1 hour before or 2 hours after meals.

Some forms of SAMe tend to degrade quickly at any temperature above freezing. Look for a temperature-stable form in a coated tablet. Store away from moisture.

Overdosage

No information on overdosage is available.

St. John's Wort

Latin name: Hypericum perforatum

Why people take it

In many—but not all—clinical trials, St. John's wort has proven to be an effective treatment for mild to moderate depressive disorders. It also has a mildly tranquilizing and sedative effect. Oily preparations of the herb are useful in the treatment of wounds, burns, blunt injuries, and inflammation of the skin.

Although its effectiveness for other ailments has not been proven, St. John's wort has also been used to treat sleep disturbances, gallbladder disorders, gastritis, bronchitis, asthma, diarrhea, bed-wetting, rheumatism, muscle pain, and gout.

What it is; how it works

St. John's wort is believed to combat depression by boosting the levels of certain chemical messengers in the brain. Like the prescription antidepressant Prozac, it seems to increase the amount of serotonin available to the nervous system. It also tends to promote higher levels of the chemical messengers norepinephrine and dopamine. In clinical trials, daily doses of 800 to 900 milligrams of St. John's wort have proven to be as effective as 20 milligrams of Prozac or 75 milligrams of the antidepressant Tofranil.

Applied to the skin, oily preparations of the herb have an antibacterial and anti-inflammatory action, though they seem to have no effect on viruses.

St. John's wort is a golden yellow perennial flower that secretes a red liquid when pinched. Cut at the start of the flowering season and processed in bunches, it must be dried quickly to preserve its oil and secretions.

This plant has been used medicinally for over 2,000 years. Ancient Greeks believed that its odor repelled evil spirits. Early Christians named the plant in honor of St. John the Baptist because they believed it released its blood-red oil on the 29th of August, the day the saint was beheaded.

Avoid if...

There are no known reasons to avoid St. John's wort at recommended dosage levels.

Special cautions

With heavy use, St. John's wort increases sensitivity to sunlight. To avoid a sunburn, patients should minimize exposure to the sun while using this medication. This herb can also cause bloating and constipation.

Possible drug interactions

Patients taking medications for HIV, the virus that causes AIDS, should not use St. John's wort. The herb is known to interfere with at least one HIV drug—Crixivan—and may reduce the effect of others, including Agenerase, Fortovase, Invirase, Norvir, and Viracept. St. John's wort should also be avoided by people taking Neoral, a drug used to keep transplant patients from rejecting their new organs. It can inhibit the drug's life-saving effect.

Research shows that St. John's wort may interact with numerous medications. The herb affects the way the body processes or breaks down many drugs; in some cases, it may speed or slow a drug's breakdown. Patients should consult their doctor before combining St. John's wort with any other medication, herb, or dietary supplement. Particular caution is warranted for people taking cyclosporine, digoxin, blood thinners, psychotropic medications, or drugs used to treat cancer.

Patients should avoid St. John's wort while taking a prescription MAO inhibitor such as Nardil or Parnate. At least in theory, a dangerous interaction is possible.

It's also best to avoid combining St. John's wort with serotonin-boosting drugs such as Celexa, Paxil, Prozac, and Zoloft. The excessive levels of serotonin that may result can trigger sweating, tremors, flushing, confusion, and agitation.

Patients who use a hormonal form of contraception should remember that oral contraceptive failure has occasionally been reported in women taking St. John's wort.

Special information about pregnancy and breastfeeding

Because the effects of using St. John's wort during pregnancy and breastfeeding have not been adequately studied, caution is advised.

Available preparations and dosage

For depression, the typical dosage of standardized extract is 300 milligrams taken 3 times a day. The extract is available in tablet, capsule, and liquid form. Strengths of commercial preparations may vary. Patients should follow the manufacturer's labeling whenever available.

A treatment regimen of 4 to 6 weeks is typically recommended for depression. Patients should check with their doctor if they feel no improvement. They may need a different therapy.

Overdosage

No information on overdosage is available.

Tocotrienols

Why people take it

Tocotrienols are a form of vitamin E. In general, people take them for the same reasons they take other forms of the vitamin (see separate entry), including the prevention of Alzheimer's disease, heart disease, and cancer, particularly breast cancer.

Most scientific study has focused on the alpha-tocopherol form of vitamin E because it appears to be the most active in humans. However, proponents of tocotrienols claim that they are the "missing link" in the vitamin E story; and preliminary research does indeed suggest that they may yield impressive benefits. For example, some studies suggest that tocotrienols can lower blood cholesterol levels more effectively than alpha-tocopherol can. Others hint that tocotrienols can greatly inhibit tumor formation, especially in human breast cells. Animal studies also suggest tocotrienols may be useful for healing alcohol-induced stomach lesions.

While the evidence is promising, many questions remain. There are four different types of tocotrienols, and scientists still aren't sure which ones are best, or how much should be taken. Studies also need to be done to find out the effects of taking tocotrienols and tocopherols together. (Some researchers claim that taking the two at the same time negates some of the benefits of tocotrienols.) Whatever the case, experts agree that alpha-tocopherol is still an important form of vitamin E and should not be avoided in favor of tocotrienols.

What it is; how it works

Like other forms of vitamin E, tocotrienols seem to be potent antioxidants that protect the fats in cell membranes from oxidation, or spoilage.

Oxidation is thought to be a significant factor in many diseases, as well as the aging process. The antioxidant abilities of tocotrienols may explain why they are helpful for protecting the cardiovascular and nervous systems. How this form of vitamin E works to prevent cancer is still unknown.

The richest sources of tocotrienols are palm, rice bran, and coconut oils. Other plant-based oils, such as corn and canola, contain very little. Like all forms of vitamin E, tocotrienols are fat soluble.

Avoid if...
Aside from an allergy to them, there are no known reasons to avoid tocotrienol supplements.

Special cautions
Because tocotrienols could interfere with blood clot formation, patients who have bleeding problems—including those with hemophilia, peptic ulcers, vitamin K deficiency, a tendency to hemorrhage, or a history of stroke—should take care not to overdose. Likewise, patients should avoid tocotrienols about 1 month before and for 2 weeks after any surgery.

Because tocotrienol supplements are relatively new, there is little information on side effects. In general, the same precautions should be followed as those for vitamin E (see separate entry).

Possible drug interactions
Patients who are taking a blood-thinning drug such as aspirin or Coumadin should check with their doctor before taking tocotrienols, which could further thin the blood. In general, patients on blood thinners should not take more than 100 milligrams of tocotrienols per day. Likewise, tocotrienols should be used cautiously by patients taking antiplatelet drugs such as Aggrenox, Plavix, and Ticlid. In theory, increased bleeding could also occur if tocotrienols are taken with supplemental garlic or the herb ginkgo.

Patients taking cholesterol-lowering drugs such as Lescol, Pravachol, and Zocor should be aware that tocotrienols may further lower their cholesterol.

Certain drugs may decrease the absorption of tocotrienols or interfere with their use in the body. These include the cholesterol-lowering drugs Colestid and Questran, the antibiotics isoniazid and neomycin, the weight-loss drug Xenical, and the ulcer medication Carafate. Other products that may decrease absorption include mineral oil, the fat substitute olestra, and cholesterol-lowering supplements, especially the plant-based phytosterols and phytostanols.

Because of possible oxidation, tocotrienols should not be taken at the same time as iron supplements.

Special information about pregnancy and breastfeeding
Due to the lack of safety data, pregnant and breastfeeding women should use tocotrienol supplements only with their doctor's approval.

Available preparations and dosage
Most supplements contain a mixture of tocotrienols in liquid softgel form. Some manufacturers also offer "mixed" vitamin E supplements that contain the tocopherol forms as well.

Unlike the alpha-tocopherol form of vitamin E, there are no governmental recommendations for tocotrienols. Dosages used in clinical studies range from 200 to 300 milligrams per day, although some researchers believe that daily doses of 30 to 50 milligrams are sufficient for general disease prevention.

Tocotrienol supplements may be listed as "esterified," which means the formulation was chemically altered to make them more stable. Unesterified tocotrienols should not be taken with supplemental iron, since the combination could actually encourage oxidation. All tocotrienol supplements should be stored at cool temperatures in a dark, tightly closed bottle. They should be taken with fat to enhance absorption.

Overdosage
Little information is available on overdosage; so far, no serious side effects have been reported.

Valerian

Latin name: Valeriana officinalis
Other names: All-heal, Amantilla, Capon's Tail, Heliotrope, Setwall, Vandal Root

Why people take it
Valerian is an accepted remedy for insomnia, and appears to calm nervousness as well. Although its other uses have not been formally verified, valerian is also taken for mental strain, lack of concentration, excitability, hysteria, stress, headache, epilepsy, premenstrual syndrome, symptoms of pregnancy, problems of menopause, nerve pain, fainting, stomach cramps, colic, and uterine spasms.

What it is; how it works
The Ancient Greek physician Galen referred to valerian as "Phu," an expression of disgust at the plant's smell. In medieval times, it was given the name "All-heal," reflecting its many purported healing properties. It was also used as a spice and an ingredient in perfume.

The medicinal parts are the carefully dried underground stem and the dried root. Rigorous clinical trials have verified that extracts of the root do indeed have a sleep-inducing effect. Researchers believe that this action stems from the herb's tendency to boost levels of GABA (gamma-aminobutyric acid), one of the chemical messengers in the brain. Valerian also seems to relax muscles and discourage spasms.

This plant, which produces bright pink to white flowers, grows 20 to 40 inches in height. It is native to Europe and the temperate regions of Asia, and is cultivated in Europe, Japan, and the U.S.

Avoid if...

Valerian should not be used in people with liver disease. Unless a doctor approves, anyone with a large skin injury, an acute skin disorder, a severe infection, heart problems, or severe muscle tension should avoid using valerian extract or oil as a bath additive.

Special cautions

In rare instances, valerian can cause digestive problems or an allergic reaction. Long-term use can lead to headache, restlessness, sleeplessness, pupil dilation, and heart problems.

Because of valerian's sedative effect, it's best to avoid operating machinery or driving for several hours after taking the herb.

Possible drug interactions

Valerian should not be combined with opioid analgesics and with other sedatives, including barbiturates such as Seconal and benzodiazepine medications such as Ativan, Halcion, Librium, Valium, and Xanax. Although there is no evidence of an interaction with alcohol, it's considered best to avoid this combination as well.

Special information about pregnancy and breastfeeding

Use of valerian during pregnancy or breastfeeding is not recommended.

Available preparations and dosage

To prepare valerian tea, combine 3 to 5 grams (about 1 teaspoonful) of crushed Valerian with 150 milliliters of hot water (about two-thirds cup), steep for 10 to 15 minutes, then strain.

To make a bath additive, combine 100 grams (about one-half cup) of crushed valerian with 2 quarts of hot water for each full bath.

A variety of commercial preparations are available in capsule and tablet form. For relief of insomnia, typical doses of valerian extract range from 400 to 900 milligrams 30 minutes before bedtime. Because the potency of commercial tablets and capsules may vary, follow the manufacturer's directions whenever available.

For other forms of the herb, the following daily dosages are commonly recommended:

Powder: 15 grams (about 3 teaspoonfuls)
Tea: 2 to 3 cups daily, including 1 before bedtime

Alcohol solution: 1 to 3 milliliters (about one-half to one teaspoonful) 1
       or more times per day
Alcohol solution (1:5): 15 to 20 drops in water several times daily
Pressed juice: 1 tablespoonful 3 times daily for adults; 1 teaspoonful 3
       times daily for children

Valerian should be stored away from light. Alcohol solutions (tinctures)
and extracts must be kept in tightly closed glass containers.

Overdosage
No information on overdosage is available.

Vinpocetine

Why people take it
A so-called "smart drug," vinpocetine is said to improve memory and
mental function by increasing the blood supply to the brain. Advocates
claim it can help healthy people, as well as those with some degree of
brain impairment. It has not, however, proved capable of halting or even
slowing the progress of Alzheimer's disease. Vinpocetine has also been
described as a possible antioxidant, protecting cells from the damaging
free radicals that can oxidize (burn) tissues throughout the body, including the brain.

Some preliminary research suggests that vinpocetine may have some
protective effects in both sight and hearing. One study of patients with
mild burn trauma in the eyes showed that vinpocetine enhanced healing,
most likely as a result of increased blood flow to the damaged tissue.
Vinpocetine has also been associated with improvements seen in retinas
damaged by hepatitis B virus. Damage from acoustic trauma has been
similarly been reduced by vinpocetine treatment.

Vinpocetine is sold as a drug in Germany, Japan, Mexico, and
Portugal for the treatment of cerebrovascular disorders—ailments that
interrupt blood circulation in the brain, starving it of oxygen. In
Portugal, it's also used to treat general circulatory problems, as well as
certain disorders of the eyes and ears. The drug is approved in Australia
for the treatment of mental function disorders in the elderly and for other
disorders of the brain. Though it has never been approved in the United
States, it can be purchased here as a dietary supplement.

What it is; how it works
Like other members of the vinca alkaloid family of drugs, such as the
cancer drugs vincristine, vinblastine, and vinorelbine, vinpocetine comes
from the periwinkle plant. Limited research data show that vinpocetine
does in fact relax the blood vessels of the brain, improve cerebral blood
flow, and inhibit blood clotting to some extent. One study implies that

the drug improves memory in healthy people. Studies in animals also indicate a protective effect when the brain is deprived of oxygen.

On the other hand, a number of trials have produced less encouraging results. To date, studies in people with Alzheimer's disease or stroke have been very disappointing. Trials in people with brain dysfunction due to other causes have produced mixed results, providing no clear answers for researchers. There is currently not enough evidence to determine whether vinpocetine does or does not reduce fatalities and dependence in ischemic stroke. It's evident that additional, wide-scale studies are needed before any firm conclusions can be drawn about vinpocetine's real value and most appropriate uses.

Avoid if...

Vinpocetine should not be taken if one has ever had an allergic reaction to one of the vinca-based anticancer drugs, or to vinpocetine itself.

Special cautions

It is a good idea for patients to get periodic checkups while taking vinpocetine whatever the status of their health. Blood pressure should be checked on a regular basis. A routine blood test is recommended from time to time to ensure that the liver is breaking down the drug properly. Don't forget that outside the U.S. vinpocetine is used like a potent prescription drug. A bit of extra caution is merited.

Side effects are relatively mild. People enrolled in research studies have taken up to 60 milligrams of vinpocetine per day without suffering serious adverse reactions. Some people found that their blood pressure dropped slightly, an effect that can cause dizziness. Facial flushing has also occurred among people taking vinpocetine. Other complaints reported include temporary sleep disturbances and restlessness (usually after 10 weeks of therapy), pressure headache, dry mouth, and stomach disturbances. Minor decreases in blood sugar have been noted, too, but it has not been determined whether this effect was actually caused by vinpocetine.

Possible drug interactions

Small changes in clotting time have been reported in people who combine the blood thinner warfarin with vinpocetine. While the combination does not seem to pose a great danger, more frequent monitoring of clotting time is a good idea.

Special information about pregnancy and breastfeeding

During pregnancy and breastfeeding it's best to avoid any medication that's not absolutely necessary for short-term health. Patients should forego vinpocetine throughout this period.

Available preparations and dosage
Vinpocetine is typically sold as 5-milligram tablets. Depending on the product purchased, the label may recommend anywhere from 5 to 30 milligrams daily. Do not exceed the recommended amount.

Overdosage
There are no reports of vinpocetine overdosage.

Vitamin E

Why people take it
Vitamin E has garnered headlines in recent years for its potential to treat—and possibly help prevent—a host of devastating illnesses, including Alzheimer's disease, heart disease, peripheral nerve damage, and cancer. Researchers are particularly impressed by a study in the *New England Journal of Medicine* that showed supplemental vitamin E helped slow the progression of mild to moderate Alzheimer's disease. The results were so convincing that the American Psychiatric Association now includes the vitamin in its treatment guidelines for Alzheimer's.

The study's authors caution that one trial cannot tell the whole story, and they still don't know how vitamin E protects the brain, or whether it could stave off dementia in the first place. Also, the dose used in the study was high—2,000 International Units a day—and treatment at such high doses needs to be supervised by a doctor since, theoretically, it could cause bleeding and other problems. Even so, some researchers believe that the possible rewards of taking vitamin E seem to outweigh the risks, especially since we have so few effective treatments for Alzheimer's.

Much interest also surrounds the use of vitamin E for fighting heart disease and cancer. Unfortunately, for every reputable study that has found a link between vitamin E and lower rates of both diseases, another one comes along that casts doubt on the evidence. While nutritional surveys strongly suggest that vitamin E can help prevent heart disease and various cancers (including prostate, breast, and colon cancer), clinical trials of the supplement have been disappointing. It could be that some studies were too short or used a dosage that was too low. For now, the best course seems to be to get adequate vitamin E from food and perhaps take modest amounts of supplements.

Vitamin E also gets attention for its role in strengthening the immune system and protecting the body from environmental toxins, including air pollution, tobacco smoke, and the sun's ultraviolet rays. For the same reasons, vitamin E supplements may be somewhat beneficial for treating asthma, diabetes, cataracts, and rheumatoid arthritis. It may also help relieve muscle cramps and some of the symptoms associated with pre-menstrual syndrome, although more research is needed. Claims that vitamin E can reverse skin aging, improve athletic abilities, and enhance fertility and sexual performance have never been substantiated.

What it is; how it works

Even though vitamin E is well known as an essential nutrient, scientists aren't sure how the body uses it. Part of the confusion stems from the vitamin's many forms. Vitamin E is actually a catchall term for a family of eight naturally occurring molecules. They are divided into two main groups, the tocopherols and the tocotrienols. The best known, and the one generally found in supplements, is alpha-tocopherol. The government bases its daily-allowance recommendation on alpha-tocopherol because, so far, it seems to be the most biologically usable form in humans. This does not, however, mean that the other forms of vitamin E are insignificant. In fact, some researchers argue that certain tocotrienols (see separate entry) are more potent antioxidants, although the evidence is still being debated.

Scientists do know that vitamin E is a powerful antioxidant that protects the fats found in cell membranes throughout the body from oxidation, or spoilage. Oxidation is thought to play a role in numerous degenerative diseases as well as the aging process. For example, it is widely believed that the oxidation of "bad" LDL cholesterol leads to the formation of artery-clogging plaque. And oxidative stress has also been linked to many nervous system disorders because brain and nerve cells are rich in fats that are vulnerable to oxidation.

Although vitamin E's role as an antioxidant gets credit for most of its protective effects, it is not the vitamin's only beneficial property. This versatile nutrient also seems to act as a blood thinner and a cell-membrane stabilizer; and it plays an important role in the maintenance of a healthy immune system. A number of studies have shown that it may inhibit the development of certain cancers.

The richest sources of vitamin E, especially the tocopherol form, are vegetable and nut oils, including corn, sunflower, canola, soybean, and olive oils. Palm, rice bran, and coconut oils are high in the tocotrienols. Most nuts are high in vitamin E, as are fatty meats, unrefined cereal and grains, and wheat germ. Various fruits and vegetables—spinach, lettuce, onions, blackberries, apples, and pears—also contain this vitamin.

Vitamin E is fat soluble, which means that the body can store vitamin E for future use. Although high doses of fat-soluble vitamins could lead to toxic buildups in the body, vitamin E has proven safe even in much larger than standard doses.

Vitamin E deficiency is rare in humans but can occur in very premature infants. Individuals who may be deficient include those with cystic fibrosis, Crohn's disease, and certain rare genetic disorders. Vitamin E deficiency is also a concern for those who have had part of their gastrointestinal tract removed. People on a strict low-fat diet may be somewhat deficient since fatty nuts and oils are the best sources of vitamin E.

Avoid if...
Aside from an allergy to them, there are no known reasons to avoid vitamin E supplements.

Special cautions
Because vitamin E can prevent the formation of blood clots, patients who have bleeding problems—including those with hemophilia, peptic ulcers, vitamin K deficiency, a tendency to hemorrhage, or a history of stroke—should take care not to overdose and may need to have their bleeding time monitored. Likewise, patients should avoid vitamin E supplements about one month before and for 2 weeks after any surgery.

In general, the risk of side effects is low. Even at doses of 1,500 International Units (IU) per day, vitamin E appears to have no harmful effects. However, at doses of 2,400 IU or more bleeding problems may begin to appear. Too much vitamin E may also reduce the body's supply of vitamin A, alter the immune system, and impair sexual function.

Rare reactions to vitamin E supplements include fatigue, breast soreness, emotional disturbances, inflammation of the veins, stomach upset, altered blood fat levels, and thyroid problems.

Possible drug interactions
Patients who are taking a blood-thinning drug such as aspirin or Coumadin should check with their doctor before taking vitamin E supplements, which could further thin the blood. In general, patients taking these drugs should not exceed total daily doses of 100 milligrams of natural vitamin E or 200 milligrams of the synthetic version. Vitamin E should also be used cautiously with antiplatelet drugs such as Aggrenox, Plavix, and Ticlid. In theory, increased bleeding could also occur if vitamin E is taken with supplemental garlic or the herb ginkgo.

Certain drugs may decrease vitamin E absorption or interfere with its use in the body. These include anticonvulsants such as phenobarbital, Dilantin, and Tegretol; the cholesterol-lowering drugs Colestid and Questran; the antibiotics isoniazid and neomycin; and ulcer drugs such as Carafate. In some studies, the weight-loss drug Xenical reduced vitamin E absorption by up to 60 percent. Other products that may counter the effects of vitamin E include fiber supplements, mineral oil, the fat substitute Olestra, and cholesterol-lowering supplements, especially the plant-based phytosterols and phytostanols.

On the plus side, vitamin E may help alleviate the side effects of Cordarone, which is used to prevent abnormal heart rhythms. It may also inhibit Retrovir's harmful effects on bone marrow, and could be useful for treating the kidney damage caused by drugs used to prevent organ rejection, including the immunosuppressants Neoral and Sandimmune. Be aware, however, that in some studies vitamin E actually interfered with immunosuppressant drugs.

Because of possible oxidation, vitamin E should not be taken at the same time as iron supplements. Patients taking supplemental oils—including flaxseed, perilla, borage, blackcurrant, evening primrose, and fish oils—should take a little extra vitamin E to prevent oxidation.

The mineral selenium may boost the effectiveness of vitamin E. In addition, taking other antioxidants—such as vitamin C, glutathione, alpha-lipoic acid, and Coenzyme Q10—may help the body hold onto vitamin E.

Special information about pregnancy and breastfeeding

Pregnant women should not take more than the Recommended Dietary Allowance (RDA) of 15 milligrams (or 22 IU) of vitamin E a day. For breastfeeding women, the RDA is 19 milligrams (or 28 IU). For both cases, the RDA is measured using natural alpha-tocopherol.

Available preparations and dosage

There are several forms of vitamin E available commercially. Most consist of alpha-tocopherol in tablets, capsules, or liquid softgel form. Some manufacturers are now offering "mixed" formulations that include additional forms such as gamma-tocopherol and the tocotrienols.

Typical daily dosages for natural alpha-tocopherol range from 100 to 400 milligrams, with a recommended upper limit of 1,000 milligrams per day. The dosages for synthetic alpha-tocopherol are double that amount, since this form is not as easily stored by the body. Patients can spot the synthetic version by checking the letters listed *before* "alpha-tocopherol." The natural form lists "d," as in d-alpha-tocopherol, while the synthetic version lists "dl," as in dl-alpha-tocopherol. The RDA set by the government is much lower than the doses used in studies: 15 milligrams of natural alpha-tocopherol a day for adults.

Vitamin E is measured in milligrams or International Units (IU), with 1 milligram of alpha-tocopherol equal to approximately 1.5 IU. Therefore, to convert from milligrams to IU, multiply by 1.5. For example, the RDA for vitamin E is 15 milligrams or about 22 IU.

Vitamin E is often listed as "esterified," which means it was chemically altered to make it more stable. Unesterified vitamin E should not be taken with supplemental iron, since the combination could actually encourage oxidation. All vitamin E supplements should be stored at cool temperatures in a dark, tightly closed bottle.

Overdosage

There are no reports of overdosage with vitamin E in any form. However, extremely high doses (2,400 IU or more per day) could theoretically cause bleeding problems due to the vitamin's clot-preventing ability.

Zinc

Why people take it

Because zinc is vital for overall body function, a deficiency could lead to a host of problems. Low levels have been linked to poor brain function, delayed wound healing, a weak immune system, infertility, alcoholism, and anorexia. People who may benefit from zinc supplements include those who do not consume enough calories, vegetarians, some older infants and children with impaired growth, and people who suffer from alcoholism or digestive diseases that cause malabsorption and diarrhea. Vegetarians may need as much as 50 percent more zinc than meat eaters, since zinc is poorly absorbed from plant foods.

If taken during pregnancy, zinc may prevent certain birth defects and ensure proper fetal growth. Preliminary research suggests that zinc may be helpful for people with immune system problems such as rheumatoid arthritis and HIV. It may also slow vision loss due to macular degeneration.

Some evidence suggests that zinc helps fight the common cold. In clinical trials, patients using zinc every 2 hours at the first sign of a cough or sniffle reduced their suffering by nearly 3 days. The trick is to use zinc in the form of throat lozenges or nasal spray, since these methods are thought to work by directly interfering with cold viruses in the nose and throat. Zinc capsules or tablets can also be taken to improve overall immunity, but this probably only works in people who have a zinc deficiency.

Some enthusiasts believe zinc could be beneficial for treating a wide range of other illnesses. The list includes Alzheimer's disease, attention deficit disorder, benign prostatic hyperplasia, bladder infection, cataracts, diabetes, Down's syndrome, and even baldness. While there is no doubt that a true zinc deficiency can lead to numerous problems, no credible evidence shows that zinc supplementation can benefit these conditions.

What it is; how it works

Zinc is an essential mineral that is found in almost every cell in the body. It stimulates the activity of some 100 enzymes, and plays an important role in regulating gene expression. It is needed to support normal growth and development during pregnancy, childhood, and adolescence. An adequate supply is needed for normal sperm production. Zinc is also important for maintaining a healthy immune system, healing cuts and wounds, and maintaining a normal sense of taste and smell.

How zinc works is somewhat of a mystery. Scientists do know that the mineral is needed to activate T-lymphocytes, a type of white blood cell that fights infection. Advocates suggest that it may also interfere with the replication of cold viruses. Some research suggests that zinc acts as an antioxidant and a cell-membrane stabilizer, which could explain why it's helpful for brain function.

Zinc is widely distributed in foods. Oysters are a particularly rich source, although red meat and poultry provide the majority of zinc in the American diet. Other sources include beans, nuts, certain seafood, whole grains, fortified breakfast cereals, and dairy products. Zinc absorption is greater from a diet high in animal protein than a diet rich in plant proteins, including soy. This is because plant-based compounds called phytates can decrease zinc absorption.

Even borderline zinc deficiency can have profound negative effects. General signs of zinc deficiency include growth retardation, hair loss, diarrhea, delayed sexual maturation and impotence, eye and skin lesions, and loss of appetite. There is also some evidence that weight loss, delayed healing of wounds, taste abnormalities, and mental lethargy can occur. Remember, however, that some of these symptoms can also result from a variety of medical conditions other than zinc deficiency.

Avoid if...
Aside from an allergy to the ingredients in a supplement, there are no known reasons to avoid zinc.

Special cautions
Zinc causes few problems in doses up to 30 milligrams a day. Higher doses may cause stomach problems, including pain, nausea, and vomiting. Other reactions include headache, drowsiness, and a metallic taste.

Possible drug interactions
Advise patients that zinc supplements could decrease the absorption of certain antibiotics, including penicillin, tetracycline, and quinolones such as Cipro and Floxin. The mineral could also decrease absorption of bone-building drugs such as Actonel, Fosamax, and Didronel. Likewise, these same drugs could inhibit the absorption of zinc.

Certain minerals can decrease zinc absorption, including phosphorus, calcium, and iron. Products that contain phosphates, such as the drug K-Phos and certain potassium supplements, also may decrease zinc levels. On the other hand, too much zinc can cause a copper deficiency.

Special information about pregnancy and breastfeeding
Pregnant women should not exceed the Recommended Dietary Allowance (RDA) of 11 milligrams of zinc a day. Nursing mothers can take up to 12 milligrams.

Available preparations and dosage

Zinc supplements are available in several forms as tablets, capsules, lozenges, and nasal sprays; the most common preparations use zinc gluconate and zinc picolinate. A typical dose is 15 milligrams per day, although daily RDA requirements are somewhat lower, at 8 milligrams for women and 11 milligrams for men. For colds, the usual dosage is 13 to 23 milligrams of zinc gluconate every 2 hours for a week or two (but no longer).

For best absorption, zinc should not be taken with food or beverages that contain caffeine, tea, oxalic acid (such as spinach, sweet potatoes, rhubarb, and beans), and phytic acid (unleavened bread, seeds, nuts, grains, and soy). Taking zinc supplements with foods rich in amino acids, especially meat, may enhance absorption.

Overdosage

The recommended upper limit for zinc intake by adults is 40 milligrams a day. Sustained megadoses can lead to nausea and vomiting. Intakes of more than 150 milligrams per day can cause copper deficiency, reduce "good" HDL cholesterol levels, and depress the immune system.

Appendices

Prescription Drugs with Potential for Abuse

Over 500 legal prescription drug products—many of them psychotherapeutic—pose at least some danger of physical or psychological dependence leading to abuse. Such drugs are subject to the Controlled Substances Act of 1970, which assigns each drug to one of four categories of risk. Listed on the following pages are both branded and generic products that fall under the Act. The meaning of their assignments is as follows:

CII = **High Potential for Abuse:** Use may lead to severe physical or psychological dependence. Prescriptions must be written or confirmed in writing. No renewals are permitted.

CIII = **Some Potential for Abuse:** Use may lead to low-to-moderate physical dependence or high psychological dependence. Prescriptions may be oral or written. Up to five renewals are permitted within six months.

CIV = **Low Potential for Abuse:** Use may lead to limited physical or psychological dependence. Prescriptions may be oral or written. Up to five renewals are permitted within six months.

CV = **Subject to State and Local Regulation:** Abuse potential is low; in some areas a prescription may not be required.

The classifications in this section are based on information from the Thomson Healthcare *Red Book*® database. This list should not be considered comprehensive; when in doubt, consult the product's FDA-approved prescribing information.

Category CII

4-Dihydrotestosterone
Actiq
Adderall
Adderall XR
Alfenta
Alfentanil
Alfentanil HCl Novation
Amobarbital Sodium
Amphetamine Salt Combo
Amytal Sodium
APAP/Oxycodone
Aspirin/Oxycodone
Astramorph PF
Atropine And Demerol
Avinza
B & O Supprettes 15A
B & O Supprettes 16A
Biphetamine
Bupivacaine HCl/Fentanyl Citrate/
  Sodium Chloride
Bupivacaine HCl/Hydromorphone HCl/
  Sodium Chloride
Cesamet
Cocaine HCl
Codeine Phosphate
Codeine Sulfate
Combunox
Concerta
Daytrana
Demerol HCl
Demerol/APAP
Depodur
Desoxyn
Desoxyn Gradumet
Dexedrine
Dexedrine Spansules
Dextroamphetamine Saccharate-Amph
  Aspartate-Dextroamphetamine
  Sulfate-Amphetamine Sulfate
Dextroamphetamine Sulfate
Dextrose/Morphine Sulfate
Dextrostat
Dilaudid
Dilaudid-5
Dilaudid-HP
Diphenoxylate HCl
Dolophine HCl
Droperidol/Fentanyl Citrate
Duragesic
Duramorph
Endocet
Endodan
Eth-Oxydose

Fentanyl
Fentanyl Citrate
Fentanyl Citrate/Sodium Chloride
Fentanyl Oralet
Focalin
Focalin XR
Glutethimide
Hydrocodone Bitartrate
Hydromorphone HCl
Hydromorphone HCl/Sodium
  Chloride
Hydrostat IR
Infumorph 200
Infumorph 500
Innovar
Kadian
Levo-Dromoran
Levorphanol Tartrate
Mepergan
Meperidine HCl
Meperidine HCl/Promethazine HCl
Meperidine HCl/Sodium Chloride
Meperitab
Meprozine
Metadate CD
Metadate ER
Methadone DISP
Methadone HCl
Methadone HCl Concentrate
Methadone HCl Intensol
Methadose
Methadose DISP
Methamphetamine HCl
Methylin
Methylin ER
Methylphenidate HCl
Methylphenidate HCl ER
Morphine Sulfate
Morphine Sulfate/Sodium Chloride
MS Contin
MS/L Concentrate
Narvox
Nembutal Sodium
Numorphan HCl
Opana
Opana ER
Opium
Oramorph SR
Orlaam
Oxy IR
Oxycodone HCl
Oxycodone HCl CR
Oxycontin
Oxycontin ER

Oxydess
Oxyfast
Palladone
Pentobarbital Sodium
Percocet
Percodan
Percolone
Rescudose
Ritalin
Ritalin LA
Ritalin-SR
RMS
Roxanol
Roxicet
Roxicodone
Roxiprin
Secobarbital Sodium
Seconal Sodium
Spancap No. 1
Sublimaze
Sufenta
Sufentanil Citrate
Sufentanil Citrate Novaplus
Tuinal
Tylox
Ultiva

Category CIII

Adipost
A-G Tussin
Anadrol-50
Anaplex HD
Androderm
Androgel
Android
Anexsia
Anodynos-DHC
Anolor DH 5
Anorex-SR
APAP/Butalbital/Caffeine/Codeine
APAP/Codeine
APAP/Codeine #2
APAP/Codeine #3
APAP/Codeine #4
APAP/Dichloralphenazone/
   Isometheptene
APAP/Hydrocodone
APAP/Hydrocodone ES
Appecon
Aspirin/Codeine
Aspirin/Butalbital/Caffeine
Aspirin/Butalbital/Caffeine/Codeine
Aspirin/Carisoprodol/Codeine
Atuss G

Atuss HD
Atuss HX
Azdone
Bancap HC
Ban-Tuss HC
Bertuss SF
Bontril
Bontril PDM
Bromcomp HC
Bromphenex HD
Brompheniramine/Hydrocodone/
   Pseudoephedrine HCl
Bromplex HD
Brontex Tablets
Brovex HC
B-Tuss
Buprenex
Buprenorphine HCl
Busodium
Butabarbital Sodium
Butalbital Compound
Butalbital Compound/Codeine
Carbinoxamine/Hydrocodone/PSE
Ceta Plus
Codafed Expectorant
Codal-DH
Codamine
Codamine Pediatric
Codeine Phosphate/Guaifenesin
Codiclear DH
Codimal DH
Codituss DH
Co-Gesic
Coldcough HC
Coldcough XP
Coldtuss
Co-Tussin
Cotuss-V
Coughtuss
Chlorpheniramine/Hydrocodone/
   Pseudoephedrine
Chlorpheniramine/Hydrocodone/
   Phenylephrine
Cytuss HC
Damason-P
Deca-Durabolin
De-Chlor G
De-Chlor HC
De-Chlor HD
De-Chlor MR
De-Chlor NX
Decotuss-HD
Delatestryl
Depo-Testosterone

Dequibolin-100
Detuss
Didrex
Dihistine
Dihydro-CP
Dihydro-GP
Dihydrotestosterone
Dital
Ditussin-HC
Dolacet
Dolagesic
Dolfen
Dolorex Forte
Donatussin DC
Drituss HD
Duradal HD
Duradal HD Plus
Dynatuss HC
Dynatuss HCG
Echotuss-HC
ED-TLC
ED-Tuss HC
Endacof HC
Endacof XP
Endacof-Plus
Endagen-HD
Endal HD
Endal HD Plus
Endotuss-HD
Enplus-HD
Entex HC
Entuss Expectorant
Exo-Tuss
Fioricet/Codeine
Fiorinal
Fiorinal/Codeine
First-Testosterone
First-Testosterone MC
Fluoxymesterone
Flutuss HC
Fortabs
Genecof-HC
Genecof-XP
Gentex HC
Giltuss HC
G-Tuss
Gua-HC
Guaifenesin-Hydrocodone Bitartrate
Guapetex HC
Guiadex DH
H-C Tussive
H-C Tussive-D
Hexatussin
Highland HC

Histerone-100
Histerone-50
Hist-HC
Histinex D
Histinex HC
Histinex PV
Hist-Plus
Histussin-D
Histussin-HC
Hi-Tuss HC
Homatropine/Hydrocodone
Hybolin Decanoate
Hybolin-Improved
Hycet
Hycodan
Hyco-DH
Hycomal DH
Hycomed
Hycomine Compound
Hycomine Pediatric
Hyco-Pap
Hycophen
Hycosin Expectorant
Hycotab
Hycotuss Expectorant
Hydex-PD
Hydone
Hydro GP
Hydro PC
Hydro PC II
Hydro PC II Plus
Hydro Pro
Hydro Pro D Liquid
Hydrocet
Hydrocodone
Hydrocodone Bitartrate/Ibuprofen
Hydrocodone Compound
Hydrocodone CP
Hydrocodone GF
Hydrocodone HD
Hydrocodone PA
Hydrocodone PA Pediatric
Hydrocodone/Homatropine
Hydrocodone/Ibuprofen
Hydrocodone/Pot Guai
Hydro-Coff
Hydrocof-HC
Hydro-DP
Hydrofed
Hydrogesic
Hydromet
Hydromide
Hydron CP
Hydron EX

Hydron KGS
Hydron PSC
Hydropane
Hydrophed
Hydrophene DH
Hydrotropine
Hydro-Tuss
Hydro-Tussin DHC
Hydro-Tussin EXP
Hydro-Tussin HC
Hydro-Tussin HD
Hydro-Tussin HG
Hydro-Tussin XP
Hyfed
Hy-KXP
Hypamine
Hyphed
Hy-PHEN
Hyphen-HD
Hytan
Hytussin
Ide-Cet
Idenal
Iodal HD
Iogreen
Iotussin D
Iotussin HC
Isoclor Expectorant
Isollyl
Isollyl/Codeine
Jaycof Expectorant
Jaycof-HC
Jaycof-XP
Kabolin
Ketalar
Ketamine HCl
KG-Dal HD
KG-Fed Expectorant
KGS-HC
KG-Tuss HD Expectorant
KG-Tussin
Kwelcof
Laniroif
Levall 5.0
Liquicough HC
Liqui-Tuss HD
Liquitussin HC
Lorcet
Lorcet 10/650
Lorcet Plus
Lorcet-HD
Lortab
Lortab 10/500
Lortab 2.5/500

Lortab 5/500
Lortab 7.5/500
Lortab ASA
Lortab Liquid
Lortuss HC
Marcof Expectorant
Margesic #3
Margesic-H
Marinol
Maxidone
Maxi-Tuss HC
Maxi-Tuss HCG
Maxi-Tuss HCX
Maxi-Tuss SA
Maxitussin HC
M-Clear
M-Clear JR
Medcodin
Med-Hist EXP
Med-Hist-HC
Medipain 5
Meditest
Medtuss HD
Megagesic
Megamor
Melfiat
M-End
M-End Max
Metestone
Methitest
Methyltestosterone
Metra
Mintuss EX
Mintuss G
Mintuss HC
Mintuss HD
Mintuss MR
Mintuss MS
Mintuss NX
Morcomine
Nalex DH
Nalex Expectorant
Nandrolate
Nandrolone Decanoate
Nandrolone Phenpropionate
Narcof
Nariz-HC
Nasatuss
Norcet
Norco
Notuss
Notuss PD
N-Tussin
Nucochem Expectorant

Nucodine Expectorant
Nucofed Expectorant
Nucofed Pediatric
Nucotuss Expectorant
Nuco-Tuss Pediatric
Nudal HD
Obalan
Obezine
Oncet
Oreton Methyl
Oxandrin
Oxandrolone
PDM GG
Panacet 5/500
Panasal 5/500
Pancof
Pancof EXP
Pancof HC
Pancof XP
Panlor
Panlor DC
Panlor SS
Panlor-DC
Panlor-SS
Para-Hist HD
Paregoric
Parzine
P-D Tuss HD
Pediatex HD
Pentothal
Phanatuss-HC Diabetic Choice
Phena-HC
Phenaphen/Codeine
Phenaphen-650/Codeine
Phendal-HD
Phendiet
Phendiet-105
Phendimet
Phendimetrazine Bitartrate
Phenylephrine HD
Phrenilin/Caffeine/Codeine
Plegine
Pneumotussin
Pneumotussin 2.5
Pneumotussin HC
Poly Hist HC
Polygesic
Poly-Tussin
Poly-Tussin HD
Poly-Tussin XP
Prelu-2
Pri-Andriol LA
Primotest Forte
Procet

Pro-Clear
Pro-Cof
Pro-Cof D
Prolex DH
Propain HC
Propatuss Expectorant
Pro-Red
Protex
Protex D
Protuss
Protuss-D
PSE BPM HD
PT 105
P-Tuss
P-V-Tussin
Pyregesic-C
Qrp Tussin
QRP-105
Q-Tuss HC
Qual-Tussin DC
Quindal HD
Quindal HD Plus
Quintex HC
Q-V Tussin
Relacon-HC
Relacon-HC NR
Relasin-HC
Reprexain
Rexigen Forte
Rhinacon DH
Rindal HD
Rindal HD Plus
Rindal HPD
Ro-Codone
Rolatuss/Hydrocodone
Ru-Tuss/Hydrocodone
Shotest
Simuc-HD
Soma Compound/Codeine
Spantuss HD
SRC Expectorant
S-T Forte
S-T Forte 2
Stabec-105
Stagesic
Stagesic-10
Stanozolol
Stanozolol Micronized
Statobex
Statuss Green
Striant
Suboxone
Subutex
Surital

Su-Tuss HD
Synalgos-DC
T-Cypionate
T-E Cypionate
Teslac
Testa-C
Testamone-100
Testaspan
Test-Estro-Cypionate
Testex
Testim
Testoderm
Testoderm TTS
Testolin
Testone L.A.
Testopel Pellets
Testosterone
Testosterone Cypionate
Testosterone Cypionate/Estradiol
Testosterone Enanthate
Testosterone Enanthate Estradiol VA
Testosterone Micronized
Testosterone Propionate Micronized
Testred
Testred Cypionate 200
Testrin-P.A.
Testro AQ
Testro-L.A.
T-Gesic
Thiopental Sodium
Touro HC
Triaminic-DH Expectorant
Triant-HC
Trimal DH
Tri-Vent HC
Tusana-D
Tusdec-HC
Tussadur-HD
Tussafed-HC
Tussafed-HCG
Tussafin Expectorant
Tussanil DH
Tuss-AX
Tuss-DS
Tussend Expectorant
Tuss-ES
Tusset
Tussgen Expectorant
Tuss-HC
Tussigon
Tussinate
Tussin-V

Tussionex Pennkinetic
Tusso-DF
Tuss-PD
Tuss-PV
Tuss-S
Tylenol/Codeine #1
Tylenol/Codeine #2
Tylenol/Codeine #3
Tylenol/Codeine #4
Ugesic
Uni Cof EXP
Uni Tuss HC
Uni-Lev 5.0
Uni-Tricof HC
Uni-Tuss HC
Valertest No. 1
Vanacet
Vanacon
Vanex Expectorant
Vanex-HD
Vendone
Ventuss Syrup
Vetuss HC
Vicoclear
Vicodin
Vicodin ES
Vicodin HP
Vicodin Tuss Expectorant
Vicoprofen
Vigorex
Vi-Q-Tuss
Virilon
Virilon IM
Vitussin Expectorant
Vortex
Wehless
Wehless Timecelles
Weightrol
Welltuss EXP
Welltuss HC
Well-Tuss HD
Winstrol
Xodol
Xpect-HC
X-Trozine LA
Xyrem
Z-Cof HC
Zerlor
Ztuss
Ztuss ZT
Zydone
Zymine HC

Category CIV

Actifed/Codeine
Adipex-P
Alamine-C
Alidrin
Allerfrin/Codeine
Alprazolam
Alprazolam Intensol
Alprazolam XR
Ambien
Ambien CR
Amidrine
Amitriptyline/Chlordiazepoxide
Anaids
APAP/Propoxyphene Napsylate
APAP/Pentazocine HCl
APAP/Propoxyphene HCl
Aquachloral Supprettes
Aspirin/Caffeine/Propoxyphene HCl
Aspirin/Meprobamate
Atarin
Ativan
Atti-Plex P Tablet #1
Balacet 325
Barbital Sodium
Bexophene
Brevital Sodium
Butorphanol Tartrate
Butorphanol Tartrate Novation
Centrax
Chloral Hydrate
Chlordiazepoxide and Amitriptyline HCl
Chlordiazepoxide HCl
Clonazepam
Clorazepate Dipotassium
Cotanal-65
Cylert
Dalmane
Darvocet A500
Darvocet-N 100
Darvocet-N 50
Darvon
Darvon Compound 32
Darvon Compound-65
Deprol
Diastat
Diastat Acudial
Diastat Pediatric
Diastat Universal
Diazepam
Diazepam Intensol
Diethylpropion HCl
Diethylpropion HCl With
    Tartaric Acid

Dilantin-PB
Dizac
Dolene
Doral
Doxaphene Compound
Duradrin
D-Val
E-Lor
Epidrin
Epromate-M
Equagesic
Equanil
Estazolam
Ethchlorvynol
Fastin
Flurazepam HCl
Gen-Xene
Halcion
I.D.A.
Ionamin
Iso-Acetazone
Isocom
Isometheptene/Dichloralphenazone/
    APAP
Isopap
Klonopin
Klonopin Wafers
Librax
Libritabs
Librium
Limbitrol
Limbitrol DS
Lorazepam
Lorazepam Amerinet
Lorazepam Intensol
Luminal Sodium
Lunesta
Margesic 65
Margesic A-C
Mazanor
Mb-Tab
Mebaral
Mephobarbital
Meprobamate
Meprobamate Compound
Meprobamate/Aspirin
Meprogesic
Meprospan-200
Meprospan-400
Meridia
Micrainin
Midazolam HCl
Midazolam HCl Novation
Midchlor

Midrin
Migquin
Migraine Capsules
Migrapap
Migratine
Migrazone
Migrend
Migrex
Migrin-A
Miltown
Miltown 600
Mitran
Mitride
Motofen
Naloxone HCl/Pentazocine
Niravam
Novaplus Butorphanol Tartrate
Novaplus Lorazepam
Novaplus Midazolam HCl
Obenix
Obephen
Oby-Cap
Oby-Trim
Oxazepam
P.E.T.N./Phenobarbital
Panshape M
Paral
Paraldehyde
Paxipam
PC-CAP
Pemoline
Phenobarbital Sodium
Phentercot
Phentermine HCl
Phentermine/Resin
Phentride
Phentrol
Placidyl
Pondimin
Poxi
PP-Cap
Prazepam
Probate
Pro-Fast HS
Pro-Fast SA
Pro-Fast SR
Pronap-100

Propacet 100
Propoxacet
Propoxacet-N 100
Propoxycon
Propoxyphene/Aspirin/Caffeine
Propoxyphene Compound-65
Propoxyphene HCl
Propoxyphene Napsylate
Prosom
Provigil
Redux
Restoril
Rexin
Sanorex
Serax
Sodium Barbital
Sodium Phenobarbital
Solfoton
Somnote
Sonata
Stadol
Stadol NS
Talacen
Talwin Compound
Talwin Lactate
Talwin NX
Tara-30
T-Diet
Temazepam
Tenuate
Tenuate Dospan
Tepanil Ten-Tab
Teramine
Trancot
Tranxene T-Tab
Tranxene-SD
Triazolam
Truxaphen
Valium
Valrelease
Va-Zone
Versed
Wygesic
Xanax
Xanax XR
Zantryl
Zetran

Category CV

Alphen Expectorant
Ambenyl
Ambophen
Amogel PG
Antitussive/Decongestant Expectorant
Aprodine/Codeine
Atrohist Plus
Atropine Sulfate/Diphenoxylate HCl
Baltussin
Ban-Tuss C
Bio-Tuss C
Biotussin AC
Biotussin DAC
Bitex Liquid
Bromanate DC
Bromanyl
Bromodiphenhydramine HCl/Codeine
Bromotuss/Codeine
Bromphen DC
Bromphen DC/Codeine
Brompheniramine DC
Broncholate CS
Bron-Tuss
Calcidrine
Calcium Iodide/Codeine
Capital/Codeine
Chemdal Expectorant
Cheracol/Codeine
Cheralin
Cheratussin AC
Cheratussin DAC
Chlorpheniramine Compound
Codafed
Codafed Pediatric Expectorant
Codahistine DH
Codahistine Expectorant
Codecon-C
Codefen
Codegesic
Codegest Expectorant
Codehist DH
Codeine/Guaifenesin/Pseudoephedrine
Codeine/Phenylephrine/Promethazine
Codeine/Promethazine
Codeine/Pseudoephedrine/Triprolidine
Codimal PH
Co-Histine DH
Co-Histine Expectorant
Coldcough PD
Conex/Codeine
C-Tussin
Cycofed Pediatric Expectorant
Cyndal Expectorant

Decohistine DH
Decohistine Expectorant
Decongestant Antitussive
Deconhist
Deconsal Pediatric
Delhistine CS
Demi-Cof
Deproist/Codeine
Diabetic Tussin C Expectorant
Diamine DC
Dia-Quel
Di-Atro
Dicomal-PH
Dihistine DH
Dihistine Expectorant
Dimetane-DC
Dimotal
Dinex Grape
Diphenoxylate HCl/Atropine
Donnagel-PG
Donnapectolin-PG
Duraganidin NR
Efasin Expectorant SF
Endal Expectorant
Enditussin Expectorant
Endotuss Expectorant
En-Pain
Gani-Tuss NR
Giltuss Ped-C
Glydeine
Guaiatussin AC
Guaiatussin DAC
Guai-Co
Guaifen AC
Guaifenesin AC Expectorant
Guaifenesin/Codeine Phosphate
Guaifenesin DAC
Guaifenesin/Pseudoephedrine/Codeine
Guaituss AC Expectorant
Guaitussin AC
Guaitussin DAC
Guiatuscon AC
Guiatussin/Codeine
Halotussin AC
Halotussin DAC
Histafed C
Iocen-C
Iodinated Glycerol-Codeine
Iodur/Codeine
Iofen-C NF
Iophen
Iophen C-NR
Iophen-C
Iotuss

Kaolin-Pectin/Paregoric
Kaopectolin-PG
Kg-Fed Pediatric Expectorant
Kolephrin #1
Liqui-Histine CS
Lomanate
Lomocot
Lomotil
Lonox
Lyrica
Mallergan VC
Medent C
Medi-Tuss/Codeine
M-Phen
Multi-Hist CS
Myphetane DC
Mytussin AC
Mytussin DAC
Naldecon CX Adult
Normatane DC
Nor-Mil
Nortussin
Novadyne DH
Novagest DH
Novagest Expectorant/Codeine
Novahistine DH
Novahistine Expectorant
Novamor DH
Novatuss HC
Novatuss LA
Novatuss-C
Nucochem Pediatric Expectorant
Nucodine Pediatric
Nucofed Pediatric Expectorant
Nucotuss Pediatric Expectorant
Orahist Expectorant
Orgadin-Tuss
Oridol C
Pancof PD
Pannaz
Para-Hist
Par-Glycerol C
Pediacof
Pedituss
Phenergan/Codeine
Phenergan VC/Codeine
Phenhist DH/Codeine
Phenhist Expectorant
Phenylchlor BA
Phenylhistine
Phenylhistine DH
Phenylhistine Expectorant
Poly-CS
Poly-Histine CS
Polytine CS

Promethazine/Codeine
Promethazine VC/Codeine
Prothazine
Pro-Tuss
Pseudoephedrine/Chlorpheniramine/
  Codeine
Q-Tuss
Quindal Expectorant
Rid-A-Pain/Codeine
Rite Aid Brands
Robafen AC
Robafen DAC
Robichem AC
Robitussin-AC
Robitussin-DAC
Roganidin
Rolatuss SR
Romilar AC
Ru-Tab
Ru-Tuss
Ryna-C
Ryna-CX
Statuss
Sudatuss-2
Sudatuss-SF
Suttar-2
Suttar-SF
Terpin Hydrate/Codeine
T-Koff
Triacin C
Triacin-C
Triafed/Codeine
Triaminic EXP/Codeine
Trifed C
Trihist-CS
Triprolidine-C
Tuss Delay
Tussar SF
Tussar-2
Tusshistine CS
Tussidin NR
Tussin DAC
Tussi-Organidin
Tussi-Organidin NR
Tussi-Organidin-S
Tussi-Organidin-S NR
Tussirex
Tussi-R-Gen
Tylenol /Codeine
Uni Multihist CS
Uni-Lom
Vanex Grape
Vi-Atro
Ztuss Expectorant

Pharmacokinetics for Psychotropic Drugs

Pharmacokinetics is often described as what the body does to a drug. It refers to the movement of a drug into, through, and out of the body—the time course of its absorption, bioavailability, distribution, metabolism, and excretion. (Pharmacodynamics, on the other hand, is what a drug does to the body, which typically involves receptor binding, postreceptor effects, and chemical interactions.) Drug pharmacokinetics determines the onset, duration, and intensity of a drug's effect. The pharmacokinetics of a drug depends on patient-related factors as well as on the drug's chemical properties. General patient-related factors include sex, age, genetic makeup, kidney function, and liver function.

The information in this appendix comes from FDA-approved prescribing information only. The table lists common pharmacokinetic parameters associated with the absorption, distribution, and elimination of psychotropic drugs, including:

- Half-life ($t_{1/2}$): The time it takes for plasma concentration of the drug to reduce by 50%.

- T_{max}: The time it takes for the drug to reach the maximum plasma concentration.

- Time to steady state: The time it takes the drug to reach a plasma concentration where the amount of drug being absorbed is the same as the amount of drug being eliminated.

Pharmacokinetics for Psychotropic drugs

Brand Name (generic name)	Half-Life ($t_{1/2}$)	Time to Peak Concentration (T_{max})	Time to Steady State Concentration*	Food Effects
Abilify (aripiprazole)	75 hours (aripiprazole in extensive metabolizers); 146 hours (aripiprazole in poor metabolizers); 94 hours (dehydro-aripiprazole)	3-5 hours (aripiprazole)	14 days	Take without regard to meals.
Adderall (amphetamine)	9.77-11 hours (d-amphetamine); 11.5-13.8 hours (d-amphetamine)	3 hours (d-amphetamine and l-amphetamine)	N/A	Take without regard to meals.
Adderall XR (amphetamine)	D-amphetamine: 10 hours (adults); 11 hours (adolescents 13-17 years, ≤75 kilograms or 165 pounds); 9 hours (children 6-12 years). L-amphetamine: 13 hours (adults); 13-14 (adolescents), 11 hours (children 6-12 years).	7 hours (d-amphetamine and l-amphetamine)	N/A	Food prolongs T_{max} by 2.5 hours.
Ambien (zolpidem tartrate)	2.6 hours (zolpidem 5 mg); 2.5 hours (zolpidem 10 mg)	1.6 hours	N/A	Food prolongs T_{max} by 60%, avoid with or immediately after a meal.
Ambien CR (zolpidem tartrate)	2.8 hours	1.5 hours	N/A	Food prolongs T_{max} by 2 hours, avoid with or immediately after a meal.
Amitriptyline HCl†	24 hours	4-6 hours	N/A	Take without regard to meals.
Amitriptyline with perphenazine†	24 hours	4-6 hours	N/A	Take without regard to meals.

Drug	Half-life	Time to peak	Duration	Administration
Amoxapine†	8 hours (amoxapine); 30 hours (8-hydroxyamoxapine)	1.5 hours (amoxapine)	N/A	N/A
Anafranil (clomipramine HCl)	19-37 hours (clomipramine); 54-77 hours (desmethylclomipramine)	2-6 hours (clomipramine)	7-14 days (clomipramine)	N/A
Antabuse (disulfiram)	N/A	N/A	N/A	N/A
Aricept (donepezil)	70 hours	3-4 hours (donepezil)	15 days	Take without regard to meals.
Ativan (lorazepam)	12 hours (lorazepam); 18 hours (lorazepam glucuronide)	2 hours	N/A	N/A
BuSpar (buspirone)	2-3 hours	40-90 min	N/A	N/A
Campral (acamprosate calcium)	20-33 hours	3-8 hours	5 days	N/A
Celexa (citalopram hydrobromide)	35 hours	4 hours	7 days	Take without regard to meals.
Chantix (varenicline tartrate)	24 hours	3-4 hours	>4 days	Take after a meal with full glass of water.
Chlorpromazine†	N/A	N/A	N/A	Take without regard to meals.
Clozaril (clozapine)	8 hours (clozapine single-dose); 12 hours (clozapine at steady state)	2.5 hours (clozapine)	N/A	Take without regard to meals.
Cognex (tacrine HCl)	2-4 hours	1-2 hours	24-36 hours	Administer 1 hour before meals.
Concerta (methylphenidate HCl)	3.5 hours	6-10 hours	N/A	Take without regard to meals.
Cymbalta (duloxetine HCl)	12 hours	6 hours	3 days	Take without regard to meals.

Brand Name (generic name)	Half-Life ($t_{1/2}$)	Time to Peak Concentration (T_{max})	Time to Steady State Concentration*	Food Effects
Dalmane (flurazepam HCl)	2.3 hours (flurazepam); 47-100 hours (N1-des-alkyl-flurazepam)	30-60 min (flurazepam)	7-10 days (N1-des-alkyl-flurazepam)	Take without regard to meals.
Daytrana (methylphenidate patch)	3-4 hours	7.5-10.5 hours	N/A	N/A
Depakote (divalproex sodium)	9-16 hours	4 hours	N/A	Take without regard to meals.
Depakote ER (divalproex sodium)	9-16 hours	4-17 hours	N/A	Take without regard to meals.
Desoxyn (methamphetamine HCl)	4-5 hours	N/A	N/A	Administer 1/2 hour before meals.
Desyrel (trazodone HCl)	N/A	N/A	N/A	Administer after meals.
Dexedrine (dextroam-phetamine sulfate)	12 hours	8 hours (spansule); 3 hours (tabs)	N/A	N/A
DextroStat (dextroam-phetamine sulfate)	10.25 hours	2 hours	N/A	N/A
Doral (quazepam)	39 hours (quazepam and 2-oxo-quazepam); 73 hours (N-desalkylation-2-oxoquazepam)	2 hours (quazepam)	7 days (quazepam and 2-oxo-quazepam); 13 days (N-desalkyl-2-oxoquazepam)	N/A
Effexor (venlafaxine HCl)	5 hours (venlafaxine); 11 hours (O-desmethylvenlafaxine)	N/A	3 days (venlafaxine and O-desmethylvenlafaxine)	Take without regard to meals.
Effexor XR (venlafaxine HCl)	6 hours (venlafaxine); 11 hours (O-desmethylvenlafaxine)	N/A	3 days (venlafaxine and O-desmethylvenlafaxine)	Take without regard to meals.
EMSAM (selegiline patch)	18-25 hours (selegiline, R(-)-N-des-methylselegiline, R(-)-amphetamine, and R(-)-methamphetamine)	N/A	5 days	N/A

				Take 1 hour before meals.
Equetro (carbamazepine)	35-40 hours (carbamazepine first dose); 12-17 hours (carbamazepine repeated dosing); 34 hours (carbamazepine 10,11-epoxide)	6-26 hours (carbamazepine); 30-42 hours (carbamazepine 10,11-epoxide)	N/A	
Eskalith (lithium carbonate)	N/A	N/A	N/A	Administer after meals.
Exelon (rivastigmine)	1.5 hours	1 hour	N/A	Take with meals.
FazaClo (clozapine)	8 hours (clozapine single-dose); 12 hours clozapine multiple-dose)	2.3 hours	N/A	Take without regard to meals.
Fluvoxamine maleate†	15.6 hours (fluvoxamine)	3-8 hours	7 days	Take without regard to meals.
Focalin (dexmethylphenidate HCl)	2.2 hours	1-1.5 hours	N/A	Take without regard to meals.
Focalin XR (dexmethylphenidate HCl)	2-4.5 hours	1.5 hours (first peak); 6.5 hours (second peak)	N/A	Take without regard to meals.
Geodon (ziprasidone)	7 hours	6-8 hours (ziprasidone)	1-3 days	Take without regard to meals.
Halcion (triazolam)	1.5-5.5 hours	2 hours (triazolam)	N/A	Take without regard to meals.
Haloperidol†	N/A	N/A	N/A	N/A
Invega (paliperidone)	23 hours	24 hours	4-5 days	Take without regard to meals.
Klonopin (clonazepam)	30-40 hours	1-4 hours	N/A	Take without regard to meals.
Lamictal (lamotrigine)	Single-dose (32.8 hours); multiple dose (25.4 hours)	1.4-4.8 hours	N/A	Take without regard to meals.
Lamictal CD (lamotrigine)	Single-dose (32.8 hours); multiple dose (25.4 hours)	1.4-4.8 hours	N/A	Take without regard to meals.

Brand Name (generic name)	Half-Life ($t_{1/2}$)	Time to Peak Concentration (T_{max})	Time to Steady State Concentration*	Food Effects
Lexapro (escitalopram oxalate)	27-32 hours	5 hours	7 days	Take without regard to meals.
Librium (chlordiazepoxide)	24-48 hours	N/A	N/A	Take without regard to meals.
Limbitrol (amitriptyline with chlordiazepoxide)	N/A	N/A	N/A	Take without regard to meals.
Lithium carbonate	24 hours	N/A	N/A	Take 1 hour after meals.
Lithobid (lithium carbonate)	24 hours	N/A	N/A	Take 1 hour after meals.
Lunesta (eszopiclone)	6 hours	1 hour	N/A	Avoid with or immediately after a fatty meal.
Maprotiline HCl†	51 hours	12 hours	N/A	Take without regard to meals.
Mebaral (mephobarbital)	N/A	N/A	N/A	Take without regard to meals.
Meprobamate†	N/A	N/A	N/A	Take without regard to meals.
Metadate CD (methylphenidate HCl)	6.8 hours	1.5 hours (first peak); 4.5 hours (second peak)	N/A	Food delays early peak by 1 hour.
Metadate ER (methylphenidate HCl)	3.4 hours	4.7 hours	24 hours	Increase in C_{max} and AUC when administered with food.

Methylin (methylphenidate HCl)	2.7 hours	1-2 hours	N/A	Fatty food delays peak by 1 hour.
Moban (molindone HCl)	24-36 hours	1.5 hours	N/A	Take without regard to meals.
Namenda (memantine)	60-80 hours	3-7 hours	N/A	Take without regard to meals.
Nardil (phenelzine sulfate)	11.6 hours	43 minutes	N/A	Take without regard to meals.
Navane (thiothixene)	N/A	N/A	N/A	Take without regard to meals.
Nefazodone HCl†	2-4 hours (nefazodone); 1.5-4 hours (hydroxynefazodone); 4-8 hours (meta-chlorophenylpiperazine); 18 hours (triazole-dione)	1 hour (nefazodone)	4-5 days (nefazodone and metabolites)	Take without regard to meals.
Nembutal sodium (pentobarbital sodium)	15-50 hours	15 minites (IV); 20-60 minites (oral, rectal)	N/A	Take without regard to meals.
Niravam (alprazolam orally disintegrating tablet)	12.5 hours (alprazolam, alpha-hydroxyalprazolam, 4-hydroxyalprazolam)	1.5-2 hours	N/A	Food prolongs Tmax by 2 hours.
Norpramin (desipramine HCl)	N/A	N/A	N/A	Take without regard to meals.
Oxazepam†	8.2 hours	3 hours	N/A	Take without regard to meals.
Pamelor (nortriptyline HCl)	N/A	N/A	N/A	Take without regard to meals.
Parnate (tranylcypromine sulfate)	N/A	N/A	N/A	Take without regard to meals.

Brand Name (generic name)	Half-Life (t$_{1/2}$)	Time to Peak Concentration (T$_{max}$)	Time to Steady State Concentration*	Food Effects
Paxil (paroxetine HCl)	21 hours	5.2 hours	10 days	Take without regard to meals.
Paxil CR (paroxetine HCl)	15–20 hours	6–10 hours	14 days	Take without regard to meals.
Perphenazine†	N/A	N/A	N/A	Take without regard to meals.
Pexeva (paroxetine mesylate)	33.2 hours	8.1 hours	13 days	Take without regard to meals.
Phenergan (promethazine HCl)	4–6 hours	N/A	N/A	Food decreased T$_{max}$ by approximately 2 hours.
Phenobarbital†	N/A	N/A	N/A	N/A
Prochlorperazine†	N/A	N/A	N/A	Take without regard to meals.
Prolixin (fluphenazine HCl)	N/A	N/A	N/A	Take without regard to meals.
ProSom (estazolam)	10–24 hours	2 hours		Take without regard to meals.
Provigil (modafinil)	15 hours (after multiple doses of modafinil)	2–4 hours	2–4 days	Take without regard to meals.
Prozac (fluoxetine HCl)	1–3 days (acute administration of fluoxetine); 4–6 days (chronic administration of fluoxetine); 4–16 days (acute & chronic administration of norfluoxetine)	6–8 hours (40 milligrams)	30 days (fluoxetine); 4-5 weeks (norfluoxetine)	Take without regard to meals.

Drug	Half-life	Time to peak	Steady state	Food
Razadyne (galantamine)	7 hours	1 hour	N/A	Take without regard to meals.
Razadyne ER (galantamine)	7 hours	4.5-5 hours	7 days	Food decreased Tmax by approximately 1.5 hours.
Remeron (mirtazapine)	20-40 hours	2 hours	5 days	Food decreased Tmax by approxi mately 1.5 hours.
Reserpine (reserpine)	5 hours (initial reserpine) 200 hours (terminal half-life reserpine)	2.5 hours	N/A	Take without regard to meals.
Restoril (temazepam)	8.8 hours	1.5 hours	3 doses	Take without regard to meals.
ReVia (naltrexone HCl)	N/A	N/A	N/A	Take without regard to meals.
Risperdal (risperidone)	3 hours (risperidone in extensive metabolizers); 20 hours (risperidone in poor metabolizers); 21 hours (9-hydroxyrisperidone in extensive metabolizers); 30 hours (9-hydroxyrisperidone in poor metabolizers)	1 hour (risperidone); 3 hours(9-hydroxyrisperidone in extensive metabolizers); 17 hours (9-hydroxyrisperidone in poor metabolizers)	1-day (risperidone in extensive metabolizers); 5 days (risperidone in poor metabolizers) (9-hydroxyrisperidone in extensive metabolizers)	Take without regard to meals.
Risperdal Consta (risperidone)	3-6 days (risperidone & 9-hydroxy-risperidone)	N/A	4-6 weeks after 4 injections	Take without regard to meals.
Risperdal M-Tab (risperidone)	3 hours (risperidone in extensive metabolizers); 20 hours (risperidone in poor metabolizers); 21 hours (9-hydroxyrisperidone in extensive metabolizers); 30 hours (9-hydroxy-risperidone in poor metabolizers)	1-hour (risperdone); 3 hours (9-hydroxyrisperidone in extensive metabolizers); 17 hours (9-hydroxyrisperi-done in poor metabolizers)	1-day (risperidone in extensive metabolizers); 5 days (risperidone in poor metabolizers) (9-hydroxyrisperidone in extensive metabolizers)	Take without regard to meals.

Brand Name (generic name)	Half-Life ($t_{1/2}$)	Time to Peak Concentration (T_{max})	Time to Steady State Concentration*	Food Effects
Ritalin (methylphenidate HCl)	N/A	1.9 hours (methylphenidate in children)	N/A	Take without regard to meals.
Ritalin LA (methylphenidate HCl)	1.5-4 hours (methylphenidate 20 mg in children); 3-4.2 hours (methylphenidate 20 mg in adults)	1-3 hours (first peak of methylphenidate 20 milligrams in children); 1.3-4 hours (first peak of methylphenidate 20 milligrams in adults); 5-11 hours (second peak of methylphenidate 20 milligrams in children); 4.3-6.5 hours (second peak of methylphenidate 20 milligrams in adults)	N/A	Take without regard to meals.
Ritalin SR (methylphenidate HCl)	N/A	4.7 hours (methylphenidate in children)	N/A	Take without regard to meals.
Rozerem (ramelteon)	1-2.6 hours	0.75 hours	N/A	Take without regard to meals.
Sarafem (fluoxetine HCl)	1-3 days (acute administration of fluoxetine); 4-6 days (chronic administration of fluoxetine); 4-16 days (acute & chronic administration of norfluoxetine)	6-8 hours (fluoxetine)	30 days (fluoxetine) 4-5 weeks (norfluoxetine)	Do not take after high-fat meal.
Seconal (secobarbital sodium)	28 hours	N/A	N/A	Take without regard to meals.
Seroquel (quetiapine fumarate)	6 hours	1.5 hours	2 days	Take without regard to meals.

Seroquel XR (quetiapine fumarate)	7 hours (quetiaoine); 9-12 hours (N-desalkyl quetiapine)	6 hours	2 days	Take without regard to meals.
Sinequan (doxepine HCl)	N/A	N/A	N/A	Take without regard to meals.
Sonata (zaleplon)	1 hour	1 hour	N/A	High fat meal decreased T_{max} by 2 hours.
Strattera (atomoxetine HCl)	5.2 hours (extensive metabolizers [EM] atomoxetine); 21.6 hours (poor metabolizers [PM] atomoxetine); 6-8 hours (EM 4-hydroxyatomoxetine & N-desmethylatomoxetine); 34-40 hours (PM N-desmethylatomoxetine)	N/A	N/A	Do not take after high-fat meal.
Suboxone (buprenorphine and naloxone)	37 hours (buprenorphine) & 1.1 hours (naloxone)	N/A	N/A	Take without regard to meals.
Surmontil (trimipramine maleate)	N/A	N/A	N/A	Take without regard to meals.
Symbyax (olanzapine)	24-54 hours (olanzapine); 1-3 days (acute administration fluoxetine); 4-6 days (chronic administration fluoxetine); 4-16 days (acute & chronic administration of norfluoxetine)	4 hours (olanzapine); 6 hours (fluoxetine)	1 week (olanzapine) 4-5 weeks (fluoxetine)	Take without regard to meals.
Thioridazine HCl†	N/A	N/A	N/A	Take without regard to meals.
Tofranil (imipramine HCl)	N/A	N/A	N/A	Take without regard to meals.
Tranxene (clorazepate dipotassium)	N/A	N/A	N/A	Take without regard to meals.

Brand Name (generic name)	Half-Life (t$_{1/2}$)	Time to Peak Concentration (T$_{max}$)	Time to Steady State Concentration*	Food Effects
Trifluoperazine HCl†	N/A	N/A	N/A	Take without regard to meals.
Trihexyphenidyl HCl†	N/A	N/A	N/A	Administer before or after meals
Valium (diazepam)	N/A	N/A	N/A	Take without regard to meals.
Vistaril (hydroxyzine HCl)	N/A	N/A	N/A	Take without regard to meals.
Vivactil (protriptyline HCl)	16 days	8-12 hours	N/A	Take without regard to meals.
Vivitrol (naltrexone)	5-10 days (naltrexone and 6-beta-naltrexol)	Initial peak in 2 hours (naltrexone) & second peak in 2-3 days (vivitrol)	4 weeks	Take without regard to meals.
Vyvanse (lisdexamfetamine dimesylate)	<1 hour	1 hour	N/A to meals.	Take without regard
Wellbutrin (bupropion)	21 hours (bupropion); 20 hours (hydroxybupropion: active metabolite; 33 hours (erythrohydrobupropion); 37 hours (threohydrobupropion)	2 hours (bupropion); 3 hours (hydroxybupropion)	8 days (bupropion)	Take without regard to meals.
Wellbutrin SR (bupropion)	22 hours (bupropion); 20 hours (hydroxybupropion: active metabolite; 33 hours (erythrohydrobupropion); 37 hours (threohydrobupropion)	3 hours (bupropion); 6 hours (hydroxybupropion)	8 days (bupropion)	Take without regard to meals.

	Half-life	Time to peak	Steady state*	
Wellbutrin XL (bupropion)	21 hours (bupropion); 20 hours (hydroxybupropion: active metabolite); 33 hours (erythrohydrobupropion); 37 hours (threohydrobupropion)	2 hours (bupropion); 3 hours (hydroxybupropion)	8 days (bupropion)	Take without regard to meals.
Xanax (alprazolam)	11.2 hours (alprazolam, 4-hydroxyalprazolam & alpha-hydroxyalprazolam)	1-2 hours (alprazolam)	N/A	Take without regard to meals.
Xanax XR (alprazolam)	10.7-15.8 hours	1-2 hours (alprazolam)	N/A	Take without regard to meals.
Zoloft (sertraline HCl)	26 hours (sertraline); 62-104 hours (N-desmethylsertraline)	4.5-8.4 hours (sertraline)	7 days (sertraline)	Take without regard to meals.
Zyban (bupropion HCl)	21 hours (bupropion); 20 hours (hydroxybupropion: active metabolite); 33 hours (erythrohydrobupropion); 37 hours (threohydrobupropion)	3 hours (bupropion); 6 hours (hydroxybupropion)	N/A	Take without regard to meals.
Zyprexa (olanzapine)	21-54 hours	6 hours	7 days	Take without regard to meals.
Zyprexa Intramuscular (olanzapine)	21-54 hours	6 hours	7 days	Take without regard to meals.
Zyprexa Zydis (olanzapine)	21-54 hours	6 hours	7 days	Take without regard to meals.

*Steady state can be estimated by multiplying the half-life by 5.
†Generic name; no brand is available.
All information based on the pharmacokinetics section of FDA-approved prescribing information.
N/A = Not available.

Indices

Psychotropic Drugs Indexed by Brand and Generic Name

Listed here are all psychotropic drugs profiled in the first section of the book. Cross-referenced generic names are shown in italics.

Psychotropic Drugs Indexed by Indication

Use this index to determine which drugs are available for a specific psychological problem. Both brand and generic names are listed; the cross-referenced generic names are shown in italics. Only medications profiled in the first section of the book are included.

Agitation
    Amitriptyline with Perphenazine

Alcohol dependence
    Acamprosate. See Campral
    Antabuse
    Campral
    Disulfiram. See Antabuse
    Naltrexone injection. See Vivitrol
    Naltrexone tablets. See ReVia
    ReVia
    Vivitrol

Alcohol withdrawal
    Chlordiazepoxide. See Librium
    Clorazepate. See Tranxene
    Diazepam. See Valium
    Librium
    Oxazepam
    Tranxene
    Valium

Alzheimer's disease
    Aricept
    Cognex
    Donepezil. See Aricept
    Exelon
    Galantamine. See Razadyne
    Memantine. See Namenda
    Namenda
    Razadyne
    Rivastigmine. See Exelon
    Tacrine. See Cognex

Anxiety disorders
    Alprazolam. See Xanax
    *Alprazolam orally disintegrating
        tablets. See* Niravam
    *Amitriptyline with Chlordiazepoxide.
        See* Limbitrol
    Amitriptyline with Perphenazine
    Ativan
    BuSpar
    Buspirone. See BuSpar
    Chlordiazepoxide. See Librium
    Clorazepate. See Tranxene
    Cymbalta

Diazepam. See Valium
Doxepin. See Sinequan
Duloxetine. See Cymbalta
Effexor
Escitalopram. See Lexapro
Lexapro
Librium
Limbitrol
Lorazepam. See Ativan
Maprotiline
Mebaral
Mephobarbital. See Mebaral
Meprobamate
Nardil
Niravam
Oxazepam
Paroxetine. See Paxil
Paxil
Pexeva. *See* Paxil
Phenelzine. See Nardil
Prochlorperazine
Sertraline. See Zoloft
Sinequan
Tranxene
Trifluoperazine
Valium
Venlafaxine. See Effexor
Vistaril
Xanax
Zoloft

**Attention Deficit
Hyperactivity Disorder**
    Adderall
    Amphetamines. See Adderall
    Atomoxetine. See Strattera
    Concerta. *See* Ritalin
    Daytrana
    Desoxyn
    Dexedrine
    Dexmethylphenidate. See Focalin
    Dextroamphetamine. See Dexedrine
    DextroStat. *See* Dexedrine
    Focalin
    Lisdexamfetamine. See Vyvanse
    Metadate. *See* Ritalin

Methamphetamine. *See* Desoxyn
Methylin. *See* Ritalin
Methylphenidate. See Ritalin
Methylphenidate patch. See Daytrana
Ritalin
Strattera
Vyvanse

Bed-wetting
Imipramine. See Tofranil
Tofranil

Behavior problems in children, severe
Chlorpromazine
Haloperidol
Thorazine. *See* Chlorpromazine

Bipolar disorder
Abilify
Aripiprazole. See Abilify
Carbamazepine. See Equetro
Chlorpromazine
Depakote
Divalproex. See Depakote
Doxepin. See Sinequan
Equetro
Eskalith. *See* Lithium Carbonate
Lamictal
Lamotrigine. See Lamictal
Lithium Carbonate
Lithobid. *See* Lithium Carbonate
Maprotiline
Olanzapine. See Zyprexa
Olanzapine and fluoxetine.
  See Symbyax
Sinequan
Symbyax
Thorazine. *See* Chlorpromazine
Zyprexa

Bulimia
Fluoxetine. See Prozac
Prozac

Depression
Amitriptyline
Amitriptyline with Chlordiazepoxide.
  See Limbitrol
Amitriptyline with Perphenazine
Amoxapine
Aventyl. *See* Pamelor
Bupropion. See Wellbutrin
Celexa
Citalopram. See Celexa
Cymbalta

Desipramine. See Norpramin
Desyrel
Doxepin. See Sinequan
Duloxetine. See Cymbalta
Effexor
Emsam
Escitalopram. See Lexapro
Fluoxetine. See Prozac
Imipramine. See Tofranil
Lexapro
Limbitrol
Maprotiline
Mirtazapine. See Remeron
Nardil
Nefazodone
Norpramin
Nortriptyline. See Pamelor
Pamelor
Parnate
Paroxetine. See Paxil
Paxil
Pexeva. *See* Paxil
Phenelzine. See Nardil
Protriptyline. See Vivactil
Prozac
Remeron
Selegiline skin patch. See Emsam
Sertraline. See Zoloft
Sinequan
Surmontil
Tofranil
Tranylcypromine. See Parnate
Trazodone. See Desyrel
Trimipramine. See Surmontil
Venlafaxine. See Effexor
Vivactil
Wellbutrin
Zoloft

Diabetic peripheral neuropathy
Cymbalta
Duloxetine. See Cymbalta

Hyperactivity
See Attention Deficit Hyperactivity
  Disorder

Insomnia
Ambien CR
Dalmane
Doral
Estazolam. See ProSom
Eszopiclone. See Lunesta
Flurazepam. See Dalmane
Halcion

Psychotropic Drugs Indexed by Category

This index allows you to identify all the psychotropic alternatives in a particular pharmacological category. Remember, though, that even closely related drugs may differ in their therapeutic action and adverse effects. Both brand and generic names are listed; the cross-referenced generic names are shown in italics. Only medications profiled in the first section of the book are included.

ANTIANXIETY AGENTS

Benzodiazepines and combinations

Alprazolam. See Xanax
Alprazolam orally disintegrating tablets. See Niravam
Amitriptyline with *Chlordiazepoxide. See* Limbitrol
Ativan
Chlordiazepoxide. See Librium
Clonazepam. See Klonopin
Clorazepate. See Tranxene
Dalmane
Diazepam. See Valium
Doral
Estazolam. See ProSom
Flurazepam. See Dalmane
Halcion
Klonopin
Librium
Limbitrol
Lorazepam. See Ativan
Niravam
Oxazepam
ProSom
Quazepam. See Doral
Restoril
Temazepam. See Restoril
Tranxene
Triazolam. See Halcion
Valium
Xanax

Miscellaneous antianxiety agents

BuSpar
Buspirone. See BuSpar
Doxepin. See Sinequan
Effexor
Hydroxyzine. See Vistaril
Meprobamate
Paroxetine. See Paxil
Paxil
Sinequan
Venlafaxine. See Effexor
Vistaril

ANTIDEPRESSANTS

Miscellaneous antidepressants

Bupropion. See Wellbutrin
Cymbalta
Duloxetine. See Cymbalta
Desyrel
Effexor
Maprotiline
Mirtazapine. See Remeron
Nefazodone
Remeron
Trazodone. See Desyrel
Venlafaxine. See Effexor
Wellbutrin

Monoamine oxidase inhibitors (MAOIs)

Emsam
Nardil
Parnate
Phenelzine. See Nardil
Selegiline. See Emsam
Tranylcypromine. See Parnate

Selective serotonin reuptake inhibitors (SSRIs)

Celexa
Citalopram. See Celexa
Escitalopram. See Lexapro
Fluoxetine. See Prozac
Fluvoxamine
Lexapro
Paroxetine. See Paxil
Paxil
Pexeva. *See* Paxil
Prozac
Sarafem. *See* Prozac
Sertraline. See Zoloft
Zoloft

Tricyclic antidepressants and combinations

Amitriptyline
Amitriptyline with Chlordiazepoxide. See Limbitrol
Amitriptyline with Perphenazine

964

Amoxapine
Anafranil
Aventyl. *See* Pamelor
Clomipramine. See Anafranil
Desipramine. See Norpramin
Doxepin. See Sinequan
Imipramine. See Tofranil
Limbitrol
Norpramin
Nortriptyline. See Pamelor
Pamelor
Protriptyline. See Vivactil
Sinequan
Surmontil
Tofranil
Trimipramine. See Surmontil
Vivactil

ANTIMANIC AGENTS
Carbamazepine. See Equetro
Depakote
Divalproex. See Depakote
Equetro
Eskalith. *See* Lithium carbonate
Lithium
Lithobid. *See* Lithium carbonate

ANTIPSYCHOTIC AGENTS
Miscellaneous antipsychotic agents
Abilify
Aripiprazole. See Abilify
Clozapine. See Clozaril
Clozaril
FazaClo ODT. *See* Clozaril
Geodon
Haloperidol
Invega
Moban
Molindone. See Moban
Navane
Olanzapine. See Zyprexa
Paliperidone. See Invega
Quetiapine. See Seroquel
Risperdal
Risperidone. See Risperdal
Seroquel
Thiothixene. See Navane
Ziprasidone. See Geodon
Zyprexa

Phenothiazines and combinations
Chlorpromazine
Fluphenazine
Perphenazine
Prochlorperazine
Thioridazine
Thorazine. *See* Prochlorperazine
Trifluoperazine

CENTRAL NERVOUS SYSTEM STIMULANTS
Amphetamines
Adderall
Amphetamines. See Adderall
Desoxyn
Dexedrine
Dextroamphetamine. See Dexedrine
DextroStat. *See* Dexedrine
Lisdexamfetamine. See Vyvanse
Methamphetamine. See Desoxyn
Vyvanse

Miscellaneous central nervous system stimulants
Concerta. *See* Ritalin
Daytrana
Dexmethylphenidate. See Focalin
Focalin
Metadate CD, Metadate ER.
  See Ritalin
Methylin, Methylin ER. *See* Ritalin
Methylphenidate. See Ritalin
Methylphenidate patch. See Daytrana
Ritalin

CHOLINESTERASE INHIBITORS (ALZHEIMER'S DISEASE)
Aricept
Cognex
Donepezil. See Aricept
Exelon
Galantamine. See Razadyne
Razadyne
Rivastigmine. See Exelon
Tacrine. See Cognex

DEPENDENCY TREATMENT AGENTS
Acamprosate. See Campral
Antabuse
Buprenorphine/Naloxone.
  See Suboxone

Psychotropic Herbs and Supplements Indexed by Indication

This index identifies the nutritional supplements and herbs generally deemed most promising for specific mental and emotional problems. These products are profiled in Section 6. Although many of them are also used for a variety of nonpsychological ailments, only their psychotropic effects are reflected here.

Mental Health Internet Resources

General Resources

Community Psychology Net
www.cmmtypsych.net

FreeMedicalJournals.com: Full-Text Articles
www.freemedicaljournals.com

Psychology.info
www.psychology.info

Psych Web
www.psychwww.com

Government Resources

National Institute of Mental Health (NIMH)
www.nimh.nih.gov

National Library of Medicine
www.nlm.nih.gov

National Mental Health Information Center
www.mentalhealth.org

Organizations

American Psychological Association (APA)
www.apa.org

Association for Psychological Science (APS)
www.psychologicalscience.org

National Association of Social Workers (NASW)
www.naswdc.org

National Association of State Mental Health Program Directors
www.nasmhpd.org

Patient Resources

Administration for Children and Families (ACF)
www.acf.dhhs.gov

National Empowerment Center (NEC)
www.power2u.org

National Mental Health Consumers' Self-Help Clearinghouse
www.mhselfhelp.org

Psychotherapy and Treatment

Association for Behavioral and Cognitive Therapies (ABCT)
www.abct.org

American Institute for Cognitive Therapy
www.cognitivetherapynyc.com

National Association of Cognitive-Behavioral Therapists (NACBT)
www.nacbt.org

National Coalition of Creative Arts Therapies Associations (NCATA)
www.nccata.org

Society for the Exploration of Psychotherapy Integration (SEPI)
www.cyberpsych.org/sepi

Substance Abuse

American Council for Drug Education
www.acde.org

American Society of Addiction Medicine (ASAM)
www.asam.org

National Institute on Alcohol Abuse and Alcoholism (NIAAA)
www.niaaa.nih.gov

National Institute on Drug Abuse (NIDA)
www.nida.nih.gov

Substance Abuse and Mental Health Services Administration (SAMHSA)
www.samhsa.gov

U.S. Drug Enforcement Administration
www.dea.gov

Suicide and Runaways

American Foundation for Suicide Prevention
www.afsp.org

Training Institute for Suicide Assessment & Clinical Interviewing
www.suicideassessment.com

National Runaway Switchboard
www.1800runaway.org

Visual Identification Guide

VISUAL IDENTIFICATION GUIDE

Use this section to quickly verify the identity of a capsule, tablet, or other solid oral medication. More than 200 leading tablets and capsules are shown in actual size and color, organized alphabetically by brand name. Each is labeled with its generic name, as well as its strength and the name of its supplier.

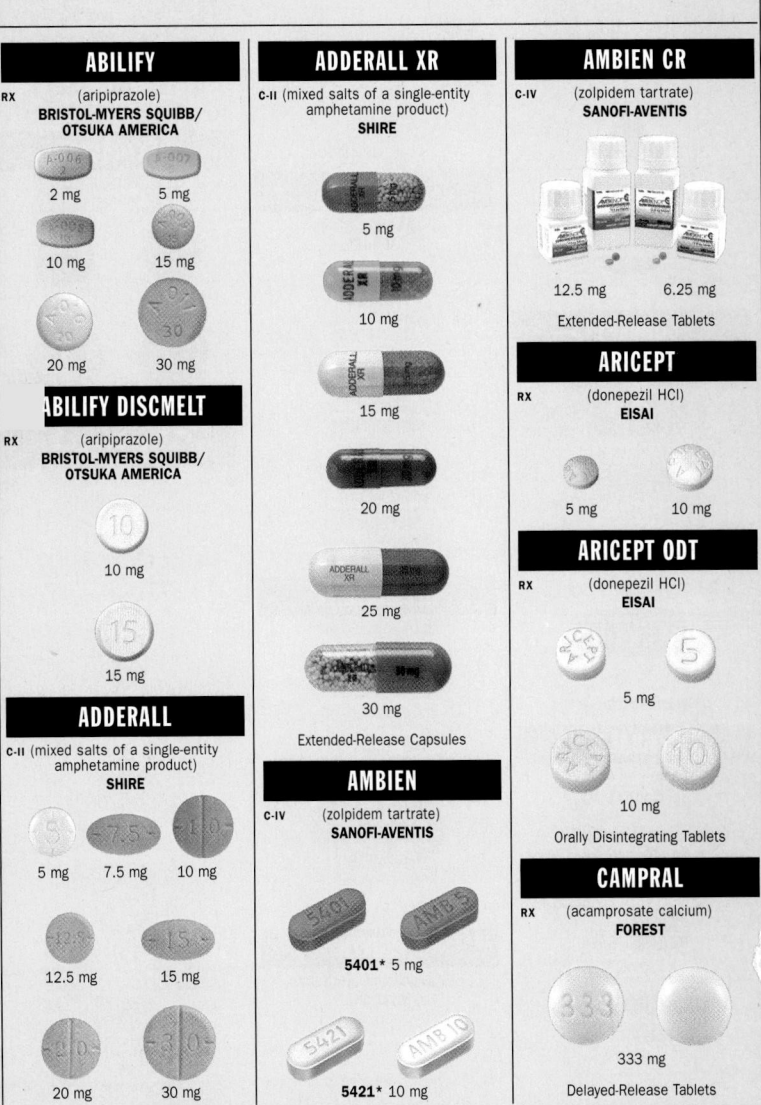

ABILIFY

RX (aripiprazole)
**BRISTOL-MYERS SQUIBB/
OTSUKA AMERICA**

2 mg   5 mg

10 mg   15 mg

20 mg   30 mg

ABILIFY DISCMELT

RX (aripiprazole)
**BRISTOL-MYERS SQUIBB/
OTSUKA AMERICA**

10 mg

15 mg

ADDERALL

C-II (mixed salts of a single-entity amphetamine product)
SHIRE

5 mg   7.5 mg   10 mg

12.5 mg   15 mg

20 mg   30 mg

ADDERALL XR

C-II (mixed salts of a single-entity amphetamine product)
SHIRE

5 mg

10 mg

15 mg

20 mg

25 mg

30 mg

Extended-Release Capsules

AMBIEN

C-IV (zolpidem tartrate)
SANOFI-AVENTIS

5401* 5 mg

5421* 10 mg

AMBIEN CR

C-IV (zolpidem tartrate)
SANOFI-AVENTIS

12.5 mg   6.25 mg

Extended-Release Tablets

ARICEPT

RX (donepezil HCl)
EISAI

5 mg   10 mg

ARICEPT ODT

RX (donepezil HCl)
EISAI

5 mg

10 mg

Orally Disintegrating Tablets

CAMPRAL

RX (acamprosate calcium)
FOREST

333 mg

Delayed-Release Tablets

* Manufacturer's Identification Code

CELEXA

RX (citalopram hydrobromide)
FOREST

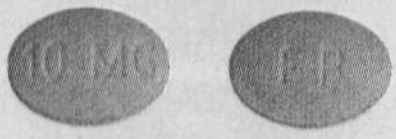

10 MG | F P
10 mg

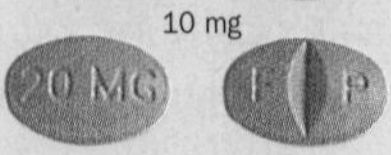

20 MG | F P
20 mg

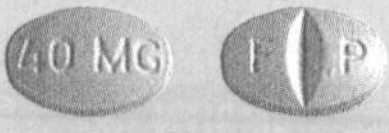

40 MG | F P
40 mg

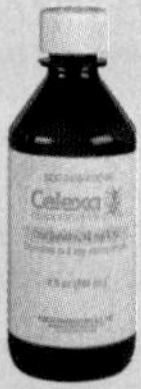

10 mg/5 mL

CONCERTA

C-II (methylphenidate HCl)
MCNEIL PEDIATRICS

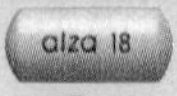

alza 18
18 mg

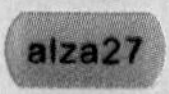

alza 27
27 mg

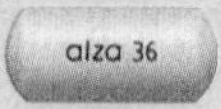

alza 36
36 mg

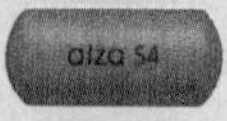

alza 54
54 mg

Extended-Release Tablets

CYMBALTA

RX (duloxetine HCl)
ELI LILLY

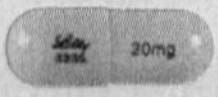

Lilly 3235 20mg
20 mg

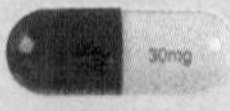

30mg
30 mg

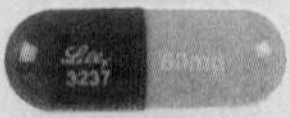

Lilly 3237 60mg
60 mg

Delayed-Release Capsules

DAYTRANA

C-II (methylphenidate
transdermal system)
SHIRE

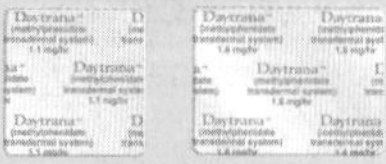

10 mg/9 hr   15 mg/9 hr

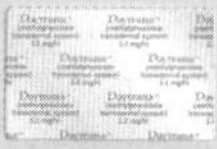

20 mg/9 hr

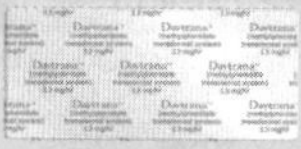

30 mg/9 hr

DEPAKOTE

RX (divalproex sodium)
ABBOTT

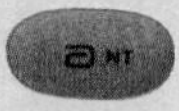

a NT
NT* 125 mg

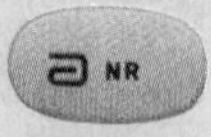

a NR
NR* 250 mg

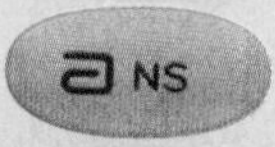

a NS
NS* 500 mg

Delayed-Release Tablets

DEPAKOTE ER

RX (divalproex sodium)
ABBOTT

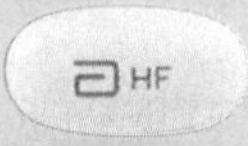

a HF
HF* 250 mg

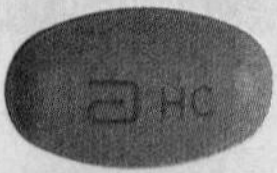

a HC
HC* 500 mg

Extended-Release Tablets

DESOXYN

C-II (methamphetamine HCl USP)
OVATION

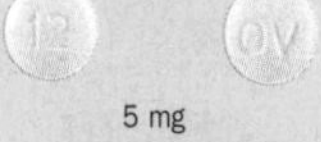

12   OV

5 mg

DEXEDRINE

C-II (dextroamphetamine sulfate)
GLAXOSMITHKLINE

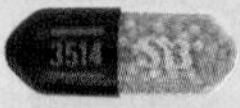

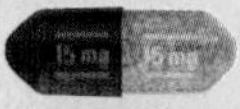

3514 SB

15 mg

15-mg Spansule®

Also available as 5-mg Spansule®
and 10-mg Spansule® capsules.

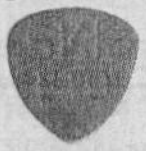

5 mg

DEXTROSTAT

C-II (dextroamphetamine sulfate)
SHIRE

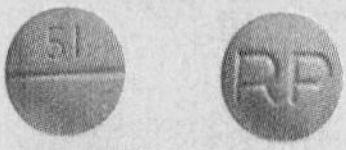

51 | RP
5 mg

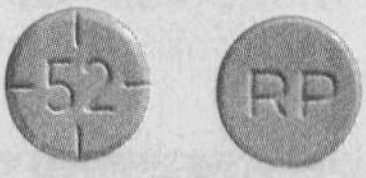

52 | RP
10 mg

EFFEXOR

RX (venlafaxine HCl)
WYETH

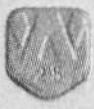

W
701** 25 mg

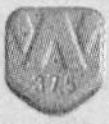

W 37.5
781** 37.5 mg

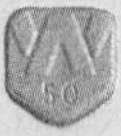

W 50
703** 50 mg

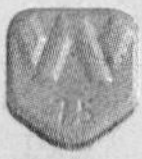

W 75
704** 75 mg

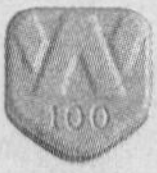

W 100
705** 100 mg

---

* Manufacturer's Identification Code   ** Product identification number on reverse side.

EFFEXOR XR

RX (venlafaxine HCl)
WYETH

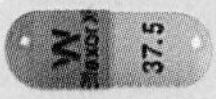

837* 37.5 mg

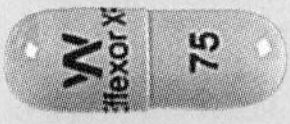

833* 75 mg

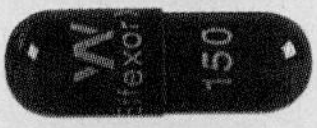

836* 150 mg

Extended-Release Capsules

EMSAM

RX (selegiline transdermal system)
BRISTOL-MYERS SQUIBB

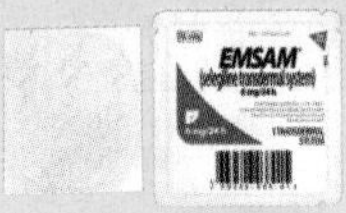

6 mg/24 hr

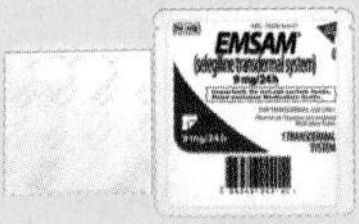

9 mg/24 hr

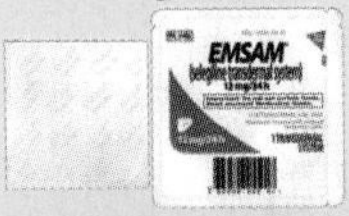

12 mg/24 hr

EQUETRO

RX (carbamazepine)
SHIRE

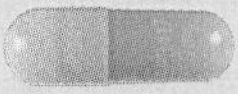

100 mg

200 mg

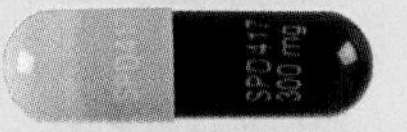

300 mg

Extended-Release Capsules

EXELON

RX (rivastigmine tartrate)
NOVARTIS

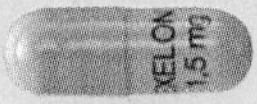

1.5 mg

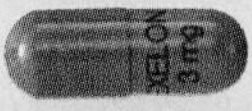

3 mg

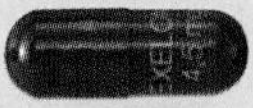

4.5 mg

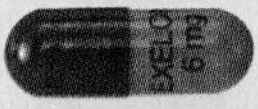

6 mg

FOCALIN

C-II (dexmethylphenidate HCl)
NOVARTIS

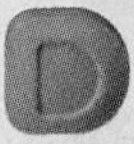

2.5 mg

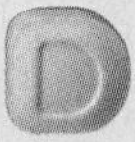

5 mg

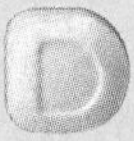

10 mg

FOCALIN XR

C-II (dexmethylphenidate HCl)
NOVARTIS

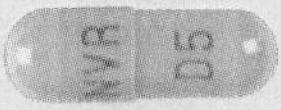

5 mg

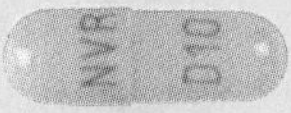

10 mg

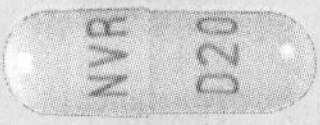

20 mg

Also available in 15-mg capsules

Extended-Release Capsules

GEODON

RX (ziprasidone HCl)
PFIZER

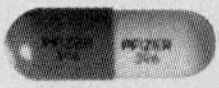

20 mg

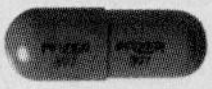

40 mg

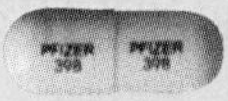

60 mg

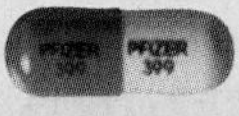

80 mg

KLONOPIN

C-IV (clonazepam)
ROCHE

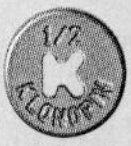

0.5 mg 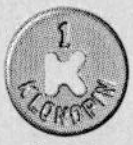   1 mg 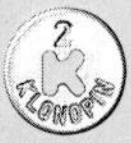   2 mg

KLONOPIN WAFERS

C-IV (clonazepam)
ROCHE

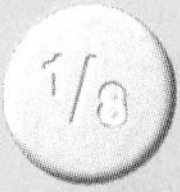

0.125 mg 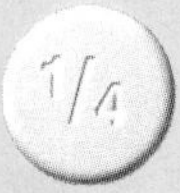   0.25 mg

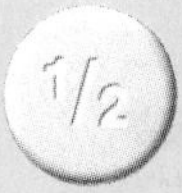

0.5 mg 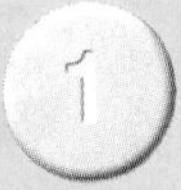   1 mg

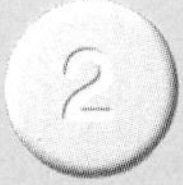

2 mg

Orally Disintegrating Tablets

* Manufacturer's Identification Code

LAMICTAL

RX (lamotrigine)
GLAXOSMITHKLINE

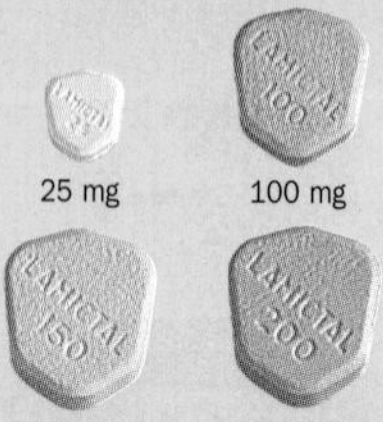

25 mg   100 mg

150 mg   200 mg

LAMICTAL CHEWABLE DISPERSIBLE TABLETS

RX (lamotrigine)
GLAXOSMITHKLINE

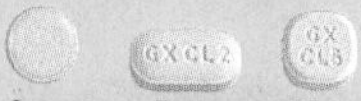

2 mg   5 mg   25 mg

LEXAPRO

RX (escitalopram oxalate)
FOREST

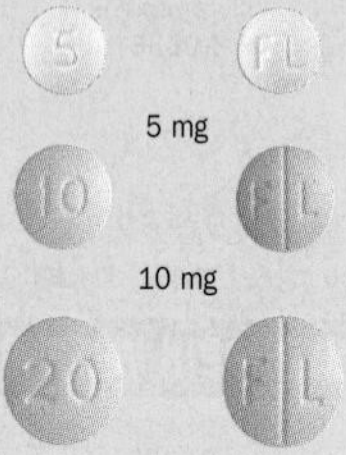

5 mg

10 mg

20 mg

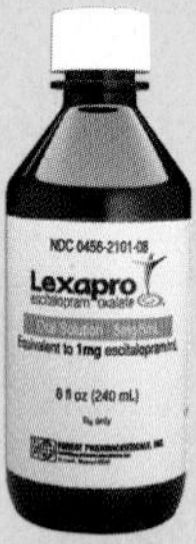

Lexapro
escitalopram oxalate
NDC 0456-2101-08
8 fl oz (240 mL)

5 mg/5 mL

LITHOBID

RX (lithium carbonate USP)
JDS

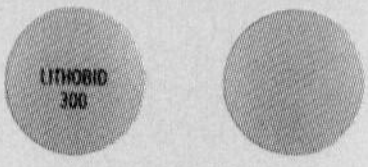

LITHOBID 300

300 mg

LUNESTA

C-IV (eszopiclone)
SEPRACOR

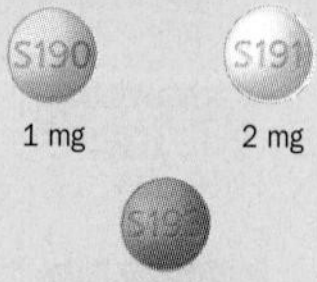

S190   S191
1 mg   2 mg

S193
3 mg

METADATE CD

C-II (methylphenidate HCl, USP)
UCB

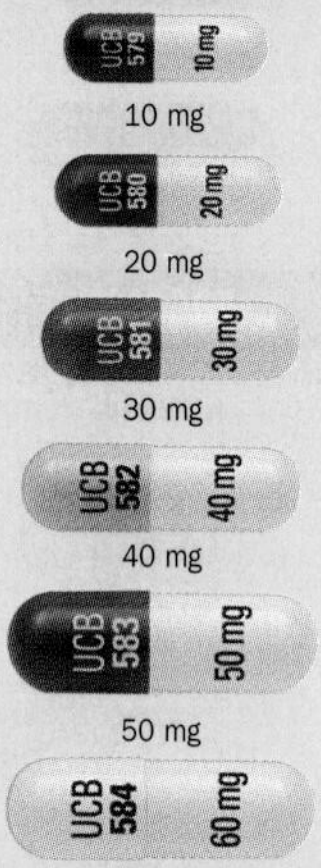

UCB 579 10 mg
10 mg

UCB 580 20 mg
20 mg

UCB 581 30 mg
30 mg

UCB 582 40 mg
40 mg

UCB 583 50 mg
50 mg

UCB 584 60 mg
60 mg

Extended-Release Capsules

NAMENDA

RX (memantine HCl)
FOREST

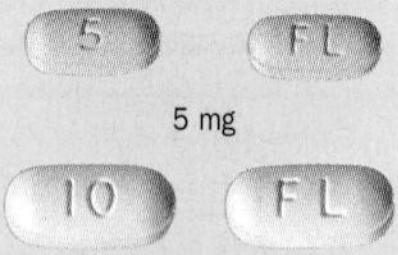

5   FL
5 mg

10   FL
10 mg

Namenda

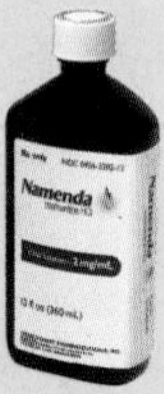

2 mg/mL

NIRAVAM

C-IV (alprazolam)
SCHWARZ

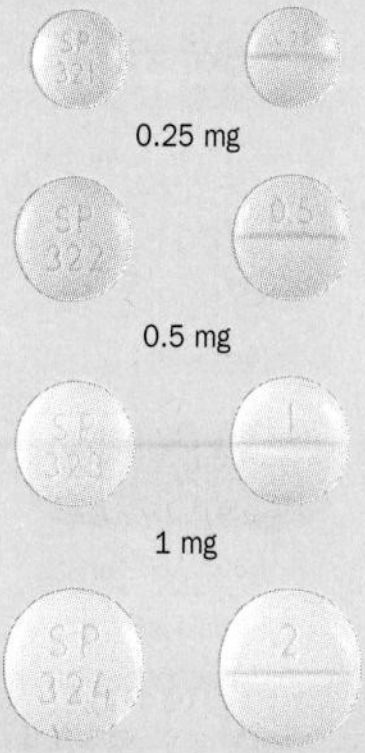

SP 321
0.25 mg

SP 322   0.5
0.5 mg

SP 323   1
1 mg

SP 324   2
2 mg

Orally Disintegrating Tablets

PAXIL

RX (paroxetine HCl)
GLAXOSMITHKLINE

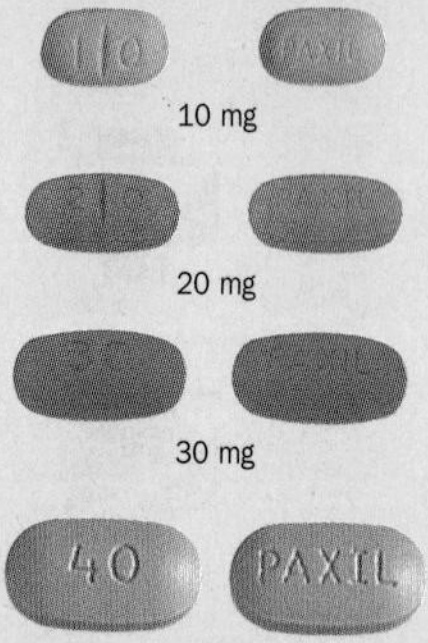

10   20
10 mg

20 mg

30 mg

40   PAXIL
40 mg

PAXIL CR

RX (paroxetine HCl)
GLAXOSMITHKLINE

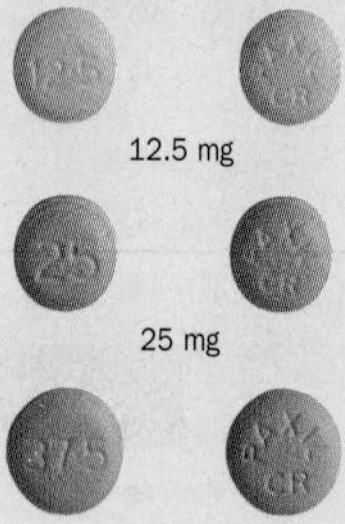

12.5
12.5 mg

25
25 mg

37.5
37.5 mg

PAXIL ORAL SUSPENSION

RX (paroxetine HCl)
GLAXOSMITHKLINE

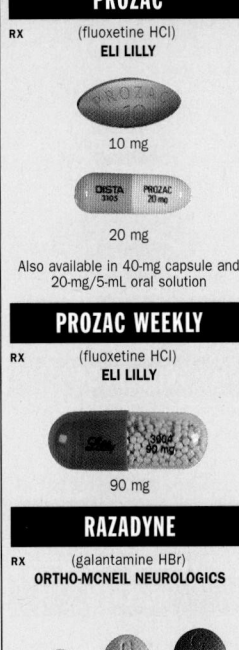

10 mg/5 mL
250 mL

PEXEVA

RX (paroxetine mesylate)
JDS

10 mg   20 mg

30 mg

40 mg

PROVIGIL

C-IV (modafinil)
CEPHALON

100 mg

PROVIGIL

200 mg

PROZAC

RX (fluoxetine HCl)
ELI LILLY

10 mg

20 mg

Also available in 40-mg capsule and
20-mg/5-mL oral solution

PROZAC WEEKLY

RX (fluoxetine HCl)
ELI LILLY

90 mg

RAZADYNE

RX (galantamine HBr)
ORTHO-MCNEIL NEUROLOGICS

4 mg   8 mg   12 mg

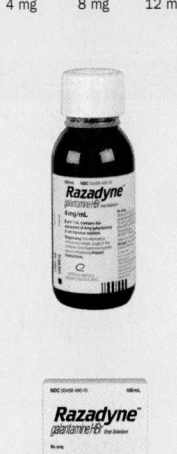

4 mg/mL

RAZADYNE ER

RX (galantamine HBr)
ORTHO-MCNEIL NEUROLOGICS

8 mg

16 mg

24 mg

Extended-Release Capsules

RESTORIL

C-IV (temazepam capsules, USP)
MALLINCKRODT

7.5 mg

15 mg

22.5 mg

30 mg

RISPERDAL CONSTA

RX (risperidone)
JANSSEN

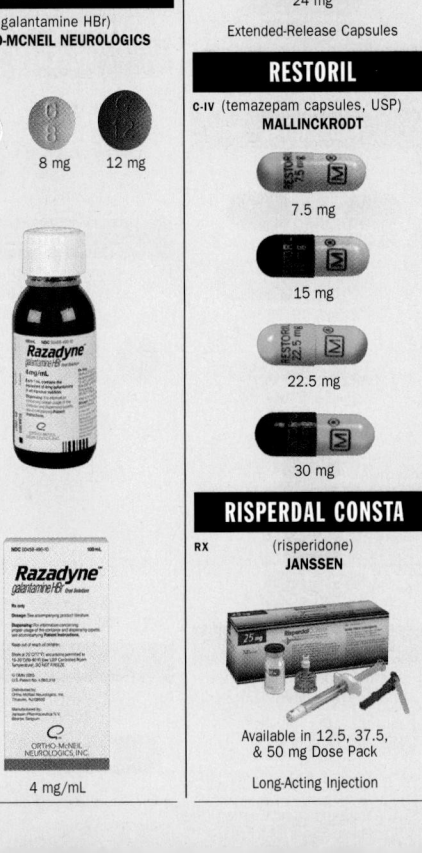

Available in 12.5, 37.5,
& 50 mg Dose Pack

Long-Acting Injection

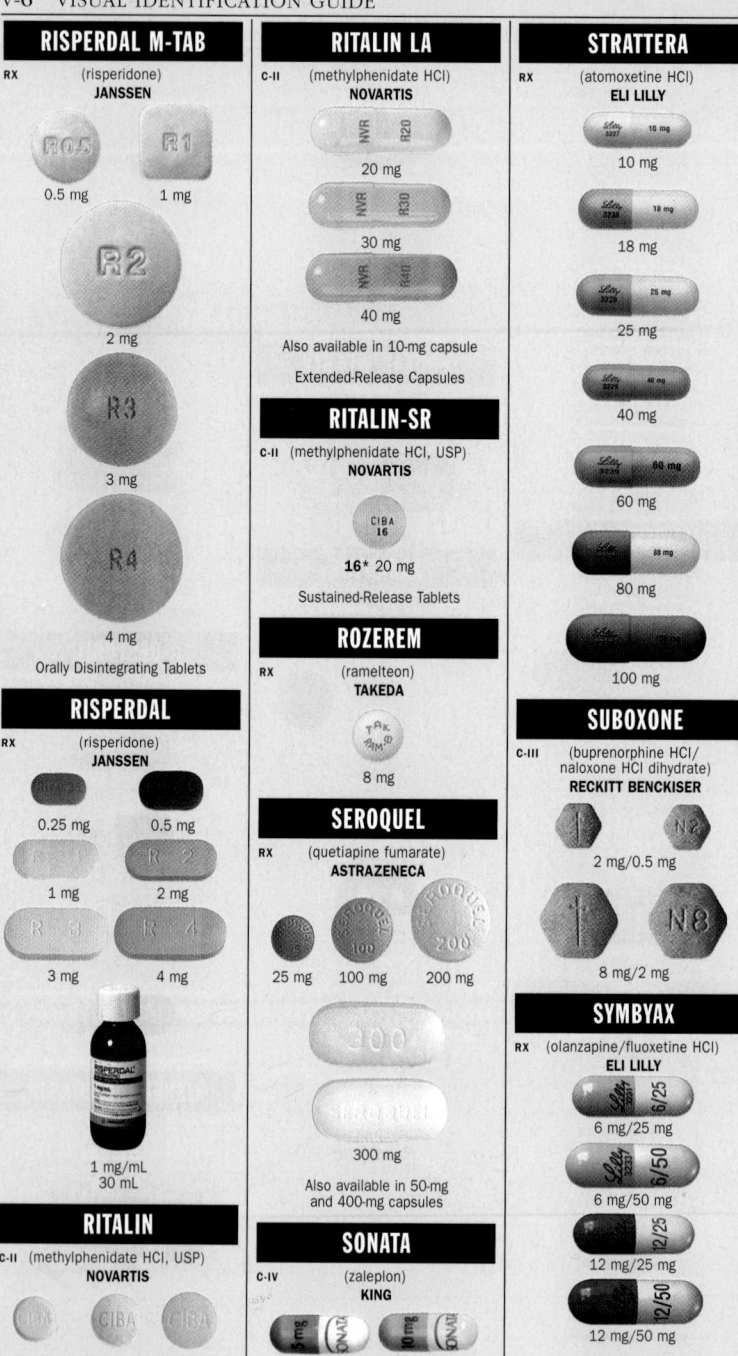

RISPERDAL M-TAB

RX   (risperidone)
JANSSEN

0.5 mg   1 mg

2 mg

3 mg

4 mg

Orally Disintegrating Tablets

RISPERDAL

RX   (risperidone)
JANSSEN

0.25 mg   0.5 mg

1 mg   2 mg

3 mg   4 mg

1 mg/mL
30 mL

RITALIN

C-II   (methylphenidate HCl, USP)
NOVARTIS

7* 5 mg   **3*** 10 mg   **34*** 20 mg

RITALIN LA

C-II   (methylphenidate HCl)
NOVARTIS

20 mg

30 mg

40 mg

Also available in 10-mg capsule

Extended-Release Capsules

RITALIN-SR

C-II   (methylphenidate HCl, USP)
NOVARTIS

CIBA
16

16* 20 mg

Sustained-Release Tablets

ROZEREM

RX   (ramelteon)
TAKEDA

8 mg

SEROQUEL

RX   (quetiapine fumarate)
ASTRAZENECA

25 mg   100 mg   200 mg

300 mg

Also available in 50-mg
and 400-mg capsules

SONATA

C-IV   (zaleplon)
KING

5 mg   10 mg

STRATTERA

RX   (atomoxetine HCl)
ELI LILLY

10 mg

18 mg

25 mg

40 mg

60 mg

80 mg

100 mg

SUBOXONE

C-III   (buprenorphine HCl/
naloxone HCl dihydrate)
RECKITT BENCKISER

2 mg/0.5 mg

8 mg/2 mg

SYMBYAX

RX   (olanzapine/fluoxetine HCl)
ELI LILLY

6/25 mg

6/50 mg

12/25 mg

12/50 mg

Also available in 3 mg/25 mg capsule

* Manufacturer's Identification Code